# Cardiology Board Review

# Cardiology Board Review

**Second Edition**

*Ramdas G. Pai, MD, FRCP (Edin), FACC*
University of California Riverside School of Medicine
Riverside, CA, USA

*Padmini Varadarajan, MD, FACC*
University of California Riverside School of Medicine
Riverside, CA, USA

*With contributions from Patrick Bagdasaryan, Percy Genyk, Chris Hauschild, Gagan Kaur, Ashis Mukherjee, Balaji Natarajan, Chirag Patel, Mandira Patel, Prashant Patel, Ravi Rao, Prabhdeep Sethi, Jarmanjeet Singh, Vrinda Vyas*

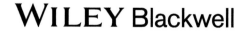
**WILEY** Blackwell

This edition first published 2023
© 2023 John Wiley & Sons Ltd

*Edition History*
Wiley-Blackwell (1e, 2018)

The right of Ramdas G. Pai and Padmini Varadarajan to be identified as the authors of this work has been asserted in accordance with law.

*Registered Offices*
John Wiley & Sons, Inc., 111 River Street, Hoboken, NJ 07030, USA
John Wiley & Sons Ltd, The Atrium, Southern Gate, Chichester, West Sussex, PO19 8SQ, UK

For details of our global editorial offices, customer services, and more information about Wiley products visit us at www.wiley.com.

Wiley also publishes its books in a variety of electronic formats and by print-on-demand. Some content that appears in standard print versions of this book may not be available in other formats.

*Library of Congress Cataloging-in-Publication Data applied for*
ISBN 9781119814948 (paperback) | ISBN 9781119814955 (adobe pdf) | ISBN 9781119814962 (epub)

Cover Design: Wiley
Cover Images: © Luis Alvarez/DigitalVision/Getty Images; smolaw/Shutterstock.com

Set in 10/12pt WarnockPro by Straive, Pondicherry, India
Printed and bound by CPI Group (UK) Ltd, Croydon, CR0 4YY

C9781119814948_020323

# Contents

# List of Contributors

**Patrick Baghdasaryan, MD**
Cardiology Fellow
University of California Riverside School of
Medicine
CA, USA

**Percy Genyk**
Cardiology Fellow
University of California Riverside School of
Medicine
CA, USA

**Christopher Hauschild, MD**
Department of Pharmacy
Loma Linda University Medical Center
Loma Linda
CA, USA

**Gagan Kaur, MD**
Cardiology Fellow
University of California Riverside School
of Medicine
CA, USA

**Ashish Mukherjee, MD, FACC, FSCAI**
Clinical Professor, Health Sciences
Program Director, Interventional Cardiology
Pulse Cardiology
University of California Riverside School
of Medicine
CA, USA

**Balaji Natarajan, MD**
Interventional Cardiology Fellow
University of California Riverside School of
Medicine
CA, USA

**Ramdas G. Pai, MD, FRCP(Edin), FACC**
Professor and Chairman of Medicine
Chair of Clinical Sciences
Director of Cardiovascular Fellowship
Program
University of California Riverside School
of Medicine
Riverside
CA, USA

**Chirag Patel, MD**
Cardiology Fellow
University of California Riverside School
of Medicine
CA, USA

**Mandira Patel, MD**
Cardiology Fellow
University of California Riverside School
of Medicine
CA, USA

**Prashanth Patel, MD, FACC**
Interventional cardiology
Pulse Cardiology, San Bernardino
CA, USA

**Ravi Rao, MD**
Cardiology Fellow
University of California Riverside School
of Medicine
CA, USA

**Prabhdeep S. Sethi, MD**
Associate Clinical Professor,
Health Sciences
Pulse Cardiology
University of California Riverside School
of Medicine
CA, USA

**Jarmanjeet Singh, MD**
Cardiology Fellow
University of California Riverside School
of Medicine
CA, USA

**Padmini Varadarajan, MD, FACC**
Professor of Medicine
Chief of Cardiology
Vice Chair of Internal Medicine
Associate Program Director of Cardiology
Fellowship and Internal Medicine Residency
Programs
University of California Riverside School
of Medicine
CA, USA

**Vrinda Vyas, MD**
Cardiology Fellow
University of California Riverside School
of Medicine
CA, USA

**Lily Yam, PharmD**
Department of Pharmacy
Loma Linda University Medical Center
Loma Linda
CA, USA

# Preface

The second edition of the Cardiology Board Review has been revised and updated and is a comprehensive review of major topics in Cardiology. This book will be very useful for those preparing for initial and recertification exams in Cardiology. It has been edited by Internationally acclaimed teaching physicians with an expertise in major topics in Cardiology.

The book is divided into chapters organized in a question-and-answer format making it easy to prepare for the Board examination. The answers are explained in detail, accompanied by references to major trials and some clinical pearls. The book also highlights a special section on electrocardiograms which are of high resolution. Sections on various imaging modalities like Chest X-Ray, echocardiography, cardiac computed tomography, and cardiac magnetic resonance imaging are also included. Questions not typically encountered in other board review books such as racial disparities in medicine and cardiac emergencies are provided to aid with detailed preparation. Finally, the book also facilitates comprehensive and critical review of cardiovascular medicine to enhance one's diagnostic and therapeutic skills.

# History and Physical Examination

# 1

**1.1.** A 25-year-old woman presents for routine follow up. She has a 2/6 ejection systolic murmur best heard in the second left intercostal space with normal S1. The S2 is split during inspiration only, and P2 intensity is normal. No apical or parasternal heave. The murmur diminishes during expiration and standing up. What is the likely cause of the murmur?
A. Physiological or normal
B. Atrial septal defect (ASD)
C. Bicuspid aortic valve
D. Hypertrophic obstructive cardiomyopathy (HOCM)

**1.2.** A 29-year-old pregnant woman was found to have a systolic murmur best heard in the second left intercostal space. It is rough and there was a palpable thrill in the same area and in the suprasternal notch. Patient is asymptomatic and has normal exercise tolerance. What is the likely explanation for the murmur?
A. Pulmonary stenosis (PS)
B. Normal flow murmur due to increased cardiac output
C. Posterior mitral leaflet prolapse causing an anteriorly directed jet
D. Mammary soufflé

**1.3.** A 22-year-old patient has a hypoplastic radial side of the forearm and fingerized thumb. What might this be associated with?
A. ASD
B. Tetralogy of Fallot
C. Coarctation of aorta
D. Ebstein's anomaly

**1.4.** A 28-year-old man presented with a history of shortness of breath on exertion. On examination, the pulse rate was 76 bpm and blood pressure (BP) 126/80 mmHg. The left ventricular apex was prominent and forceful. The S1 and S2 were normal, but there was a 2/6 ejection systolic murmur best heard in the third right intercostal space. There was no appreciable variation with respiration, but there was an increase in intensity with the Valsalva maneuver and on standing up. It seemed to be less prominent on squatting. There was no audible click. This patient is likely to have?
A. Valvular aortic stenosis
B. Hypertrophic obstructive cardiomyopathy (HOCM)
C. Mitral valve prolapse (MVP)
D. Innocent murmur

*Cardiology Board Review*, Second Edition. Ramdas G. Pai and Padmini Varadarajan.
© 2023 John Wiley & Sons Ltd. Published 2023 by John Wiley & Sons Ltd.

**1.5.** A 36-year-old asymptomatic woman was found to have a systolic murmur best heard in the apex, but also in the aortic area. It was mid to late systolic and was associated with a sharp systolic sound. What is the likely cause of the murmur?
A. Posterior mitral leaflet prolapse
B. Anterior mitral leaflet prolapse
C. Valvular aortic stenosis
D. Aortic subvalvular membrane

**1.6.** A 78-year-old man with hypertension and diabetes mellitus presented with exertional shortness of breath of 6months' duration. Examination revealed a 4/6 crescendo-decrescendo or ejection systolic murmur best heard in the second right intercostal space. The first component of the second sound was soft. The murmur was also heard along the right carotid artery. What is this patient likely to have?
A. Mild aortic stenosis
B. Moderate or severe aortic stenosis
C. Pulmonary stenosis
D. MR

**1.7.** A thrill and a continuous machinery murmur in the left infraclavicular area is indicative of what?
A. Patent ductus arteriosus (PDA)
B. Increased flow due to left arm arteriovenous (AV) fistula for dialysis
C. Venous hum
D. Pulmonary AV fistula

**1.8.** Which of the following is not a feature of aortic coarctation?
A. A continuous murmur on the back
B. Lower blood pressure in the legs compared with an arm
C. Radiofemoral delay
D. Pistol shot sounds on femoral arteries

**1.9.** A 22-year-old newly immigrant woman was referred to the high-risk pregnancy clinic because of clubbing and cyanosis. Examination in addition revealed a parasternal heave, 4/6 ejection systolic murmur in the third left intercostal space, normal jugular venous pressure (JVP), and oxygen saturation of 75%. What will you recommend after confirmation of the diagnosis?
A. Continue pregnancy with sodium restriction
B. Continue pregnancy, but deliver at 28 weeks
C. Advise termination of pregnancy
D. Perform percutaneous ASD closure and continue pregnancy

**1.10.** What is the cause of murmur in ASD?
A. Continuous due to flow across the defect
B. Ejection systolic due to increased flow across the pulmonary valve
C. Mid-diastolic due to increased flow across the tricuspid valve
D. Continuous murmur over lung fields due to increased flow in lungs

**1.11.** What is a systolic click that disappears on inspiration likely to be due to?
A. Pulmonary valvular stenosis
B. Bicuspid aortic valve

C. MVP

D. Pulmonary hypertension

**1.12.** A 36-year-old woman presented with an 8-month history of progressive exertional dyspnea. Physical examination revealed a heart rate of 74 bpm, regular, BP 126/78 mmHg, with no pedal edema. JVP and carotid upstroke were normal. Cardiac auscultation revealed normal S1, an accentuated P2 with narrow splitting of S2, an ejection click, and a 2/6 ejection systolic murmur. What is the likely diagnosis?

A. Pulmonary hypertension

B. PS

C. Aortic stenosis

D. ASD

**1.13.** Causes of prominent "a" wave in jugular venous pulsations include all of the following except which option?

A. PS

B. Pulmonary hypertension

C. Tricuspid stenosis

D. Aortic stenosis

E. ASD

**1.14.** What is a 6-year-old Amish boy in Pennsylvania with short stature, polydactyly, short limbs, absent upper incisor teeth with dysplasia of other teeth, and a systolic murmur most likely to have?

A. ASD

B. Ventricular septal defect

C. Aortic coarctation

D. PS

**1.15.** Which of the following describes a ventricular septal defect murmur?

A. Holosystolic

B. Ejection systolic

C. Systolic-diastolic

D. None of the above

**1.16.** Clubbing and cyanosis in lower limbs, but not upper limbs, is indicative of which of the following?

A. PDA with coarctation of the aorta

B. PDA with pulmonary hypertension

C. Ventricular septal defect Eisenmenger's

D. ASD Eisenmenger's with coarctation of aorta

**1.17.** A 46-year-old man presented with progressive fatigue and leg swelling. He had no significant past medical history except a front-on collision in a car he was driving. Examination revealed 2+ edema, raised JVP, and an enlarged liver, which seemed to expand during systole. What is the likely diagnosis?

A. Severe tricuspid stenosis

B. Severe tricuspid regurgitation (TR)

C. Constrictive pericarditis

D. Restrictive cardiomyopathy

**1.18.** A 23-year-old has a mid-diastolic rumble and sharp early diastolic sound. What is the likely explanation?

A. Mitral stenosis

B. Constrictive pericarditis

C. Restrictive cardiomyopathy

D. Bicuspid aortic valve

**1.19.** A 28-year-old man has history of progressive fatigue and exertional shortness of breath over the previous 6 months. Examination revealed a raised JVP that seemed to increase with inspiration and a sharp precordial sound in early diastole. What is the most likely diagnosis?

A. Right ventricular infarct

B. Tricuspid stenosis

C. Constrictive pericarditis

D. Restrictive cardiomyopathy

**1.20.** A 66-year-old woman with left breast cancer post mastectomy, radiation, and chemotherapy was admitted with shortness of breath, heart rate of 120 bpm, and BP of 90/60 mmHg. On slow cuff deflation during BP measurement, Korotkoff's sounds started at 90 mmHg during expiration only and throughout the respiratory cycle at a cuff pressure of 70 mmHg. An echocardiogram was obtained. What is this likely to show?

A. Akinesis of the left anterior descending area

B. Thick pericardium

C. Large pericardial effusion

D. Large, globally hypokinetic left ventricle.

**1.21.** Features of restrictive cardiomyopathy may include all of the following except?

A. Raised JVP

B. Loud S3

C. Kussmaul's sign

D. A diastolic knock in the pulmonary area

**1.22.** Pulsus paradoxus despite tamponade may not be present in which of the following?

A. ASD

B. Aortic stenosis

C. Mitral stenosis

D. Old age

**1.23.** Pulsus paradoxus may occur in all of the following except?

A. Tamponade

B. Status asthmaticus

C. Pulmonary embolism

D. Aortic stenosis

**1.24.** A Square sign during Valsalva maneuver occurs in which of the following?

A. HOCM

B. MVP

C. Aortic stenosis

D. Congestive heart failure

**1.25.** An abnormal Schamroth's test may be found in all of the following except?

A. Tetralogy of Fallot
B. Subacute bacterial endocarditis
C. Left atrial myxoma
D. Aortic stenosis

**1.26–1.31.** For the jugular vein or RA pressure tracings shown in Figures 1.26–1.31, match with an appropriate clinical scenario from the following choices:

A. Normal
B. Pericardial constriction
C. Restrictive cardiomyopathy
D. ASD
E. Tricuspid stenosis
F. TR
G. Cardiac tamponade
H. Superior vena cava syndrome
I. Heart failure
J. PS

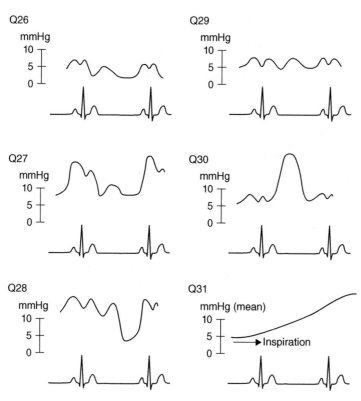

Figures 1.26–1.31

**1.132–1.37.** For the jugular vein or RA pressure tracings shown in Figures 1.32–1.37, match with an appropriate clinical scenario from the following choices:

  **A.** Normal
  **B.** Pericardial constriction
  **C.** Restrictive cardiomyopathy
  **D.** ASD
  **E.** Tricuspid stenosis
  **F.** TR
  **G.** Cardiac tamponade
  **H.** Superior vena cava syndrome
  **I.** Heart failure
  **J.** PS
  **K.** Complete heart block

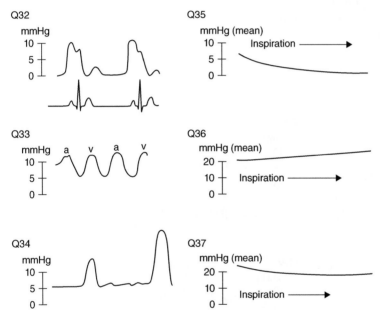

Figures 1.32–1.37

**1.138–1.45.** For the carotid pulse or arterial pressure tracings shown in Figures 1.38–1.45, match with an appropriate clinical scenario from the following choices:

  **A.** Normal
  **B.** Constriction
  **C.** Aortic stenosis
  **D.** AR
  **E.** Mitral stenosis
  **F.** Mixed aortic stenosis and AR
  **G.** Cardiac tamponade
  **H.** HOCM
  **I.** Heart failure
  **J.** Complete heart block
  **K.** MR
  **L.** Premature ventricular contraction (PVC)

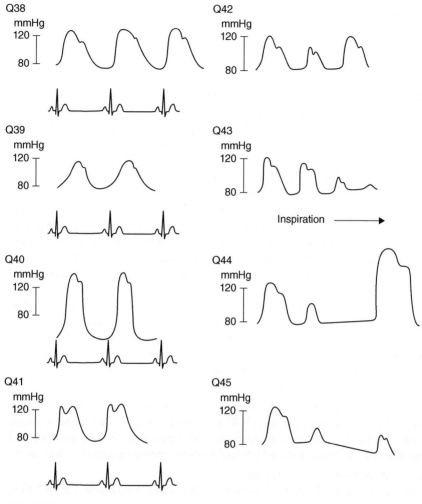

**Figures 1.38–1.45**

## Answers

**1.1.** A. Physiological or normal.

The murmur is <3/6 in intensity and diminishes with standing, when venous return is less, indicating a flow murmur. S2 split during inspiration only is physiological. During inspiration, increased venous return and pulmonary flow prolongs right ventricular (RV) ejection. This delays P2. The S2 split will be fixed with a similar gap during both inspiration and expiration. Characteristics of a physiological systolic murmur include being 2/6 in intensity or less, diminution during standing and normal physiological split.

**1.2.** A. Pulmonary stenosis (PS).

A murmur associated with a thrill indicates it is pathological and not just due to increased cardiac output. A thrill in the suprasternal notch is pathognomonic of PS. Valvular PS would be associated with an ejection click which diminishes with inspiration. Left parasternal heave would be indicative of RV hypertrophy (RVH) secondary to pressure overload on the RV imposed by PS. Murmur because of posterior mitral leaflet prolapse may be heard in the aortic area as the mitral regurgitation jet may hug the ascending aorta and the murmur may be transmitted along that. Mammary soufflé occurs in lactating women because of increased blood flow to the breast and the murmur is continuous.

**1.3. A. ASD.**

The features are suggestive of Holt-Oram syndrome. They can also have unequal arm length, various other deformities of the hand, VSD and varying degrees of atrioventricular conduction disturbances. Cardiac anomalies are present in 75% of patients with Holt-Oram syndrome which is a genetic defect.

**1.4. B. HOCM.**

In HOCM, the left ventricular (LV) outflow obstruction is dynamic and is increased by an increase in LV contractility or a reduction in LV size. Standing, Valsalva maneuver, and amyl nitrite inhalation reduce venous return, reduce LV filling, reduce LV size and increase systolic anterior motion of the anterior mitral leaflet (SAM), resulting in increased LV outflow tract (LVOT) obstruction. Squatting kinks the leg arteries, raising peripheral resistance and hence an increase in LV volume through an increase in afterload. This increase in LV size reduces SAM and LV outflow obstruction. Valvular aortic stenosis murmur intensity is flow dependent, and hence reduction in venous return with standing or Valsalva maneuver as well as an increase in peripheral resistance with squatting would diminish the murmur. In mitral valve prolapse (MVP), an increase in LV volume would reduce prolapse, and a reduction in LV volume would lengthen the murmur by producing earlier prolapse. MVP is generally associated with a mid-systolic click.

**1.5. A. Posterior mitral leaflet prolapse.**

The systolic click and late systolic murmur indicate MVP. In anterior leaflet prolapse, the mitral regurgitation (MR) jet is directed posteriorly and murmur may be conducted to the axilla. In posterior leaflet prolapse, the jet is anterior wall hugging, along the aortic root, which facilitates its conduction to the aortic area.

**1.6. B. Moderate or severe aortic stenosis.**

This is a classic aortic stenosis murmur with carotid conduction. Soft A2 (first component of S2 indicates significant aortic stenosis). Features of severe aortic stenosis are late-peaking murmur, absent A2, paradoxic splitting of S2, (i.e. split during expiration instead of inspiration), and a slow-rising carotid pulse (pulsus parvus et tardus).

**1.7. A. Patent ductus arteriosus (PDA).**

Though the other conditions can produce continuous murmurs, they are not associated with a thrill or machinery character. Pulmonary AV fistula results in a continuous murmur over the lung fields. The venous hum is due to flow in the jugular veins and gets less by assuming the supine position. The murmur due to AV fistula created for hemodialysis is heard on the side of the fistula in the clavicular area due to increased venous flow – this can be temporarily silenced by transient pressure over the fistula.

**1.8. D. Pistol shot sounds on femoral arteries.**

Pistol shot sounds occur in severe aortic regurgitation (AR). Others are features of aortic coarctation. Continuous murmur on the back is due to chest wall arterial collaterals bypassing aortic coarctation. Radiofemoral delay and lower BP in the leg are due to obstruction in the aorta and collateral dependent flow in the lower extremities. In severe coarctation, the flow in the abdominal aorta would be non-pulsatile and continuous.

**1.9.** C. Advise termination of pregnancy.

The findings are typical of tetralogy of Fallot, and the murmur is due to PS. Murmur of ASD is due to flow and softer and not associated with clubbing or cyanosis unless associated with Eisenmenger's syndrome. Tetralogy of Fallot is associated with extremely high risk, and the pregnancy should be terminated. Other very high-risk cardiac conditions include severe pulmonary hypertension, severe LV dysfunction or prior history of peripartum cardiomyopathy, and severe left-sided obstructive valvular diseases.

**1.10.** B. Ejection systolic due to increased flow across the pulmonary valve.

Flow across the defect and the lungs does not produce murmurs. The gradient across ASD is less than 1 mmHg and does not produce turbulence to produce a murmur. It takes a torrential shunt to produce a mid-diastolic flow murmur across the tricuspid valve as the tricuspid aortic valve area of 7–8 cm² (compared to 5 cm² for the mitral valve and about 3.5 cm² for pulmonary and aortic valves). Flow murmurs are generated across smaller valves.

**1.11.** A. Pulmonary valvular stenosis.

In severe PS, due to low pulmonary artery (PA) pressure, an increase in venous return to right ventricle during inspiration may open the pulmonary valve before systole, eliminating the ejection click.

**1.12.** A. Pulmonary hypertension.

This is suggested by loud P2. In pulmonary hypertension, P2 moves closer to A2 due to higher pulmonary valve closure pressure, and S2 may be single when PA pressure approaches systemic pressure. Ejection click and soft ejection systolic murmur may occur because of PA dilation. Other features of pulmonary hypertension may include a palpable PA in the second left intercostal space, a palpable P2 or diastolic knock, parasternal heave due to RVH and a prominent "a" wave in jugular venous pulsation due to RVH resulting in accentuated right atrial (RA) systole. PS results in a louder murmur and diminished P2. ASD results in wide, fixed, splitting of S2.

**1.13.** E. ASD.

A prominent "a" wave occurs due to forceful right atrial systole against some resistance, and this can occur against stenotic tricuspid valve, hypertrophied RV (PS and pulmonary hypertension) or hypertrophied ventricular septum (aortic stenosis, hypertrophic cardiomyopathy, or hypertension). In ASD, a defect in the atrial septum would not allow a prominent "a" wave, even in the presence of pulmonary hypertension, as the right atrium would decompress into the left atrium during atrial systole.

**1.14.** A. ASD.

ASD, or common atrium as part of Ellis-van Creveld syndrome (EVC) or mesoectodermal or chondroectodermal dysplasia, is an autosomal recessive inheritance disorder that occurs in the old-order Amish population. The *EVC* gene is on chromosome number 4, short arm. It is a form of ciliopathy. Other ciliopathies that result in abnormal organogenesis include Bardet-Biedl syndrome, polycystic kidney and liver disease, Alstrom syndrome, Meckel-Gruber syndrome, and some forms of retinal degeneration, and so on.

**1.15.** A. Holosystolic as the pressure gradient between LV and RV is throughout LV isovolumic contraction, ejection and isovolumic relaxation. On echo-Doppler, there may also be a presystolic left-to-right flow associated with left atrial systole.

**1.16.** B. PDA with pulmonary hypertension.

In PDA Eisenmenger's, the shunt reversal through PDA causes desaturation in the lower part of the body only, resulting in central cyanosis and clubbing in lower extremities and not upper extremities (differential cyanosis). In ASD and VSD, Eisenmengers, cyanosis and clubbing involve both the upper and lower extremities. In PDA without suprasystemic pulmonary hypertension, the flow will be from the aorta to pulmonary artery only and no desaturated blood comes to the aorta.

**1.17.** B. Severe tricuspid regurgitation (TR).

Liver that is pulsatile (expansile) in systole is indicative of a powerful right atrial "V" wave, and this suggests severe TR. This can also be seen in the jugular venous pulsation. Sternal compression during the motor vehicle accident likely caused a flail tricuspid valve and severe TR. Liver pulsation in tricuspid stenosis is presystolic. Liver pulsations are not seen in constriction or restriction.

**1.18.** A. Mitral stenosis.

This is typical mitral stenosis with pliable leaflets, which causes opening snap (OS). The A2–OS interval is a good measure of mitral stenosis severity. Normally, 70–100 ms (same as isovolumetric relaxation time). Less than 70 ms indicates high left atrial pressure, suggesting severe mitral stenosis. In constrictive pericarditis, you can get a pericardial knock which is a sharp protodiastolic sound that occurs a little later. Restrictive cardiomyopathy produces S3 due to high left atrial pressure and is generally later and is a dull sound like a thud and best heard with the bell of the stethoscope. S3 is due to rapid deceleration of the early passive filling wave across the mitral valve.

**1.19.** C. Constrictive pericarditis.

A rise in JVP is paradoxical (Kussmaul's sign), and sharp protodiastolic sound is a pericardial knock – classic features of constriction. Kussmaul's sign occurs due to lack of transmission of negative intrathoracic pressure to the right atrium through the rigid pericardium. Hence, the increased venous return during inspiration causes a rise in RA pressure. In tricuspid stenosis, inspiratory increase in venous return may not readily empty into the right ventricle, causing a paradoxical rise in JVP with inspiration. Kussmaul's sign can occur in an RV infarct but occurs in the setting of inferior myocardial infarction. Restrictive cardiomyopathy may be associated with S3, which is less sharp (a thud), but no venous paradox.

**1.20.** C. Large pericardial effusion.

This is typical cardiac tamponade with classic paradoxic pulse, hypotension, and tachycardia. Constriction causes venous paradox.

**1.21.** C. Kussmaul's sign.

As the pericardium is normal in restrictive cardiomyopathy, inspiratory negative intrathoracic pressure is transmitted to the pericardial space and cardiac
chambers, and hence the venous paradox does not occur. Diastolic knock is palpable with loud P2; a feature of pulmonary hypertension that it is common in restrictive LV physiology.

**1.22.** A. ASD.

Pulsus paradoxus may not be present when LV filling is not affected by phase of
inspiration due to lack of interventricular dependence, as in ASD, or LV filling
from other sources, such as severe AR or MR.

**1.23.** D. Aortic stenosis.

**1.24.** D. Congestive heart failure.

See the explanation in Box 1.1 Clinical Pearls. This is because though a Valsalva
maneuver reduces left-sided venous return, it does not affect LV stroke volume as
it is already well filled and beyond the peak of Starling's curve. An increase in
intrathoracic pressure is transmitted to the aorta, causing an increase in aortic
pressure.

**1.25.** D. Aortic stenosis.

This test is named after a South African cardiologist for diagnosis of clubbing.
In clubbing, the angle between the nail and nail fold is >165° and when nails of the
fingers from both sides are apposed, the gap between them disappears. Clubbing
is seen in cardiac conditions (in addition to a variety of pulmonary diseases), in
subacute bacterial endocarditis, congenital cyanotic heart diseases, and left atrial
myxoma.

**1.26.** A. Normal.

Note the mean RA pressure of <5 mmHg and the "a" wave due to atrial systole
is slightly higher than the "V" wave, which occurs because of RA filling on the
closed tricuspid valve. A smaller "V" wave indicates a compliant right atrium.
The sharp "C" wave that coincides with the QRS complex of the electrocardiogram is due to a combination of tricuspid valve closure and transmitted carotid
impulse.

**1.27.** E. Tricuspid stenosis.

Note the large "a" wave as the RA contracts against a stenosed tricuspid valve;
the gradient is reflected as a large "a" wave. Note the mean RA pressure is also
slightly elevated commensurate with trans tricuspid gradient. In conditions causing RVH (pulmonary hypertension, PS, aortic stenosis with septal hypertrophy),
the "a" wave may be prominent due to noncompliant RV (RV fourth heart sound),
but mean RA pressure may not be high unless there is heart failure.

**1.28.** B. Pericardial constriction.

Note the elevated RA pressure with rapid "Y" descent.

**1.29.** D. ASD.

In ASD, the "a" and "V" waves would be of similar height because the defect
leads to equilibration of the LA and RA pressures.

**1.30.** F. TR.

The large "V" wave is due to TR filling up the RA during systole. When the "V" wave pressure is about 25–30 mmHg, it may become palpable to the examining finger and associated with an expansile liver.

**1.31.** B. Pericardial constriction.

The increasing mean RA pressure with inspiration is the venous paradox or Kussmaul's sign. This is due to dissociation between intrathoracic and intrapericardial pressures because of a thick pericardium. During inspiration, the intrathoracic pressure drops, increasing venous return to the right atrium, but the intrapericardial and intra-RA pressure does not drop and returning blood increases the pressure further. Kussmaul's sign can occur even in acute pericarditis and RV infarcts; the latter invoking pericardial restraint.

**1.32.** J. PS.

Note a large "a" wave with near-normal mean RA pressure. Contrast this with tricuspid stenosis.

**1.33.** G. Cardiac tamponade.

Note the raised RA pressure with prominent "X" and "Y" troughs.

**1.34.** K. Complete heart block.

The intermittent large waves are "cannon a" waves when atria and ventricles happen to contract simultaneously due to AV dissociation.

**1.35.** A. Normal.

The RA pressure is <5 mmHg and drops with inspiration.

**1.36.** H. Superior vena cava syndrome.

Note the high JVP which does not drop on inspiration as the superior vena cava is blocked and the jugular vein is not in communication with right atrial hemodynamics or pulsatile changes. In contrast to constriction, the JVP in superior vena cava syndrome is nonpulsatile. It would be high in both.

**1.37.** I. Heart failure.

High JVP that drops with inspiration.

**1.38.** A. Normal.

This is the typical normal tracing. Note the fairly rapid upstroke, pulse pressure of about 40 mmHg, dicrotic notch and dicrotic wave.

**1.39.** C. Aortic stenosis.

Note the very slow rise, attributable to high blood flow velocity across the valve which converts pressure to kinetic energy.

**1.40.** D. AR.

Note the rapid upstroke, rapid downstroke (water-hammer pulse), wide pulse pressure, and low diastolic pressure due to peripheral vasodilation. This can also occur in PDA and large AV fistulae.

**1.41.** F. Mixed aortic stenosis and AR.

This is called pulsus bisferiens or double pulse. Can also occur in HOCM.

**1.42.** I. Heart failure.

This is pulsus alternans. Alternating strong and weak pulse with regular RR interval due to alternating stronger and weaker myocardial contraction with every other beat attributable to altered calcium handling by contractile proteins. It is a sign of severe systolic dysfunction.

**1.43.** G. Cardiac tamponade.

A BP drop with inspiration is called pulsus paradoxus. An inspiratory drop of >10 mmHg may indicate tamponade.

**1.44.** L. Premature ventricular contraction (PVC).

With appropriate increase in pulse pressure in the post PVC beat, because of a combination of increased preload due to a long filling period and increased contractility due to the force-frequency relationship.

**1.45.** H. HOCM.

In this patient, after PVC, instead of an augmented pulse there is a smaller pulse volume. This is due to the fact that increased contractility in the post-PVC beat increases dynamic LVOT obstruction and reduces stroke volume. This is called Brockenbrough phenomenon on cardiac catheterization. This contrasts with valvular aortic stenosis, where pulse pressure increases after a PVC.

---

**Box 1.1   Clinical Pearls**

- Loud S1 occurs when the mitral valve closes forcefully from an open position against the transmitral gradient or prematurely and occurs in mitral stenosis, short pulmonary regurgitation (PR) interval, and hyperdynamic circulation.
- S1 is soft in MR, with a long PR interval, and severe AR. In severe AR, the mitral valve may move toward closure in presystole.
- P2 can be loud in pulmonary hypertension (higher pulmonary valve closure sound) and dilated PA (better P2 transmission).
- S2 may be paradoxically split when aortic valve closure is delayed and comes after P2 as in left bundle branch block, severe aortic stenosis, severe LV dysfunction, and PDA (increased transaortic flow). S2 is split in expiration and not in inspiration when RV filling and ejection time are increased.
- The only right-sided sound/murmur is attenuated by inspiration is pulmonary ejection click of valvular PS as an inspiratory increase in venous return to the right ventricle in the presence of RVH may cause an increase on RV end diastolic pressure high enough to open the pulmonary valve as the PA pressure is lower.
- A Carey Coombs murmur is a mid-diastolic mitral murmur due to mitral valvulitis in rheumatic fever.
- An Austin Flint murmur is a mitral mid-diastolic murmur heard in severe AR. Potential explanations include: AR jet causing an anterior mitral leaflet vibration, or mitral/AR jet interaction or an AR jet causing a partial diastolic closure of anterior mitral leaflet.
- A Graham Steel murmur is an early diastolic murmur of PR that occurs in severe pulmonary hypertension. A higher PA diastolic pressure causes turbulence of the PR jet and the murmur.
- A mid-diastolic murmur of mitral stenosis is best heard with the bell without much pressure as it is a low-frequency murmur and better heard in the left lateral position. Presystolic accentuation indicates atrial contraction.

- A tapping apex typically occurs in mitral stenosis and it is palpable S1.
- Maneuvers are helpful in evaluating murmurs. Inspiration increases right-sided venous return and augments right-sided murmurs. Standing reduces venous return and, after three or four beats, LV filling as well reducing its size. This may augment an HOCM murmur and lengthen an MR murmur of MVP. Squatting kinks limb arteries and increases afterload. This may reduce murmurs of valvular aortic stenosis through reduced stroke volume and an HOCM murmur through an increase in LV volume and shorten a murmur of MVP through increasing LV volume and reducing prolapse.
- The Valsalva maneuver involves expiration against a closed glottis, increasing the intrathoracic pressure. There are four phases of heart rate and BP response. The normal response includes the following:
  - Phase 1. Early during the Valsalva maneuver, pressure on the intrathoracic aorta and pulmonary veins emptying into left heart transiently increases filling, stroke volume, and BP with reflex slowing of heart.
  - Phase 2. With a continued Valsalva maneuver, LV filling diminishes and lowers stroke volume and BP, resulting in compensatory tachycardia. Reflex peripheral vasoconstriction slowly increases BP and lowers the heart rate.
  - Phase 3. With release of the Valsalva maneuver, pressure on the aorta drops, and BP drops with some increase in heart rate.
  - Phase 4. The left ventricle fills, with an increase in stroke volume with continued peripheral vasoconstriction causing BP to overshoot the baseline value. This will reflexively reduce the heart rate below the baseline.
  Phase 2 is used in dynamic auscultation.
- In HOCM, the Valsalva maneuver results in a smaller left ventricle size causing increased LVOT obstruction and an increase in murmur intensity.
- In MVP, reduced LV volume with phase 2 Valsalva results in earlier and greater prolapse and the MR murmur lengthens.
- A heaving apex denotes LV hypertrophy; forceful apical lift signifies LV volume overload, tapping apex loud S1, and bifid apex with presystolic lift LV occurs due to a combination of LVH with a forceful atrial kick causing S4 as it occurs in hypertrophic cardiomyopathy.
- Left parasternal or precordial bulge indicates RVH occurring before the rib cage ossifies (young age), and parasternal lift or heave indicates RVH starting after childhood.
- A downward tug on the larynx held up with fingers after deglutition indicates aortic arch aneurysm. Also called tracheal tug or Oliver's sign, this occurs with every heartbeat.
- A large, sharp systolic wave in jugular venous pulsation during systole is the cannon wave. This occurs when the right atrium contracts over a closed tricuspid valve, as in complete heart block (intermittent) or junctional or idioventricular rhythm with retrograde ventriculoatrial conduction.

ECG diagnostic criteria are listed in Box 2.1.

For the tracings in the questions/figures in this section, please analyze carefully and list the important findings and possible clinical setting. Answers are found at the end of the chapter.

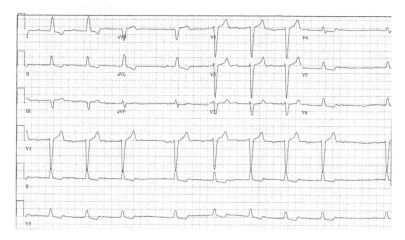

**Figure 2.1**

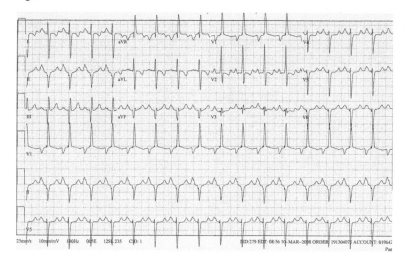

**Figure 2.2**

*Cardiology Board Review*, Second Edition. Ramdas G. Pai and Padmini Varadarajan.
© 2023 John Wiley & Sons Ltd. Published 2023 by John Wiley & Sons Ltd.

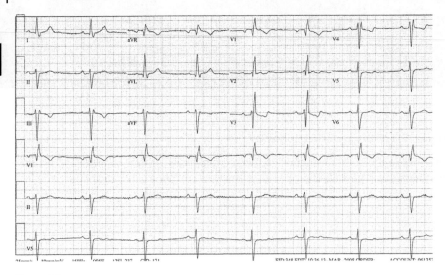

**Figure 2.3**

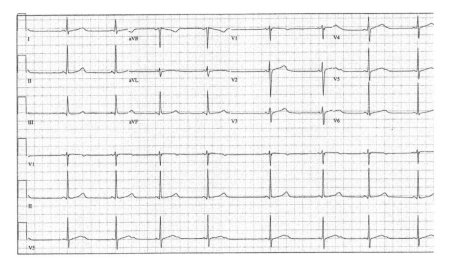

**Figure 2.4**

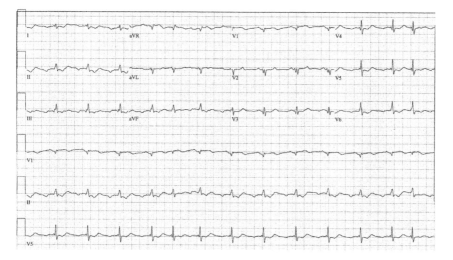

Figure 2.5

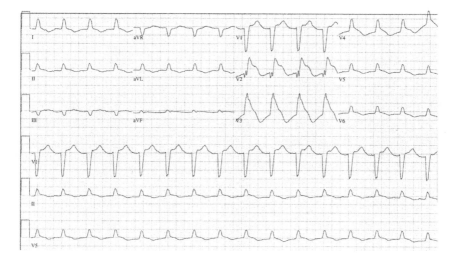

Figure 2.6

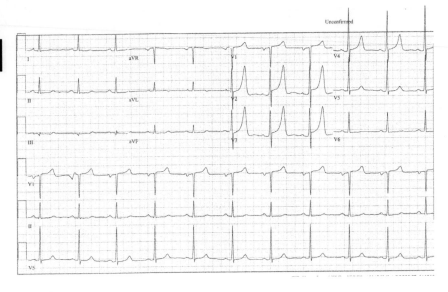

**Figure 2.7**

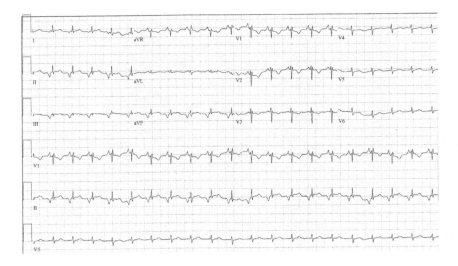

**Figure 2.8**

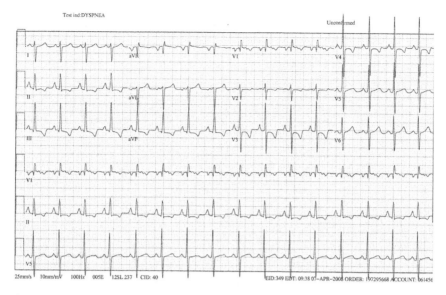

**Figure 2.9**

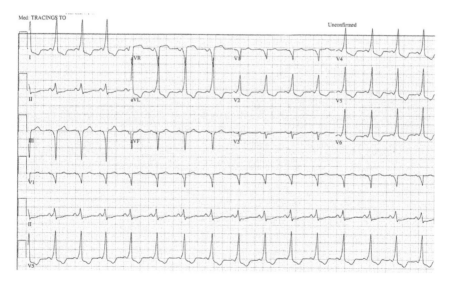

**Figure 2.10**

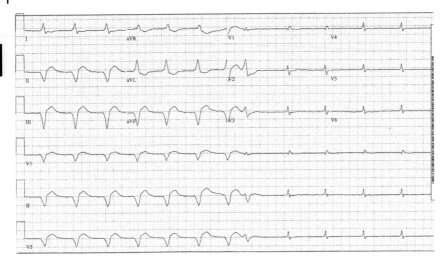

**Figure 2.11**

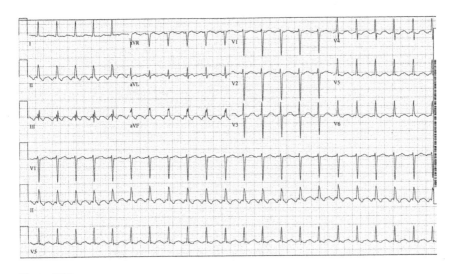

**Figure 2.12**

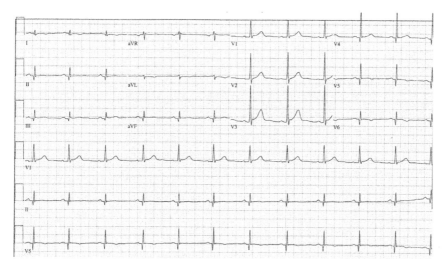

**Figure 2.13**

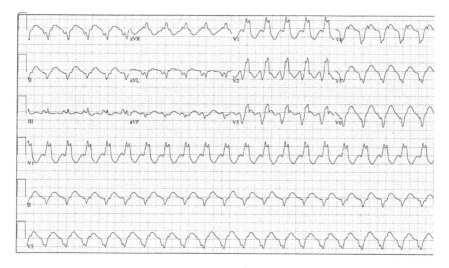

**Figure 2.14**

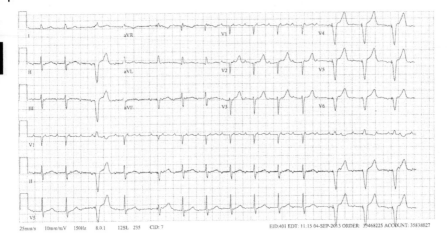

**Figure 2.15**

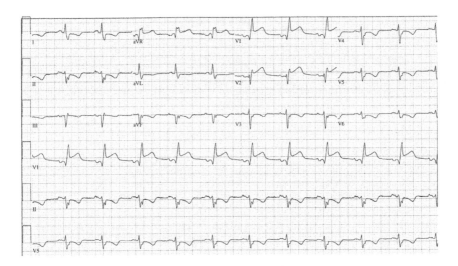

**Figure 2.16**

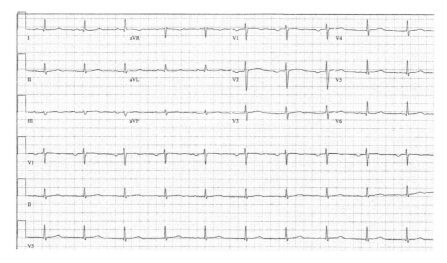

**Figure 2.17**

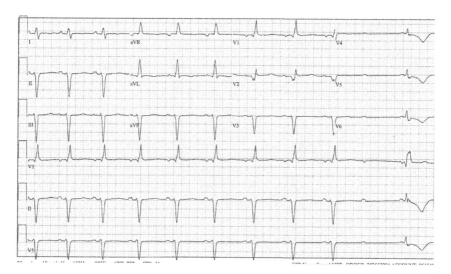

**Figure 2.18**

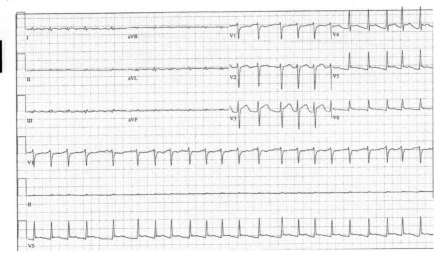

**Figure 2.19**

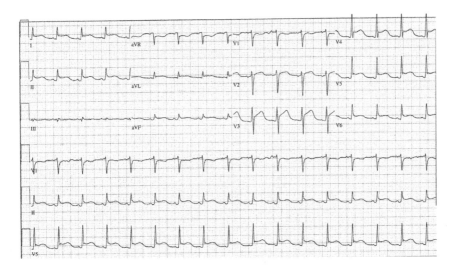

**Figure 2.20**

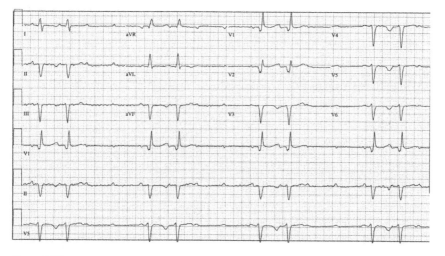

**Figure 2.21**

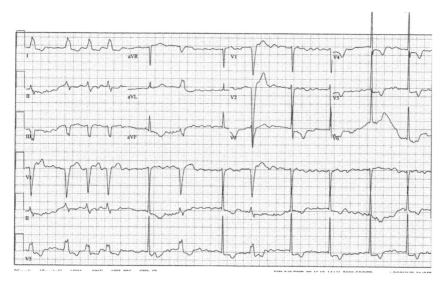

**Figure 2.22**

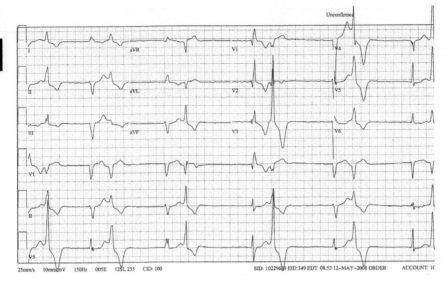

**Figure 2.23**

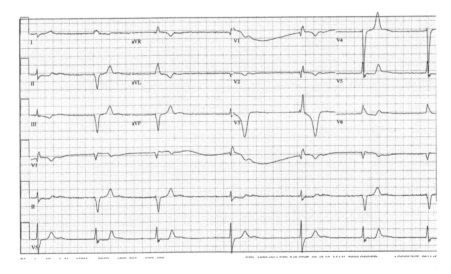

**Figure 2.24**

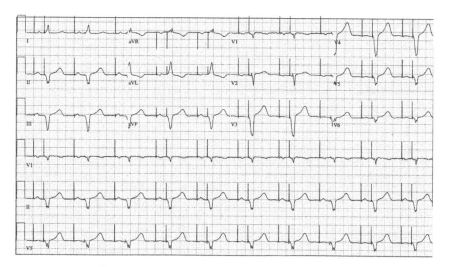

**Figure 2.25**

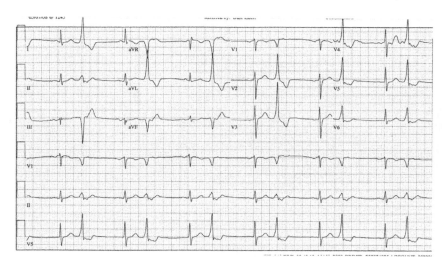

**Figure 2.26**

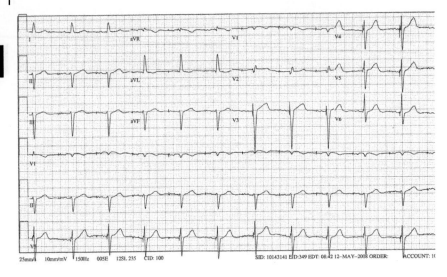

**Figure 2.27**

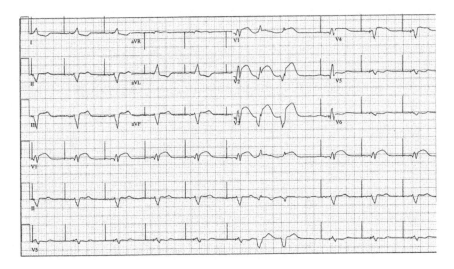

**Figure 2.28**

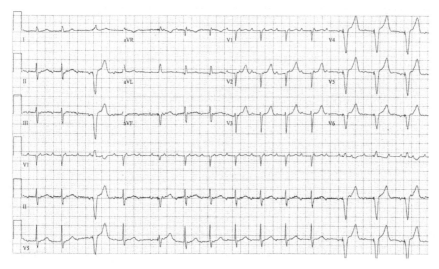

**Figure 2.29**

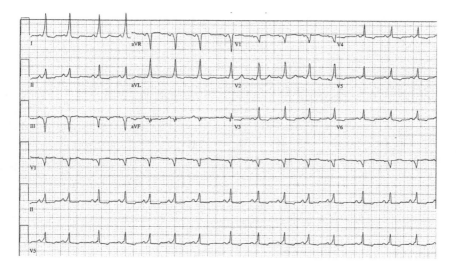

**Figure 2.30**

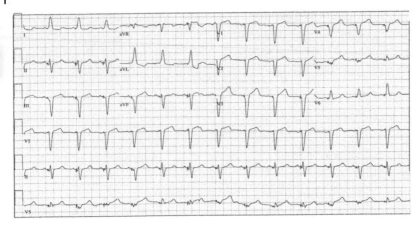

**Figure 2.31**

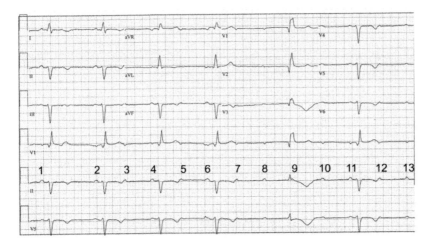

**Figure 2.32**

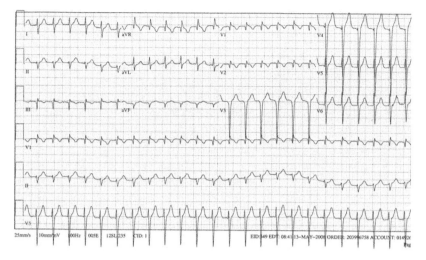

**Figure 2.33**

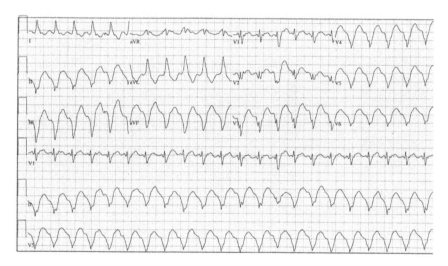

**Figure 2.34**

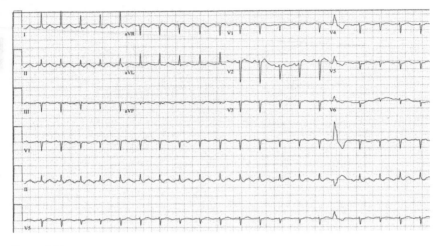

**Figure 2.35**

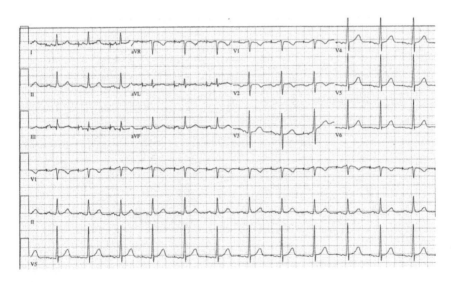

**Figure 2.36**

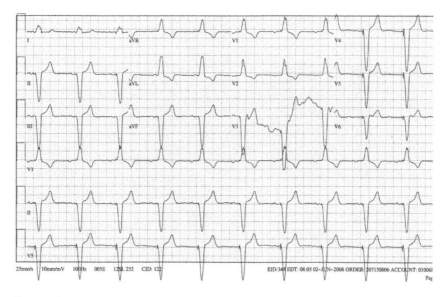

**Figure 2.37**

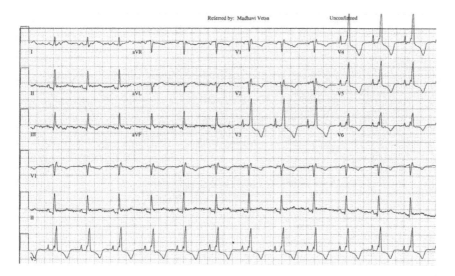

**Figure 2.38**

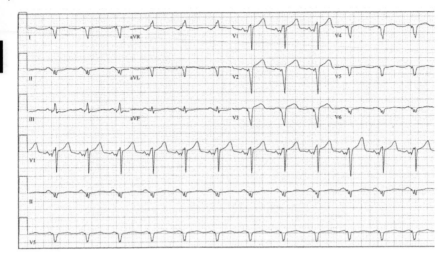

**Figure 2.39**

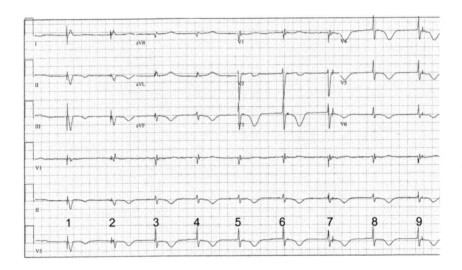

**Figure 2.40**

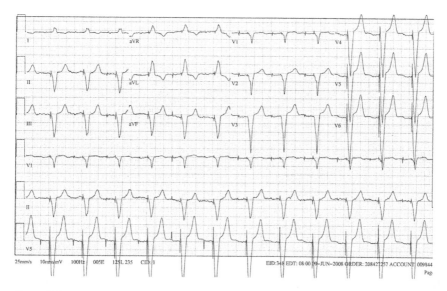

**Figure 2.41**

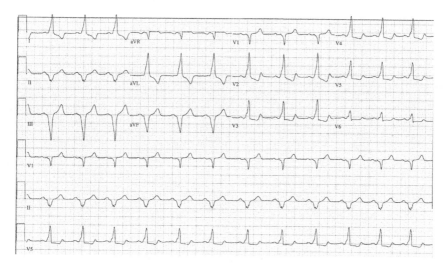

**Figure 2.42**

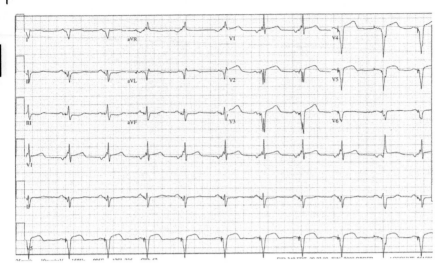

**Figure 2.43**

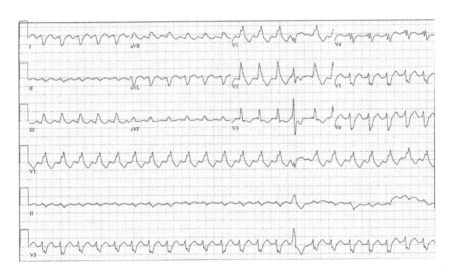

**Figure 2.44**

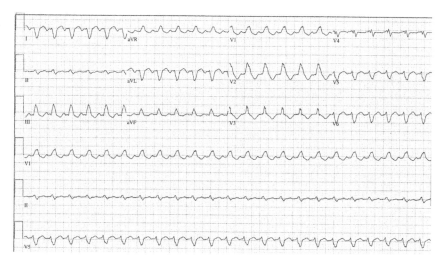

**Figure 2.45**

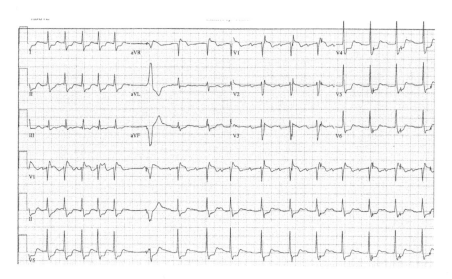

**Figure 2.46**

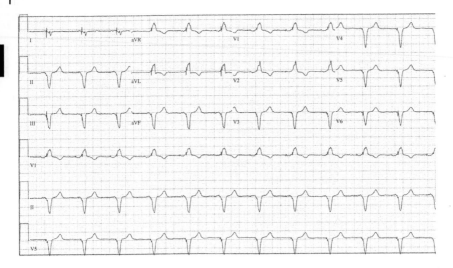

**Figure 2.47**

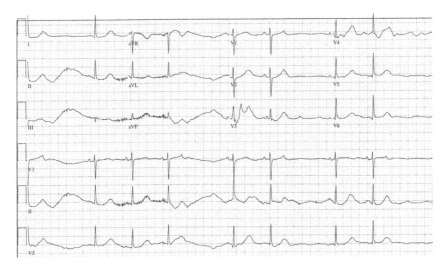

**Figure 2.48**

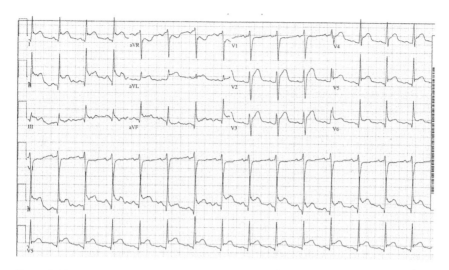

**Figure 2.49**

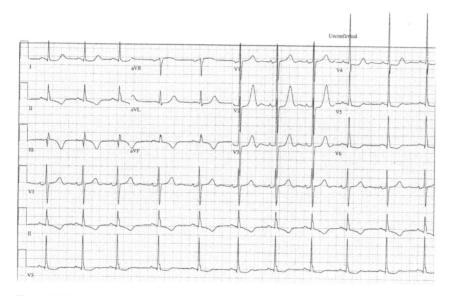

**Figure 2.50**

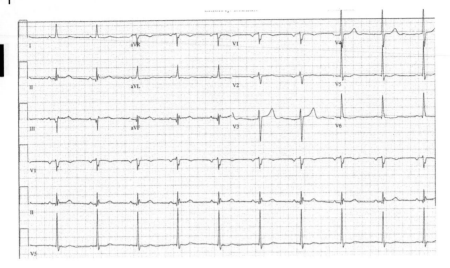

**Figure 2.51**

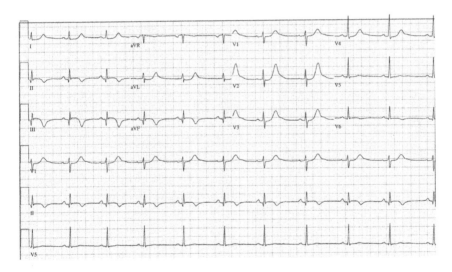

**Figure 2.52**

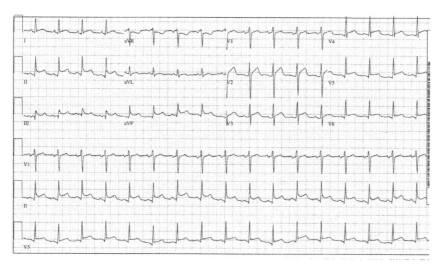

Figure 2.53

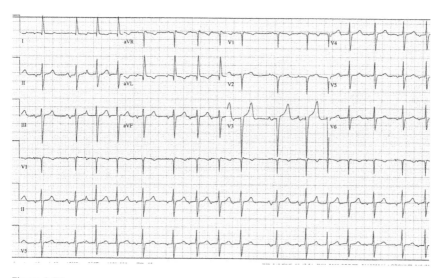

Figure 2.54

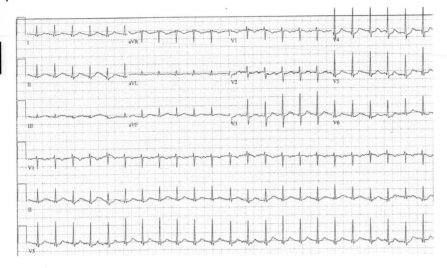

Figure 2.55

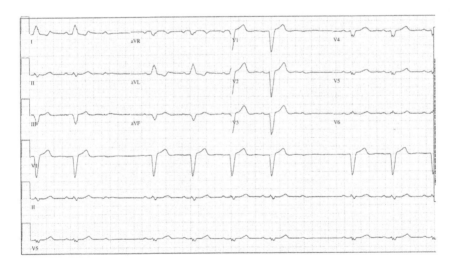

Figure 2.56

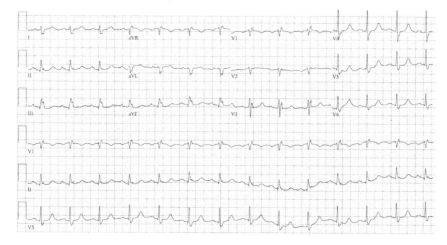

**Figure 2.57**

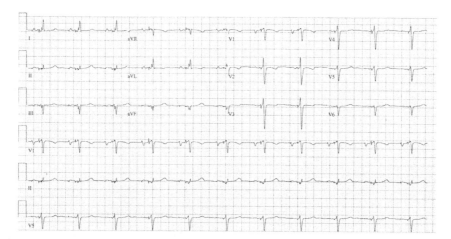

**Figure 2.58**

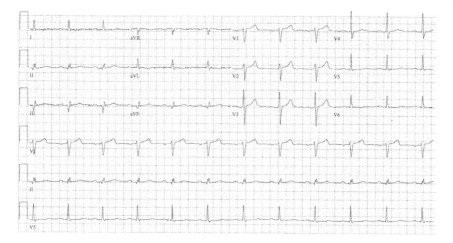

**Figure 2.59**

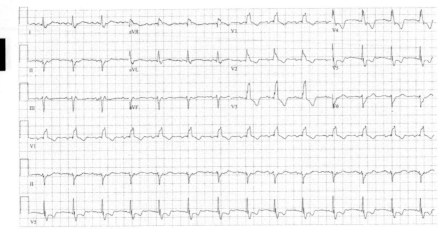

**Figure 2.60**

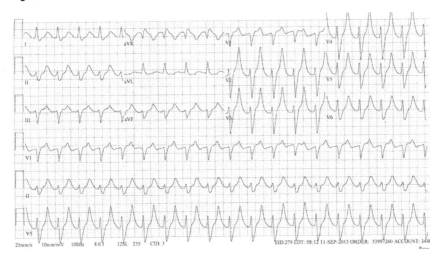

**Figure 2.61**

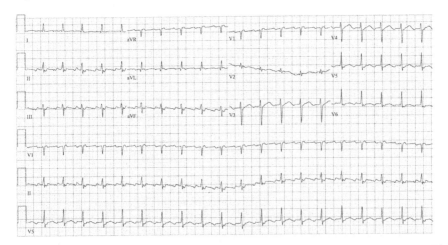

**Figure 2.62**

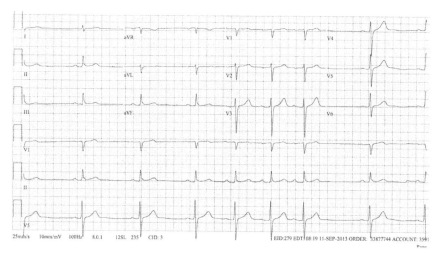

**Figure 2.63**

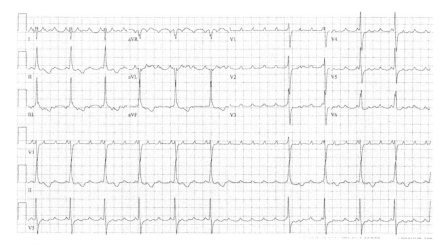

**Figure 2.64**

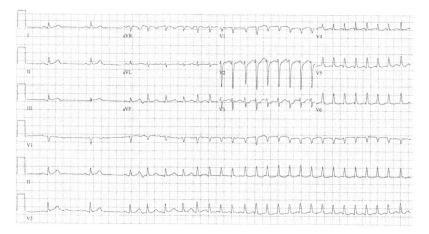

**Figure 2.65**

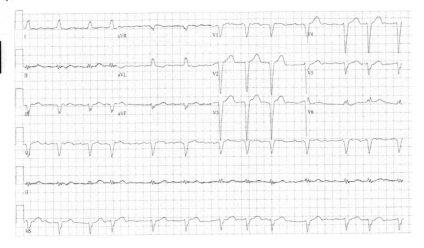

**Figure 2.66**

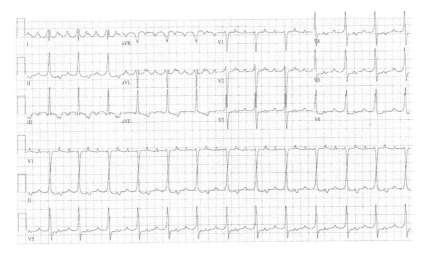

**Figure 2.67**

## Answers

**2.1.** Second-degree atrioventricular (AV) block, Mobitz type I (AV Wenckebach). Note increasing PR interval and PR interval being the shortest after a dropped beat. Also, note that the patient has intraventricular conduction delay (IVCD) and lateral T-wave inversion. Despite IVCD, it is less likely to be trifascicular block as AV Wenckebach is generally a nodal rather than infra-Hisian phenomenon.

**2.2.** Right ventricular (RV) hypertrophy (RVH) with strain and biatrial enlargement. R in V1 > 5 mm with right axis deviation and ST–T changes in right chest leads support RVH. P wave amplitude >3 mm supports right atrial enlargement and P-terminale in V1 > 1 × 1 box supports left atrial enlargement.

**2.3.** Sinus rhythm with bifascicular block. Note the right bundle branch block (RBBB) and left axis deviation with mean QRS axis less than −30° suggesting left anterior fascicular block (LAHB). Also note the peak of R wave is earliest in III, followed by II, and then I, indicating late activation of left ventricular (LV) lateral wall supplied by anterior fascicle. The inferior wall is supplied by posterior fascicle and R wave peaks early in these leads.

**2.4.** Sinus arrhythmia with short PR interval suggesting Lown-Ganong-Levine syndrome. Note that there is no delta wave or QRS prolongation indicating Wolff-Parkinson-White (WPW) syndrome. In Lown-Ganong-Levine syndrome, the accessory pathway is atrio-Hisian, shortening the PR interval. In WPW syndrome, AV preexcitation of a portion of ventricular myocardium results in delta wave and QRS prolongation.

**2.5.** Atrial fibrillation. Note the absence of P wave and irregularly irregular ventricular response. Also note the low QRS voltage (<5 mm in limb and < 10 mm in chest leads), which should raise the suspicion of chronic obstructive pulmonary disease, pericardial effusion, or diffuse myocardial disease.

**2.6.** Acute anterior ST elevation myocardial infarction (STEMI). Note hyperacute, tombstone ST elevation in V2 and V3.

**2.7.** Hyperkalemia. Note the peaked, tall T waves in V2 and V3.

**2.8.** Junctional tachycardia. P waves are inverted in inferior leads with superior axis indicating junctional or low atrial origin.

**2.9.** RVH. qR in V1 with right axis deviation and strain pattern in right chest leads is suggestive of RVH.

**2.10.** WPW syndrome (? Posteroseptal).

**2.11.** Seven beats of accelerated idioventricular rhythm, followed by a fusion beat and then accelerated junctional rhythm. This is suggestive of digoxin toxicity.

**2.12.** Atrial flutter with 2 : 1 conduction. Flutter waves are clearly visible in inferior leads.

**2.13.** Posterior myocardial infarction. Note the tall R waves in V1 and V2 with upright T wave associated with Q waves inferolaterally. In RVH, one would expect to see strain pattern in right chest leads.

**2.14.** Ventricular tachycardia. Broad complexed tachycardia with RBBB morphology with left rabbit ear, QRS duration of 200 ms and indeterminate axis – all suggestive of ventricular tachycardia (VT) rather that supraventricular tachycardia (SVT) with aberrancy.

**2.15.** Atypical atrial flutter with 3 : 1 conduction, intermittent RV pacing (third and last three beats) and one fusion complex (fifth beat).

**2.16.** Acute anterior STEMI. Note Q waves and ST elevation of 3–4 mm in V1 and V2.

**2.17.** Sinus rhythm with low QRS voltage (<5 mm in limb leads or <10 mm in chest leads). Consider pericardial effusion, emphysema.

**2.18.** Nonconducted P (second from right) followed by a P associated with a ventricular escape beat showing T-wave inversion. Consistent with Mobitz type II AV block. Also note the anterior Q wave, RBBB and LAFB - a substrate for trifascicular block.

**2.19.** Atrial fibrillation with rapid ventricular response. Also note the low QRS voltage and diffuse ST elevation, suggesting pericarditis with effusion which may result in atrial fibrillation through atrial irritation.

**2.20.** Acute pericarditis. Note diffuse concave-up ST elevation and PR segment depression in most of the leads and reciprocal PR segment elevation and ST depression in aVR.

**2.21.** Episodes of complete heart block. Note >1 nonconducted P in a row. Note old inferior and acute anterior STEMI and mechanism of heart block is likely to be infra-Hisian with high risk of lack of escape rhythm.

**2.22.** Premature ventricular contractions (PVCs), three-beat VT (beats 2–4), accelerated idiojunctional rhythm (fairly regular narrow complex with no preceding P at a rate of 65 bpm, beats 9–12), Afib (lack of a P wave), short QT interval. These are highly indicative of digoxin toxicity. Digoxin toxicity blocks AV node and promotes subsidiary pacemakers at a faster rate.

**2.23.** Junctional rhythm with ventricular bigeminy.

**2.24.** Junctional rhythm with RBBB (beats 1, 4, and 5) with intermittent V-pacing (beats 2, 3, 6, and 7). Note a small pacer spike, changed QRS morphology upright in I, and different T wave morphology with paced beats.

**2.25.** Dual-chamber pacing.

**2.26.** Ventricular bigeminy.

**2.27.** Atrial pacing, ventricular tracking with ventricular pseudofusion. The V-spike before QRS is coincidental and QRS has normal conducted morphology. Lengthening AV delay will conserve the battery.

**2.28.** Dual chamber pacing with ventricular couplet (beats 7 and 8).

**2.29.** Atrial flutter with 2 : 1 conduction and intermittent V-pacing.

**2.30.** WPW syndrome.

**2.31.** Dual-chamber pacer with atrial sensing and V-pacing producing a slightly fused complex. Only very initial part of QRS is slightly slurred, indicating pacer-induced depolarization and the rest of the QRS is normally conducted. Also, note LAFB.

**2.32.** High-grade AV block. The P waves are numbered. The atrial rate is about 86 bpm, and between 1 and 2 (rate 43) a P wave is dropped, indicating 2 : 1 sino-atrial block (produced by a nonconducted premature atrial contraction [PAC] between 1 and 2 through concealed retrograde conduction. The PAC is deforming the ST segment). Then, there is 2 : 1 A : V block till 7 followed by two successive Ps being dropped (complete AV block) with a ventricular escape beat at 9 burying a P wave.

**2.33.** Narrow complex regular tachycardia at a rate of 150 bpm without a discernible P wave. Likely paroxysmal SVT and possible atrioventricular nodal reentry tachycardia.

**2.34.** Broad complex tachycardia at a rate of 140 bpm, suggestive of VT. Note the negative concordance in chest leads, superior axis, QRS duration of >200 ms, and slow upstroke of QRS complex – all suggestive of VT.

**2.35.** Atrial flutter with 2 : 1 conduction. Note a clear flutter waves in lead II. There is a single PVC.

**2.36.** Atrial paced rhythm with normal AV conduction and normal QRS.

**2.37.** Atrial sensed and ventricular paced rhythm. Note that QRS is upright in V1, suggesting probable LV rather than RV pacing. The patient has a biventricular (BiV) pacer.

**2.38.** WPW syndrome. Note the delta waves in V4 and V5.

**2.39.** Dual-chamber pacer with atrial tracking and V-pacing producing fusion QRS complexes with initial portion due to pacing and remainder being conducted.

**2.40.** VOO pacing with pacer competing with junctional rhythm producing fully paced beat (1), fusion complex (2), pseudofusion (3), and lack of sensing (5–9). Also note QT prolongation. T-wave inversion can occur because of repolarization memory secondary to V-pacing.

**2.41.** Dual-chamber pacing.

**2.42.** WPW syndrome, probably posteroseptal pathway because of inferior Q waves, positive delta waves in anterolateral leads, and rapid transition from V1 to V2.

**2.43.** BiV pacer with atrial and LV pacing. Note that QRS is negative in lateral leads and positive in V1, indicating LV pacing.

**2.44.** Broad complex tachycardia at a rate of 140 bpm with QRS duration of 160 ms, RBBB pattern with right rabbit ear and right axis deviation and rapid upstroke of initial part of QRS (in V5/V6) with broadening of latter part suggesting SVT with aberrancy. Note that the PVC did not reset the rhythm.

**2.45.** Broad complex tachycardia with monophasic RBBB pattern in V1, right axis deviation, and QRS duration of 160 ms. No P waves seen. Note the rapid rise of QRS voltage in V5 and V6. The patient had SVT with aberrancy.

**2.46.** Atrial fibrillation for the first five beats, then V-pacing for a beat followed by sinus rhythm with first-degree AV block and lack of V-sensing in last three beats. Also note an acute anterior STEMI.

**2.47.** BiV pacer. Patient is paced in atrium and left ventricle, producing RBBB QRS morphology.

**2.48.** Blocked PACs. The pauses are due to nonconducted PACs which occurred on the T wave and during the refractory period of AV node. This does not signify AV nodal disease. When there are pauses, always look for nonconducted PACs. Also note QT prolongation.

**2.49.** Acute inferolateral STEMI. Note reciprocal ST depression in aVR; in pericarditis, there is reciprocal ST and PR segment elevation in aVR.

**2.50.** BiV hypertrophy. R in V1 is >5 mm and R/S in V1 is 1, suggesting RVH. R in V5 plus S in V2 is 35 mm, and ST depression in V5 and V6 suggests LV hypertrophy (LVH).

**2.51.** Normal electrocardiogram.

**2.52.** Acute inferior STEMI with near-complete ST segment resolution and inferior Q waves.

**2.53.** Acute inferolateral STEMI.

**2.54.** Multifocal atrial tachycardia. Note three different P wave morphologies and average rate >100 bpm.

**2.55.** Sinus tachycardia.

**2.56.** Intermittent dropped QRSs without progressive PR prolongation suggesting second-degree Mobitz type II AV block. Also note the patient has left bundle branch block (LBBB), further supporting that the mechanism of AV block is likely infra-Hisian rather than intranodal. High risk of complete heart block.

**2.57.** Bifascicular block. The patient has RBBB and right axis deviation, suggesting left posterior fascicular block. Note the peaks of R wave in leads II and III follow lead I, suggesting activation spreading from lateral to inferior wall, the region of posterior fascicle.

**2.58.** Dual-chamber pacing, but QRS is native rather than paced. The V-spike comes before QRS, but QRS is narrow and has near-normal morphology.

**2.59.** Inferior myocardial infarction, age undetermined, possibly recent (slight ST elevation in leads III and aVF).

**2.60.** Bifascicular block with RBBB and LAFB. Also note the absence of r in leads V1 to
V4, indicating anterior myocardial infarction. Hence, the likely mechanism is diffuse conduction system disease through ischemia and signifies high risk due to the
infra-Hisian mechanism and extent of myocardial involvement.

**2.61.** Severe hyperkalemia with near sine wave appearance: Note peaked T waves, QRS
prolongation, and absent P waves.

**2.62.** Atrial flutter with 2 : 1 conduction. The atrial rate is 240 bpm and ventricular rate
is 120 bpm.

**2.63.** Marked respiratory sinus arrhythmia. Note that the P wave morphology is constant and cyclical changes in P-P intervals are consistent with frequency of respiration. It is a marker of vagotonia and seems to be more marked in the young and
at slow heart rates.

**2.64.** Atrial tachycardia with variable block.

**2.65.** Paroxysmal atrial fibrillation with rapid ventricular response.

**2.66.** Atypical atrial flutter with variable block and IVCD of LBBB morphology.

**2.67.** Atrial tachycardia with 3 1 conduction. Atrial rate is about 225 bpm, and this
could also be slow flutter because of antiarrhythmic therapy.

---

**Box 2.1    ECG Diagnostic Criteria**

**Normal Sinus P Wave**

- P wave duration <120 ms
- Amplitude ≤2.5 mm
- P wave axis between 45° and 75° in frontal plane

**Criteria for Left Atrial Enlargement**

- P wave duration >120 ms in lead II
- Notched P wave in lead II with inter-notch distance >40 ms (P-mitrale)
- P-terminale in V1 > 0.04 mm
- P wave axis between +45° and −30° in frontal plane (left axis deviation)

**Criteria for Right Atrial Enlargement**

- P wave amplitude >2.5 mm in lead II (P-pulmonale)
- Area under initial positive part of P wave in V1 > 0.06 mm
- P wave axis > 75° in frontal plane (right axis deviation)

**Criteria for LVH**

- Sokolov criteria: S in V1 plus R in V5 or V6 > 35 mm; R in a VL > 11 mm
- Cornell criteria: S in V3 plus S in V1 ≥ 28 mm for men and ≥20 mm for women
- Romhilt-Estes criteria (LVH if 5 points): R wave in any limb lead ≥20 mm, or S in V1 or
  V2 ≥ 30 mm, or R in V5 or V6 ≥ 30 mm (3 points); left atrial abnormality (3 points); ST-T

changes without digoxin (3 points) or with digoxin (1 point); QRS axis $< -30°$ (2 points); QRS duration >90 ms (1 point); intrinsicoid deflection in V5 or V6 > 50 ms (1 point)

## Criteria for RVH

- R in V1 $\geq$ 7 mm
- QR in V1
- R/SinV1 > 1 with R at least 5 mm
- R/Sin V5 or V6 < 1
- $S_1Q_3T_3$ pattern (pulmonary embolism)
- $S_1S_2S_3$ pattern

## Criteria for BiV Hypertrophy

- Tall R in both left and right chest leads
- LVH with right axis deviation
- LVH with deep S in V5 or V6
- LVH with shift of precordial transition (R/S = 1) to the left of V4

## Criteria for LAFB

- QRS axis $< -45°$ with rS in inferior leads (i.e. no inferior Q waves) and qR in high lateral leads plus QRSd <120 ms

## Criteria for Left Posterior Fascicular Block

- QRS axis > 120° with RS in high lateral leads and qR in inferior leads plus QRSd <120 ms

## Criteria for LBBB

- Broad notched R wave in lateral leads, absent q in left-sided leads (septal activation will be right to left), QRSd $\geq$ 120 ms

## Criteria for RBBB

- Broad notched R wave in V1 and V2 with right rabbit ear, deep slurred S in left-sided leads (reciprocal of R'), QRSd $\geq$ 120 ms

## Causes of Tall R Wave in VI

- RVH (generally with right axis deviation and secondary ST-T changes or right atrial enlargement)
- True posterior infarct (generally with upright T, inferior or lateral Q)
- Hypertrophic obstructive cardiomyopathy (due to septal depolarization)
- Duchenne muscular dystrophy
- RBBB
- WPW syndrome with posterior or lateral pathways
- Heart shifted to right

## Causes of Q Waves

- Normal in V1/V2 and III (in lead III will disappear with deep breath which makes heart vertical)
- Myocardial infarction
- Myocardial infiltration (sarcoid, amyloid)
- Myocarditis
- WPW syndrome
- LBBB results in Q in V1/V2
- Hypertrophic obstructive cardiomyopathy (septal hypertrophy causing Q in lateral leads)

## Causes of ST Elevation

- Normal variant (early repolarization, generally V1–V4)
- Myocardial injury (convex up)
- LV aneurysm (persistent beyond 6months)
- Pericarditis (concave up, diffuse, ST and PR elevation in aVR, PR depression)
- Brugada syndrome
- Hyperkalemia ("dialyzable current of injury")
- Type IC antiarrhythmic agents
- LVH and LBBB (in right chest leads as reciprocal of ST depression on left chest leads)

## Hyperkalemia

- Peaked T wave (early sign)
- Increased QRS duration
- Absent P wave
- Sine wave morphology in late stage

## Hypercalcemia

- Shortened QT interval

## Hypocalcemia

- QT lengthening (especially ST segment lengthening)

# Chest X-Ray in Cardiology

**3**

3.1. A 52-year-old African-American male was admitted with complaints of short-ness of breath and edema. He has a history of methamphetamine use. A chest X-ray (Figure 3.1a) was performed in the emergency room (ER). What does the chest X-ray show?

A. Cardiomegaly
B. Cardiomegaly, automatic implantable cardioverter-defibrillator (AICD) lead and generator
C. Normal findings
D. Cardiomegaly, AICD lead and generator, left pleural effusion

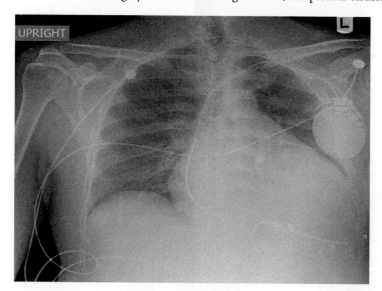

**Figure 3.1a**

3.2. An 84-year-old male was admitted with shortness of breath. He was diagnosed with left pleural effusion. He underwent thoracentesis. A few hours later, he developed increasing oxygen requirements. A chest X-ray was done (see Figure 3.2a). What does it show?

A. Pulmonary edema
B. Right apical pneumothorax
C. Left apical pneumothorax
D. Right-sided pneumonia

*Cardiology Board Review*, Second Edition. Ramdas G. Pai and Padmini Varadarajan.
© 2023 John Wiley & Sons Ltd. Published 2023 by John Wiley & Sons Ltd.

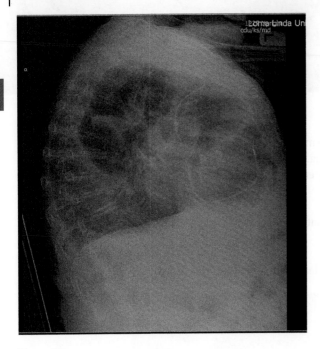

Figure 3.2a

3.3. A 59-year-old male was admitted with a history of subarachnoid hemorrhage. A PA chest X-ray (Figure 3.3a) was performed in the ER. What does the chest X-ray show?

A. Normal chest X-ray

B. Prosthetic valve in the mitral position

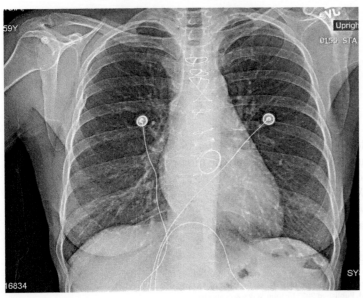

Figure 3.3a

C. Prosthetic valve in the aortic position

D. Prosthetic valves in the aortic and mitral positions

3.4. A 75-year-old male presented to the ER with complaints of shortness of breath. A chest X-ray (Figure 3.4a) was performed in the ER. What does the X-ray show?

A. Left pleural effusion

B. Right pleural effusion

C. Consolidation

D. Pulmonary edema

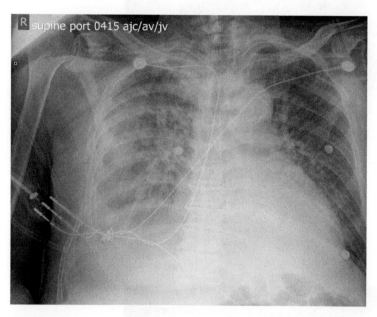

Figure 3.4a

3.5. A 59-year-old Pakistani male presented to the ER with complaints of headache. He had a computed tomography (CT) scan of his head, which showed evidence of subdural hemorrhage. He also had a chest X-ray (Figure 3.5a) in the ER. What does the X-ray show?

A. Bioprosthetic valve in the aortic position

B. Bileaflet mechanical prosthesis in the mitral position

C. Bioprosthetic valve in the mitral position

D. No prosthetic valve is seen

3.6. A 56-year-old male presented to the ER with complaints of shortness of breath on exertion, cough with whitish expectoration, and pedal edema. In the ER, he had a chest X-ray (see Figure 3.6a). What is the most important finding on the X-ray?

A. Pneumothorax

B. Right pleural effusion only

C. Left pleural effusion

D. Bilateral pleural effusion

E. No abnormality seen

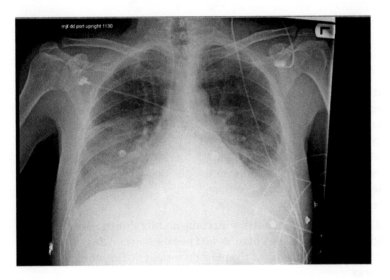

Figure 3.5a

Figure 3.6a

3.7. A 39-year-old male presented to the hospital after a cardiac arrest at home. He was brought to the hospital and had a chest X-ray (Figure 3.7). What does the chest X- ray show?

A. Normal heart size
B. Cardiomegaly
C. Left pneumothorax
D. Right pneumothorax

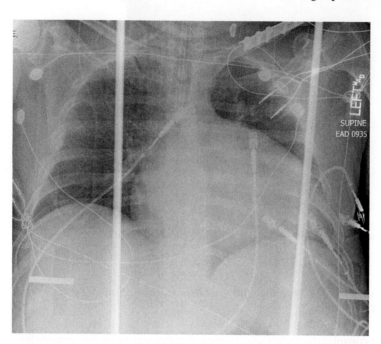

Figure 3.7

3.8. A 51-year-old male came to the hospital with complaints of fatigue and cough. He had a chest X-ray (see Figure 3.8a) in the ER. What does his chest X-ray show?

A. Normal aortic size
B. Prominent aortic knob
C. Prominent main pulmonary artery
D. Prominent left bronchus

3.9. The patient in Question 3.8 then had an echocardiogram. He had mild tricuspid regurgitation, velocity of 4.7 m/s, elevated right atrial pressure of 20 mmHg, and estimated pulmonary artery systolic pressure of 110 mmHg. What are these findings suggestive of?

A. Primary pulmonary hypertension
B. Pulmonary vascular congestion
C. Right-to-left shunt
D. None of the above

3.10. A 69-year-old male was admitted to the hospital complaining of shortness of breath. His initial chest X-ray showed pulmonary edema and he was started on intravenous diuretics. Two days later, he complained of feeling feverish,

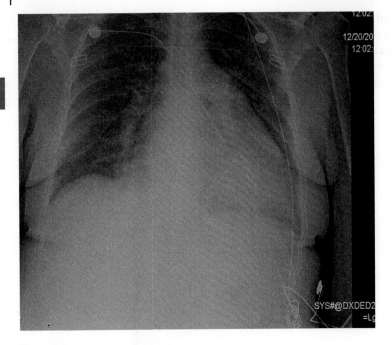

Figure 3.8a

temperature was 101°F, with chills and greenish expectoration. What does the repeat chest X-ray (Figure 3.10a) show?
A. Pulmonary edema
B. Right hilar consolidation with superimposed pulmonary vascular congestion
C. Left hilar consolidation
D. Right hilar consolidation

3.11. A 62-year-old male was admitted with complaints of shortness of breath. What does the chest X-ray in Figure 3.11a show?
A. Left atrial enlargement
B. Right ventricular enlargement
C. Left ventricular enlargement
D. Right atrial and right ventricular enlargement

3.12. An 80-year-old female patient has a history of long-standing systolic murmur at the base. She had a chest X-ray (Figure 3.12a). What is the most important finding?
A. Marked enlargement of main pulmonary artery
B. Marked enlargement of the aorta
C. Marked enlargement of the right pulmonary artery
D. Marked enlargement of the main pulmonary artery and left pulmonary artery

3.13. What does the blue arrow point to on the chest X-ray in Figure 3.13?
A. Enlarged left atrium
B. Aortic knob
C. Enlarged pulmonary artery
D. None of the above

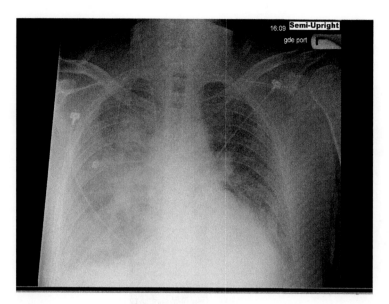

Figure 3.10a

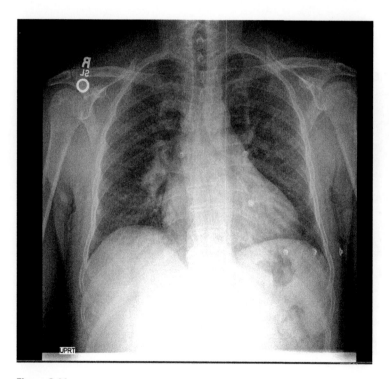

Figure 3.11a

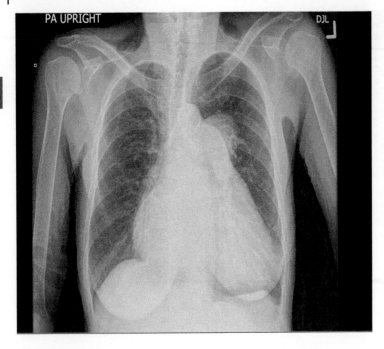

Figure 3.12a

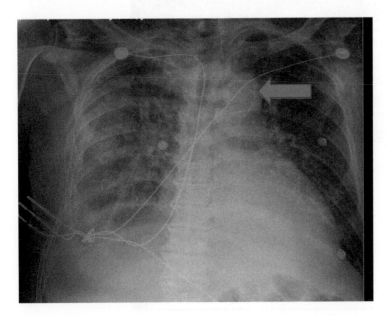

Figure 3.13

**3.14.** What structure indicated by the blue arrow in Figure 3.14 forms the cardiac boundary:

A. Ascending aorta
B. Arch of the aorta

C. Right pulmonary artery
D. Superior vena cava

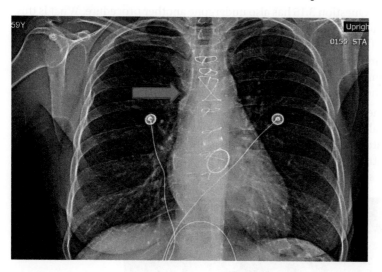

Figure 3.14

**3.15.** Figure 3.15a shows a 93-year-old female patient with a history of shortness of breath who has undergone what procedure?

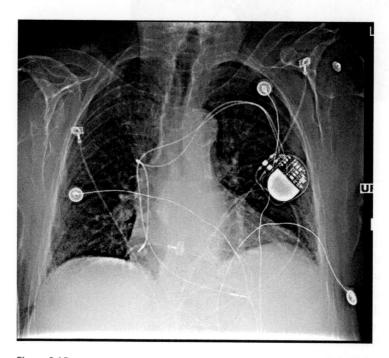

Figure 3.15a

A. Surgical replacement of mitral valve
B. Surgical replacement of aortic valve
C. Transaortic valve replacement (TAVR)
D. None of the above

3.16. The patient in Question 3.15 has also undergone another procedure. What is this other procedure?
  A. Permanent single-chamber pacemaker
  B. Dual-chamber pacemaker
  C. Dual-chamber AICD
  D. None of the above

3.17. What does the blue arrow in Figure 3.17 point to?
  A. Right atrial pacer lead
  B. Right ventricular pacer lead
  C. Right ventricular implantable cardioverter-defibrillator (ICD) lead
  D. Coronary sinus lead

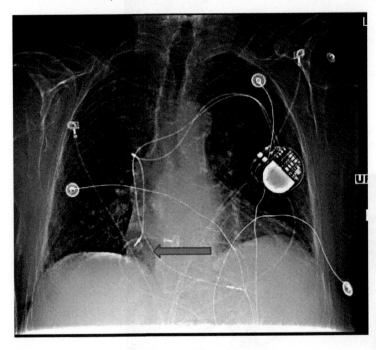

Figure 3.17

3.18. What does the blue arrow in Figure 3.18 point to?
  A. Right atrial pacer lead          C. Right atrial ICD lead
  B. Right ventricular ICD lead       D. Coronary sinus lead

3.19. What does the blue arrow in Figure 3.19a point to?
  A. Right atrial pacer lead
  B. Right ventricular ICD lead
  C. Right atrial ICD lead
  D. Coronary sinus lead

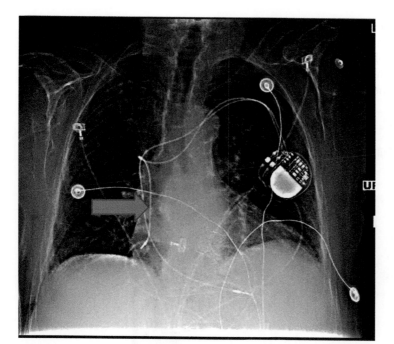

Figure 3.18

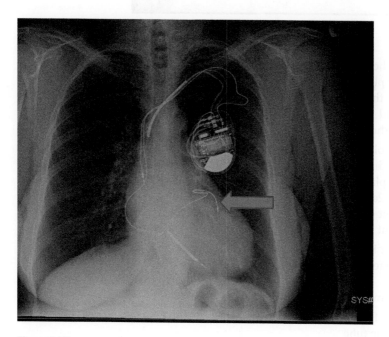

Figure 3.19a

3.20. What does the blue arrow in Figure 3.20 point to?
 A. A pacer lead
 B. Catheter placed through left subclavian vein
 C. Arterial line
 D. None of the above

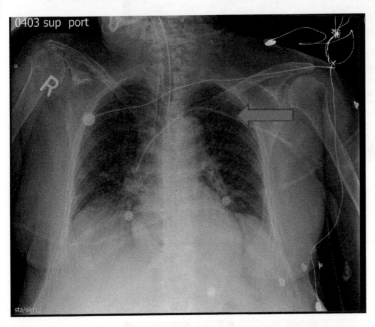

Figure 3.20

3.21. What does the blue arrow in Figure 3.21 point to?
 A. Catheter placed through right internal jugular vein
 B. Catheter through right subclavian vein
 C. Pacer lead
 D. None of the above

3.22. An 86-year-old male with history of chronic obstructive pulmonary disease (COPD) is admitted to the hospital. After one day, he was noted to be hypoxic. He also complained of feeling feverish and increasingly short of breath. Referring to Figure 3.22a, what procedure did he undergo?
 A. Placement of central line
 B. Placement of a pacer
 C. Endotracheal intubation (ET)
 D. Thoracentesis

3.23. The arrow in Figure 3.23 points to which landmark on the chest X-ray from the patient in Question 3.22?
 A. Carina
 B. Main pulmonary artery
 C. Esophagus
 D. Aorta

3.24. The arrow in Figure 3.24 points to what structure on the chest X-ray?
 A. Nasogastric tube
 B. Percutaneous endoscopic gastrostomy tube
 C. Central venous catheter
 D. None of the above

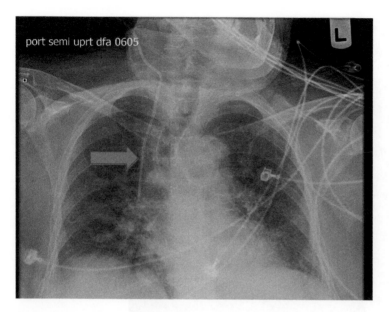

Figure 3.21

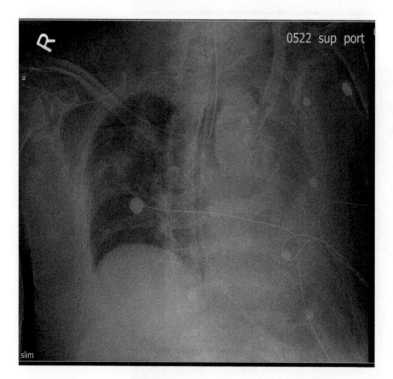

Figure 3.22a

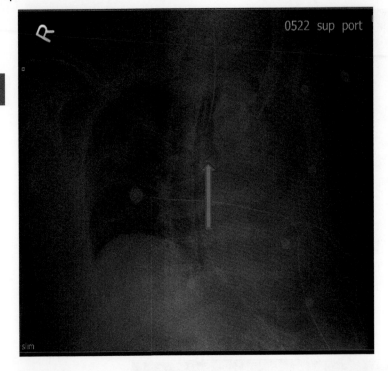

Figure 3.23

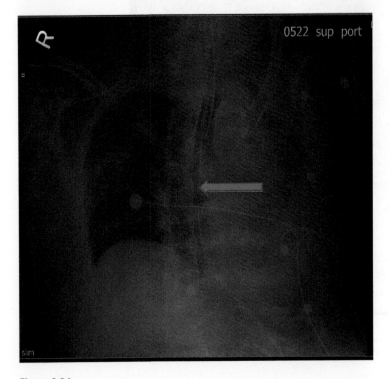

Figure 3.24

**3.25.** A 59-year-old Hispanic female patient was admitted to the hospital with complaints of fever and shortness of breath. A chest X-ray was performed (see Figure 3.25a) and she had which of the following procedures performed?
  A. Pericardiocentesis
  B. Placement of a catheter in the right pleural space
  C. Placement of a catheter in the left pleural space
  D. Right paracentesis

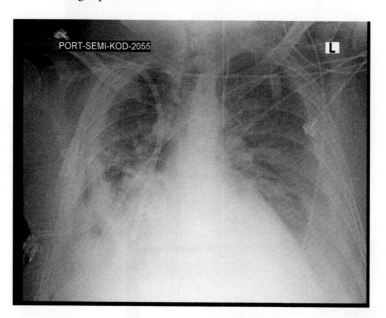

Figure 3.25a

**3.26.** The chest X-ray in Figure 3.26a shows which of the following:
  A. Dextroposition
  B. Dextrocardia
  C. Levocardia
  D. Mesocardia

**3.27.** A 69-year-old male with a history of heart transplant 10 years previously is complaining of low-grade fever, fatigue, and loss of appetite. He had a chest X-ray (see Figure 3.27a) as part of his work up. What does this chest X-ray show?
  A. Normal chest X-ray
  B. A rounded opacity in the right lower lobe
  C. Patchy consolidation in the left lower lobe
  D. Multiple lung nodules

**3.28.** Plethoric lung fields on chest X-ray are seen in all of the following except:
  A. Atrial septal defect (ASD)
  B. Ventricular septal defect (VSD)
  C. Patient ductus arteriosus (PDA)
  D. Mitral stenosis

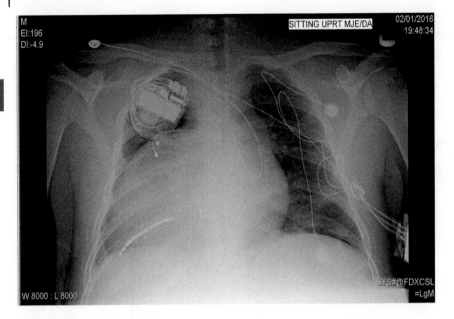

Figure 3.26a

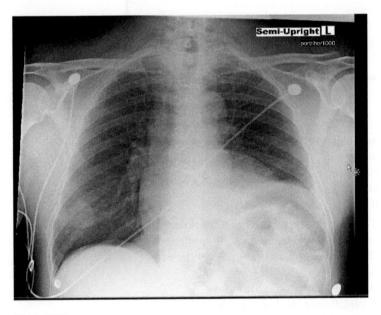

Figure 3.27a

3.29. What is peripheral pulmonary artery pruning a feature of?
  A. Pulmonary hypertension
  B. Pulmonary stenosis
  C. Acute pulmonary embolism
  D. Pulmonary regurgitation

3.30. Dilated main pulmonary artery (jug handle appearance) in a patient with Eisenmenger's syndrome is indicative of:
  A. ASD Eisenmenger's
  B. VSD Eisenmenger's
  C. PDA Eisenmenger's

3.31. Straightened left heart border is classically seen in which of the following:
  A. Mitral stenosis
  B. Aortic stenosis
  C. ASD
  D. PDA

3.32. Coeur en Sabot is a feature of which of the following:
  A. Tetralogy of Fallot
  B. Aortic coarctation
  C. Dilated cardiomyopathy
  D. Hypertrophic cardiomyopathy

3.33. Snowman appearance is a classic description of which of the following:
  A. Partial anomalous pulmonary venous drainage
  B. Total anomalous pulmonary venous drainage
  C. Ebstein's anomaly
  D. ASD

3.34. Scimitar sign is seen in which of the following:
  A. Partial anomalous pulmonary venous drainage
  B. Total anomalous pulmonary venous drainage
  C. Ebstein's anomaly
  D. ASD

3.35. An increase in subcarinal angle due to lifting of the left bronchus is a feature of which of the following:
  A. Left ventricular hypertrophy
  B. Left atrial dilation
  C. Right atrial dilation
  D. Pulmonary ectasia

## Answers

3.1. D. Cardiomegaly, AICD lead, left pleural effusion.
  The cardiomediastinal ratio is increased, which is indicative of cardiomegaly (red arrow in Figure 3.1b). There is also an AICD lead in the right ventricle (blue arrow in Figure 3.1b). The left costophrenic angle is blunted, which is suggestive of the presence of pleural effusion.

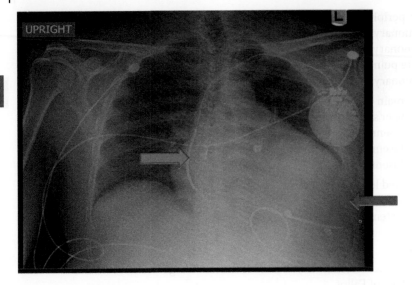

Figure 3.1b

**3.2.** C. Left apical pneumothorax.

The patient had thoracentesis, which then caused left apical pneumothorax: blue arrow in lateral view (Figure 3.2b); multiple arrows in posteroanterior (PA) view (Figure 3.2c). The pneumothorax was drained with a chest tube.

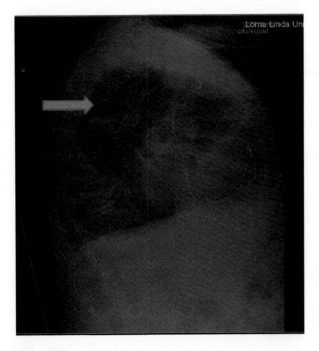

Figure 3.2b

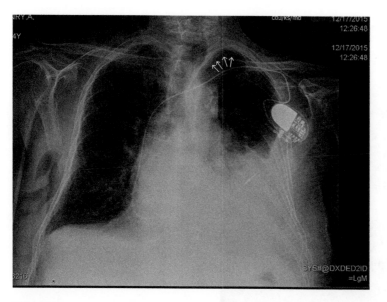

Figure 3.2c

**3.3.** D. Prosthetic valves in the aortic and mitral positions.

Chest X-rays (Figures 3.3b and 3.3c) show two mechanical valve prosthetic rings: one in the aortic (red arrow) and another in the mitral position (blue arrow). Mitral is to the left of the midline, caudal, and posterior.

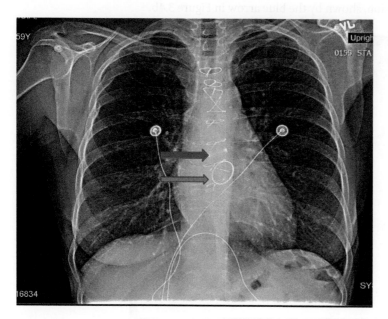

Figure 3.3b

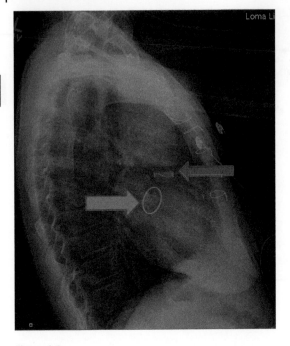

Figure 3.3c

3.4. B. Right pleural effusion.

　　The right costophrenic angle is blunted. The lower to middle lung zones are indistinct and markings are obscured. Chest X-ray shows the presence of right pleural effusion, shown by the blue arrow in Figure 3.4b.

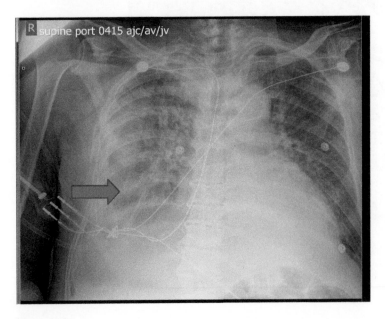

Figure 3.4b

**3.5.** B. Bileaflet mechanical prosthesis in the mitral position.

Chest X-ray shows sternal wires indicative of previous surgery (red arrow in Figure 3.5b). There is a bileaflet mechanical prosthesis in the mitral position (blue arrow in Figure 3.5b). The patient's international normalized ratio was 13 and probably caused the subdural hemorrhage.

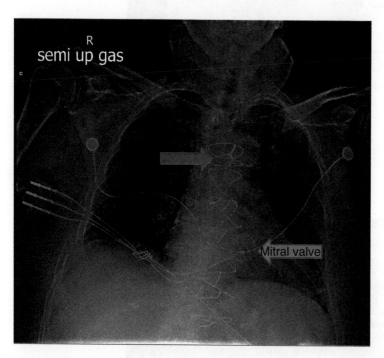

Figure 3.5b

**3.6.** D. Bilateral pleural effusion.

Chest X-ray shows blunting of both costophrenic angles, which is indicative of bilateral pleural effusion (blue arrows in Figure 3.6b).

**3.7.** B. Cardiomegaly.

The patient's chest X-ray shows increased cardiomediastinal ratio, which is suggestive of cardiomegaly.

**3.8.** C. Prominent main pulmonary artery.

The main pulmonary artery is enlarged and is prominent (blue arrow in Figure 3.8b). The red arrow points to the left pulmonary artery, which has a pruned appearance in the peripheral lung zones.

**3.9.** A. Primary pulmonary hypertension.

The patient is young and has a prominent main pulmonary artery on the chest X-ray. His echocardiogram (ECG) reveals pulmonary hypertension. The lungs fields are not plethoric. Given the findings on chest X-ray and echocardiogram, he has primary pulmonary hypertension.

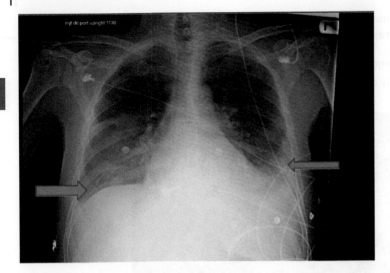

Figure 3.6b

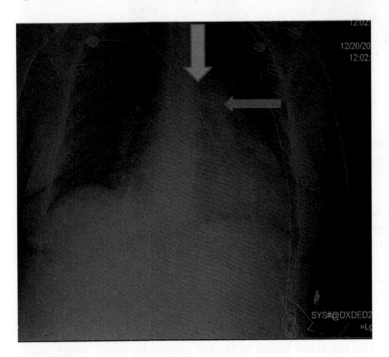

Figure 3.8b

3.10. B. Right hilar consolidation with superimposed pulmonary vascular congestion.
Chest X-ray shows increased pulmonary vascular congestion. But the more striking finding is the presence of right hilar consolidation (blue arrow in Figure 3.10b) suggestive of pneumonia. The less likely differential diagnosis is unilateral right pulmonary edema.

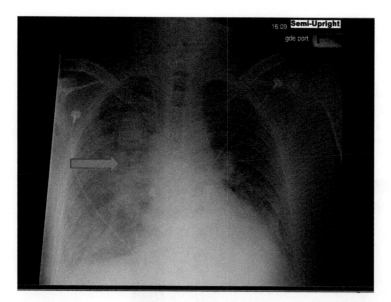

Figure 3.10b

**3.11.** D. Right atrial and right ventricular enlargement.

This patient's chest X-ray shows enlargement of both right atrium (blue arrow in Figure 3.11b) and right ventricle, as evidenced by lifted apex (red arrow). Enlargement of the right ventricle usually causes the apex to be rounded and

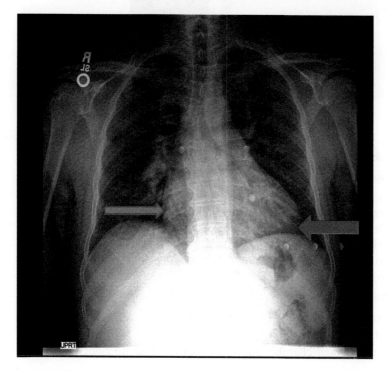

Figure 3.11b

uplifted, as shown by the red arrow. This patient had an echocardiogram (ECG) which showed enlargement of the right-sided chambers without any signs of a shunt. He then underwent a transesophageal echocardiogram, which revealed a sinus venosus atrial septal defect (ASD).

3.12. D. Marked enlargement of the main and left pulmonary artery.

In Figure 3.12b, the red arrow points to the enlarged main pulmonary artery and the blue arrow points to the enlarged left pulmonary artery. This is suggestive of pulmonary valve stenosis.

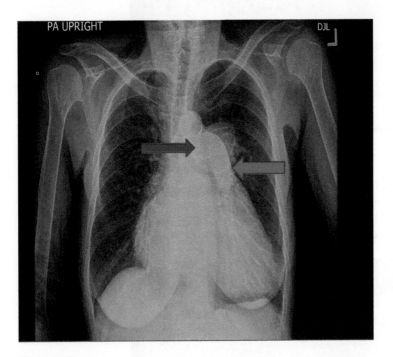

PA UPRIGHT                                                    DJL

**Figure 3.12b**

3.13. B. Aortic knob.

3.14. D. Superior vena cava.

3.15. C. Transaortic valve replacement.

This patient with complaints of shortness of breath had severe aortic stenosis. She then underwent a transaortic valve replacement. The bioprosthetic valve is shown by the blue arrow in Figure 3.15b. This is an Edwards valve and has a titanium mesh to hold the leaflets and not just the sewing ring. Also note there are no sternotomy wires.

3.16. B. Dual-chamber pacemaker.

3.17. B. Right ventricular pacer lead.

3.18. A. Right atrial pacer lead.

This patient has a dual-chamber pacemaker with leads in the right atrium and right ventricle.

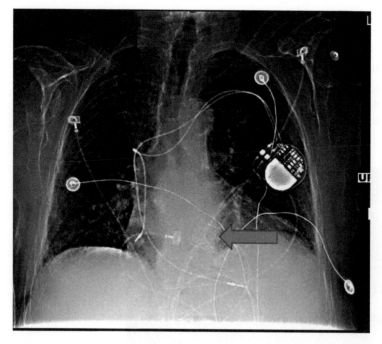

Figure 3.15b

**3.19.** D. Coronary sinus lead.

In this patient's chest X-ray, three leads are visible. In Figure 3.19b, the blue arrow points to the coronary sinus lead. The lead in the right ventricle is thicker than a regular pacing lead and is indicative of an ICD lead (red arrow). The third lead is the right atrial lead (yellow arrow).

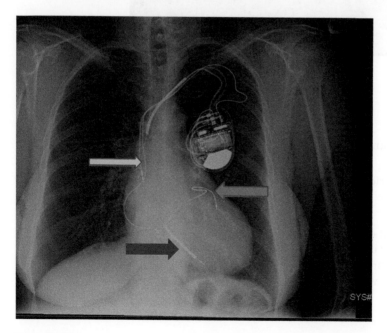

Figure 3.19b

**3.20.** B. Catheter placed through left subclavian vein.

There is a catheter that has been placed through a left subclavian approach and is terminating at the lower level of the superior vena cava.

**3.21.** A. Catheter placed through right internal jugular vein.

**3.22.** C. Endotracheal intubation.

The patient was tachypneic and hypoxic. He had emergent endotracheal intubation and was started on mechanical ventilation. The blue arrow in Figure 3.22b points to the endotracheal tube.

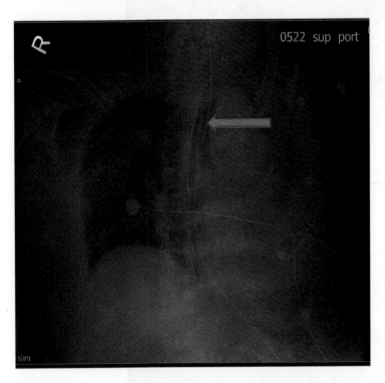

Figure 3.22b

**3.23.** A. Carina.

The endotracheal tube (ET) can be seen terminating about 1 cm above the carina.

**3.24.** A. Nasogastric tube.

The arrow points to the nasogastric tube, which is terminating below the diaphragm.

**3.25.** B. Placement of a catheter in the right pleural space.

The arrow in Figure 3.25b points to the catheter in the right pleural space. The right costophrenic angle is still obscured. The patient probably had right pleural effusion that was drained by placement of a right pleural catheter.

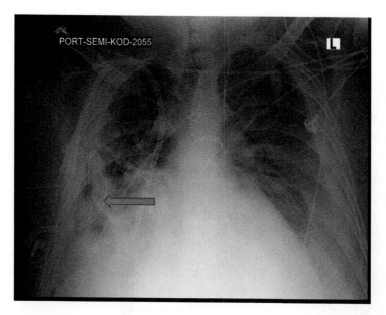

Figure 3.25b

3.26. B. Dextrocardia.

This is a portable chest X-ray. The most striking feature is that the apex of the heart is pointing to the right. This is called dextrocardia. In dextroposition, the apex still points to the left but the heart itself is shifted to the right. The arrow in Figure 3.26b points to the apex of the heart, which is pointing to the right.

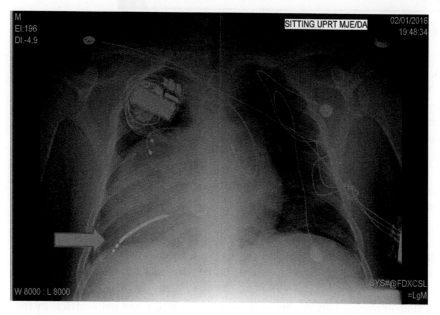

Figure 3.26b

**3.27.** B. A rounded opacity in the right lower lobe.

The rounded opacity in the right lower lobe is shown by the arrow in Figure 3.27b. Since this patient's status is post-heart transplant, he is prone to opportunistic infections such as aspergillosis, norcardiosis, and coccidiomycosis. He underwent a CT scan of the lung which again demonstrated the rounded opacity in the right lower lobe. He underwent CT-guided biopsy and pathology was positive for *Norcardia*. Also note the elevated left hemidiaphragm, which may suggest left phrenic nerve palsy.

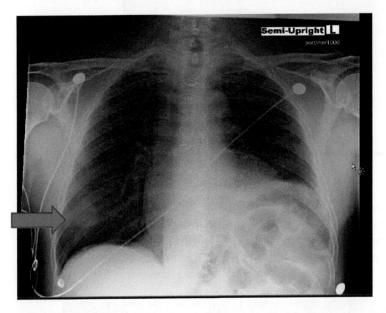

Figure 3.27b

**3.28.** D. Mitral stenosis.

Plethoric lung fields are indicative of increased pulmonary blood flow and are seen in left-to-right shunts such as ASD, VSD, and PDA. The pulmonary artery branches are prominently seen up to peripheral lung fields and flow is significantly increased.

**3.29.** A. Pulmonary hypertension.

Peripheral vasoconstriction, along with dilated central pulmonary arteries, results in this appearance in pulmonary hypertension. In pulmonary stenosis, lung fields are oligemic.

**3.30.** A. ASD Eisenmenger's.

A severely dilated main pulmonary artery is a feature of large ASD. In large VSDs, as pulmonary artery pressure does not regress during childhood, the pulmonary artery tends to have thicker walls and hence does not dilate as much.

**3.31.** A. Mitral stenosis.

Filling of the bay between the main pulmonary artery and left ventricle by the dilated left atrial appendage in mitral stenosis causes straightening of left heart border.

**3.32.** A. Tetralogy of Fallot.

This is due to right ventricular hypertrophy, which lifts the apex up mimicking the wooden boots of Danish farmers.

**3.33.** B. Total anomalous pulmonary venous drainage.

**3.34.** A. Partial anomalous pulmonary venous drainage.

Partial anomalous pulmonary venous drainage from the right upper pulmonary vein to inferior vena cava results in a scimitar-shaped shadow along the right heart border. Diagnosis is confirmed by transesophageal echocardiography.

**3.35.** B. Left atrial dilation.

This is typically seen in mitral stenosis due to severe left atrial enlargement. A dilated left atrium may also show as a double-atrial shadow near right atrial border with acute angulation with right hemidiaphragm, pressure on left recurrent laryngeal nerve causing hoarseness of voice (Ortner's syndrome), and dysphagia due to pressure on esophagus. Pressure on the esophagus is best appreciated by performing a barium swallow.

# Stress Testing and Risk Stratification of Asymptomatic Subjects

**4**

4.1. A 45-year-old male comes to your office for evaluation of chest pain. He reports substernal chest pressure that lasts a few minutes, does not radiate to his shoulder or jaw, occurs with exertion sometimes, and is relieved on its own in a few minutes. His risk factors include hypertension controlled on hydrochlorothiazide and amlodipine. He was also a 20-pack-a-year smoker but quit one month previously. His electrocardiogram (ECG) shows no abnormalities. To evaluate his chest pain, what should the next step be?
   A. Coronary angiography
   B. Exercise stress echocardiogram
   C. Exercise stress test
   D. No testing needed at this time

4.2. The patient walked for five minutes on the treadmill (Bruce protocol) and had to stop the test due to substernal chest pressure. His peak stress blood pressure (BP) dropped to 90 mmHg from a resting pressure of 130 mmHg. His stress ECG shows 4 mm downsloping ST depressions in the anterior chest leads that last 5 minutes into recovery. He is nauseous and diaphoretic. What is the next step in his evaluation?
   A. Nothing at present
   B. Adenosine myocardial perfusion imaging (MPI)
   C. Coronary angiogram to evaluate for obstructive CAD
   D. Modify medical therapy

4.3. A 55-year-old male comes to your office for evaluation of chest pain. He reports no cardiac risk factors other than hypercholesterolemia. He describes his chest pain as a discomfort, in the central chest that occurs at rest, lasts a few minutes, and is relieved with aspirin. A resting ECG done in the office reveals preexcitation. What does the next step in his evaluation include?
   A. Exercise stress test
   B. Coronary angiogram
   C. Referral to an electrophysiologist
   D. Exercise myocardial perfusion

4.4. In the evaluation of a patient with chest pain and right bundle branch (RBBB) on ECG, which of the following is true regarding exercise stress testing?
   A. Stress test is not useful in patients with RBBB
   B. Stress testing should always be combined with imaging

*Cardiology Board Review*, Second Edition. Ramdas G. Pai and Padmini Varadarajan.
© 2023 John Wiley & Sons Ltd. Published 2023 by John Wiley & Sons Ltd.

C. Stress testing can be undertaken without affecting the predictive value of stress ECG

D. None of the above

4.5. A 50-year-old women presents to the emergency room (ER) with complaints of chest pain. Her chest pain started three days prior to presentation and radiates to her jaw, occurs with exertion, and is relieved with rest. Her risk factors include hypertension and hypercholesterolemia. Her ECG at presentation is normal. Three sets of cardiac biomarkers drawn at presentation and then eight hours apart are negative. What is the best next recommended step?

Chapter 4

A. She is at low risk for ischemia; hence, discharge her home with advice regarding risk factor modification

B. Refer her for coronary angiography

C. Order a pharmacological stress nuclear study

D. Order an exercise stress test

4.6. Which of the following is not a contraindication to exercise ECG stress testing?

A. A 75-year-old male with complaints of chest pain and one episode of frank syncope. On examination, he has slow-rising carotid pulse and a harsh 3/6 ejection systolic murmur with radiation to both carotids.

B. A 35-year-old female with complaints of shortness of breath. On examination, jugular venous pressure is elevated, 15 cm $H_2O$, S3 gallop, and 2+ pedal edema. She has recently delivered her second baby.

C. A 68-year-old male with complaints of chest pain. He describes it as a sharp substernal chest pain, worse on deep inspiration. He gives a history of hip replacement two weeks previously.

D. A 44-year-old male with complaints of chest pain brought on by exertion, started a month previously. Physical examination is unremarkable except for an elevated BP of 140/78 mmHg. His ECG shows first-degree atrioventricular block and incomplete RBBB.

E. A 65-year-old male presents to the ER with exertional chest pain. Pain started 24 hours prior to presentation. He is currently chest-pain free. His ECG showed sinus bradycardia with Q waves in anterior chest leads V1–V4. An ECG done one month previously at his doctor's office was completely normal.

4.7. Which is an indication to stop an exercise treadmill test?

A. Drop of >10 mmHg from baseline BP despite an increase in workload with associated features of ischemia

B. Sustained ventricular tachycardia

C. Moderate to severe angina

D. Signs of cyanosis or pallor

E. All of the above

4.8. Which of the following is a class III indication for exercise stress testing without imaging (echo or nuclear perfusion)?

A. Patients with a high pretest probability of having CAD

B. Preexcitation on baseline ECG

C. Left ventricular hypertrophy with <1 mm ST depression on baseline ECG

D. Patient with vasospastic angina

**4.9.** A 45-year-old male is being evaluated by his primary care physician as part of his executive health checkup. He reports no risk factors and is asymptomatic. His baseline ECG shows no resting abnormalities. He is able to walk for 14 minutes (13.5 METS on a Bruce protocol). He reaches an exercise heart rate of 185 bpm, has no angina, and has no ST segment changes on his ECG. What would his Duke treadmill score be?

A. 9                                C. 2

B. 14                               D. 3.4

**4.10.** Based on the test results in Question 4.9, what is the next most appropriate step?

A. Stress imaging study

B. Computed tomography (CT) angiography

C. Coronary angiography

D. No further testing

E. Repeat testing in one year

**4.11.** Which one of the following is a class I recommendation in assessing asymptomatic adults with no known CAD?

A. Genomic testing

B. Obtain global risk score (Framingham)

C. Assessment of lipoprotein and apolipoprotein

D. Measurements of natriuretic peptides

**4.12.** Which one of the following is a class I recommendation in assessing asymptomatic adults with no known CAD?

A. Genomic testing

B. Obtain family history

C. Assessment of lipoprotein and apolipoprotein

D. Coronary CT angiogram

**4.13.** Measurement of C-reactive protein (CRP) is not recommended in which of the following?

A. In men over 50 years of age with a low-density lipoprotein (LDL) of <130 mg/dl

B. In women over 60 years with an LDL <130 mg/dl not on hormone replacement therapy (HRT), and without diabetes or chronic kidney disease

C. In asymptomatic high-risk adults

D. In asymptomatic intermediate-risk men 50 years of age and younger or women 60 years old and younger

**4.14.** With one exception, the following are class III recommendations in assessing low-risk asymptomatic adults with no known history of CAD. Which is the exception?

A. Coronary CT angiogram

B. Magnetic resonance imaging (MRI) for plaque detection

C. Measurement of coronary calcium score

D. Resting ECG

**4.15.** In patients with diabetes mellitus, which of the following is not recommended?

A. Stress echocardiogram

B. Stress MPI

C. Coronary calcium score measurement

D. Measurement of hemoglobin A1C

**4.16.** In asymptomatic women, all of the following except one are not recommended. Which is the exception?

A. Obtaining a global risk score

B. Obtaining natriuretic peptides

C. MRI for plaque detection

D. Measurement of lipoprotein

**4.17.** Stress MPI is recommended in which of the following situations?

A. In the assessment of a low-risk individual

B. In the assessment of an intermediate-risk individual

C. In an asymptomatic adult with diabetes mellitus

D. None of the above

**4.18.** Which of the following is not true?

A. Echocardiography (ECG) is recommended to detect left ventricular hypertrophy in patients with hypertension

B. ECG is recommended in risk assessment of asymptomatic adults without hypertension

C. A resting ECG is reasonable in asymptomatic adults with hypertension

D. All of the above

**4.19.** Which of the following is a class III indication in the assessment of asymptomatic adults?

A. Measurement of arterial stiffness

B. Obtaining a resting ECG

C. Obtaining an ECG in a patient with hypertension

D. Stress MPI in an individual with diabetes mellitus

**4.20.** Which of the following is not indicated regarding assessment of an asymptomatic adult with diabetes mellitus

A. Measurement of hemoglobin A1C

B. Stress MPI

C. Testing for microalbuminuria

D. Coronary CT angiogram

**4.21.** The thallium scan in Figure 4.21 (study 2 is a 4 hour redistribution) is from a 47-year-old man presenting with chest pain and ejection fraction (EF) of 35%. The coronary angiogram showed origin occlusion of LAD with collaterals from the right. The rest of the vessels were normal. What would you do?

A. Refer for single-vessel coronary artery bypass grafting with possible left internal mammary artery to left anterior descending (LAD) artery

B. Perform a positron emission tomography scan for viability

C. Refer for implantable cardioverter-defibrillator

D. None of the above

**4.22.** A 55-year-old man with diabetes and prior myocardial infarction with a right coronary artery (RCA) stent presented with chest pain. His cardiac markers were normal and EF on echo was 45% with inferior wall hypokinesis. The results of a stress Sestamibi scan are shown in Figure 4.22. What would you recommend?

A. Coronary angiography

B. Undertake a stress echo

C. Perform stress perfusion scan in six months

D. Medical management only at this point

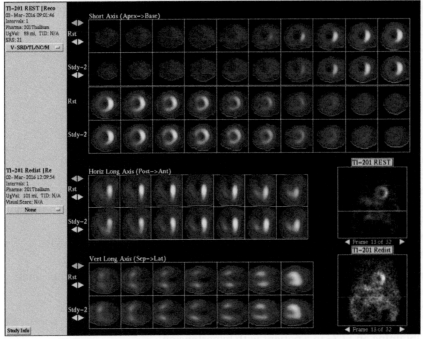

Figure 4.21

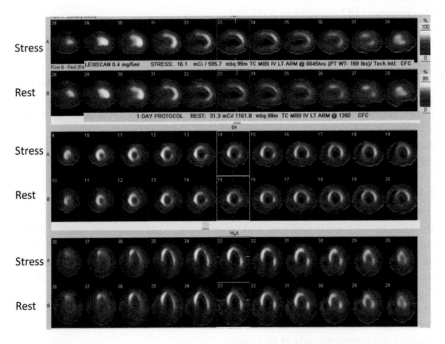

Figure 4.22

4.23. A 67-year-old man with hypertension and diabetes presented with central chest pain lasting 30 minutes. There were no ECG changes, and cardiac markers were negative. The results of a stress perfusion study are shown in Figure 4.23. What will you recommend?

A. Coronary angiography

B. Medical management only

C. Perform stress echo

D. None of the above

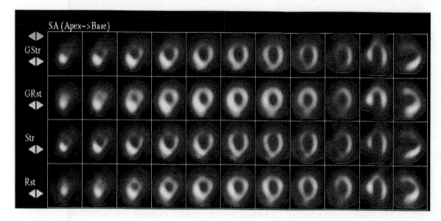

Figure 4.23

4.24. What is the stress perfusion image shown in Figure 4.24 suggestive of?

A. Reversible ischemia of large LAD area

B. Infarct of LAD area

C. Ischemia of RCA area

D. Ischemia of circumflex area

4.25. What does the stress perfusion image in Figure 4.25 show?

A. Reversible apical perfusion defect

B. Reversible defect of entire LAD area

C. Inferior wall ischemia

D. Apical infarct

4.26. What is the stress perfusion scan in Figure 4.26 suggestive of?

A. Perfusion defect in LAD area

B. Ischemia of inferior wall

C. Apical infarct

D. Normal rest and stress perfusion

4.27. The results of stress perfusion only are shown in Figure 4.27 (no rest perfusion shown). What are the results indicative of?

A. Normal stress perfusion and normal left ventricular wall motion

B. Normal perfusion with inferior hypokinesis

C. Anterior perfusion defect with normal wall motion

D. Inferior perfusion defect with inferior hypokinesis

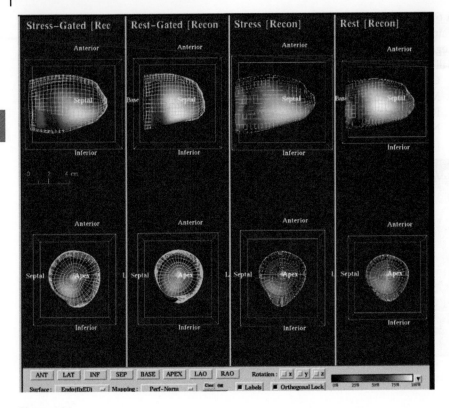

Figure 4.24

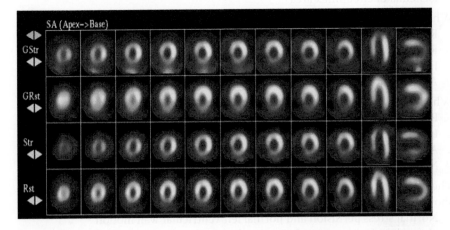

Figure 4.25

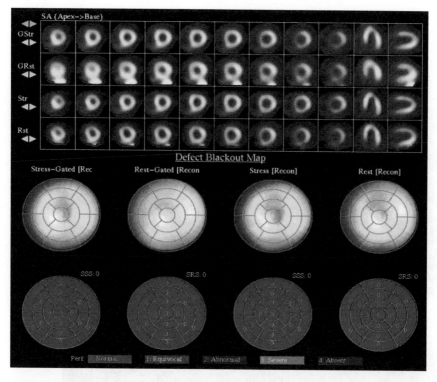

Figure 4.26

Ung =Ungated; ED = End-diastole; ES = Endsystole

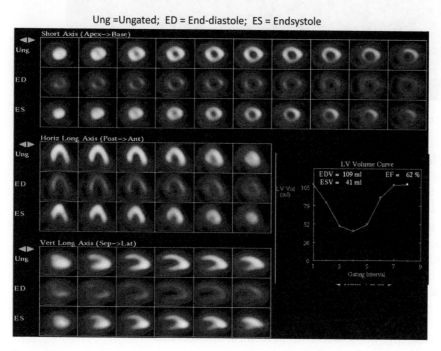

Figure 4.27

4.28. What is the rest/stress perfusion study shown in Figure 4.28 indicative of?
   A. Inferior wall infarction
   B. Inferior wall ischemia
   C. Inferior and anterior ischemia
   D. Anterior wall infarct with minor reversibility

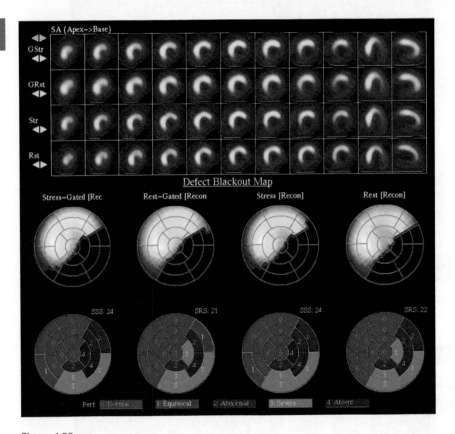

Figure 4.28

4.29. What is the patient whose rest/stress perfusion test results are shown in Figure 4.29 likely to have?
   A. Severe LAD artery lesion
   B. Left main lesion
   C. Circumflex lesion
   D. RCA lesion

4.30. A 66-year-old diabetic presented to the ER with chest pain. The resting ECG showed nonspecific ST-T changes, and cardiac markers were negative. The patient was on metformin, aspirin, atorvastatin, and lisinopril, with a heart rate of 68 bpm and BP of 123/78 mmHg. Cardiac examination was normal. The patient's nuclear stress test is shown in Figure 4.30. What will be a next logical step?
   A. Admit for further observation
   B. Refer for coronary angiography
   C. Discharge home and continue medical management
   D. Perform an echocardiogram

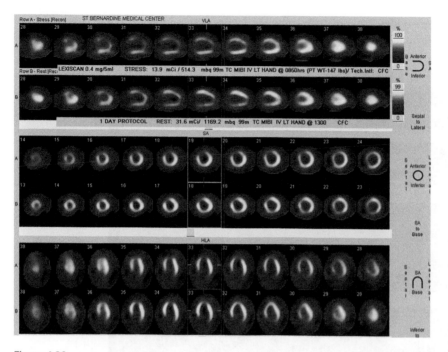

Figure 4.29

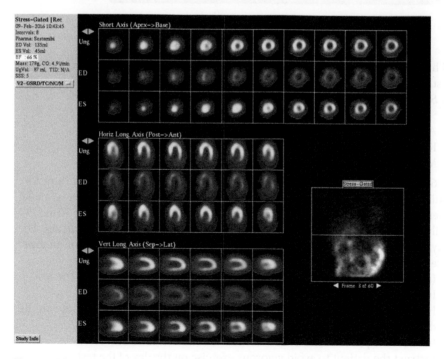

Figure 4.30

**4.31.** The vasodilator stress study shown in Figure 4.31 is indicative of what?

A. Normal perfusion

B. Ischemia in LAD area

C. Ischemia in RCA area

D. Ischemia in circumflex area

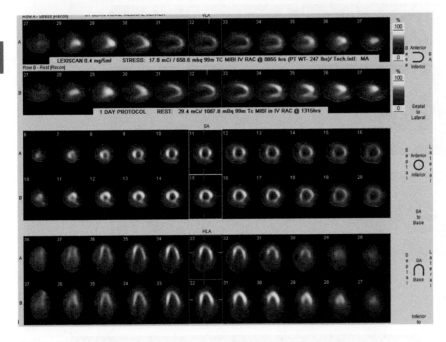

Figure 4.31

**4.32.** Which of the following is not an absolute contraindication to exercise stress testing?

A. Severe aortic stenosis

B. >3 mm ST-segment depression at rest

C. Acute myopericarditis

D. Known severe left main disease

E. Mobitz type 2 AV block

**4.33.** A 68-year-old man presents with new chest discomfort of 2 months duration, while climbing two flights of stairs. He denies any dyspnea, orthopnea, pedal edema. One week previously, he was started on isosorbide mononitrate 30 mg PO daily, and metoprolol 50 mg PO twice daily by his primary care physician. His physical examination is normal. Which of the following instructions for an exercise stress test is false?

A. Instruct the patient to hold metoprolol for at least 24 hours prior to the test

B. Instruct the patient to avoid caffeine

C. Instruct the patient to hold his morning dose of isosorbide mononitrate on the day of the test

D. Instruct the patient to continue all medications

E. Instruct the patient to avoid vigorous exercise on the day of the test

4.34. When should an exercise stress test not be stopped?
  A. A decrease in the systolic blood pressure by 10 mmHg
  B. 1 mm ST elevation in the anterior precordial leads
  C. Patient would like to terminate the test due to fatigue
  D. Mobitz type one second-degree heart block
  E. Isolated premature ventricular contractions

4.35. A 66-year-old man with an intermediate pre-test probability of having ischemic heart disease is scheduled for stress testing. Which of the following is not recommended?
  A. Exercise stress with nuclear myocardial perfusion imaging if able to exercise but uninterpretable ECG
  B. Exercise echocardiography if able to exercise but ECG is uninterpretable
  C. Pharmacological stress with nuclear myocardial perfusion imaging if able to exercise and the ECG is interpretable
  D. Exercise ECG if able to exercise and ECG is interpretable

4.36. Each of the following is an appropriate indication for the use of either stress MPI or stress echocardiography in patients with chest pain except:
  A. Resting ECG ST-segment depression greater than 1 mm
  B. LBBB
  C. Previous revascularization with PTCA or surgery
  D. Physical deconditioning

## Answers

4.1. C. Exercise stress test.
   This patient has atypical chest pain. He has risk factors that warrant further testing. His ECG shows no resting abnormalities. If the patient is able to exercise, the first step in his evaluation should be exercise stress testing. According to the American College of Cardiology (ACC)/American Heart Association (AHA) 2002 guidelines (Gibbons et al. 2002), if a patient has stable chest pain, has- low to intermediate risk of unstable angina, has symptoms that warrant a diagnosis of coronary artery disease (CAD), is able to exercise, and has an interpretable ECG, then exercise stress testing is the first step.

4.2. C. Coronary angiogram to evaluate for obstructive CAD.
   This patient has several high-risk features on his stress test. He walked only five minutes on a Bruce protocol, having to stop due to chest pain. He had significant ST depression at a low level of stress that was accompanied by a drop in his systolic BP. These features point to significant CAD. He should be referred for a coronary angiogram.

4.3. D. Exercise myocardial perfusion.
   This patient's resting ECG shows preexcitation. According to the ACC/AHA guidelines (Gibbons et al., 2002), class III indications for exercise stress test alone without imaging include preexcitation (Wolff-Parkinson-White) syndrome, electronically paced ventricular rhythm, greater than 1 mm resting ST depression, and complete left bundle branch block.

Chapter 4

| Cardiology Board Review

**4.4.** C. Stress testing can be undertaken without affecting the predictive value of stress ECG.

With exercise, ST depression usually occurs with RBBB in leads V1–V3. But in leads V4–V6 or the inferior leads, ST changes with stress are similar to those of a normal resting ECG (without RBBB). Hence, the presence of RBBB on resting ECG does not reduce the sensitivity, specificity, or predictive value of the stress ECG in the diagnosis of ischemia.

**4.5.** D. Order an exercise stress test.

This patient has intermediate probability for CAD based on age, gender, and symptoms. Women have a lower prevalence of obstructive CAD; an exercise stress test, which is used to detect focal stenosis, is less sensitive and specific in women. Women tend to have resting ST and T wave changes which can become more pronounced with stress, causing decreased accuracy when used to detect focal disease. Despite the lower accuracy of exercise stress ECG testing, the 2005 ACC/AHA guidelines on the Role of Noninvasive Testing in the Clinical Evaluation of Women Suspected with Coronary Artery Disease recommends an exercise ECG as the first test of choice in women with intermediate risk and normal baseline ECG. In women, other parameters, such as poor exercise capacity, low heart rate recovery, and failure to reach target heart rate, are more predictive of outcome than ST changes with stress.

**4.6.** D. A 44-year-old male with complaints of chest pain brought on by exertion, started one month previously. Physical examination is unremarkable except for an elevated BP of 140/78 mmHg. His ECG shows first-degree atrioventricular block and incomplete RBBB.

The patient in D can safely undergo stress testing. Contraindications to exercise stress ECG testing include severe symptomatic aortic stenosis (scenario A), decompensated heart failure (scenario B), acute pulmonary embolism (scenario C), and within two days of an acute myocardial infarction (scenario E).

**4.7.** E. All of the above.

The scenarios listed are all absolute indications to stop the treadmill test. In addition, ST elevation >1 mm in leads without Q waves, the patient's desire to stop, and technical difficulties in monitoring ECG or BP are all absolute indications to stop the exercise treadmill test.

**4.8.** B. Preexcitation on the baseline ECG.

It is a class III indication to use an exercise stress test in patients with preexcitation, paced ventricular rhythm, greater than 1 mm resting ST depression, and complete left bundle branch block. It is a class IIa indication to perform an exercise stress test in patients with vasospastic angina and class IIb to perform a treadmill stress test in patients with high pretest probability for CAD according to ACC/AHA guidelines (Gibbons et al. 2002).

**4.9.** B. 14.

Duke treadmill score is calculated as

$$\text{Exercise time (min)} - (5 \times \text{Amount of ST deviation (mm)}) - (4 \times \text{Exercise angina index})$$

(0: none; 1: if exercise angina occurred; 2: if angina was the reason to stop the test). Here, it would be $14 - (5 \times 0) - (4 \times 0) = 14$. Exercise time is based on a standard Bruce protocol.

**4.10.** D. No further testing.

A Duke treadmill score of >5.5 is suggestive of low risk of death (<1% per year) and hence no further testing is needed. Patients with an intermediate score (−10 to +4) have a mortality risk of 1–3% per year and those with a high-risk score (<−10) have a mortality risk of >3% per year.

**4.11.** B. Obtain global risk score (Framingham).

Obtaining a global risk score in asymptomatic adults without a clinical history of CAD is a class I indication. These scores are helpful in combining individual risk factor measurements into a single quantitative estimate of risk that can be used in prevention strategies. It is not recommended to perform genomic testing or measure lipoprotein or natriuretic peptides in this population; these are considered to be a class III indication (Greenland et al. 2010).

Chapter 4

**4.12.** B. Obtain family history.

Obtaining a family history of atherothrombotic coronary vascular disease is recommended in the assessment of asymptomatic adults (Greenland et al. 2010).

**4.13.** C. In asymptomatic high-risk adults.

Measurement of CRP is not recommended in asymptomatic high-risk adults (class III). In men 50 years of age and older or women of 60 years and older with an LDL of <130 mg/dl and who are not on lipid-lowering therapy, hormone replacement therapy (HRT), or immunosuppressive therapy, without clinical CAD, diabetes mellitus, chronic kidney disease, severe inflammatory conditions, or contraindications to statin therapy, CRP can be used to select patients for statin therapy (class IIa). It is also deemed reasonable to measure CRP in asymptomatic intermediate-risk men younger than 50 or women younger than 60, for assessment of CAD risk (class IIb) (Greenland et al. 2010).

**4.14.** D. Resting ECG.

A resting ECG may be reasonable in the assessment of asymptomatic adults with no history of hypertension or diabetes mellitus (class IIb). It is a class III indication to obtain coronary CT angiogram, coronary calcium score, or MRI for plaque detection in low-risk asymptomatic individuals (Greenland et al. 2010).

**4.15.** A. Stress echocardiogram.

In asymptomatic adults with diabetes mellitus it is reasonable to measure the coronary calcium score (class IIa). It is also reasonable to measure hemoglobin A1C and stress MPI (class IIb). Stress MPI may be considered for patients with diabetes or when prior risk assessment suggests high risk, such as a coronary artery calcium of over 400 (Greenland et al. 2010).

**4.16.** A. Obtaining global risk score.

It is a class I indication to obtain a global risk score in all asymptomatic women.

**4.17.** C. In an asymptomatic adult with diabetes mellitus.

Stress MPI may be considered for advanced cardiovascular risk assessment in asymptomatic individuals with diabetes mellitus or in adults with a strong family history of CAD, or when prior risk assessment such as a coronary artery calcium score of over 400. Stress MPI is not recommended for assessment of low- or intermediate-risk asymptomatic individuals (class III) (Greenland et al. 2010).

**4.18.** B. Echocardiography (ECG) is recommended in the risk assessment of asymptomatic adults without hypertension.

It is a class III indication to perform ECG in asymptomatic adults without hypertension. A resting ECG can be obtained in patients with hypertension or diabetes (class IIa) or an ECG obtained in patients with hypertension to detect left ventricular hypertrophy (class IIb) (Greenland et al. 2010).

**4.19.** A. Measurement of arterial stiffness.

Measurement of arterial stiffness is a class III indication at the present time (Greenland et al. 2010).

**4.20.** D. Coronary CT angiogram.

It is a class III indication to obtain a coronary CT angiogram in an asymptomatic adult with diabetes (Greenland et al. 2010).

**4.21.** A. Refer for single-vessel coronary artery bypass grafting with possible left internal mammary artery to left anterior descending (LAD) artery.

Though there is no redistribution, the resting scan shows significant thallium uptake in the anterior wall and septum, indicating viability and revascularization is appropriate. There is good probability that ejection fraction (EF) will improve, obviating the need for a primary prevention implantable cardioverter-defibrillator.

**4.22.** D. Medical management only at this point.

There is only a fixed inferior wall defect attributable to an old myocardial infarction. There are no reversible defects.

**4.23.** A. Coronary angiography.

Note the fully reversible perfusion defect in the anterior wall and septum suggesting proximal LAD artery lesion. The reversible defect is >30% of the myocardium, indicating high risk.

**4.24.** A. Reversible ischemia of large LAD area.

**4.25.** A. Reversible apical perfusion defect.

**4.26.** D. Normal rest and stress perfusion.

**4.27.** A. Normal stress perfusion and normal left ventricular wall motion.

**4.28.** A. Inferior wall infarction.

Inferior wall infarction is indicated by the fixed perfusion deficit.

**4.29.** A. Severe LAD artery lesion.

**4.30.** C. Discharge home and continue medical management.

The patient has normal perfusion without any ischemia, normal left ventricular wall motion, and normal EF. This indicates a low risk profile.

**4.31.** B. Ischemia in LAD area.

**4.32.** B. >3 mm ST-segment depression at rest is a *relative* contraindication to exercise stress testing. Other options are all absolute contraindications.

**4.33.** D. It is preferred to hold antianginal medications to minimize their anti-ischemic impact so that the test sensitivity may not be compromised. Caffeine is an antagonist of adenosine receptors and thus blocks the effect of adenosine and regadenoson. It should not be consumed for at least 12 hours prior to test if there is a possibility of the patient undergoing a vasodilator stress if the exercise stress test is inconclusive. Vigorous exercise on the day of the test may be avoided so that the patient is able to achieve maximum exercise potential and reach the target heart rate.

4.34. E. 2002 ACC/AHA guidelines state that stress tests should be stopped when premature ventricular contractions occur in pairs with increasing frequency, or when at least three-beat ventricular tachycardia occurs but not for isolated premature ventricular contractions. Other indications for an exercise stress test to be terminated include ST-segment elevation >1 mm in precordial or inferior leads that do not have a resting Q wave, any decrease in systolic blood pressure during exercise, ST depression ≥2 mm, the onset of second-degree or third-degree AV block, other patient-related factors such as dyspnea, fatigue, musculoskeletal pain, and increasing angina.

4.35. C. Patients with an intermediate pretest probability of CAD benefit the most from stress testing. The choice of stress test depends on whether the patient can exercise and whether the resting ECG can be interpreted. The ACC/AHA SIHD guidelines recommend standard exercise ECG testing for interpretable ECG in a patient who has moderate exercise capacity.

Exercise with nuclear myocardial perfusion imaging or ECG is recommended for patients with an intermediate to high pretest probability whose ECG is uninterpretable and who have moderate exercise capacity. Pharmacological stress with nuclear myocardial perfusion imaging or echocardiography is not recommended for patients who have an interpretable ECG and at least moderate physical functioning.

4.36. B. Both exercise myocardial perfusion imaging or exercise echocardiography is appropriate in a patient with resting ST-segment depression greater than 1 mm, preexcitation on the resting ECG, or previous revascularization, assuming the patient can exercise. In a patient who is unable to exercise, either dobutamine echocardiography or myocardial perfusion imaging is appropriate. However, in patients with LBBB, pharmacological myocardial perfusion imaging is preferred to dobutamine echocardiography.

## References

Gibbons, R.J., Balady, G.J., Bricker, J.T. et al. (2002). ACC/AHA 2002 guideline update for exercise testing: summary article. A report of the American College of Cardiology/American Heart Association task force on practice guidelines (committee to update the 1997 exercise testing guidelines). *Circulation* 106: 1883–1892.

Greenland, P., Alpert, J.S., Beller, G.A. et al. (2010). 2010 ACCF/AHA guideline for assessment of cardiovascular risk in asymptomatic adults: executive summary. A report of the American College of Cardiology Foundation/American Heart Association task force on practice guideline. *Circulation* 122: 2748–2764.

# Echocardiography

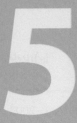

5.1. Which of the following manipulations will increase the echocardiographic frame rate (see Box 5.1)?
A. Increase depth
B. Increase transmit frequency
C. Decrease sector angle
D. Increase transmit power

5.2. The lateral resolution increases with:
A. Decreasing transducer diameter
B. Reducing power
C. Beam focusing
D. Reducing transmit frequency

5.3. Axial resolution can be improved by which of the following manipulations?
A. Reducing beam diameter
B. Beam focusing
C. Reducing gain
D. Increasing transmit frequency

5.4. Which of the following is associated with continuous-wave Doppler compared with pulsed-wave Doppler?
A. Aliasing
B. Range specificity
C. Ability to record higher velocities
D. All of the above

5.5. An intraoperative transesophageal echocardiogram (TEE) revealed mitral regurgitation (MR) with the following measurements: regurgitant jet area $4\,cm^2$, proximal isovelocity surface area (PISA) radius 0.8 cm at a Nyquist limit of 50 cm/s at a heart rate of 82 bpm and arterial blood pressure 80/40 mmHg (see Box 5.2). What does this represent?
A. Mild MR
B. Moderate MR
C. Severe MR

5.6. With one exception, for a given regurgitant volume, all but one of the following result in a reduction in the jet size. Which is the exception?
A. Fast heart rate
B. Doubling the sector angle
C. Increasing the imaging depth
D. Increasing the blood pressure

*Cardiology Board Review*, Second Edition. Ramdas G. Pai and Padmini Varadarajan.
© 2023 John Wiley & Sons Ltd. Published 2023 by John Wiley & Sons Ltd.

5.7. A patient has an LV outflow tract (LVOT) velocity of 1 m/s, time velocity integral (TVI) of 25 cm, LVOT diameter of 2 cm, aortic transvalvular velocity of 1.5 m/s, and heart rate 70 bpm. What is the cardiac output of this patient?

A. 5.5 l/min

B. 4.5 l/min

C. 6.3 l/min

D. Cannot be determined based on the data given

5.8. A patient with aortic stenosis (AS) has an LVOT diameter of 2 cm, LVOT velocity (V1) of 2.5 m/s, and transaortic valve velocity (V2) of 5 m/s; two-dimensional examination showed moderate systolic anterior motion (SAM) of the mitral leaflet. How would you describe the valvular AS in this patient?

A. Mild

B. Moderate

C. Severe

D. Cannot be calculated based on data given

5.9. In a patient with isolated aortic regurgitation (AR), the following measurements were obtained: transmitral flow 80 cm³/beat, flow across aortic valve 140 cm³/beat, TVI of AR signal 100 cm. How would you describe the AR in this patient?

A. Mild

B. Moderate

C. Severe

D. Cannot be determined

5.10. The presence of severe AR in a patient with mitral stenosis (MS) is likely to do which of the following to the calculated mitral valve area by the pressure half-time method?

A. Overestimate the valve area

B. Underestimate the valve area

C. Have no effect

5.11. What is this patient in Figure 5.11 likely to have?

A. Severe AS

B. Severe MR

C. Severe pulmonary hypertension

D. Mild AS

5.12. For the patient in question 5.11, the LVOT diameter was 2 cm and the LVOT velocity by pulse Doppler was 1 m/s. What is the aortic valve area by the continuity equation?

A. 0.2 cm²

B. 0.3 cm²

C. 0.5 cm²

D. 0.8 cm²

5.13. Figure 5.13 is the continuous wave signal obtained from the pulmonary valve at the mid to proximal esophageal location. What is this patient likely to have?

A. Wide-open pulmonary regurgitation (PR)

B. Mild PR

C. Severe valvular pulmonary stenosis (PS)

D. Severe subvalvular PS

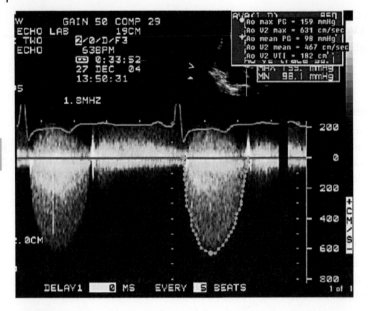

Figure 5.11

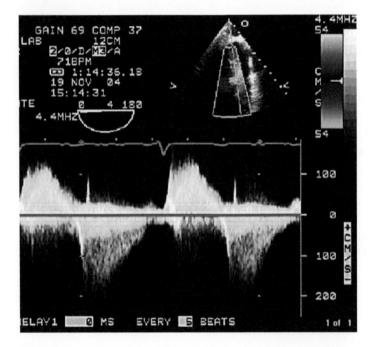

Figure 5.13

5.14. The pulmonary vein flow shown in Figure 5.14 is indicative of what?
   A. Elevated LA pressure with normal end diastolic pressure (EDP)
   B. Elevated LA pressure with elevated EDP
   C. Abnormal LV relaxation with normal EDP
   D. Elevated LV EDP with normal LA pressure

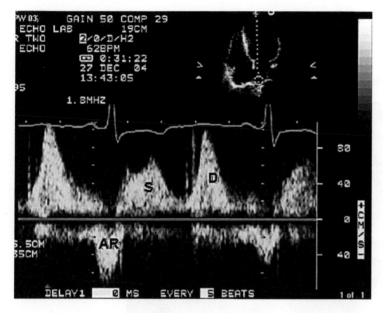

Figure 5.14

5.15. The mitral flow pattern shown in Figure 5.15 is suggestive of what?
   A. Normal LA pressure
   B. High LA pressure
   C. Atrial mechanical failure
   D. Abnormal LV relaxation with normal LA pressure

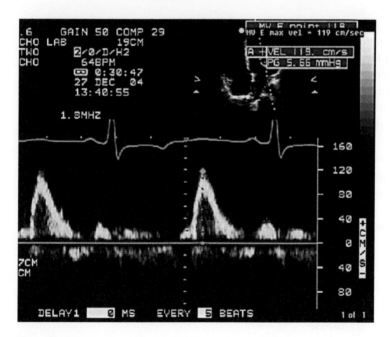

Figure 5.15

5.16. What condition does the patient in Figure 5.16 have?
   A. Mitral atresia
   B. Tricuspid atresia
   C. Transposition of great vessels with atrial baffle
   D. Epstein's anomaly

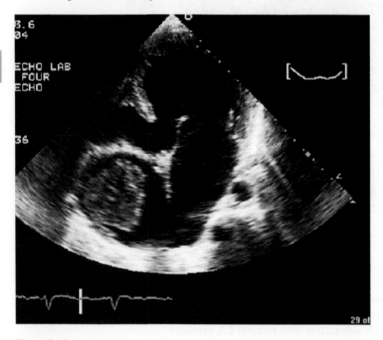

Figure 5.16

5.17. Which of the following does the patient in Figure 5.17 have?
   A. Prominent Eustachian valve
   B. Ostium secundum ASD
   C. Ostium primum ASD
   D. Sinus venosus ASD

5.18. What type of flow was recorded from the mid-esophageal position in Figure 5.18?
   A. Mitral flow                           C. Superior vena cava flow
   B. Pulmonary vein flow                   D. Flow across ASD

5.19. The patient in Question 5.17 with secundum atrial septal defect (ASD) has ASD dimensions of the defect 3 cm × 2 cm, tricuspid valve insufficiency (TVI) of flow across the defect is 39 cm, and heart rate of 70/s. What is the approximate shunt flow across the ASD?
   A. 12.8 l/min
   B. 3 l/min
   C. 7 l/min
   D. Cannot be calculated

5.20. What is the cause of the patient's mitral valve problem shown in Figure 5.20?
   A. Rheumatic heart disease
   B. Degenerative valve disease
   C. Fen-phen valvulopathy
   D. Ischemic heart disease

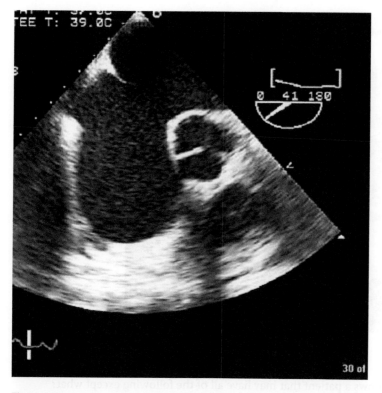

Figure 5.17

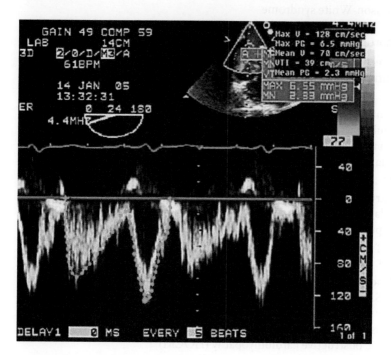

Figure 5.18

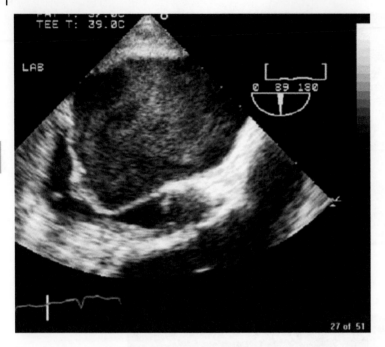

Figure 5.20

5.21. Figure 5.21 shows a patient that may have all of the following except what?
   A. Atrial septal defect
   B. Wolf-Parkinson-White syndrome
   C. TR
   D. Bicuspid aortic valve

5.22. The M-mode echocardiogram in Figure 5.22 is suggestive of what?
   A. Normal mitral valve motion      C. Severe AR
   B. MS                              D. High LA pressure

5.23. What is the image shown in Figure 5.23 suggestive of?
   A. Mitral annuloplasty
   B. Catheter in the coronary artery
   C. Biventricular pacemaker or implantable cardioverter-defibrillator (ICD)
   D. An artifact

5.24. What is the structure denoted by the arrow in Figure 5.24?
   A. LA appendage
   B. Left lower pulmonary vein
   C. Left upper pulmonary vein
   D. Right lower pulmonary vein

5.25. The patient shown in Figure 5.25 has what condition?
   A. Valvular AS
   B. Subvalvular AS
   C. Endocarditis
   D. Hypertrophic obstructive cardiomyopathy (HOCM)

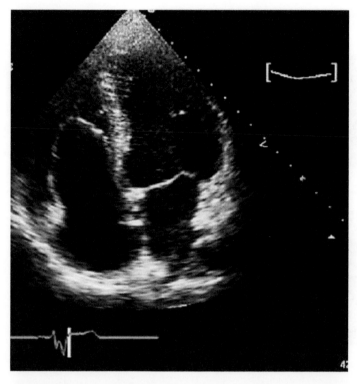

Figure 5.21

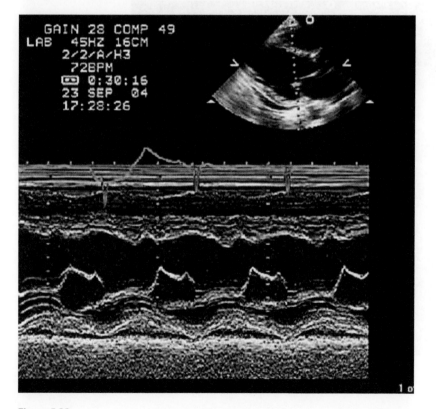

Figure 5.22

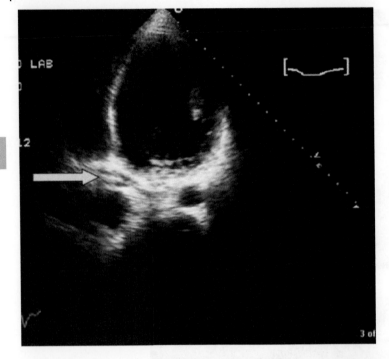

Figure 5.23

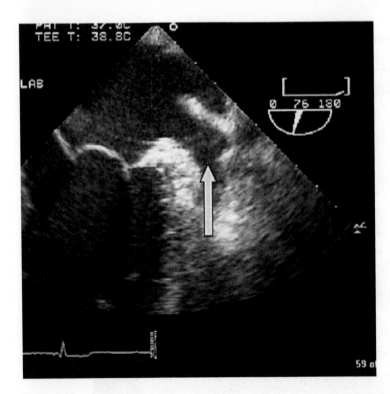

Figure 5.24

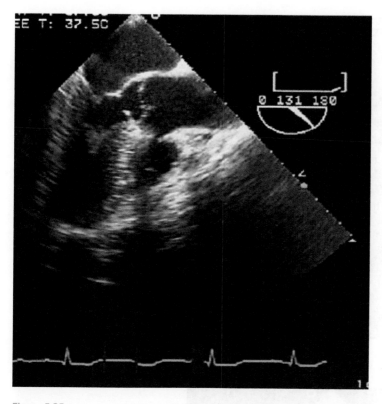

Figure 5.25

5.26. The cause of dyspnea in the patient in Figure 5.26 is likely to be due to what?
   A. Left heart failure
   B. Primary pulmonary hypertension
   C. Chronic obstructive pulmonary disorder
   D. None of the above

5.27. Figure 5.27 shows an end systolic frame in a patient with shortness of breath. What is the most likely diagnosis?
   A. Ebstein's anomaly
   B. Hypertrophic cardiomyopathy
   C. ASD
   D. Dilated cardiomyopathy

5.28. What is the most likely mechanism of MR in the patient in Figure 5.28?
   A. P2 tethering
   B. P2 prolapse
   C. Bileaflet mitral valve prolapse
   D. None of the above

5.29. A 19-year-old patient was stabbed in the precordial area. Examination revealed a loud systolic murmur (Figure 5.29). What is the most likely cause of this murmur?
   A. Penetrating injury to the interventricular septum
   B. Mitral valve prolapse
   C. HOCM
   D. None of the above

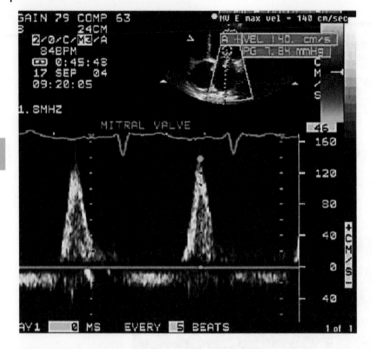

Figure 5.26

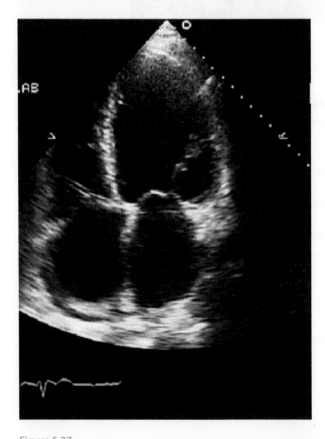

Figure 5.27

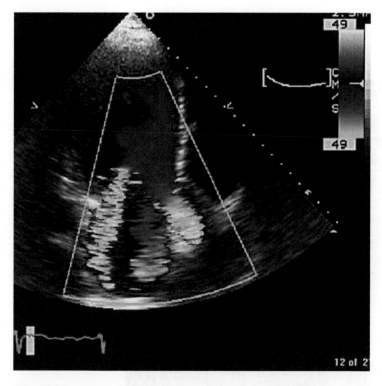

Figure 5.28

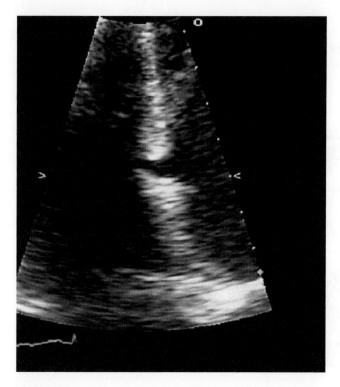

Figure 5.29

5.30. What is the continuous-wave Doppler signal in Figure 5.30 suggestive of?

A. AS and AR

B. MS and MR

C. VSD flow

D. Aortic flow in a patient with coarctation

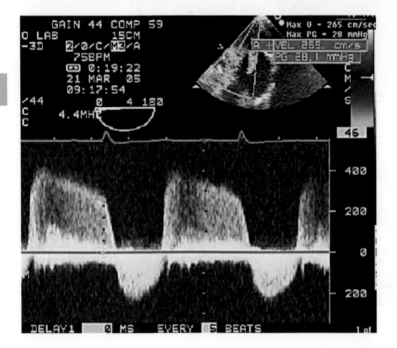

Figure 5.30

5.31. The continuous wave signal in Figure 5.31 was obtained from the mid-transesophageal location. What is it indicative of?

A. AS and AR

B. MS and MR

C. VSD flow

D. None of the above

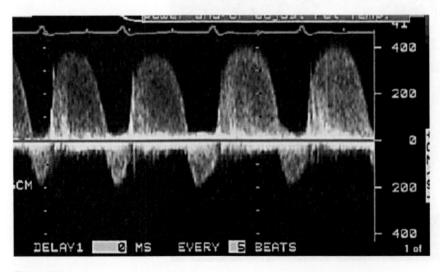

Figure 5.31

5.32. Figure 5.32 shows a TEE image from the mid-esophagus of a late diastolic frame of the aortic valve. What is this patient most likely to have?

A. Severe AR          C. HOCM

B. Severe AS          D. Ascending aortic dissection

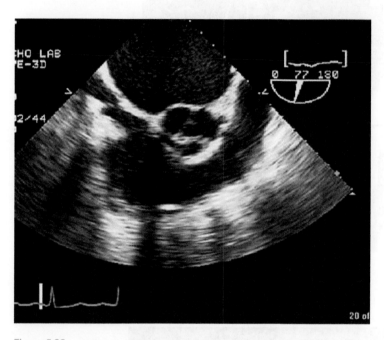

Figure 5.32

5.33. What is the patient in Figure 5.33 most likely to have?

A. Acute severe MR          C. Severe MS and mild MR

B. Chronic severe MR          D. None of the above

5.34. The patient in Figure 5.34 had *Staphylococcus aureus* endocarditis of the aortic valve. What is the most likely cause?

A. Central venous catheter-associated infection

B. Dental work

C. Immunosuppressed state

D. Intravenous drug use

5.35. What is the image of the aortic valve in Figure 5.35 suggestive of?

A. Aortic valve vegetation

B. Node of Arantius

C. Lambl's excrescences

D. Ascending aortic dissection causing prolapse of the noncoronary cusp

5.36. What is the most likely cause of the signal shown in Figure 5.36?

A. HOCM

B. Critical valvular AS

C. Acute MR

D. None of the above

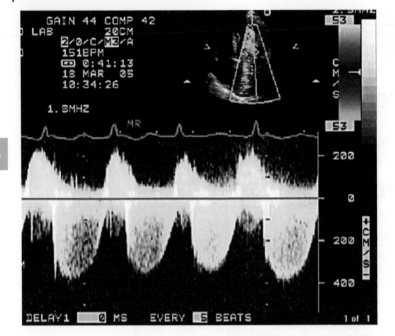

Figure 5.33

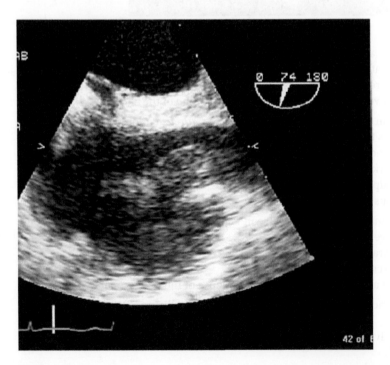

Figure 5.34

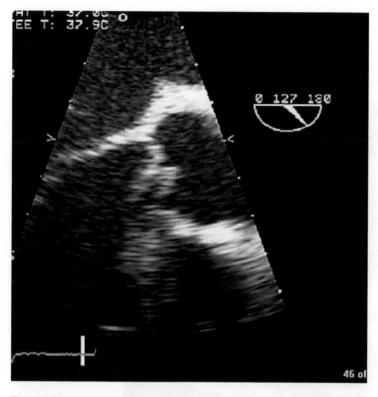

Figure 5.35

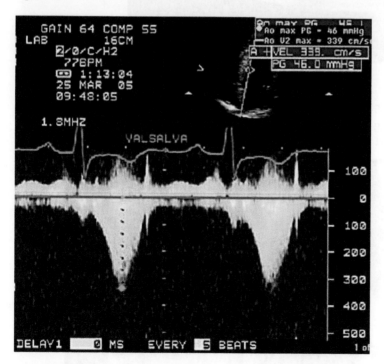

Figure 5.36

5.37. What is the image shown in Figure 5.37 suggestive of?
   A. Bioprosthetic tricuspid valve
   B. Carcinoid valvulopathy of tricuspid valve
   C. Tricuspid annuloplasty ring
   D. Large tricuspid vegetation

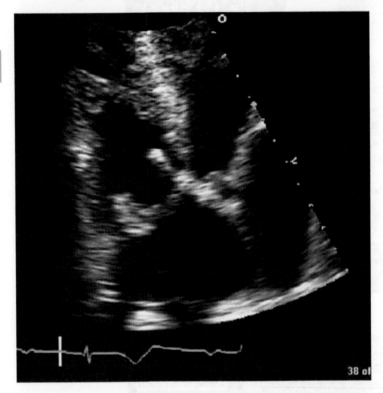

Figure 5.37

5.38. What is the 65-year-old patient with MR in Figure 5.38 likely to have?
   A. An opening snap
   B. Third heart sound
   C. Fourth heart sound
   D. Summation gallop

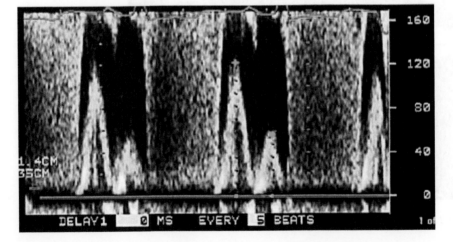

Figure 5.38

5.39. What is the continuous-wave Doppler signal in Figure 5.39 consistent with?
   A. Critical AS
   B. Severe MR
   C. Maladie de Roger
   D. None of the above

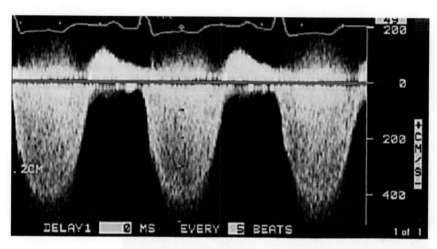

Figure 5.39

5.40. The TR signal in Figure 5.40 was obtained from TEE. The clinically estimated right atrial (RA) pressure in this patient was 20 mmHg and there is no PS. What would the PA systolic pressure in this patient be?
   A. 30 mmHg
   B. 50 mmHg
   C. 80 mmHg
   D. Cannot be calculated

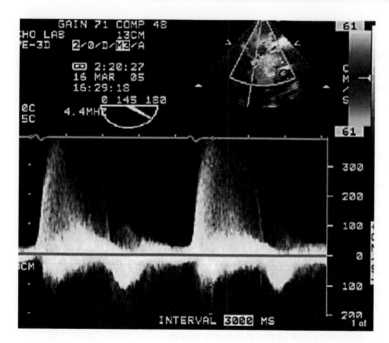

Figure 5.40

5.41. What condition is the patient in Figure 5.41 likely to have?
- A. Acute severe AR
- B. Mild AR
- C. MS
- D. None of the above

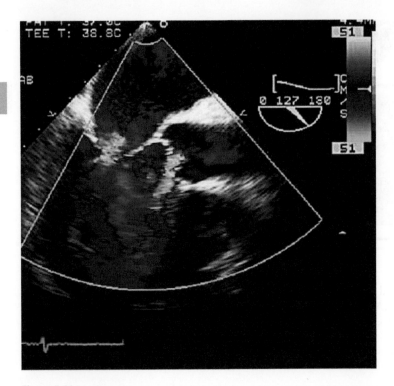

Figure 5.41

5.42. The transmitral flow in Figure 5.42 is obtained from the esophageal transducer location from a patient with *S. aureus* bacteremia and acute hemodynamic decompensation. The patient is in sinus rhythm. What is the most likely cause of his decompensation?
- A. Acute MR
- B. Acute AR
- C. Rupture of the ventricular septum
- D. None of the above

5.43. The pulse-wave Doppler flow signal in the descending thoracic aorta on a TEE shown in Figure 5.43 is indicative of what?
- A. Coarctation of the aorta
- B. Middle aortic syndrome
- C. Severe AR
- D. HOCM

5.44. What is the likely cause of heart failure in the 30-year-old man shown in Figure 5.44?
- A. Noncompaction of the left ventricle
- B. Hemochromatosis
- C. Cardiac amyloid
- D. Hypertrophic cardiomyopathy

5.45. What is the structure indicated by the arrow in Figure 5.45?
- A. IVC-RA junction
- B. Superior vena cava
- C. Anomalously draining right upper pulmonary vein
- D. ASD

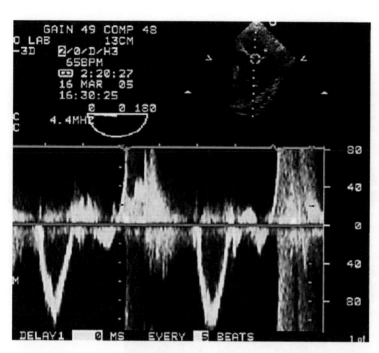

Figure 5.42

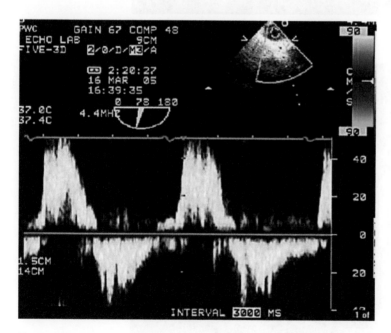

Figure 5.43

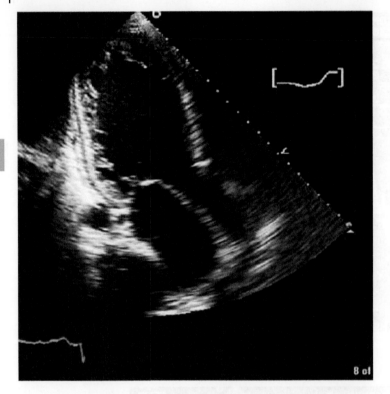

Figure 5.44

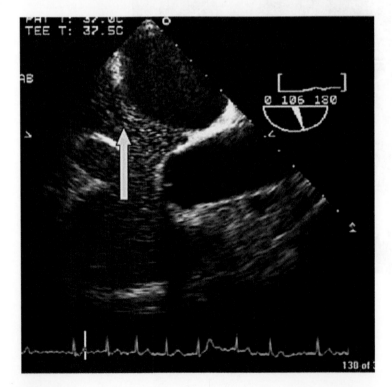

Figure 5.45

5.46. What is the approximate MR flow rate of the patient in Figure 5.46 (PISA radius of 0.9 cm, aliasing velocity of 38 cm/s)?

A. ~200 cm³/s

B. ~200 cm³/min

C. ~100 cm³/min

D. ~100 cm³/s

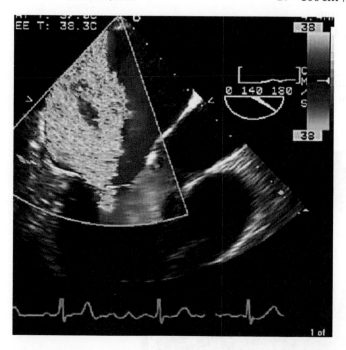

Figure 5.46

5.47. What is the likely diagnosis of the patient in Figure 5.47?

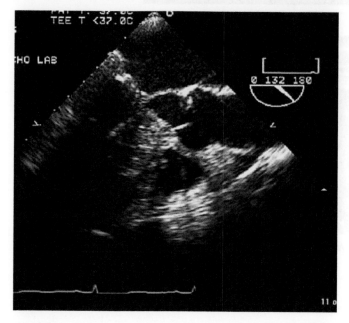

Figure 5.47

A. An early diastolic murmur
B. Late-peaking systolic ejection murmur with absent A2 component of S2
C. Late-peaking systolic murmur increased by Valsalva's maneuver and normal A2
D. Mid-diastolic murmur

5.48. What is the most likely diagnosis of the patient in Figure 5.48?
A. HOCM
B. Severe AS
C. Mitral valve prolapse
D. None of the above

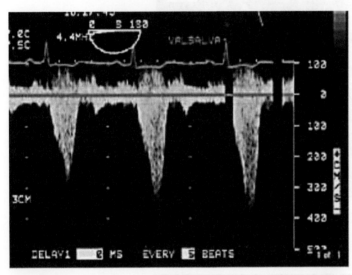

At rest

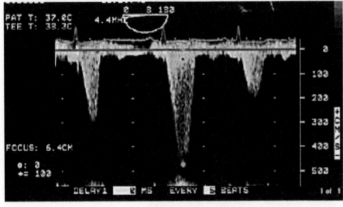

With Valsalva

Figure 5.48

5.49. What is the most likely diagnosis of the patient in Figure 5.49?
- A. Apical HOCM
- B. Hypertensive heart disease
- C. Endomyocardial fibrosis
- D. None of the above

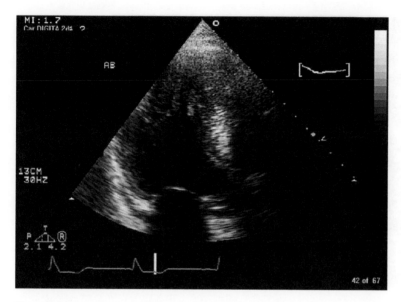

Figure 5.49

5.50. The appearance of the atrial septum in the patient in Figure 5.50 is due to what?
- A. ASD repair with a pericardial patch
- B. ASD closure device
- C. PFO closure device
- D. None of the above

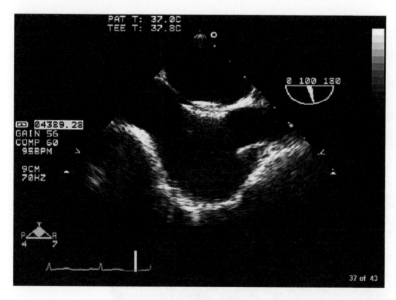

Figure 5.50

**5.51.** What does Figure 5.51 show?

A. Normal native tricuspid valve

B. Normal bioprosthetic valve

C. Vegetation on a bioprosthetic valve

D. Avulsion of the tricuspid valve

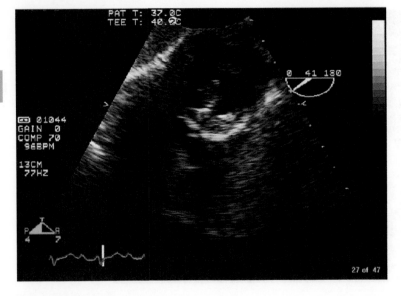

Figure 5.51

**5.52.** A 31-year-old woman with no other medical history had two episodes of transient ischemic cerebral attacks, the first one after a long duration of air travel and the second one during straining in the restroom. From the TEE image in Figure 5.52, what is the most likely cause of this patient's attacks?

A. Paradoxical embolism

B. Vagally mediated atrial fibrillation

C. LA thrombus

D. None of the above

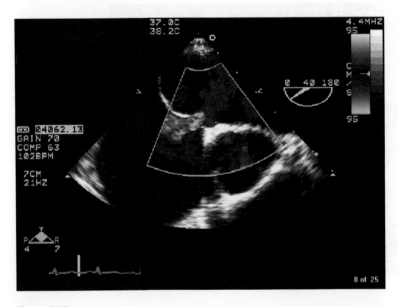

Figure 5.52

5.53. A 35-year-old patient with AIDS and bicuspid aortic valve has *Staphylococcus* bacteremia. What is the parasternal long-axis color flow image in Figure 5.53 suggestive of?
   A. Right coronary artery flow
   B. Pulmonary vegetation
   C. Fistulous communication between aorta and right ventricle
   D. None of the above

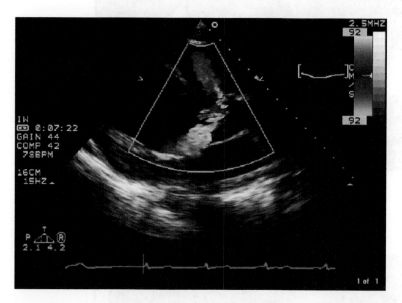

Figure 5.53

5.54. What are the patient's bilateral *Staphylococcus* lung abscesses shown in Figure 5.54 likely due to?
   A. Tricuspid valve endocarditis
   B. Pulmonary valve endocarditis
   C. Catheter-related infection of superior vena cava and right atrium
   D. None of the above

5.55. What is the structure indicated by the arrow in Figure 5.55?
   A. Coronary sinus
   B. IVC
   C. ASD
   D. None of the above

5.56. Describe the amount of TR in the patient in Figure 5.56.
   A. Mild                          C. Severe
   B. Moderate                   D. Cannot quantify

5.57. Which of the following is the patient in Question 5.56 likely to have?
   A. Normal PA pressure
   B. Mild pulmonary hypertension
   C. Moderate or severe pulmonary hypertension

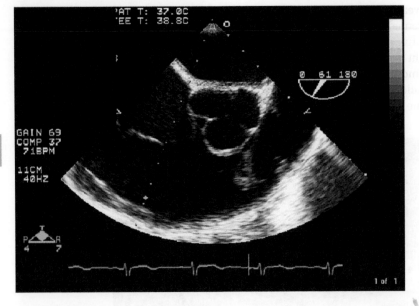

Figure 5.54

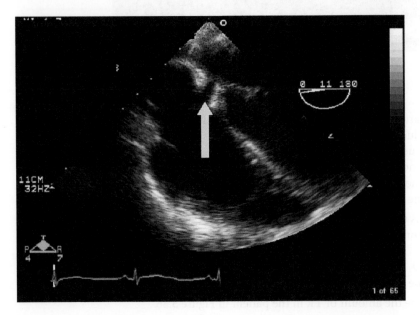

Figure 5.55

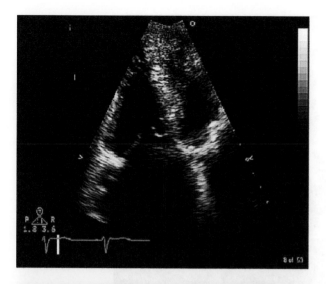

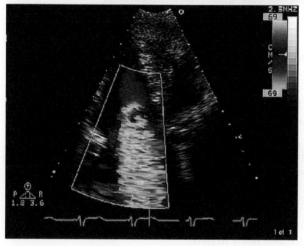

Figure 5.56

5.58. What is the likely type of surgical procedure performed on the mitral valve of the patient in Figure 5.58?
A. Mitral annuloplasty
B. Alfieri procedure
C. Replacement with a bioprosthetic valve
D. Replacement with a mechanical valve

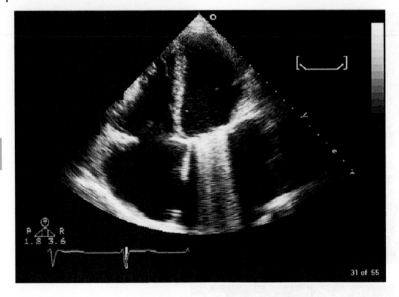

Figure 5.58

5.59. What intervention can potentially change the mitral inflow pattern seen in the images in Figure 5.59?
   A. Diuresis
   B. Control of severe hypertension
   C. Correction of severe anemia
   D. All of the above

5.60. What is the abnormality shown in Figure 5.60?
   A. Thoracic aortic aneurysm
   B. Cor triatriatum
   C. Artifact
   D. Dilated left PA

5.61. What is the patient in Figure 5.61 likely to have?
   A. Mitral valve prolapse
   B. Elevated LV EDP
   C. HOCM
   D. Severe AR

5.62. What does the mitral valve motion in the patient in Figure 5.62 suggest?
   A. Atrial fibrillation
   B. Elevated LV EDP
   C. Mitral valve prolapse
   D. Severe AR

5.63. What is the aortic valve m-mode in Figure 5.63 suggestive of?
   A. AS
   B. HOCM
   C. Congestive heart failure
   D. Hypertension

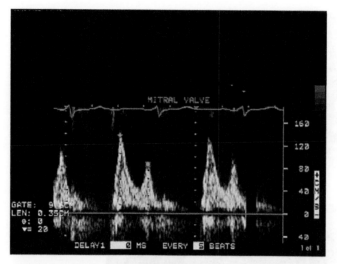

Before

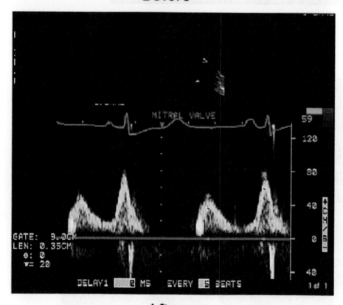

After

Figure 5.59

Chapter 5

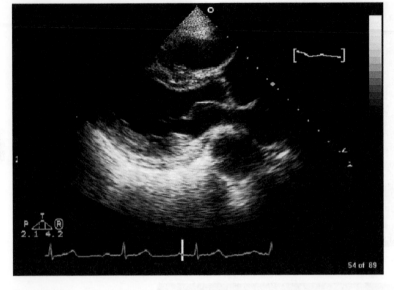

Figure 5.60

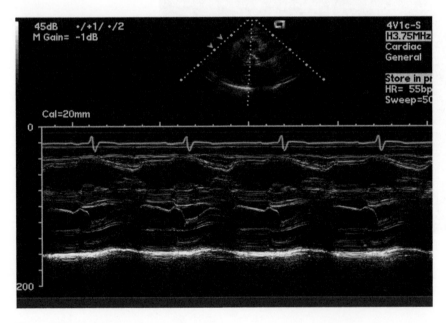

Figure 5.61

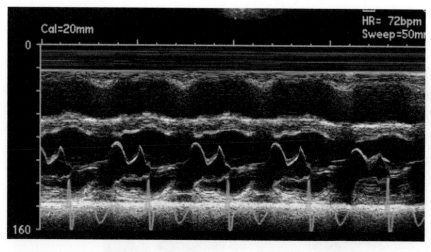

Figure 5.62

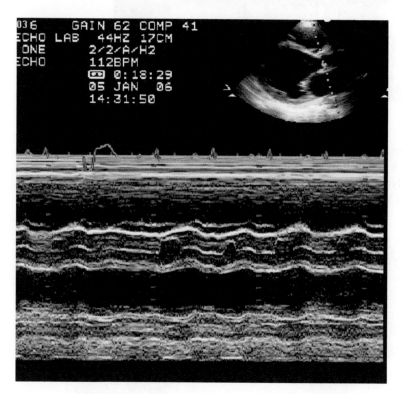

Figure 5.63

**5.64.** What is the patient in Figure 5.64 likely to have?

A. Mild AR

B. MS with high LA pressure

C. Acute severe AR

D. Severe MR

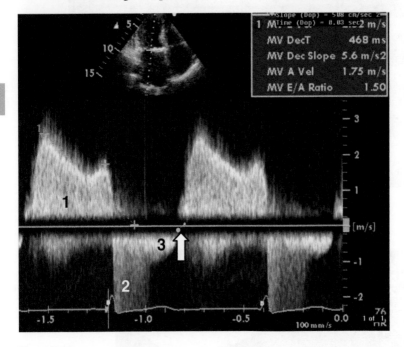

Figure 5.64

**5.65.** The patient in Figure 5.65 has MS with which of the following?

A. High LA pressure

B. Hyperdynamic LV

C. Severe LV systolic dysfunction

D. MR

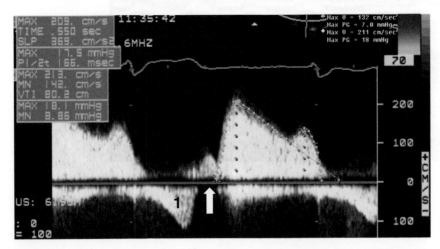

Figure 5.65

5.66. What is the continuous-wave Doppler signal in Figure 5.66 suggestive of?

A. Severe AR          C. Pulmonary hypertension

B. MS                D. Severe PR

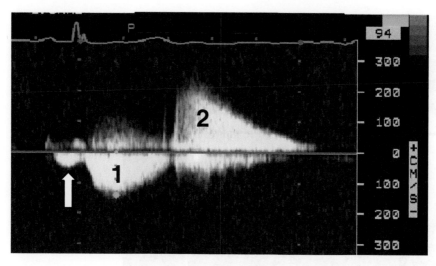

Figure 5.66

5.67. What is the continuous-wave signal in Figure 5.67 from a 22-year-old woman with a history of heart surgery during infancy indicative of?

A. Severe AS          C. Severe PS and PR

B. Severe PS          D. Severe pulmonary hypertension

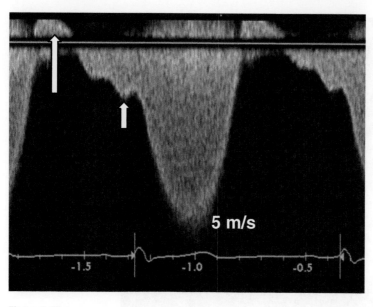

Figure 5.67

5.68. What was the signal in Figure 5.68 obtained from?
- A. Apical window
- B. Parasternal window
- C. Suprasternal window
- D. Subcostal window

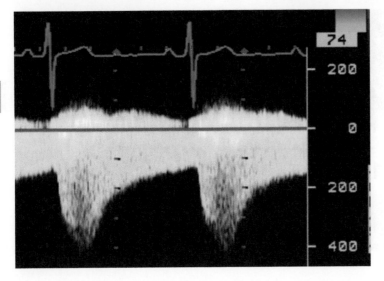

Figure 5.68

5.69. What condition does the patient in Figure 5.69 have?
- A. PA branch stenosis
- B. PR
- C. Patent ductus arteriosus (PDA)
- D. None of the above

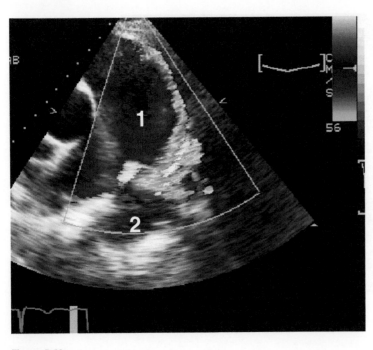

Figure 5.69

5.70. In Figure 5.70, the flow obtained on TEE from the descending thoracic aorta is indicative of what?

A. Aortic coarctation

B. PDA

C. Normal flow in intercostal artery

D. Severe AR

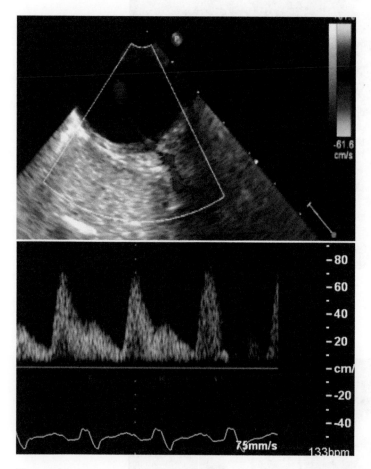

Figure 5.70

5.71. In Figure 5.71, the flow from this subcostal view is indicative of what?

A. Large ASD

B. Severe MR

C. MS

D. Tricuspid stenosis

5.72. Figure 5.72 is a recording of flow across the pulmonary valve using pulsed-wave Doppler in a patient with severe dyspnea. What is the likely diagnosis?

A. Pulmonary hypertension

B. PS

C. PR

D. Large ASD

5.73. Figure 5.73 shows a patient with what condition?

A. LV systolic dyssynchrony

B. LV diastolic dyssynchrony

C. Good LV synchrony

D. None of the above

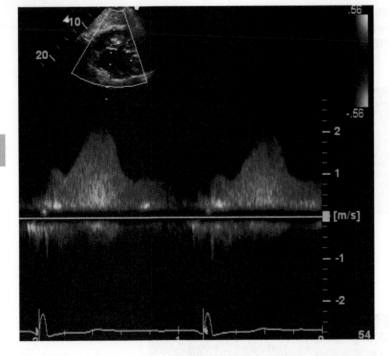

Figure 5.71

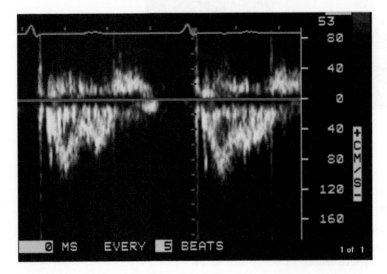

Figure 5.72

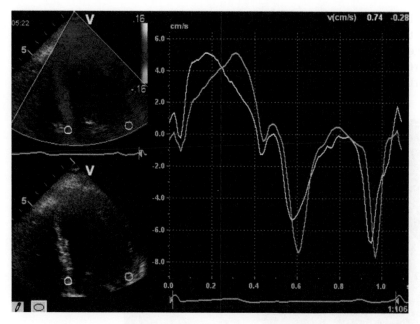

Figure 5.73

5.74. In Figure 5.74, what are the signals from the septum and LV lateral wall of?
   A. LV strain
   B. Strain rate
   C. Velocity
   D. None of the above

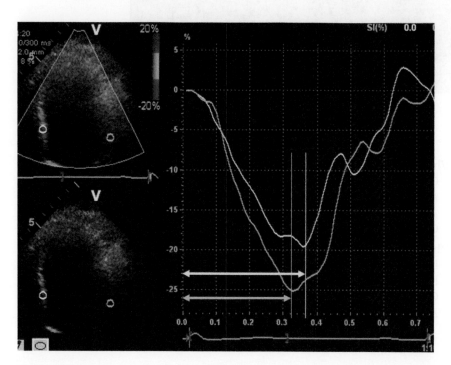

Figure 5.74

5.75. In the TEE image in Figure 5.75, what does the downward-pointing arrow refer to?
   A. Aortic valve
   B. Vegetation on the aortic valve
   C. Aortic subvalvular membrane
   D. Aortic dissection

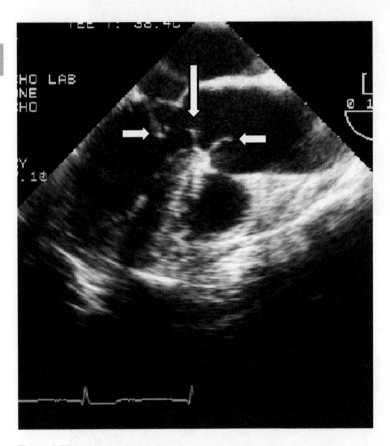

Figure 5.75

5.76. What does the arrow on the TEE image in Figure 5.76 point to?
   A. Coronary artery
   B. Aortic valve ring abscess
   C. Artifact
   D. Coronary sinus

5.77. What is depicted for the patient in Figure 5.77?
   A. Dilated coronary sinus and dextrocardia
   B. Dilated coronary sinus and levocardia
   C. Cor triatriatum
   D. Aneurysm of circumflex coronary artery

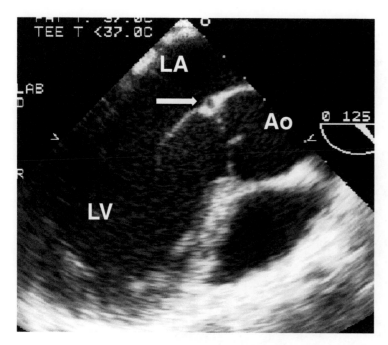

Figure 5.76

(a)

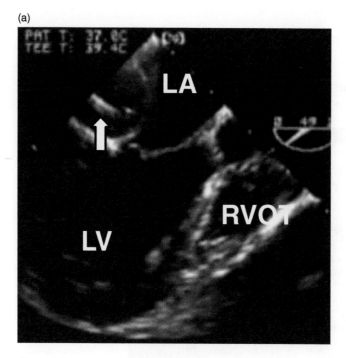

Figure 5.77

(b)

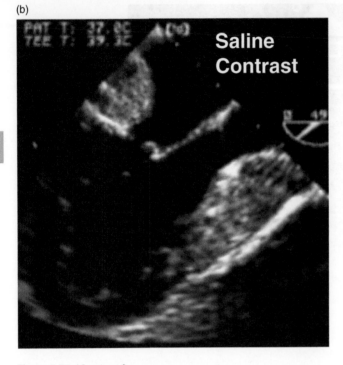

Figure 5.77 (*Continued*)

5.78. What does the arrow point to in Figure 5.78? (DTA: descending thoracic aorta)
   A. Aortic aneurysm
   B. IVC
   C. Dilated azygos vein
   D. Mirror image artifact

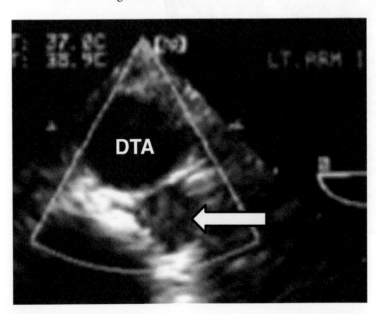

Figure 5.78

5.79. This 23-year-old patient had neonatal heart transplantation for hypoplastic left heart syndrome. The left ventricular function was normal. The following signal was obtained from the suprasternal window. What does this indicate? (Figure 5.79)
   A. Coarctation of the aorta
   B. Patent ductus arteriosus
   C. Stenosis of pulmonary trunk stenosis at anastomotic site
   D. Aortic stenosis

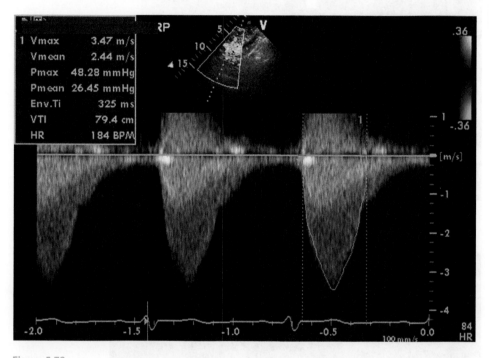

Figure 5.79

5.80. This is 58-year-old patient undergoing routine surveillance echocardiogram after a heart transplant 5 years earlier. What does the arrow indicate? (Figure 5.80)
   A. Aortic dissection
   B. Right coronary artery
   C. Left coronary artery
   D. Sinus of Valsalva fistula to RV

5.81. This patient had a heart transplant seven years earlier and presents with shortness of breath. The parasternal long axis view is shown. What does the arrow point to? (Figure 5.81)
   A. Left atrial anastomotic line
   B. Pericardium anterior to loculated pericardial effusion
   C. Hiatus hernia
   D. Descending aortic dissection

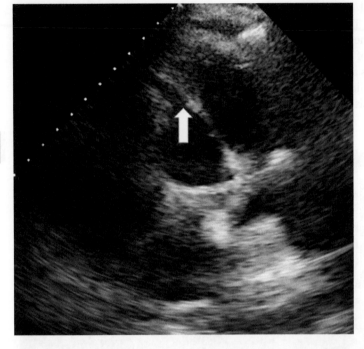

Figure 5.80

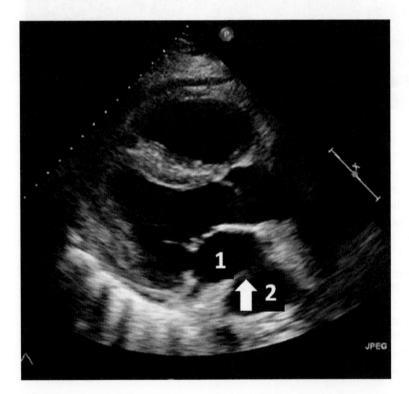

Figure 5.81

5.82. What is the structure denoted by "$" in these 2 apical views? (Figure 5.82)
- A. Left atrial myxoma
- B. Left atrial thrombus
- C. Thombosed descending aorta
- D. Hiatus hernia

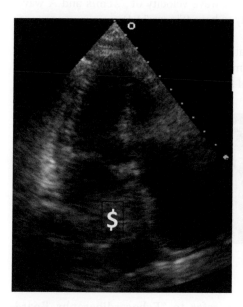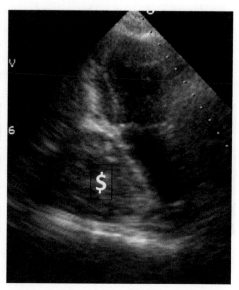

Figure 5.82

5.83. This 71-year-old woman presented with heart failure. She had edema and a raised jugular venous pressure (JVP) of 20 cm of water. Images from subcostal view are shown. The possible cause of her heart failure is (Figure 5.83):
- A. Severe mitral stenosis
- B. Severe aortic stenosis
- C. Severe mitral regurgitation
- D. Severe tricuspid regurgitation

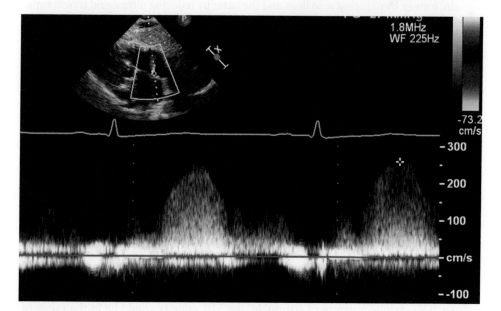

Figure 5.83

5.84. This 77-year-old patient presented with exertional shortness of breath. The echocardiogram (ECG) revealed normal left ventricular wall motion with an ejection fraction (EF) of 65% and normal valvular function. The transmitral flow showed an E-wave velocity of 90 cm/s, A wave velocity of 72 cm/s and A wave duration of 110 ms. This patient is likely to have (Figure 5.84):

A. Normal left atrial pressure
B. Normal left atrial pressure and elevated LVEDP
C. Elevated left atrial pressure and normal LVEDP
D. Elevated left atrial pressure, elevated LVEDP and increased Tau

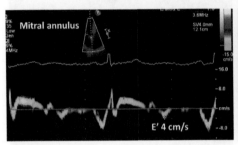 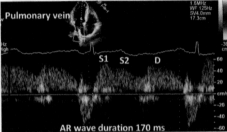

Figure 5.84

**For additional questions on echos, please refer to "Echocardiography Board Review" by Pai and Varadarajan.**

## Answers

5.1. C. Decrease sector angle.

Increase in frame rate occurs with reducing sector angle and reducing depth, the former by reducing scan lines and the latter by reducing ultrasound transit time. It is independent of transmit frequency and power.

5.2. C. Beam focusing.

Focusing increases lateral resolution. Increasing transducer diameter and increasing frequency also increase lateral resolution.

5.3. D. Increasing transmit frequency.

Increasing the transmit frequency will reduce the wavelength and hence the spatial pulse length. This will increase the pulse repetition frequency and the axial resolution. Beam diameter and focusing have no effect on axial resolution.

5.4. C. Ability to record higher velocities.

Aliasing and range specificity are properties of pulsed-wave Doppler. Continuous-wave Doppler is not associated with range ambiguity. Continuous-wave Doppler will also permit recording of higher velocities than pulsed-wave Doppler will, as it is not limited by the pulse repetition frequency as transmitted ultrasound is continuous.

5.5. C. Severe MR.

The jet area underestimates the severity of MR as the driving pressure is low. The regurgitant flow rate is approximately 200 cm³/s. Because of low left ventricular (LV) systolic pressure of 80 mmHg, the MR velocity would be in the range of

4 m/s (400 cm/s) assuming a left atrial (LA) pressure of 16 mmHg. Hence, the effective regurgitant orifice (ERO) area would be about 200/400, or 0.5 cm². Hence, in an intraoperative setting, it is important to bring up the blood pressure before performing MR quantitation.

5.6. D. Increasing the blood pressure.

Underestimation of MR can occur due to undersampling in the setting of low frame rate (increasing sector angle and depth) and high heart rates. Increasing blood pressure will increase the driving pressure across the mitral valve, and hence the jet size will increase because of a combination of an increase in regurgitation as well as higher kinetic energy in the jet imparted by higher driving pressure. Jet size is proportional to its kinetic energy. Wall-hugging jets tend to be smaller than free jets because of loss of jet energy to the wall.

5.7. A. 5.5 l/min.

The stroke volume equals the cross-sectional area multiplied by the TVI of the LVOT, which is $3.14 \times 1 \times 1 \times 25 = 78$ cm³. Cardiac output equals stroke volume multiplied by heart rate: $78 \times 70 = 5.5$ l/min.

5.8. D. Cannot be calculated based on data given.

In a patient with serial stenosis in close proximity, the continuity equation cannot be applied because of difficulty in obtaining precise subvalvular velocity and cross-sectional area of the flow in the LVOT. In a person without SAM the cross-sectional area of subvalvular flow is roughly equal to the cross-sectional area of the LVOT. Subvalvular obstruction will result in flow streams such that the cross-sectional area of flow is less than the anatomical LVOT area.

5.9. C. Severe.

Regurgitant volume is $140 - 80 = 60$ cm³/beat and regurgitant fraction is $60/140 = 43\%$. ERO area is regurgitant volume/TVI of aortic signal: $60/100 = 0.6$ cm². The regurgitant fraction in AR depends not only on ERO, but diastolic period and driving pressure. Hence, the ERO area is a more reliable index of AR volumetric severity. An ERO area of $\geq 0.4$ cm² is indicative of severe AR.

5.10. A. Overestimate the valve area.

In the presence of severe AR, the pressure half-time is decreased due to a rise in LV diastolic pressure produced by AR. Hence, in the calculation of mitral valve area by the pressure half-time method, the valve area will be overestimated or MS severity will be underestimated. Pressure half-time is decreased due to an increase in late LV diastolic pressure, causing a reduction in the LA-LV pressure gradient.

5.11. A. Severe AS.

This is an AS signal. Please pay attention to the onset of the signal, which is some time after the onset of QRS indicative of signal arising during ejection. Typically, a peak gradient >80 mmHg and a mean gradient of 40 mmHg are indicative of severe AS, though these are flow dependent. Valve area is a better indicator of severity of AS. MR signal starts with QRS. Tricuspid regurgitation (TR) signal in severe pulmonary hypertension also starts with QRS. (See Box 5.3.)

5.12. C. 0.5 cm².

By the continuity equation $A1 \times V1 = A2 \times V2$. Hence, the aortic valve area ($A2 = A1 \times V1/V2$) is approximately $3.14 \times 1 \times 1 \times 1/6 = 0.5$ cm².

**5.13.** A. Wide-open pulmonary regurgitation (PR).

Note the rapid deceleration of the PR signal with rapid equilibration of late diastolic pulmonary artery (PA) and right ventricular (RV) pressures. The increased systolic flow velocity is due to increased flow secondary to wide-open PR. Note that from this TEE view, you are looking at the pulmonary valve from above (i.e. the PA side), unlike a parasternal short-axis view.

**5.14.** B. Elevated LA pressure with elevated EDP.

The rapid D-wave deceleration with time <170 ms indicates high LA pressure. In addition, the S wave is smaller than the D wave. The atrial reversal wave duration is about 220 ms. The normal duration is about 80–100 ms. This is due to increased duration of atrial systole having to pump against elevated LV EDP. Pulmonary vein atrial regurgitation duration greater than mitral A-wave duration is indicative of high LV EDP.

**5.15.** B. High LA pressure.

This inflow pattern shows a high E/A ratio. The deceleration time is also short, suggestive of high LA pressure. In pure atrial mechanical failure, the E wave is normal, with diminished mitral A-wave amplitude.

**5.16.** B. Tricuspid atresia.

The atretic tricuspid valve is shown. There was no atrial septal defect (ASD), and outflow from right atrium was through right atrium to PA shunt. The patient also had a superior vena caval-right PA shunt. Both were patent. This would need low pulmonary vascular resistance and low PA pressure. This patient has a nonrestrictive ventricular septal defect (VSD), and hence RV systolic pressure would be the same as LV systolic pressure and to maintain low PA pressure, the RV outflow should be minimal or nonexistent. In this patient, this was accomplished surgically with banding of the PA.

Right atrial thrombus in this patient with tricuspid atresia is due to stasis.

**5.17.** B. Ostium secundum ASD.

Primum ASD would be in the lower part of the septum and may involve anterior mitral leaflet and A-V conduction. Sinus venosus ASD is in the upper septum near the superior vena cava and may also be associated with anomalous drainage of the right upper pulmonary vein. There is also a rare type of sinus venosus ASD in the vicinity of the inferior vena cava (IVC). In unroofed coronary sinus, the shunt is from left-to-right atrium through a posterior defect into the coronary sinus such that flow goes through the coronary sinus into the right atrium.

**5.18.** D. Flow across ASD.

This biphasic flow with a systolic-early diastolic component and LA contraction is typical of ASD flow. Pulmonary vein flow and superior vena cava flow would be triphasic, with distinct systolic and diastolic flows with reversal and atrial contraction. Mitral flow only has diastolic components with early and late diastolic components.

**5.19.** A. 12.8 l/min.

The shunt flow per beat can be calculated as the product of the TVI of the shunt flow and the anatomic area of the defect. This would be $39 \times 3.14 \times 1.5 \times 1 \, \text{cm}^3/\text{beat}(183 \, \text{cm}^3)$. This multiplied by the heart rate gives the shunt flow per minute.

5.20. A. Rheumatic heart disease.

The patient has classic rheumatic MS. The anterior leaflet is thin with a hockey stick appearance in diastole, which occurs due to commissural fusion. In degenerative MS, there is severe annular calcification, which extends into the leaflets causing stenosis. In fen-phen valvulopathy, the leaflets are thick and fibrosed and may result in both MS and MR. Ischemic involvement of the left ventricle without papillary muscle rupture causes restriction of closure and functional MR and not MS. Also, note the severe smoke-like echo or spontaneous echo contrast in the left atrium and layered thrombus in the body of the left atrium at the top of the image.

5.21. D. Bicuspid aortic valve.

This patient has Epstein's anomaly. Note the downward displacement of the septal leaflet of the tricuspid valve compared with the mitral leaflet attachment. A displacement of >8 mm/m² is suggestive of Epstein's. The septal leaflet may be large, sail-like, and adherent to the ventricular septum. This is frequently associated with ASD, right-sided accessory pathway, and TR, but not with bicuspid aortic valve.

5.22. A. Normal mitral valve motion.

This M mode is suggestive of normal mitral valve motion. There is normal mitral valve opening with greater early diastolic opening compared with opening associated with LA contraction. Valvular MS would cause mitral leaflet thickening, reduced opening and reduced ejection fraction (EF) slope, and paradoxical anterior motion of the posterior leaflet during diastole because of commissural fusion. Severe AR may cause fluttering of the anterior mitral leaflet and premature closure of the anterior mitral leaflet as the mitral valve opening is flow dependent. Features of high LA pressure will include predominant early opening, rapid EF slope, and a smaller opening with atrial contraction mirroring the transmitral inflow pattern.

5.23. C. Biventricular pacemaker or implantable cardioverter-defibrillator (ICD).

The arrow here depicts a lead in the coronary sinus and is consistent with a biventricular pacemaker.

5.24. A. LA appendage.

The structure denoted by the arrow is the LA appendage. This is separated from the left upper pulmonary vein, which is to the posterior with a ridge popularly known as the "coumadin ridge" because of the potential to be misinterpreted as a thrombus. Because this ridge is echo reflective, sometimes one can see thrombus-like artifacts in the appendage as mirror image artifacts. Though the appendage is clearly visualized here, this view alone is not sufficient to rule out a thrombus. Multiple tomographic views have to be obtained through the appendage in its entirety as the appendage may have multiple lobes.

5.25. B. Subvalvular AS.

The structure attached to the septum below the aortic valve is a classic subaortic membrane. Occasionally, vegetations can be seen here due to seeding from the aortic valve. This is a diastolic frame, and hence aortic valve opening cannot be evaluated.

**5.26.** A. Left heart failure.

The mitral inflow shown here is indicative of high LA pressure. Though the patient is in atrial fibrillation with only E wave, the E wave deceleration is very rapid, with a deceleration time of 100 ms.

**5.27.** D. Dilated cardiomyopathy.

There is a four-chamber dilatation. There is no increase in wall thickness to suggest HOCM. In ASD, both the right ventricle and right atrium will be dilated due to volume overload with normal LA and LV size. The tricuspid valve position is normal and hence does not support the diagnosis of Ebstein's anomaly.

**5.28.** A. P2 tethering.

This is an apical long-axis view, showing A2 and P2 scallops of the mitral valve. The MR jet is directed posterolaterally toward P2, consistent with P2 tethering. A similar jet direction can also occur in A2 prolapse, but both leaflets coapt distal to the plane of the mitral annulus. Bileaflet prolapse of equal magnitude will result in a central jet.

**5.29.** A. Penetrating injury to the interventricular septum.

A defect is seen in the ventricular septum. This patient had a penetrating injury to the septum. The image does not support the presence of mitral valve prolapse or hypertrophic septum.

**5.30.** A. AS and AR.

Unlike the MR signal, the AS signal occupies only the ejection period and is absent during the isovolumic contraction time. Hence, the signal starts a few milliseconds after the QRS. The diastolic velocity is too high for MS. This order of gradient and LA pressure would be incompatible with life. VSD flow is predominantly systolic with a presystolic component caused by atrial contraction. The gradient across a coarctation is systolic; the duration increases with greater degrees of stenosis and there may be a diastolic gradient. However, both the systolic and diastolic components will be in the same direction.

**5.31.** B. MS and MR.

Note that in TEE, from a mid-esophageal location, the MR jet is directed toward the transducer.

**5.32.** A. Severe AR.

The aortic leaflets are thickened with rolled-up edges and a central coaptation defect in end diastole. This anatomy would be associated with wide-open AR, as the regurgitant orifice is visible by anatomic imaging. AS cannot be diagnosed by a diastolic frame. HOCM typically causes mid-systolic closure of the aortic valve, best visualized by M mode. Aortic dissection may cause AR by one of several mechanisms: dilatation of sino-tubular junction, leaflet tethering, extension of hematoma into the aortic leaflet causing it to prolapse, or as a result of a primary problem such as bicuspid aortic valve or annulo-aortic ectasia.

**5.33.** B. Chronic severe MR.

The MR signal density is more than 60% of the mitral inflow signal. This correlates with a volume of regurgitation. In addition, the mitral inflow velocity is increased without a slow deceleration. A slow deceleration would indicate significant MS. Despite severe MR, the profile of the MR signal is quite rounded without the rapid deceleration that would typically be seen in acute severe MR, because of the large LA V wave, the so-called "V wave cutoff sign." Note that the heart rate is

151 bpm. At rapid heart rates, MR may be grossly underestimated by color Doppler due to limited temporal resolution and continuous-wave Doppler is very helpful.

5.34. A. Central venous catheter-associated infection.

This bicaval transesophageal view shows a large mass in the superior vena cava, which is typically associated with a central catheter-associated thrombus or vegetation. This is the most likely cause of his sepsis and endocarditis. In addition, there is a possible defect at the superior portion of the fossa ovalis, suggesting a patent foramen ovale (PFO). This patient had a large PFO by color and contrast echocardiography, allowing paradoxical embolization of the bacterial mass to cause left-sided endocarditis, escaping the protective filtration mechanism offered by the lung.

5.35. A. Aortic valve vegetation.

The mass on the aortic valve is suggestive of mass on the left ventricular side of the aortic valve. This is suggestive of vegetation. Also, there is prolapse of the non-coronary cusp, causing significant AR, and this is due to leaflet destruction with endocarditis. The other mechanism for prolapse could be a bicuspid aortic valve with prolapse of the larger cusp. Node of Arantius, as the name suggests, is a nodular thickening of the central portion of the leaflet edge and is best visualized from the short-axis view of the valve. Lambl's excrescences are thin, filamentous structures attached to the leaflet margin. There is no evidence of aortic dissection or intramural hematoma in this patient.

5.36. A. HOCM.

This late-peaking dagger-shaped signal is typical of SAM caused by HOCM. This occurs due to the dynamic LVOT obstruction increasing through systole. Critical valvular AS is unlikely as, in this case, the velocity is likely to be higher (unless cardiac output is very low) and the signal contour would be more rounded. Acute MR gives rise to an early peaking signal with a rapid deceleration because of a large LA V wave, the so-called V wave cutoff sign. In LV cavity obliteration, this signal will be much later peaking, with a gradient only in the very late part of systole when there is very little blood left in the distal LV cavity.

5.37. A. Bioprosthetic tricuspid valve.

This patient has Hancock porcine bioprosthetic tricuspid valve. The struts of the bioprosthetic valve are well seen. An annuloplasty ring would be seen as a small, rounded structure in cross-section at the tricuspid annulus only.

5.38. B. Third heart sound.

The mitral inflow is suggestive of high LA pressure. The mitral E/A ratio is >2 and deceleration time is 60 ms, indicating very high LA pressure. The calculated E-wave deceleration calculated from the E-wave amplitude and its time (velocity/time) is about $20 \, m/s^2$. A rate of deceleration of $>8-9 \, m/s^2$ is likely to result in S3. Age is relevant, as such a filling pattern in young children is normal because they have extremely efficient LV relaxation, which would result in physiological S3. S4 results from a prominent atrial-filling wave in a stiff ventricle and, in a summation gallop, the E and A waves are fused. This patient has no MS, and hence opening snap is unlikely.

5.39. B. Severe MR.

The temporal continuity of the systolic signal with the inflow signal suggests its origin at the mitral valve. The AS signal would occupy only the ejection period, being separated from the mitral inflow signal by isovolumic contraction and relaxation periods. A small VSD may result in a holosystolic signal, but generally has a presystolic component associated with LA systole and, generally, this flow is directed toward the transducer from most of the imaging windows.

5.40. C. 80 mmHg.

The TR velocity is 4 m/s, yielding an RV-RA systolic gradient of 64 mmHg. With an RA pressure of 20 mmHg, the RV systolic pressure would be about 80 mmHg, which would be the same as the PA systolic pressure in the absence of significant PS.

5.41. A. Acute severe AR.

The late diastolic frame in Figure 5.41 shows diastolic MR. There is also AR by color. The mitral valve is closed prematurely. This combination of findings is consistent with acute severe AR. A smaller AR jet in late diastole was due to late diastolic equilibration of aortic and LV pressures. Diastolic MR results from the receipt of AR volume in a left ventricle with high operating end-diastolic stiffness.

5.42. B. Acute AR.

The Doppler flow suggests premature closure of the mitral valve with lack of A wave despite being in sinus rhythm. This is pathognomonic of acute AR causing rapidly rising LV diastolic pressure due to failure to accommodate a large acute volume overload. In acute AR, the left atrium would still be contracting, but would be unable to eject against an acute increase in afterload. Pulmonary vein flow profile in this patient would show a prominent AR wave, and the tricuspid inflow would still have the A wave. Acute MR and VSD would not eliminate the A wave unless the patient had a recent episode of atrial fibrillation and the atrium is stunned.

5.43. C. Severe AR.

A prominent holodiastolic flow reversal suggesting retrograde flow in the aorta is seen. This flow would also cause Duroziez's murmur by physical examination due to the turbulence produced by partial occlusion by the finger, which would produce a diastolic murmur in the proximal femoral artery. Coarctation and middle aortic syndrome diminish pulsatility in the distal aortic flow and the flow becomes continuous due to flow through collaterals. Though HOCM can produce mid-systolic closure of the aortic valve, it does not produce any flow disturbance in the distal aorta.

5.44. A. Noncompaction of the left ventricle.

The inferolateral wall of the left ventricle in this patient is heavily trabeculated; noncompacted (trabeculated) to compacted wall thickness ratio is more than 2 : 1. This is highly indicative of noncompaction of LV myocardium, which is a developmental disorder causing congestive heart failure. In the other three conditions, the LV myocardium would be thicker, either due to infiltration or increased myocardial mass.

5.45. A. IVC-right atrium junction.

Part of the proximal IVC is seen with entry of saline contrast, in the longitudinal plane from a TEE. With this orientation, caudal structures are seen on the left and cephalad structures are seen on the right. This patient has a prominent Eustachian valve and, in a patient with a prominent Eustachian valve, in a low esophageal view, where the left atrium is not seen, this junction may be mistaken for an ASD. This patient was referred from an outside facility with that mistaken diagnosis from a TEE.

5.46. A. ~200 cm³/s.

The regurgitant flow rate equals $2\pi r^2$ times the Nyquist limit. Here, the PISA radius is 0.9 cm and the Nyquist limit is 38 cm/s. Regurgitant flow rate is $2 \times 3.14 \times 0.9^2 \times 38 \approx 200$ cm³/s.

5.47. C. Late-peaking systolic murmur increased by Valsalva's maneuver and normal A2.

This patient clearly has SAM of the anterior mitral leaflet causing LVOT obstruction. As the SAM increases in late systole, the gradient velocity and turbulence are more in late systole, causing a late peaking late systolic murmur. SAM is increased by LV volume reduction and vasodilatation. A2 is preserved in these patients, in contrast to patients with severe AS, who may also have late-peaking systolic murmur.

5.48. A. HOCM.

This patient has HOCM with dynamic LVOT obstruction caused by SAM, which causes a late-peaking systolic gradient, increased by Valsalva's maneuver and amyl nitrate inhalation. The gradient would also be increased by positive inotropic agents and vasodilators and decreased by an increase in afterload, with vasoconstrictors or handgrip. In addition to HOCM, SAM can occur in volume-depleted states with small left ventricle cavity and also after surgical mitral valve repair in patients with long anterior and posterior leaflets, especially if a small annuloplasty ring is used.

5.49. A. Apical HOCM.

This patient has disproportionately thickened LV apical myocardium typical of apical HOCM. This results in a spade-shaped LV cavity in diastole. These patients also have giant T-wave inversions in their chest leads. In hypertensive heart disease, LV hypotension is more uniformly distributed. Endomyocardial fibrosis causes apical obliteration due to endocardial thickening rather than myocardial thickening.

5.50. C. PFO closure device.

The image shows two parallel discs sandwiching the upper atrial septum. The RA disc is larger than the LA disc. This is suggestive of an Amplatzer PFO closure device. In an ASD closure device, the LA disc is larger than the RA disc. Patch repair of the septum will not show the triple-layer morphology as seen here.

5.51. C. Vegetation on a bioprosthetic valve.

This is a short-axis view of the tricuspid valve, best obtained from a proximal gastric location, with clockwise probe rotation at about 20–30°. The sewing ring of the prosthetic valve is clearly seen here, and there is a mass attached to the leaflets, indicative of vegetation.

5.52. A. Paradoxical embolism.

Figure 5.52 shows the interatrial septum with a large PFO in its typical location. The color flow shows left-to-right flow. This flow would reverse under situations of increased RA pressure, such as straining, coughing, and right heart failure. The orientation of the opening is favorable for thrombi originating in the IVC region to traverse the PFO to the left atrium even in the absence of raised RA pressure.

5.53. C. Fistulous communication between aorta and right ventricle.

In addition to the fistulous communication, Figure 5.53 also shows AR. Fistulous communications generally result from rupture of an aortic root abscess. This may result in communications to the right atrium, right ventricle, PA, or the LVOT. Other local complications include abscess of mitral aortic intervalvular fibrosa, leaflet aneurysm, and perforation of the anterior mitral leaflet. One may also get an abscess in the ventricular septum, causing a VSD after rupture.

5.54. B. Pulmonary valve endocarditis.

This is a mid-esophageal image showing the aortic valve in short axis in the center and the RV inflow and outflow wrapped around it akin to the short axis of the aortic valve from a parasternal view. There is a large mass attached to the pulmonary valve consistent with vegetation. This is the likely source of his lung abscesses.

5.55. A. Coronary sinus.

Figure 5.55 is a low esophageal view partially cutting through the posterior A–V groove showing the coronary sinus.

5.56. C. Severe.

This is severe as judged by jet size, vena contract, and PISA radius. In addition, the two-dimensional image shows lack of tricuspid leaflet coaptation, leading to wide-open TR. The mechanism is tricuspid annular dilatation, and hence is functional, probably secondary to previous pulmonary hypertension due to mitral valve disease resulting in RV and RA dilatation, thus stretching the tricuspid annulus. This is repairable with tricuspid annuloplasty. Also note the partially seen mitral prosthesis. TR quantitations by using the three components of the jet are not well validated.

5.57. C. Moderate or severe pulmonary hypertension.

In patients with wide-open TR, the tricuspid valve may be fairly nonrestrictive, allowing right ventricle and right atrium to behave virtually as a single chamber during systole. In such a situation, the TR pressure gradient cannot reliably be calculated using the simplified Bernoulli equation as a considerable amount of energy may be expended in causing acceleration of the TR jet. In addition, RA pressure may be very high, leading to underestimation of PA pressure. In this example, one can count the number of aliases to estimate the TR velocity at the vena contracta. There are four aliases, corresponding to a velocity of 69 cm/s × 4; that is, 2.76 cm/s. Though the pressure gradient is 30 mmHg, the patient is likely to have very high RA pressure (i.e. 20–30 mmHg), and because of wide-open TR, the TR pressure gradient would have underestimated the pressure gradient. Hence, the PA systolic pressure is at least moderate but more likely to be in the severe range in the absence of PS. In such patients, careful examination of the pulmonary regurgitant jet to obtain an estimate of PA diastolic pressure would be helpful.

5.58. D. Replacement with a mechanical valve.

This prosthesis is probably a bileaflet valve in view of the two areas of reverberations seen in the left atrium. A bioprosthetic valve would show struts in the periphery and thin leaflets in the center, unless calcified. An annuloplasty ring is an echo-dense structure at the base of the mitral leaflet on the LA side with intact leaflets. This ring can be partial or complete. An Alfieri stitch can be central or asymmetric and is simply a stitch that focally unites the tips of anterior and posterior leaflets and converts the mitral orifice into a double orifice, best seen in short-axis view.

5.59. D. All of the above.

Pre-intervention mitral flow is indicative of high LA pressure. This pattern is seen despite a heart rate of 92 bpm, as faster heart rates result in atrial predominance of ventricular filling. Post intervention, the mitral flow is suggestive of impaired left ventricular relaxation, which is consistent with normal or low mean LA pressure. Note that the heart rate is slower at 62 bpm. This patient had dilated cardiomyopathy with severe functional MR, which responded to diuresis and afterload reduction with a reduction of LV size and elimination of MR. Uncontrolled hypertension will reduce LV ejection performance, increase LV size, and give rise to MR, as myopathic ventricles are exquisitely sensitive to afterload. As these patients have little or no functional reserve, anemia has a serious and deleterious effect on hemodynamics because of a reduction in oxygen-carrying capacity and a demand for higher cardiac output.

5.60. A. Thoracic aortic aneurysm.

The thoracic aorta runs posterior to the left atrium, is rounded, and on dynamic imaging is pulsatile. Turning the imaging plane by 90° would show the long axis of the descending aorta. The membrane of cor triatriatum separates the pulmonary venous chamber from the lower part of the atrium and is best seen from parasternal long-axis and apical views. The location is across the left atrium. Left PA is not seen in the posterior mediastinum.

5.61. C. HOCM.

Note the SAM of the anterior mitral leaflet starting in midsystole. The SAM narrows the LV outflow tract in a dynamic manner, producing LV outflow obstruction and gradient. Elevated LV EDP is not an unreasonable response as deceleration of mitral A wave is slow, though not a classical B hump. Mitral valve prolapse results in late systolic sagging of the mitral valve, not anterior motion. Severe AR with a posteriorly directed jet on to the anterior mitral leaflet results in diastolic fluttering.

5.62. B. Elevated LV EDP.

Note the prominent B hump after the A point of mitral valve motion. In atrial fibrillation, there is loss of A wave. Also see explanation for Question 5.61.

5.63. C. Congestive heart failure.

This is typical of pulsus alternans, which occurs in severe systolic heart failure. Note there is reduced opening and duration of opening of the aortic valve with every other beat, and this results from reduced stroke volume with every other beat. Also note that, in this instance, pulsus alternans was triggered by a premature ventricular complex. In AS, there is leaflet thickening and reduced opening.

In HOCM, there may be midsystolic closure of the aortic valve. Hypertension does not produce any characteristic changes in aortic valve motion.

5.64. B. MS with high LA pressure.

The diastolic signal "1" is that of MS, and this patient is in sinus rhythm as there is an A wave. The peak diastolic gradient is about 30 mmHg and mean gradient is 18 mmHg at a heart rate of 76 bpm, and this indicative of severe MS. The arrow points to isovolumic relaxation time (IVRT), which was 30 ms, indicating high LA pressure or large LA "V" wave. Partial MR velocity is indicated by "2", as it is contiguous with ending of the MS signal, and "3" indicates LV outflow and the gap between that and mitral inflow, which is indicated by the arrow in IVRT.

5.65. B. Hyperdynamic LV.

Systolic signal denoted by "1" is not MR but due to LV cavity obliteration as it is late peaking and hence indicates a hyperdynamic LV. It also occurs during ejection phase, unlike an MR signal. IVRT indicated by the arrow is 110 ms (time between small marks is 200 ms and two vertical lines is 1 s), and this indicates normal LA pressure. IVRT is the Doppler equivalent of the auscultatory A2–OS interval; that is, interval between aortic component of second heart sound and opening snap in MS. A short A2-OS interval indicates severe MS.

5.66. D. Severe PR.

Signal "2" is early diastolic following an ejection flow "1" suggestive of origin at a semilunar valve. The arrow points to forward flow across the semilunar valve with atrial systole, and this can occur only at the pulmonary valve with normal PA pressure. If the PA pressure is high, atrial systole cannot generate a forward flow even when there is late diastolic equilibration of pressures between PA, right ventricle, and right atrium. For the same reason, you do not get forward flow across the aortic valve in severe AR as aortic diastolic pressure is too high and high LV diastolic pressure may cause premature closure of the mitral valve. The diastolic flow is of low velocity and ends in mid-diastole, indicating severe PR with normal PA pressure.

5.67. C. Severe PS and PR.

This patient in fact had a bovine jugular non-valved conduit between the right ventricle and PA for pulmonary atresia in a foreign country during infancy and presented with shortness of breath and edema. As the conduit has become too small for her body size and flow requirements, it was functionally stenotic, resulting in a very high systolic gradient. The longer arrow points to the PR signal. The PR is severe and it also rapidly decelerates with equilibration of pressures between PA and right ventricle. The shorter arrow indicates forward flow with RA systole; this indicates normal PA pressure.

5.68. C. Suprasternal window.

This is a classic flow because of severe coarctation of the aorta with systolic and diastolic components. The signals are negative or flow is going away from the transducer. This signal is obtained from the suprasternal window.

5.69. C. Patent ductus arteriosus (PDA).

This is a typical PDA flow obtained from a parasternal short-axis basal view with clockwise rotation of the probe to show PA and branches. Dilated main PA is indicated by "1" and "2" arch/descending aortic junction from which flow is occurring into PA. Note this is a diastolic frame (see marker on electrocardiogram) and flow is into the main PA; hence, not left PA branch stenosis.

5.70. A. Aortic coarctation.

Note that the flow is into the aortic lumen throughout the cardiac cycle, indicative of retrograde flow in the intercostal artery. This occurs in collateral dependent distal perfusion as it occurs in severe aortic coarctation. This patient had interrupted aorta. In severe AR, holodiastolic retrograde flow occurs in the aortic lumen.

5.71. B. Severe MR.

This flow is across the foramen ovale due to excessive stretching produced by high atrial pressures. The flow is from left to right atrium, and note that the highest velocity is in late systole, indicative of a large LA "V" wave which occurs in severe MR. In large ASD, flow will be nonrestrictive across the defect, resulting in very low or transient pressure gradients.

5.72. A. Pulmonary hypertension.

This is a typical "flying W sign" associated with pulmonary hypertension. Midsystolic deceleration occurs due to rapidly returning reflected pressure waves secondary to a stiffer PA that occurs when it operates under high pressure. These is no PR signal and no continuous-wave signal to assess if there is a gradient across the pulmonary valve. The velocity of the signal is under 1 m/s, indicating normal amount of PA flow, and this is inconsistent with a large ASD. Large ASD is associated with increased PA flow.

5.73. A. LV systolic dyssynchrony.

Tissue Doppler or tissue velocity images are shown here. Focal velocity profiles of medial (yellow) and lateral annulus (green) are produced offline by placing samples in these regions. Note the peak of lateral annulus velocity is about 150 ms after the medial annulus velocity peak, suggestive of septolateral mechanical dyssynchrony. A septolateral delay of >65 ms is indicative of LV dyssynchrony. There was good diastolic synchrony, as judged by annular E wave velocity profiles.

5.74. A. LV strain.

Note the units are in percent, which is percentage shortening compared with original length. Normal myocardial strain is 15–20%, very similar to percentage sarcomeric shortening during contraction of cardiac muscle cell.

5.75. C. Aortic subvalvular membrane.

This is a classic example of membranous subaortic stenosis. Also note part of this circumferential membrane on the LV side of the anterior mitral leaflet. The image also shows the aortic valve (left-pointing arrow) and the SAM of the anterior mitral leaflet (right-pointing arrow).

5.76. A. Coronary artery.

This was anomalous circumflex coronary artery originating from right coronary artery with a retroaortic course between the aorta and left atrium. Note that it is small and perfectly circular unlike an abscess, which tends to have irregular edges and inflammatory thickening or other sequelae around it. One can study the course of the vessel by imaging this structure in different imaging planes. Coronary sinus would be in the posterior atrioventricular (AV) groove.

5.77. A. Dilated coronary sinus and dextrocardia.

Note opacification of the structure at the AV groove with saline contrast, indicating anomalous connection of left or right or entire superior vena cava into coronary sinus (as it is not specified which arm was injected). Also note a pacemaker lead in the coronary sinus. At an angle of 49°, the LVOT is on the right side, indicating dextrocardia. This view is typically obtained at 120–140° with levocardia – sort of a mirror image.

5.78. C. Dilated azygos vein.

This is a typical appearance. This patient had an interrupted IVC, and the IVC drained through the azygos vein into the superior vena cava. The IVC does not relate to the thoracic aorta. A mirror image artifact looks like a duplicate image of the DTA.

5.79. A. Coarctation of aorta.

The systolic signal going away from the transducer from the suprasternal notch is typical of coarctation as the blood flows away from the transducer. The mean gradient is over 20 mmHg and there is a diastolic gradient indicating severe coarctation. The signal from aortic stenosis will be directed toward the transducer, hence positive and will not have a diastolic component. The pulmonary anastomotic site can get stenosed as well and this signal is directed mostly up and posteriorly and best recorded from parasternal short axis view. The PDA flow would be from the distal arch to left pulmonary artery origin and will be away from suprasternal notch, continuous (unless these is pulmonary hypertension) and is best recorded from the parasternal short axis view of the main pulmonary artery showing the branches.

5.80. B. Right coronary artery (RCA).

This is the typical location of RCA. The left coronary artery originates at 3 or 4 o'clock position in this view. Aortic dissection will have a linear shadow inside the aortic lumen.

5.81. A. Left atrial anastomosis between donor and recipient atria. 1 is the donor atrium and 2 is the recipient atrium which is connected to the pulmonary veins.

5.82. D. Hiatus hernia. Note that it is retrocardiac and extrinsically compresses the left atrium. This is the typical location posterior to the left atrium. This can be diagnosed by giving a carbonated drink to the patient. The release of gas will make it look bright on echo imaging.

5.83. C. Severe mitral regurgitation. Note the patent formaen ovale with left-to-right flow (red jet). The CW signal is across this defect and has peak velocity of 2.5 m/s, peaking in end-systole. The flow is entirely left to right indicating that LA pressure is higher than RA pressure throughout the cardiac cycle – in other words, higher than 20 cm of water which is about 15 mmHg (200 mm $H_2O$ divided by specific gravity of mercury 13.6). Hence, the left atrial "V" wave pressure is about 40 mmHg. A large "V" wave indicates severe mitral regurgitation. In severe AS and MS, you may get left atrial pressure augmentation during atrial systole. In severe TR, there would be a large right atrial "V" wave and this may reverse the flow across the atrial septum during ventricular systole.

5.84. D. Elevated left atrial pressure, elevated LVEDP and increased Tau. Note the following: The septal E' velocity is reduced (<8 cm/s) indicating impaired LV relaxation – the gold standard measure for this on invasive hemodynamics using high-fidelity LV pressure tracing is Tau or constant of isovolumic LV pressure decay. In impaired relaxation, Tau is increased. The E/E' ratio in this patient is 90/4 = 22.5; increased (>15) indicating high LA pressure. The AR wave duration in pulmonary vein (170 ms) exceeds mitral A wave duration (110 ms) by 60 ms indication high LVEDP (>30 ms, original study by Rossvol and Hatle.

---

**Box 5.1   Key Practical Pearls**

- Higher transducer frequency results in better resolution, but reduced penetration. Better color-flow images are obtained at lower transducer frequency.
- To increase frame rate, reduce depth or sector angle and eliminate color flow if you can. Reduce the color-flow box width to as narrow as possible to increase frame rate.
- Regurgitant jets are underestimated at low frame rates and low gain. Wall-hugging jets are smaller for a given severity due to loss of kinetic energy at the jet-wall interface. Jet size depends on kinetic energy contained in the jet, and hence is a function of both regurgitant flow rate and driving pressure.
- In AS assessment: zoom LVOT and clean up to see LVOT boundaries clearly, obtain VI to minimize spectral dispersion and V2 from multiple windows. For peak velocity of VI, get the peak but, for TVI, trace through modal velocity.
- In obtaining pressure half-time in MS, ignore the initial rapid ski slope, which is affected markedly by LV relaxation and recoil. Mean gradient depends on heart rate: lower at lower heart rate due to longer diastolic filling time. Mean gradient should be given along with heart rate.
- A transesophageal echocardiogram (TEE) has a higher spatial resolution than a transthoracic echocardiogram (TTE) because of higher carrier frequency.
- In the performance of TEE, obtain key information first to answer the clinical question, just in case the patient becomes intolerant of the procedure and the procedure needs to be abandoned. For example, when the question is "rule out acute aortic dissection", examine the ascending aorta first as its involvement mandates emergency ascending aortic repair. Then, look at pericardial effusion, LV function, AR and its mechanism, extent of dissection, entry point location, coronary and arch vessel involvement, and so on. In suspected endocarditis, examine the left- and then right-sided valves first in a comprehensive fashion from midaortic location, which is most tolerable for the patient.

---

**Box 5.2   Key Guideline Summaries**

- Echocardiographic criteria for severe MR include jet area to LA area ratio >40%, jet area >10 cm², vena contracta diameter ≥7 mm, regurgitant volume ≥60 cm³, regurgitant fraction ≥50%, ERO area ≥0.4 cm², or systolic flow reversal in any of the pulmonary veins. There may be a large coaptation defect in the mitral valve closure mechanism. MR signal by continuous wave may be triangular, the so-called "V" wave cutoff sign due to large LA "V" wave (Zoghbi et al. 2003). In eccentric wall-hugging jets, jet size may be smaller by as much as 50% for a given regurgitant volume.

- Echocardiographic sign of severe MS is the mitral valve area <1.0 cm$^2$ with or without supporting features of mean diastolic gradient of >10 mmHg or PA systolic pressure of >50 mmHg (Baumgartner et al. 2009).
- Echocardiographic criteria for severe AS include aortic valve area <1.0 cm$^2$, indexed valve area <0.6 cm$^2$, V2 > 4 m/s, mean gradient >40 mmHg, or velocity ratio (V1/V2) <0.25 (Baumgartner et al. 2009).
- Severe AS with low gradient is said to exist when AV area <1 cm$^2$ and mean gradient <30 mmHg and can occur in those with both normal and low ejection fraction (EF) and is associated with high mortality which is reduced by AVR. Low dose dobutamine echo can be used in these patients to differentiate from pseudo severe AS (increase in AV area with an increase in cardiac output), true severe AS (mean gradient increases with increase in stroke volume, but AV area remains unchanged), or evaluate for contractile reserve (EF and cardiac output increase).
- Echocardiographic criteria for severe AR include jet height to LVOT diameter ratio ≥65%, jet area to LVOT area ≥60%, vena contracta diameter >6 mm, regurgitant volume ≥60 cm$^3$, regurgitant fraction ≥50%, ERO area ≥0.3 cm$^2$, or prominent holodiastolic flow reversal in the descending aorta. AR pressure half-time may be <200 ms (Zoghbi et al. 2003).
- Echocardiographic criteria for severe TR include jet area >10 cm$^2$, vena contracta diameter >7 mm, PISA radius >9 mm at a Nyquist limit of 50–60 cm/s, or systolic flow reversal in the hepatic veins. There may be a large coaptation defect in tricuspid valve closure mechanism. TR signal by continuous wave may be triangular, the so called "V" wave cutoff sign due to large RA "V" wave (Zoghbi et al. 2003).
- Criteria for severe tricuspid stenosis: mean diastolic gradient ≥5 mmHg, diastolic TVI >60 cm, pressure half-time ≥190 ms, tricuspid valve area by continuity equation ≤1.0 cm$^2$ (Baumgartner et al. 2009).
- Echocardiographic criteria for severe PR include a large jet size at origin, steep deceleration of PR signal by continuous wave often stopping in mid-diastole, increased pulmonary flow compared with systemic flow, and RV enlargement. Features are less quantitative (Zoghbi et al. 2003).
- Echocardiographic criteria for severe PS: peak systolic velocity > 4 m/s or peak systolic gradient >64 mmHg (Baumgartner et al. 2009).

---

Box 5.3   Important Clinical Trial or Outcome Data Summaries

- **Cardiac resynchronization therapy (CRT) in narrow QRS cohort study.** In the Yu et al. (2006) study, of the 102 patients with class III or IV heart failure and EF <35%, 51 had QRSd <120 ms but also had LV mechanical asynchrony by echo. Both groups had a similar response to CRT in terms of the six-minute walk test and reduction in LV volumes and MR and improvement in EF. Response rate in both groups was about 70%.

- **RethinQ trial.** In Beshai et al. (2007), 172 patients with standard indication for ICD, QRSd <130 ms, and echocardiographic evidence of LV dyssynchrony was randomized to CRT versus no CRT. Primary end point was improvement in peak oxygen consumption. There was no improvement in peak oxygen consumption with CRT. Subgroup analysis showed improvement in those with QRSd >120 ms. The six-minute walk improved significantly in those with nonischemic cardiomyopathy and New York Heart Association class improved in both groups. The trial is criticized for poor echo data quality, three different core labs, lack of standardization, three different vendors, need to drop some data, and poor reproducibility.
- **Echo-CRT trial.** In the Ruschitzka et al. (2013) study, 809 patients with heart failure class III or IV, EF <35%, QRSd <130 ms, and echo evidence of LV dyssynchrony were randomized to ICD with CRT turned on or off. Of 1680 809 patients had LV dyssynchrony. The primary end point was all-cause mortality and hospitalization for heart failure. The trial was stopped prematurely due to higher mortality in the CRT arm (hazard ratio 1.8, $p = 0.02$).

## References

Baumgartner, H., Hung, J., Bermejo, J. et al. (2009). Echocardiographic assessment of valve stenosis: EAE/ASE recommendations for clinical practice. *European Journal of Echocardiography* 10: 1–25.

Beshai, J.F., Grimm, R.A., Nagueh, S.F. et al. (2007). Cardiac-resynchronization therapy in heart failure with narrow QRS complexes. *New England Journal of Medicine* 357: 2461–2471.

Ruschitzka, F., Abraham, W.T., Singh, J.P. et al. (2013). Cardiac-resynchronization therapy in heart failure with a narrow QRS complex. *New England Journal of Medicine* 369: 1395–1405.

Yu, C.M., Chan, Y.S., Zhang, Q. et al. (2006). Benefits of cardiac resynchronization therapy for heart failure patients with narrow QRS complexes and coexisting systolic asynchrony by echocardiography. *Journal of theAmerican College of Cardiology* 48: 2251–2257.

Zoghbi, W.A., Enriquez-Sarano, M., Foster, E. et al. (2003). Recommendations for evaluation of the severity of native valvular regurgitation with two-dimensional and Doppler echocardiography. *Journal of the American Society of Echocardiography* 16: 777–802.

# Cardiac Magnetic Resonance Imaging

# 6

6.1. Magnetic resonance imaging (MRI) makes use of nuclei with unpaired spins. What is the nucleus used in image production?
- A. Hydrogen-1
- B. Carbon-13
- C. Phosphorus-31
- D. Sodium-23

6.2. What is the resonance frequency with a 1.5 T scanner?
- A. 63 MHz
- B. 42 MHz
- C. 126 MHz
- D. None of the above

6.3. How is spatial localization of signal origin achieved?
- A. Magnetic gradient
- B. Timing of received RF signal
- C. Timing of transmitted RF signal
- D. All of the above

6.4. With which of the following is cardiac MRI generally not advisable in patients?
- A. Automated implantable cardioverter defibrillator (ICD)
- B. Cerebral aneurysm clips
- C. Iron-containing foreign body in the eye that has been there for six years
- D. All of the above
- E. None of the above

6.5. What are the potential effects of a strong magnetic field in a patient with a pacer or implantable cardioverter-defibrillator (ICD)?
- A. May burn the circuits
- B. Heat generation at lead tip and tissue coagulation and rise in threshold
- C. Reset device
- D. All of the above

6.6. Gadolinium (Gd) does which of the following?
- A. Shortens T1 and increases signal on T1-weighted images
- B. Lengthens T1 and increases signal on T1-weighted images
- C. Shortens T1 and reduces signal on T1-weighted images
- D. Lengthens T1 and reduces signal on T1-weighted images

**6.7.** Which of the following can magnetic resonance (MR) coronary angiography be performed with?
   **A.** Single breath hold
   **B.** Multiple breath holds
   **C.** With the use of a navigator pulse
   **D.** None of the above

**6.8.** In the FIESTA or steady-state free precession (SSFP) MR image shown in Figure 6.8, what does "1" refer to?
   **A.** Right ventricle
   **B.** Left ventricle
   **C.** Right atrium
   **D.** Left atrium

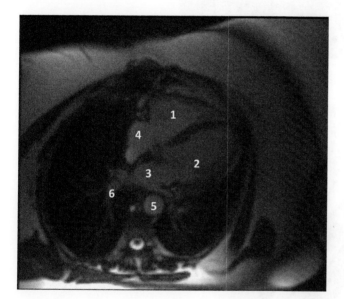

Figure 6.8

**6.9.** In the FIESTA or SSFP MR image shown in Figure 6.9, what does "2" refer to?
   **A.** Right ventricle
   **B.** Left ventricle
   **C.** Right atrium
   **D.** Left atrium

**6.10.** In the T1-weighted black blood MR image shown in Figure 6.10, what does "1" refer to?
   **A.** Right ventricle
   **B.** Left ventricle
   **C.** Right atrium
   **D.** Left atrium

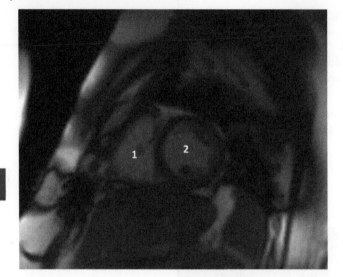

Figure 6.9

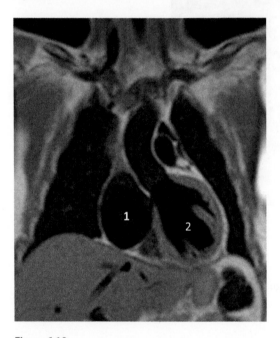

Figure 6.10

**6.11.** Figure 6.11 shows a delayed Gd-enhanced image in a patient with occluded left anterior descending (LAD) artery. What is the image indicative of?
   **A.** Scarred left ventricle anterior wall
   **B.** Scarred left ventricle inferior wall
   **C.** LAD area looks fully viable
   **D.** None of the above

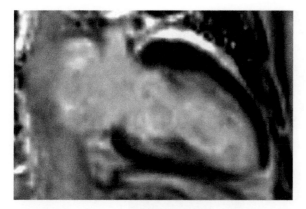

Figure 6.11

**6.12.** What does the MRA in Figure 6.12 show?
- **A.** Pulmonary artery branch stenosis
- **B.** Pulmonary infundibular stenosis
- **C.** Normal pulmonary veins
- **D.** None of the above

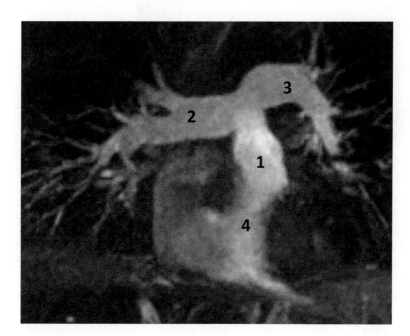

Figure 6.12

**6.13.** What does the image in Figure 6.13 show?
- **A.** T1-weighted image
- **B.** FIESTA image
- **C.** Contrast-enhanced MRA
- **D.** None of the above

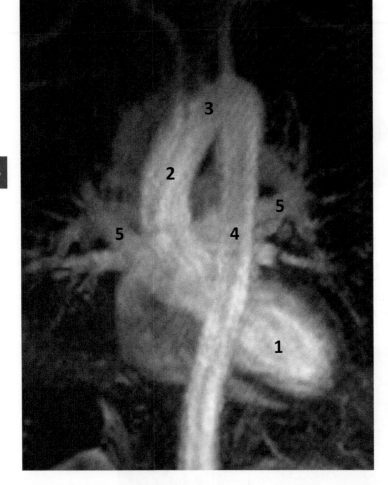

**Figure 6.13**

**6.14.** Which of the following statements about Figure 6.14 are accurate?
  A. It is a volume rendered MRA image
  B. Gd contrast was used for imaging
  C. 1, 2, and 3 refer to ascending aorta, main pulmonary artery (MPA), and pulmonary veins respectively
  D. All of the above

**6.15.** What does the arrow point to in Figure 6.15?
  A. Lipomatous atrial septum
  B. Atrial myxoma
  C. Sarcoma
  D. Artifact

**6.16.** What is the patient in Figure 6.16 likely to have?
  A. Heart failure
  B. Pneumonia
  C. Atrial septal defect
  D. Descending aortic dissection

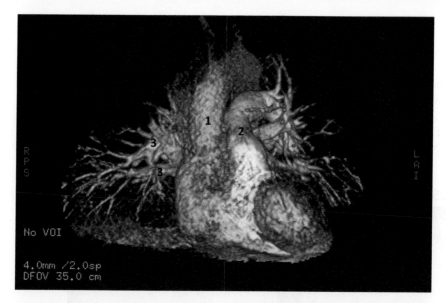

Figure 6.14

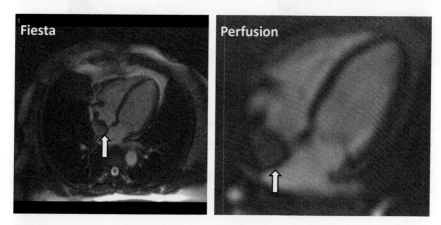

Figure 6.15

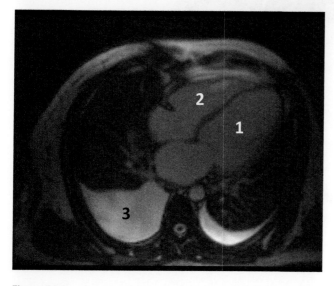

Figure 6.16

6.17. What is the patient in Figure 6.17 likely to have?
    A. Multivessel coronary artery disease
    B. Single-vessel circumflex disease
    C. Extensive myocardial scarring due to prior infarcts
    D. Normal coronary artery

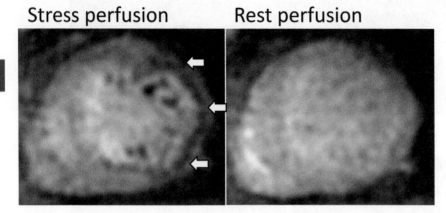

Figure 6.17

6.18. What is the patient in Figure 6.18 likely to have had?
    A. Arrhythmogenic right ventricular dysplasia (ARVD)
    B. Inferior myocardial infarction
    C. Anterior myocardial infarction
    D. Myocarditis

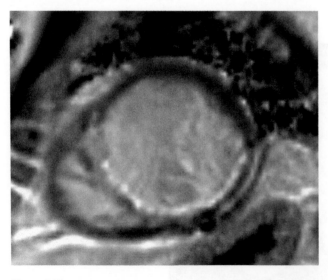

Figure 6.18

**6.19.** What is the patient in Figure 6.19 likely to have had?
   **A.** ARVD
   **B.** Inferior myocardial infarction
   **C.** Anterior myocardial infarction
   **D.** Myocarditis

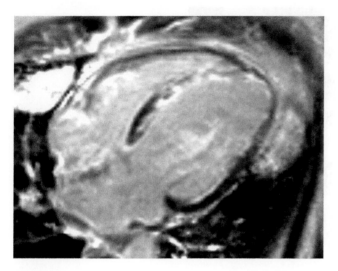

Figure 6.19

**6.20.** The patient in Figure 6.20 has severe left ventricle dysfunction. What is the etiology likely to be?
   **A.**  Left ventricle noncompaction
   **B.** Myocarditis
   **C.** Myocardial infarct with fatty replacement
   **D.** Cardiac amyloid

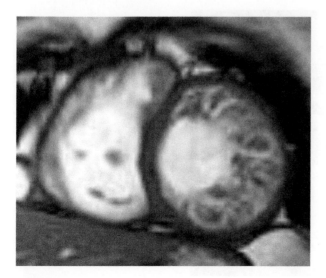

Figure 6.20

**6.21.** What is the patient in Figure 6.21 likely to have?
   A. Bicuspid aortic stenosis
   B. Aortic valve vegetation
   C. Aortic dissection
   D. None of the above

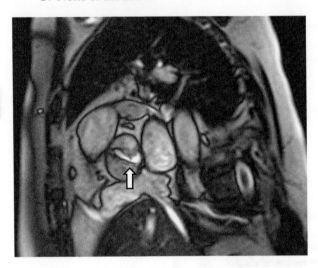

Figure 6.21

**6.22.** In the black blood cardiac MR image of the chest in Figure 6.22, what does the arrow point to?
   A. Trachea
   B. Right pulmonary artery
   C. Left pulmonary artery
   D. Aorta

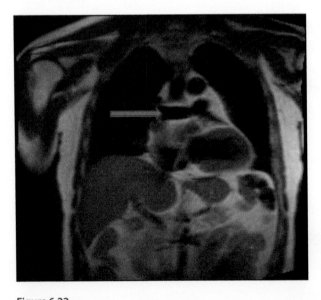

Figure 6.22

**6.23.** What structure does the arrow point to on the black blood cardiac MR image in Figure 6.23?
A. Trachea
B. Right main bronchus
C. Left main bronchus
D. Pulmonary artery

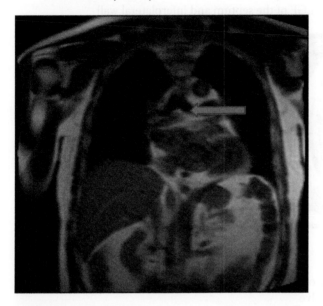

Figure 6.23

**6.24.** The 58-year-old male seen in Figure 6.24 complained of shortness of breath and palpitations (AO: aorta; LA: left atrium; LV: left ventricle). This patient probably has which of the following conditions?
A. Hypertrophic cardiomyopathy
B. Sigmoid-shaped septum
C. Normal myocardium
D. Hypertensive heart disease

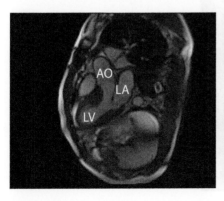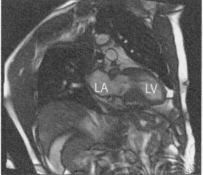

Figure 6.24

**6.25.** The regions arrowed in the inversion recovery images from the patient in Question 6.24 shown in Figure 6.25 are indicative of what? (LA: left atrium; LV: left ventricle; RA: right atrium; RV: right ventricle)
A. Normal myocardium
B. Transmural late gadolinium enhancement (LGE) of the septum
C. Subendocardial LGE of the septum and lateral wall
D. Midmyocardial patchy LGE of the septum and inferolateral wall

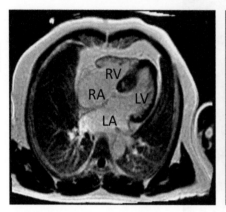
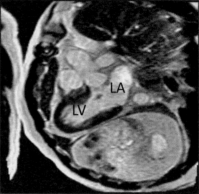

Figure 6.25

**6.26.** What does the still frame of the short-axis image in Figure 6.26a show?
A. Cleft anterior mitral valve
B. Cleft posterior mitral valve
C. Normal mitral valve
D. Mitral valve vegetation

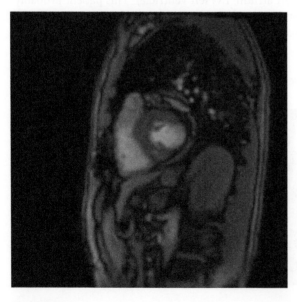

Figure 6.26a

**6.27.** What structure does the arrow point to on the bright blood cardiac MR image in Figure 6.27a?
A. Main pulmonary artery
B. Ascending aorta
C. Right pulmonary artery
D. Left pulmonary artery

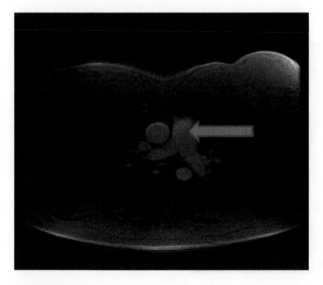

Figure 6.27a

**6.28.** What structure does the arrow point to on the bright blood cardiac MR image shown in Figure 6.28a?
A. Main pulmonary artery
B. Ascending aorta
C. Right pulmonary artery

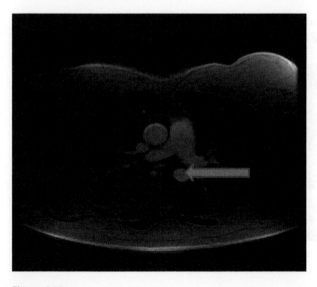

Figure 6.28a

D. Left pulmonary artery

E. Descending aorta

6.29. What structure does the arrow point to in the bright blood cardiac MR image in Figure 6.29a?

A. Superior vena cava

B. Inferior vena cava

C. Pulmonary artery

D. Aorta

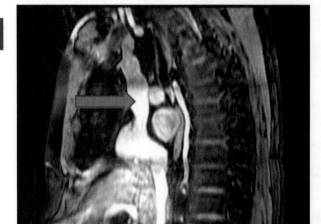

Figure 6.29a

6.30. A 50-year-old male was admitted to hospital with complaints of chest pain. The electrocardiogram (ECG) obtained at the time of admission showed 3 mm ST elevation in leads V3-V6. He was rushed to the cardiac cath lab, which showed occlusion of the distal LAD artery. He then underwent cardiac MRI to evaluate left ventricle function and scar burden. What do the inversion recovery images in Figure 6.30 show?

A. LGE of the left ventricular apex

B. Transmural LGE of the apex with an apical thrombus

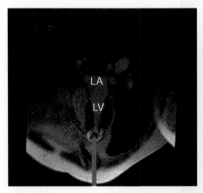 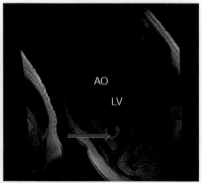

LA: left atrium; LV: left ventricle; AO: aorta

Figure 6.30

  C. Apical thrombus

  D. Subendocardial LGE of the apex

6.31. An 18-year-old female with a history of hypertension underwent a procedure. Based on the images shown in Figure 6.31, what procedure did she undergo?

  A. Aortoplasty

  B. Balloon dilatation of aorta

  C. Stent of coarctation of the aorta with restenosis

  D. Surgical anastomosis of coarctation of aorta with restenosis

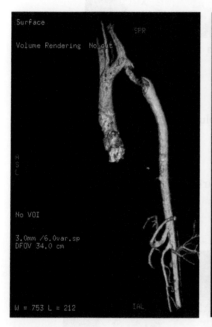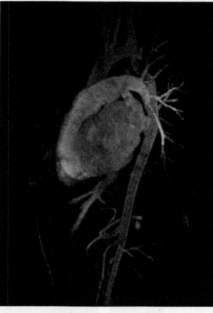

Figure 6.31

6.32. A 50-year-old female patient is referred to the cardiology clinic for complaints of substernal chest pain. She has complaints of palpitations, and a Holter monitor demonstrated premature ventricular complexes. Her family history is significant for premature coronary artery disease. Owing to orthopedic problems, she underwent a Lexiscan stress cardiac MRI. What do the perfusion images in Figure 6.32 show?

  A. Stress-induced myocardial perfusion defect in the septum, anterior and inferior walls

  B. Rest myocardial perfusion defect in the anterior and inferior walls

  C. Global stress-induced perfusion defect

  D. Artifact

Rest perfusion                    Vasodilator stress perfusion

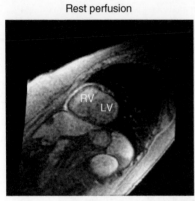 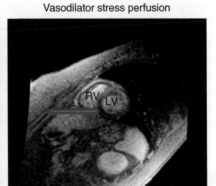

RV: right ventricle; LV: left ventricle

hapter 6

Figure 6.32

**6.33.** What do the contrast-enhanced MRA and volume-rendered image of the aorta in Figure 6.33 show?
   A. Normal aorta
   B. Dissection in the ascending aorta
   C. Dissection flap in the descending aorta starts just distal to the arch
   D. Artifact

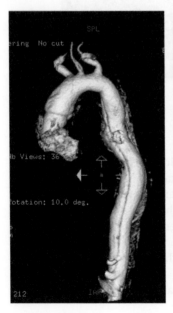 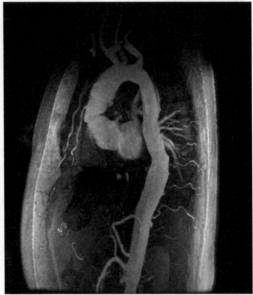

Figure 6.33

**6.34.** A 58-year-old male patient was admitted to hospital for chest pain. He has a history of hypertension and chronic smoking and his echo images were suboptimal. He underwent a cardiac MRI (Figure 6.34) to evaluate left ventricle function. What is the cause of his chest pain?
  **A.** Myocarditis
  **B.** Constrictive pericarditis
  **C.** Dissection of the aorta
  **D.** Pulmonary embolism

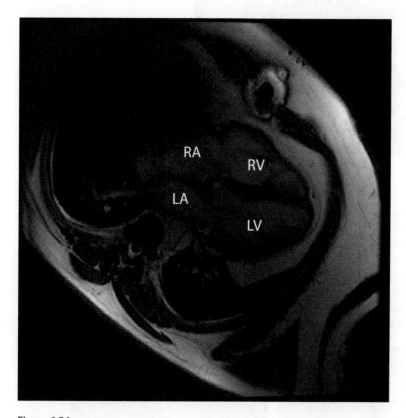

**Figure 6.34**

**6.35.** What does the still-frame long-axis view of the heart in Figure 6.35 show?
  **A.** Normal aortic and mitral valves
  **B.** Normal aortic valve
  **C.** Normal mitral valve and artifact from a prosthetic aortic valve
  **D.** None of the above

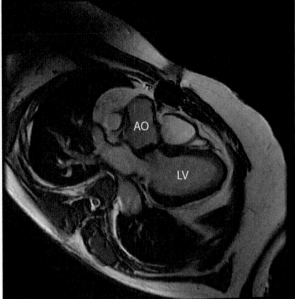

Figure 6.35

**6.36.** A 50-year-old female had a routine transthoracic echocardiogram (TTE). Her cardiologist found a mass in the right atrium. She was then referred for a cardiac MRI (see Figure 6.36) to evaluate this mass further. What is the mass is suggestive of?

**A.** Right atrial myxoma
**B.** Right atrial sarcoma
**C.** Thrombus
**D.** Lipomatous hypertrophy of the interatrial septum

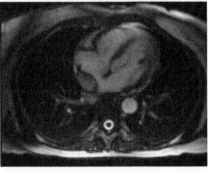
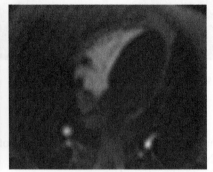

SSFP                                                          Perfusion

Figure 6.36

## Answers

**6.1.** A. Hydrogen-1.

Hydrogen-1 is most abundant in living tissues.

**6.2.** A. 63 MHz.

It is 42 MHz multiplied by the magnetic field strength $B_o$ in tesla.

**6.3.** A. Magnetic gradient.

There is a slight gradient in the $X$, $Y$, and $Z$ planes (strength of magnetic field varies from slightly above to below 1.5 T in a 1.5 T system) and this helps localize where the signal is coming from.

**6.4.** D. All of the above.

Spinal cord stimulator is also a contraindication. Coronary stents, heart valves, artificial joints, and vertebral plates are not contraindications.

**6.5.** D. All of the above.

**6.6.** A. Shortens T1 and increases signal on T1-weighted images.

The seven unpaired electrons on Gd couple with excited water spins and hasten relaxation, thereby reducing T1. This property of Gd is used for magnetic resonance angiography (MRA), first-pass perfusion, and late Gd enhancement (LGE) of the myocardial scar.

**6.7.** C. With the use of a navigator pulse.

It takes 15–20 minutes based on slice thickness and extent needed and hence needs the navigator pulse to track the diaphragm so that images can be acquired only at certain phases of the respiratory cycle.

**6.8.** A. Right ventricle.

The other numbers indicate the following structures: 2, left ventricle; 3, left atrium; 4, right atrium; 5, descending thoracic aorta; 6, pulmonary vein.

**6.9.** B. Left ventricle.

Structure "1" is the right ventricle.

**6.10.** C. Right atrium.

Structure "2" is the left ventricle. This is the coronal plane.

**6.11.** C. LAD area looks fully viable.

The scar looks white on delayed Gd-enhanced imaging. There is no evidence of scarring in this image.

**6.12.** D. None of the above.

This is a normal MRA of the pulmonary artery and branches: 1, main pulmonary artery; 2, right pulmonary artery; 3, left pulmonary artery; 4, right ventricle outflow tract.

**6.13.** C. Contrast-enhanced MRA.

This is of the aorta. The aorta looks normal. 1, left ventricle; 2–4, aorta; 5, pulmonary veins.

**6.14.** D. All of the above.

**6.15.** A. Lipomatous atrial septum.

Its location in the atrial septum and the absence of a perfusion point to a lipomatous septum. There was no delayed enhancement.

**6.16.** A. Heart failure.

Note the bilateral pleural effusions. The left ventricle seems to be dilated with thinning of the apical area. The atrial septum is intact and bowing to the right, indicating high right atrial pressure. The descending aorta (behind left atrium) is normal (1: left ventricle; 2: right ventricle; 3: left pleural effusion).

**6.17.** A. Multivessel coronary artery disease.

The dark area pointed to by the arrows is a perfusion defect during first-pass perfusion using Gd chelate. The perfusion defect is seen during vasodilator stress in the lateral wall as well as anterior and inferior walls and completely fills in during rest perfusion. A reversible perfusion defect indicates ischemia and not infarct, and extent indicates multivessel disease.

**6.18.** B. Inferior myocardial infarction.

A subendocardial scar indicates an infarct; involvement of inferior septum and inferior wall is consistent with right coronary artery lesion. In ARVD, scarring may be seen in the right ventricle wall along with a fatty deposit, dilation, aneurysm formation, and reduced function. The scar pattern in myocarditis may be patchy, midmyocardial, subepicardial, or even transmural.

**6.19.** C. Anterior myocardial infarction.

Note the scar distribution in mid and distal septum consistent with LAD artery lesion.

**6.20.** A. Left ventricle noncompaction.

Note the heavily trabeculated left ventricle with noncompacted to compacted myocardial thickness ratio of >2.5. There is a high risk of thrombus formation, and anticoagulation is recommended when there is a thrombus, embolic event, atrial fibrillation, or just EF is <40%. In cardiac amyloid, the left ventricle would be thick.

**6.21.** A. Bicuspid aortic stenosis.

The arrow in Figure 6.21 is pointing to the aortic valve. This is a FIESTA or SSFP cine sequence.

**6.22.** B. Right pulmonary artery.

**6.23.** C. Left main bronchus.

The arrow in Figure 6.23 is pointing to the left main bronchus. The carina is shown well where the trachea branches into the right and left main bronchi.

**6.24.** Hypertrophic cardiomyopathy.

This patient has hypertrophy of his anterior septum and anterior and inferior walls. The upper septum is asymmetrically hypertrophied (arrow) and points more to hypertrophic cardiomyopathy.

**6.25.** D. Midmyocardial patchy LGE of the septum and inferolateral wall.

The LGE pattern seen here is midmyocardial patchy enhancement, whereas in the setting of coronary artery disease, the LGE pattern is either subendocardial or transmural.

**6.26.** A. Cleft anterior mitral valve.

The short-axis mitral valve view shows a cleft of the anterior mitral valve (arrowed in Figure 6.26b).

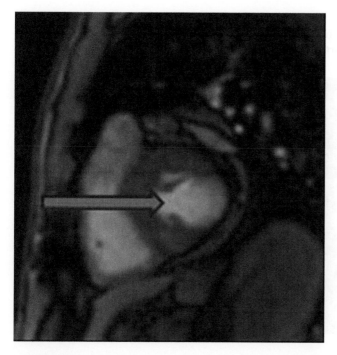

**Chapter 6**

Figure 6.26b

**6.27.** A. Main pulmonary artery.

Figure 6.27b shows the main pulmonary artery (MPA), along with the aorta (AO).

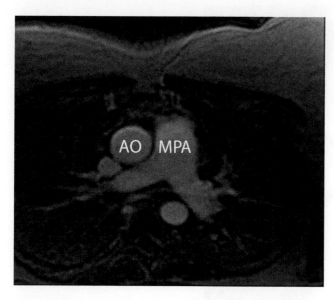

Figure 6.27b

**6.28.** E. Descending aorta.

Figure 6.28b shows the descending aorta (arrowed), along with the aorta (AO) and main pulmonary artery (MPA).

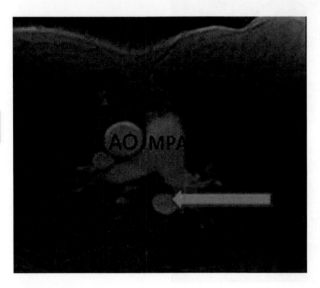

Figure 6.28b

**6.29.** A. Superior vena cava.

Figure 6.29b shows the superior vena cava (SVC), along with the right atrium (RA).

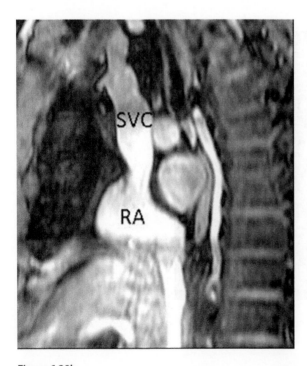

Figure 6.29b

**6.30.** B. Transmural LGE of the apex with an apical thrombus.

The red arrow in Figure 6.30 shows transmural LGE of the apex and the blue arrow an apical thrombus. Both the four- and three-chamber views show transmural scar of the apex with a dark filling defect representing thrombus. The scarred areas take up Gd that is not washed out and appears as bright areas on this sequence, whereas thrombus does not take up contrast and appears as a filling defect (LV: left ventricle; LA: left atrium; AO: aorta).

**6.31.** C. Stent of coarctation of the aorta with restenosis.

The stented segment, which measured 30 mm, is clearly seen on both images in Figure 6.31. The lumen of the stented segment is narrowed up to 50%, representing restenosis.

**6.32.** A. Stress-induced myocardial perfusion defect in the septum, anterior and inferior walls.

The arrow in Figure 6.32 shows the stress-induced perfusion defect in the septum, anterior and inferior walls (LV: left ventricle). At rest, there is homogeneous perfusion of Gd in all myocardial segments. With vasodilator stress, there is lack of perfusion in the septum, anterior and inferior walls (dark areas), representing myocardial ischemia.

**6.33.** C. Dissection flap in the descending aorta starts just distal to the arch.

The contrast-enhanced image of the aorta shows contrast in the true lumen (T), while the false lumen (F) does not enhance. The blue arrow points to the dissection flap. This patient had a type A dissection and underwent ascending aortic repair including a hemiarch.

**6.34.** C. Dissection of the aorta.

The size of the heart looks normal. Figure 6.34, a still-frame image, shows a flap in the descending aorta (arrow; LA: left atrium; LV: left ventricle; RA: right atrium; RV: right ventricle). The cause of this patient's chest pain is due to dissection of the aorta.

**6.35.** C. Normal mitral valve and artifact from a prosthetic aortic valve.

This patient has a normal mitral valve but has a prosthetic aortic valve. There is artifact from the mechanical prosthesis indicative of a mechanical aortic valve (arrow; LV: left ventricle; LA: left atrium; AO: aorta).

**6.36.** D. Lipomatous hypertrophy of the interatrial septum.

The mass is lipomatous hypertrophy of the interatrial septum. The mass is in continuity with the upper part of the interatrial septum. On the perfusion image, there is no enhancement indicative of avascularity. On T1-weighted images, this mass will appear bright and can be suppressed with fat suppression sequences (LV: left ventricle; RV: right ventricle; RA: right atrium).

# Cardiac Computed Tomography

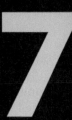

**7.1.** Which of the following scan modes is used for coronary calcium scanning?
  **A.** Prospective gated noncontrast
  **B.** Prospective gated contrast scan
  **C.** Retrospective gated noncontrast
  **D.** Retrospective gated contrast scan

**7.2.** What is the traditional slice thickness for coronary calcium screening?
  **A.** 0.625 mm
  **B.** 1 mm
  **C.** 3 mm
  **D.** 5 mm

**7.3.** Which scan mode is used for assessment of left ventricle function?
  **A.** Prospective, gated with contrast
  **B.** Retrospective, gated with contrast
  **C.** Retrospective, gated without contrast
  **D.** Prospective, gated without contrast

**7.4.** Which of the following imaging procedures is likely to be associated with lowest radiation exposure?
  **A.** Prospectively gated, electrocardiogram (ECG)-triggered cardiac computed tomography angiography (CTA)
  **B.** Retrospectively gated, cardiac CTA
  **C.** Coronary angiography
  **D.** Stress perfusion scan with sestamibi

**7.5.** Which of the following imaging procedures is likely to be associated with the highest radiation exposure?
  **A.** Retrospectively gated, cardiac CTA with dose modulation
  **B.** Retrospectively gated, cardiac CTA
  **C.** Dual-isotope myocardial perfusion scan with thallium and sestamibi
  **D.** Stress perfusion scan with sestamibi

**7.6.** Who are at the highest cancer risk with cardiac computed tomography (CT)?
  **A.** Men
  **B.** Women
  **C.** Blacks
  **D.** Caucasians

**7.7.** During cardiac CTA, which organ gets the highest radiation dose?
  **A.** Heart
  **B.** Lungs
  **C.** Esophagus
  **D.** Breast

*Cardiology Board Review*, Second Edition. Ramdas G. Pai and Padmini Varadarajan.
© 2023 John Wiley & Sons Ltd. Published 2023 by John Wiley & Sons Ltd.

**7.8.** Which of the following affects radiation dose?

    **A.** Tube voltage                      **C.** Pitch

    **B.** Tube current                    **D.** All of the above

**7.9.** Pitch is table movement divided by collimated beam width. At a pitch of 1, there is no overlap of data. At a pitch >1 there is a gap, and with a pitch <1 there is overlap. Which pitch is likely to be associated with least amount of radiation?

    **A.** 0.4                            **C.** 1.0

    **B.** 0.6                            **D.** 3.0

**7.10.** Which of the following has least amount of radiation?

    **A.** Calcium score with electron-beam CT

    **B.** Calcium score with X-ray CT

    **C.** Chest X-ray

    **D.** Cardiac MRI with gadolinium vasodilator stress

**7.11.** Which of the following 45-year-old patients presenting to the emergency room (ER) with atypical chest pain are appropriate candidates for coronary CTA?

    **A.** Patient with hypertension, diabetes mellitus, and prior left anterior descending (LAD) artery stent

    **B.** Patient with hypertension, ECG shows nonspecific ST-T changes, negative cardiac enzymes

    **C.** Patient with a prior myocardial infarction followed by coronary artery bypass grafting

    **D.** All of the above

**7.12.** Which of the following agents are appropriate to slow the heart rate for coronary CTA?

    **A.** Beta blockers

    **B.** Nondihydropyridine calcium channel blocker (e.g. diltiazem)

    **C.** Ivabradine

    **D.** All of the above

**7.13.** Which of the following is likely to reduce radiation dose the most?

    **A.** Increasing pitch by 25%

    **B.** Decreasing tube current by 25%

    **C.** Increasing tube current by 25%

    **D.** They are all similar

**7.14.** Which of the following is the best measure of radiation dose to the patient?

    **A.** CT dose index (CTDI)

    **B.** Dose-length product (DLP)

    **C.** Effective radiation dose (ERD)

    **D.** All of the above

**7.15.** What is the US legal limit for radiation dose to a pregnant woman for the entire length of pregnancy?

    **A.** 0.05 mSv

    **B.** 0.5 mSv

    **C.** 5 mSv

    **D.** 50 mSv

**7.16.** During coronary CTA to the mother, how much radiation is the fetus likely to get?
   **A.** 14 mSv
   **B.** 1.4 mSv
   **C.** 0.14 mSv
   **D.** None with shielding

**7.17.** What is the typical HU value for fat?
   **A.** −1000 HU            **C.** 0 HU
   **B.** −50 HU             **D.** 1000 HU

**7.18.** What is the typical HU threshold for calcium in a CT scan for calcium scoring?
   **A.** 100
   **B.** 130
   **C.** 0
   **D.** 400

**7.19.** Image noise can be reduced by which of the following?
   **A.** Increasing tube voltage
   **B.** Increasing tube current
   **C.** Iterative reconstruction
   **D.** All of the above

**7.20.** Which of the following statements is correct about iterative reconstruction?
   **A.** It takes longer as it makes multiples passes through the data
   **B.** It increases signal-to-noise ratio
   **C.** It can be performed on any CT scanner
   **D.** All of the above

**7.21.** What is the image pixel size of a CT image reconstruction with a field of view (FOV) of 256 mm and a 512 × 512 matrix?
   **A.** 0.5 mm × 0.5 mm
   **B.** 0.25 mm × 0.25 mm
   **C.** 2 mm × 2 mm
   **D.** None of the above

**7.22.** How can the image pixel size be increased during CT image reconstruction?
   **A.** Decreasing FOV
   **B.** Increasing matrix
   **C.** Both
   **D.** Neither

**7.23.** Spatial and temporal resolution are affected by all of the following except which?
   **A.** Detector width
   **B.** Rotation time
   **C.** Dual-source technology
   **D.** Number of detector rows

**7.24.** If a reconstructed image is noisy, how can this noise be reduced?
   **A.** Increasing slice thickness
   **B.** Reducing slice thickness
   **C.** Changing window level
   **D.** None of the above

**7.25.** Which of the following techniques may be helpful for better coronary visualization for those with calcification?
   **A.** Dual-energy CT
   **B.** Reconstruction with sharp filter
   **C.** Both
   **D.** Neither

**7.26.** How can visualization within a stent be facilitated?
   **A.** Dual-energy CT
   **B.** Reconstruction with sharp filter
   **C.** Wide window
   **D.** Thin slice
   **E.** All of the above

**7.27.** In a person presenting to the ER with chest pain and suspicion of acute coronary syndrome (ACS), which of the following are appropriate indications for coronary CTA?
   **A.** Normal ECG and biomarkers, low or intermediate probability of CAD
   **B.** Nonspecific ECG changes and normal biomarkers, low or intermediate probability of CAD
   **C.** Nondiagnostic ECG and biomarkers, low or intermediate probability of CAD
   **D.** Normal ECG and biomarkers, low or intermediate probability of CAD, unable to exercise
   **E.** All of the above

**7.28.** In a person presenting to the ER with chest pain, negative ECG and enzymes, and a history of prior coronary stent, which of the following are appropriate or possibly appropriate indications for coronary CTA?
   **A.** Left main coronary artery drug-eluting stent, 4 mm, 1 year ago
   **B.** LAD coronary artery stent two years ago 2.5 mm
   **C.** Mid right coronary artery (RCA) stent, 3.5 mm a year ago
   **D.** All of the above

**7.29.** It is appropriate to perform coronary CTA in which of the following asymptomatic patients?
   **A.** Left main coronary artery stenting with stent size >3 mm
   **B.** Left main coronary artery stenting with stent size <3 mm
   **C.** LAD bifurcation stent 4 mm size
   **D.** None of the above

**7.30.** Which of the following are reasonable indications for coronary CTA?
   **A.** Patient with ejection fraction (EF) of 30%, low to intermediate risk for CAD, to rule out ischemic etiology
   **B.** To rule out anomalous origin or coronary artery
   **C.** To monitor for CAD post heart transplant
   **D.** To check for graft patency in a patient with chest pain after prior coronary artery bypass grafting
   **E.** All of the above

**7.31.** Which of the following does the arrow in Figure 7.31 point to?
   **A.** Anomalous RCA                **C.** Normal RCA origin, calcified
   **B.** Normal RCA origin, not calcified    **D.** None of the above

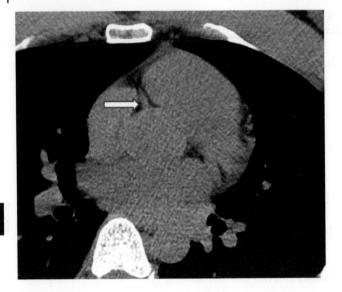

**Figure 7.31**

**7.32.** What is the arrow in Figure 7.32 pointing to?
 A. Anomalous origin of left coronary artery
 B. Normal left main coronary artery origin, not calcified
 C. Normal left main coronary artery origin, calcified
 D. Anomalous origin of RCA

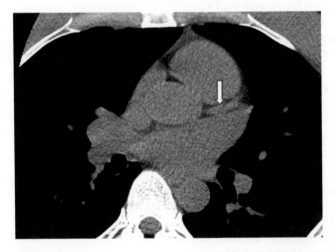

**Figure 7.32**

**7.33.** What do the numbers 1, 2, 3, and 4 correspond to in Figure 7.33?
 A. Pulmonary veins: left upper, left lower, right upper, right lower respectively
 B. Pulmonary veins: Left lower, left upper, right lower, right upper respectively
 C. Pulmonary veins: right upper, right lower, left upper, left lower respectively
 D. None of the above

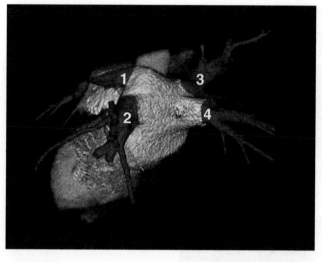

**Figure 7.33**

**7.34.** What does the number 1 correspond to in Figure 7.34?
- **A.** Left atrial appendage
- **B.** Left superior pulmonary vein
- **C.** Left inferior pulmonary vein
- **D.** Body of left atrium

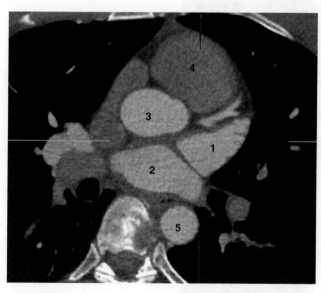

**Figure 7.34**

**7.35.** Figure 7.35 shows a volume rendered image viewed from the top. What does the number 1 refer to?
- **A.** Ascending aorta
- **B.** Pulmonary artery
- **C.** Pulmonary vein
- **D.** Body of left atrium

**7.36.** Figure 7.36 shows a volume rendered image. What does the number 1 refer to?
- **A.** LAD artery
- **B.** Diagonal artery
- **C.** Circumflex artery
- **D.** RCA

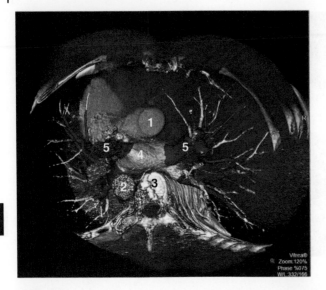

**Figure 7.35**

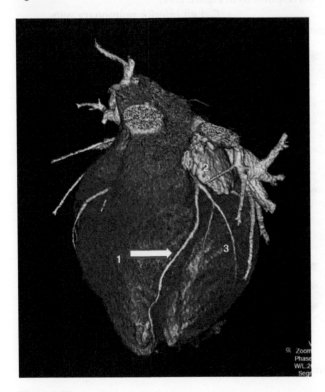

**Figure 7.36**

**7.37.** Figure 7.37 shows a volume rendered image. What does the arrow point to?

    **A.** LAD artery

    **B.** Diagonal artery

    **C.** Circumflex artery

    **D.** Right ventricle branch of RCA

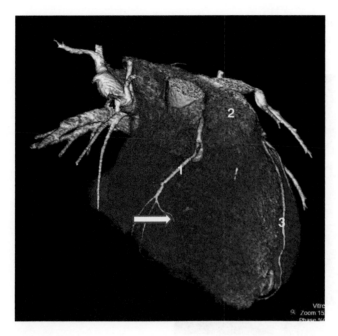

**Figure 7.37**

**7.38.** In Figure 7.38, what does the number 1 refer to?
A. RCA
B. Circumflex
C. Mitral annular calcification
D. Pericardiophrenic bundle

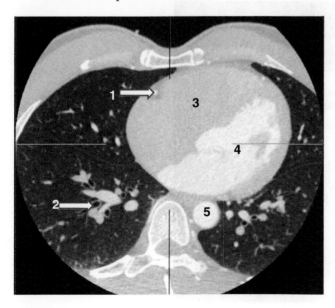

**Figure 7.38**

**7.39.** In Figure 7.39, what does the number 2 refer to?

    **A.** Ascending thoracic aorta       **C.** Inferior vena cava

    **B.** Descending aorta            **D.** Azygos vein

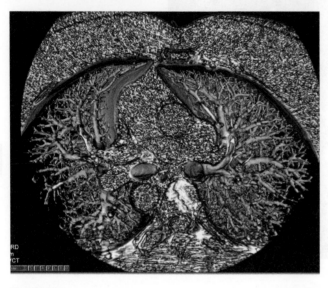

**Figure 7.39**

**7.40.** Figure 7.40 shows a volume rendered image. What does the number 1 refer to?

    **A.** Left lower pulmonary vein       **C.** Left pulmonary artery

    **B.** Left upper pulmonary vein      **D.** Right lower pulmonary vein

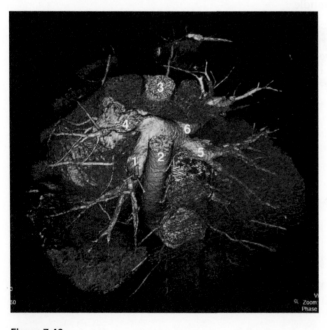

**Figure 7.40**

**7.41.** Figure 7.41 shows a volume rendered image. What does the number 1 refer to?
  **A.** LAD artery
  **B.** Left internal mammary artery
  **C.** Diagonal
  **D.** Right internal mammary artery

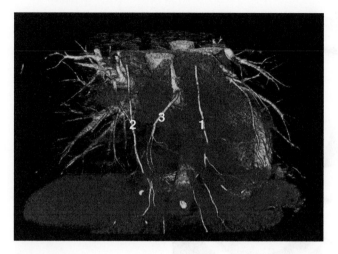

**Figure 7.41**

**7.42.** Figure 7.42 shows a volume rendered image. What does the number 1 refer to?
  **A.** LAD artery
  **B.** Left internal mammary artery
  **C.** Aorta
  **D.** Pulmonary vein

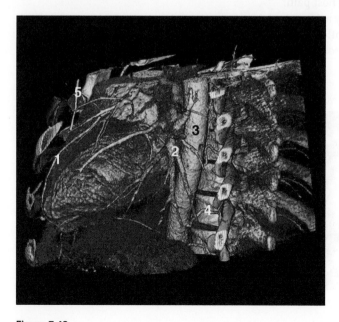

**Figure 7.42**

**7.43.** In the axial scan in Figure 7.43, what does the number 1 refer to?
  **A.** Coronary sinus
  **B.** Right coronary artery
  **C.** Circumflex coronary artery
  **D.** Anomalous left circumflex coronary artery

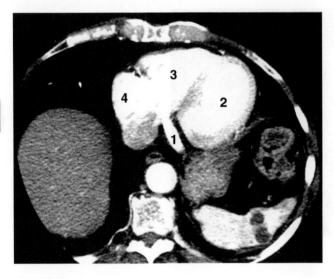

**Figure 7.43**

**7.44.** A 44-year-old man with no cardiac risk factors was seen in the ER with exertional chest pain. Axial contrast-enhanced scans are shown in Figure 7.44. What is the possible cause of his chest pain?
  **A.** Left main coronary artery stenosis
  **B.** Anomalous circumflex artery
  **C.** Anomalous RCA from left coronary cusp with interarterial course
  **D.** None of the above

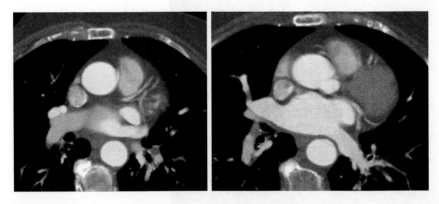

**Figure 7.44**

**7.45.** Which of the following options describes the LAD artery segment shown in Figure 7.45?
   **A.** Normal
   **B.** Has severe stenosis in the proximal segment
   **C.** Has a large mixed plaque in the cross-section shown
   **D.** Has a large soft plaque in the cross-section shown

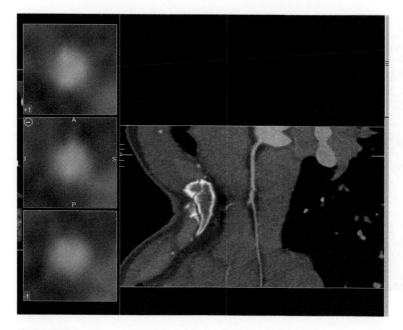

**Figure 7.45**

**7.46.** The volume rendered scan in Figure 7.46 shows what?
   **A.** Normal coronary anatomy       **C.** Anomalous RCA from left sinus
   **B.** Anomalous LCA                 **D.** Saphenous venous graft to RCA

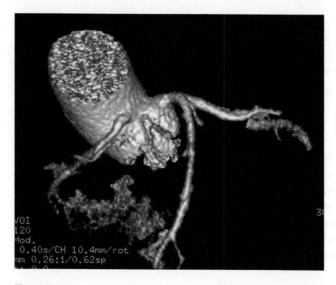

**Figure 7.46**

7.47. What can be said from the volume rendered scan shown in Figure 7.47?
   A. Has normal coronary anatomy
   B. Has severe LAD artery stenosis
   C. Need to evaluate LAD artery and other vessels using curved multiplanar reformation and centerline methods to comment about the coronaries
   D. Has moderate LAD artery stenosis, and stress test is indicated

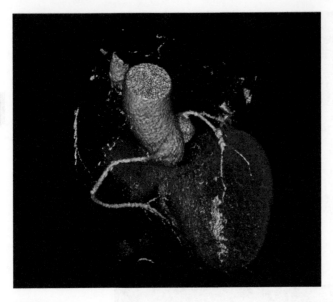

Figure 7.47

7.48. A 48-year-old patient with hypertension and diabetes mellitus was seen in the ER with atypical chest pain. Cardiac enzymes were normal. Coronary calcium distribution is shown in Figure 7.48. What would be a reasonable next step?
   A. Cancel coronary CTA in view of severe coronary calcification and order a stress test
   B. Go ahead with coronary CTA; if lesions are moderate or indeterminate, consider cardiac catheterization
   C. Cancel coronary CTA and treat with aspirin and high-intensity statin
   D. Refer for cardiac catheterization

7.49. What does the arrow in the axial scan in Figure 7.49 refer to?
   A. Coronary sinus
   B. RCA
   C. Circumflex coronary artery
   D. Anomalous circumflex artery

7.50. For transcatheter aortic valve replacement (TAVR) planning, what type of cardiac protocol is most appropriate?
   A. Noncontrast CT with cardiac gating
   B. Noncontrast CT without cardiac gating
   C. Contrast CT with cardiac gating
   D. Contrast CT without cardiac gating

hapter 7

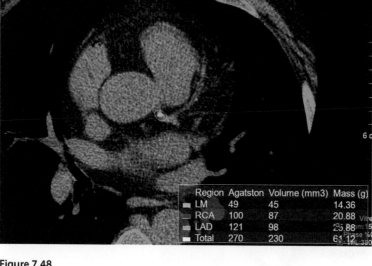

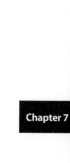

| Region | Agatston | Volume (mm3) | Mass (g) |
|--------|----------|--------------|----------|
| LM | 49 | 45 | 14.36 |
| RCA | 100 | 87 | 20.88 |
| LAD | 121 | 98 | 25.88 |
| Total | 270 | 230 | 61.12 |

**Figure 7.48**

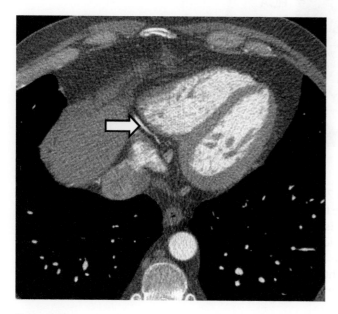

**Figure 7.49**

**7.51.** What cardiac CT measures are useful for TAVR planning?
  **A.** Aortic annulus size
  **B.** Left and right coronary height from aortic annulus
  **C.** Size of aortic sinus and sinotubular junction
  **D.** Aortic leaflet size and degree of calcification
  **E.** All of the above

**7.52.** The CT images shown in Figure 7.52 would permit which of the following?
  **A.** Size 23 mm TAVR
  **C.** 29 mm TAVR
  **B.** 26 mm TAVR
  **D.** Coronary height is too low for TAVR

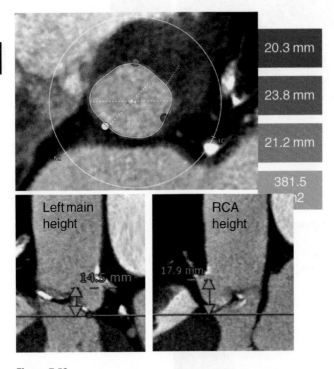

20.3 mm

23.8 mm

21.2 mm

381.5 m2

Left main height

14.5 mm

RCA height

17.9 mm

**Figure 7.52**

**7.53.** The patient in Figure 7.53 has severe calcific aortic stenosis and TAVR is being planned. Which of the following statements is correct?
  **A.** The aortic annulus is large and may need a 29 mm valve
  **B.** There is severe aortic valve calcification and this may increase the risk of coronary occlusion
  **C.** The coronary height and size of the sinus and sinotubular junction are not shown and these are important in planning
  **D.** All of the above

**7.54.** A peripheral CTA of a patient being considered for TAVR is shown in Figure 7.54 (RCFA: right common femoral artery; RCIA: right common iliac artery; REIA: right external iliac artery). Which of the following conclusions can be drawn?
  **A.** Peripheral vessels are adequate for a transfemoral approach
  **B.** Either side can be used for a transfemoral approach
  **C.** Both
  **D.** Neither

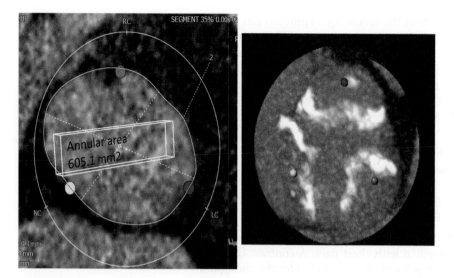

Figure 7.53

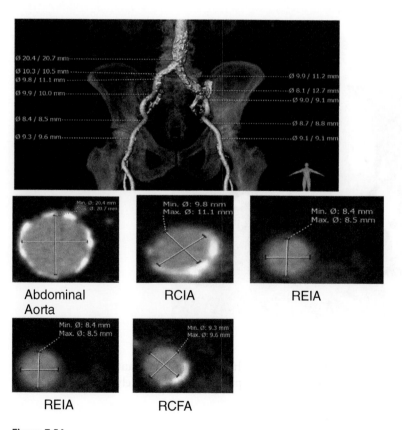

Figure 7.54

**7.55.** Which of the following techniques has the potential to evaluate the functional significance of a coronary artery lesion using cardiac CT?
   A. Dynamic CT-myocardial perfusion imaging
   B. Static CT-myocardial perfusion imaging
   C. Transluminal attenuation gradient assessment
   D. CT-fractional flow reserve
   E. All of the above
   F. None of the above

**7.56.** Which of the following characteristics is associated with a potentially severe coronary artery stenosis?
   A. Small area of stenosis
   B. Greater lesion length
   C. E. All of the above
   D. Positive remodeling
   E. F. None of the above
   F. Low-attenuation plaque <30 HU

**7.57.** A 35-year-old patient who had undergone a Bentall procedure two months earlier presented with chest pain. A contrast CT axial image is shown in Figure 7.57a. What is the likely explanation for the chest pain?
   A. Leaking pseudoaneurysm of the aorta
   B. Occluded left coronary anastomosis
   C. Occluded RCA
   D. None of the above

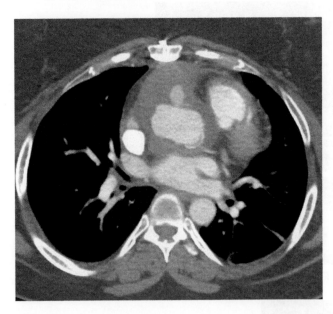

Figure 7.57a

**7.58.** The patient shown in Figure 7.58 has a recent implantable cardioverter-defibrillator and presented with chest pain. What is the likely cause of the chest pain?
   A. Right ventricular lead perforation
   B. Inferior infarct
   C. Large pericardial effusion
   D. None of the above.

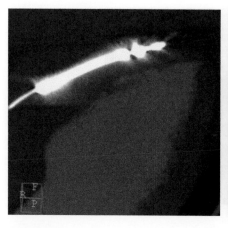
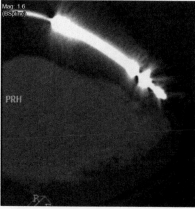

Figure 7.58

**7.59.** The RCA of the patient shown in Figure 7.59 shows what?
  **A.** Severe RCA classification        **C.** RCA stent
  **B.** Severe lesion in mid segment      **D.** Normal RCA

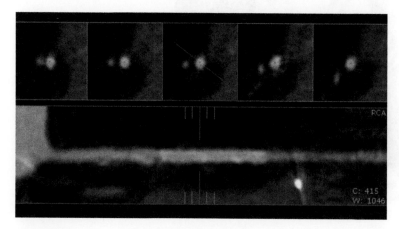

Figure 7.59

**7.60.** The LAD artery of the patient shown in Figure 7.60 is described by which of the following?
  **A.** Normal anatomy                    **C.** Mid LAD artery lesion.
  **B.** Myocardial bridging               **D.** None of the above

**7.61.** A 40-year-old truck driver passed out while loading his truck. There were no other medical problems. A chest CT (Figure 7.61a) was performed in the ER to rule out pulmonary embolism because of his leg swelling and positive D-dimer. Which of the following is a possible cause of his syncope?
  **A.** Pulmonary embolism
  **B.** Large pericardial effusion
  **C.** Anomalous origin of left coronary artery
  **D.** Anomalous origin of RCA

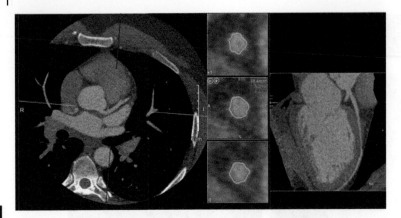

Figure 7.60

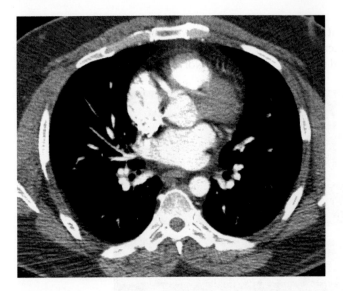

Figure 7.61a

**7.62.** What would be your recommendation to the patient in Question 7.61?
A. Reassurance
B. Exercise stress test
C. Stress echo
D. Coronary angiography and possible left coronary reimplant

**7.63.** An 83-year-old woman presented with acute central chest pain. Chest CT with contrast was obtained in the ER (Figure 7.63a). What are the images suggestive of?
A. Stanford type A aortic dissection
B. Stanford type B aortic dissection
C. Pulmonary embolism
D. Intramural hematoma

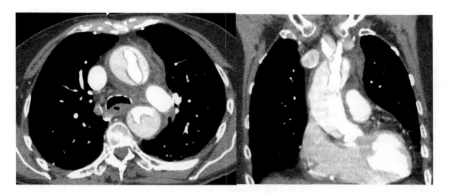

Figure 7.63a

**7.64.** This 45 -year-old truck driver presented to the ER with exertional chest pain and syncope. A CT pulmonary angiogram was performed in the ER and was negative for pulmonary embolism. What will be appropriate treatment? (Figure 7.64)

**A.** Beta blocker

**B.** Increase fluid intake

**C.** Nitrate

**D.** Coronary angiogram followed by possible coronary reimplantation

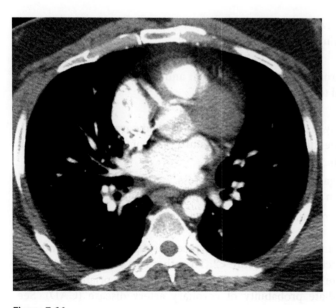

Figure 7.64

## Answers

**7.1.** A. Prospective gated noncontrast.

Prospective gating reduces radiation exposure. Contrast should not be used. Generally, a Hounsfield unit (HU) threshold of 130 units is used to detect calcium.

**7.2.** C. 3 mm.

Outcome data are based on this slice thickness.

**7.3.** B. Retrospective, gated with contrast.

For left ventricle function assessment, the left ventricle has to be opacified; scan should be gated and should have all phases.

**7.4.** A. Prospectively gated, electrocardiogram (ECG)-triggered cardiac computed tomography angiography (CTA).

This is associated with an absorbed radiation dose of about 3 mSv, compared with about 15 mSv for retrospectively gated, cardiac CTA, 7 mSv for coronary angiography, and about 15 mSv for stress perfusion scan with sestamibi.

**7.5.** C. Dual isotope myocardial perfusion scan with thallium and Sestamibi.

This is associated with a radiation exposure of about 25 mSv. Dose modulation during prospective gating reduces the radiation dose by about 40%, but prospective gating reduces it by about 85%.

**7.6.** B. Women.

The young are also at high risk as they have more years to live after radiation exposure, such that cancer phenotype can develop following DNA damage.

**7.7.** D. Breast.

Breast and skin receive the highest radiation dose, and then the lung, heart, and esophagus in descending order.

**7.8.** D. All of the above.

Radiation dose is proportional to tube current and square of tube voltage. It is inversely proportional to pitch.

**7.9.** D. 3.0.

Radiation is inversely proportional to pitch. Hence, compared with a pitch of 1, 3 is associated with one third of the radiation and a pitch of 0.4 is associated with 2.5 times the radiation.

**7.10.** D. Cardiac MRI with gadolinium vasodilator stress.

There is no radiation with MRI. It uses radiofrequency pulses.

**7.11.** B. Patient with hypertension, ECG shows nonspecific ST-T changes, negative cardiac enzymes.

This is a level 4 chest pain patient; that is, atypical chest pain with a thrombolysis in myocardial infarction (TIMI) score <2. The other two scenarios are level 3 and are appropriate for stress testing. Coronary CTA is appropriate in patients with low to intermediate probability of coronary artery disease (CAD). See Box 7.1.

**7.12.** D. All of the above.

Beta blockers in oral and intravenous form are traditionally used. In those with reactive airway disease, calcium channel blockers are an option. In those with low blood pressure who may not tolerate either of these, ivabradine, which selectively slows the sinus node without lowering blood pressure, is an option. This drug is approved for treatment of heart failure.

**7.13.** C. Decreasing tube current by 25%.

This will reduce radiation dose by about 40%, whereas A and B options reduce radiation dose by only 25%.

**7.14.** C. Effective radiation dose (ERD).

ERD is expressed in millisieverts. CTDI is the radiation dose delivered by the machine for a given scan parameter based on phantom simulation. DLP (mGy cm) takes into consideration scan length: DLP = CTDIvol × scan length. ERD = DLP × 0.014 (where 0.014 is a conversion factor) for cardiac CTA. Hence, for a DLP of 1000 mGy cm, the ERD for cardiac CT is 1000 × 0.014 = 14 mSv

**7.15.** C. 5 mSv.

50 mSv is for adult radiation workers.

**7.16.** C. 0.14 mSv.

This is very low with low risk. Even with shielding, the fetus will get some scattered radiation.

**7.17.** B. −50 HU.

Water is 0 HU, air is −1000 HU.

**7.18.** B. 130.

**7.19.** D. All of the above.

Decreasing pitch also reduces noise, but it increases radiation.

**7.20.** D. All of the above.

Multiple passes and signal averaging improve signal strength and reduce noise.

**7.21.** A. 0.5 mm × 0.5 mm.

$$\text{Pixel size} = \frac{\text{FOV}}{\text{matrix}}$$

**7.22.** C. Both.

**7.23.** D. Number of detector rows.

This affects the amount of coverage during one cardiac cycle, but not temporal or spatial resolution.

**7.24.** A. Increasing slice thickness.

This gives more photons or energy or signal. To reduce noise by half, you have to increase slice thickness fourfold, as noise is inversely proportional to the square of the number of photons.

**7.25.** C. Both.

With dual energy, you can subtract calcium from the image. Reconstruction with a sharp filter has to be performed on the scanner raw data.

**7.26.** E. All of the above.

**7.27.** E. All of the above.

**7.28.** B. LAD coronary artery stent two years ago 2.5 mm.

It is inappropriate to perform coronary CTA when stent size is <3 mm. In others with symptoms, it is of uncertain significance.

**7.29.** A. Left main coronary artery stenting with stent size ≥3 mm.

It is inappropriate to do in other asymptomatic patients. Presence of symptoms, stent size of ≥3 mm, and left main coronary artery location make coronary CTA increasingly appropriate. Use of techniques such as dual-source CT or appropriate processing with iterative processing and use of sharp filters would be helpful for better quality images.

**7.30.** E. All of the above.

**7.31.** B. Normal RCA origin, not calcified.

**7.32.** B. Normal left main coronary artery origin, not calcified.

**7.33.** A. Pulmonary veins: left upper, left lower, right upper, right lower respectively.

**7.34.** A. Left atrial appendage.

2: Body of left atrium; 3: Ascending aorta; 4: Right ventricle outflow tract, 5: Descending thoracic aorta.

**7.35.** A. Ascending aorta.

2: Descending aorta; 3: Vertebral body; 4: Roof of left atrium; 5: Pulmonary vein.

**7.36.** A. LAD artery.

2: Left atrial appendage; 3: Diagonal artery.

**7.37.** D. Right ventricle branch of RCA.

1: RCA; 2: Right ventricular outflow tract (RVOT); 3: LAD artery; 4: Right pulmonary veins.

**7.38.** A. RCA.

The RCA is in the right atrioventricular groove. The pericardiophrenic bundle would be outside the pericardium. 2: Bronchus; 3: Right ventricle; 4: Left ventricle; 5: Descending thoracic aorta.

**7.39.** A. Ascending thoracic aorta.

1: Ascending aorta.

**7.40.** A. Left lower pulmonary vein.

2: Descending thoracic aorta; 3: Ascending aorta; 4: Left upper pulmonary vein; 5: Right lower pulmonary vein; 6: Right upper pulmonary vein. Figure 7.40 is a view from the back.

**7.41.** B. Left internal mammary artery.

2: Right internal mammary artery; 3: RCA.

**7.42.** A. LAD artery.

2: Left lower pulmonary vein; 3: Descending thoracic aorta; 4: Intercostal artery; 5: Left internal mammary artery.

**7.43.** A. Coronary sinus.

2: Left ventricle; 3: Right ventricle; 4: Right atrium.

**7.44.** C. Anomalous RCA from the left coronary cusp with interarterial course.

Note that the proximal course is between the aorta and RVOT. Circumflex courses normally. No LAD artery stenosis is seen in the images in Figure 7.44.

**7.45.** A. Normal.

**7.46.** C. Anomalous RCA from the left sinus.

There is an interarterial course between the aorta and pulmonary artery (pulmonary artery not shown).

**7.47.** C. Need to evaluate LAD artery and other vessels using curved multiplanar reformation and centerline methods to comment about the coronaries.

One cannot comment about stenosis severity from volume rendered images.

**7.48.** B. Go ahead with coronary CTA; if lesions are moderate or indeterminate, consider cardiac catheterization.

Despite two risk factors, patient is at low to intermediate risk for CAD and coronary CTA (TIMI score 2 and level 4) is appropriate. Coronary calcification may impede lumen visualization, but coronary calcium score is not >400. Use of interactive processing and using a sharp filter or dual-source CT would be helpful to better evaluate calcified areas.

**7.49.** B. RCA.

Distal RCA in the right posterior atrioventricular groove.

**7.50.** C. Contrast CT with cardiac gating.

This could be prospectively gated for midsystolic phase or retrospectively gated so that systolic phase can be reconstructed. The measurements of aortic annulus should be obtained in systole and contrast is essential for blood-wall interface visualization.

**7.51.** E. All of the above.

Aortic annulus is best sized by CT. Coronary height of >10 mm assures that the aortic leaflets may not occlude coronary ostia after TAVR. The amount of calcification and length of aortic leaflets also have a bearing on the potential to occlude coronary ostia. If the aortic sinus is small and coronary height is less, the risk of coronary occlusion is high and there may be a need to wire the coronary before TAVR.

**7.52.** A. Size 23 mm TAVR.

Based on annular dimensions and area. Coronary height >10 mm is adequate.

**7.53.** D. All of the above.

**7.54.** C. Both.

The vessels are >7 mm, which would permit any delivery sheath. With the newer generation valves, even 5–6 mm vessels are adequate.

**7.55.** E. All of the above.

**7.56.** E. All of the above.

**7.57.** A. Leaking pseudoaneurysm of the aorta.

Anteriorly, as shown by the arrow in Figure 7.57b – possibly related to RCA anatomosis.

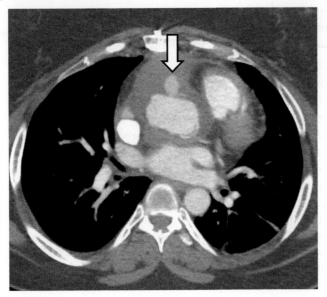

**Figure 7.57b**

**7.58.** A. Right ventricular lead perforation.

   Note that the tip of the lead is beyond the right ventricle wall and in epicardial fat or beyond.

**7.59.** C. RCA stent.

   The RCA stent is in the middle of the segment shown. CTA is not very optimal to evaluate for lesions within the stent, though the stent looks patent.

**7.60.** C. Myocardial bridging.

   Note the smooth narrowing and intramyocardial course.

**7.61.** C. Anomalous origin of left coronary artery.

   Note that the left coronary artery (arrow in Figure 7.61b) is originating from right the coronary sinus and courses in between the aorta and RVOT. This course has elevated risk of sudden death, though it is commonly found at routine autopsies. Ventricular arrhythmia brought on by exertion is a possibility.

**7.62.** D. Coronary angiography and possible left coronary reimplant.

   As the patient had syncope and is in a high-risk occupation, this is very justified. If he was asymptomatic, there would be controversy on controversial what would be the best management, but most would lean toward coronary reimplant or a graft on the coronary. Reimplant may be associated with recurrent ostial stenosis of the left main coronary artery and needs close monitoring. A stress test would be reasonable if the patient was asymptomatic and had normal left ventricular function. However, the American College of Cardiology/American Heart Association guidelines recommend surgical correction for all coronaries coursing between great vessels.

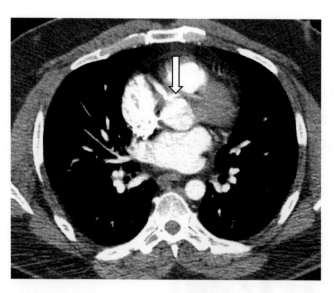

**Figure 7.61b**

**7.63.** A. Stanford type A aortic dissection.

This involves the ascending and descending aorta (DeBakey type II). The axial image on the left of Figure 7.63b shows the true lumen in the ascending aorta (blue arrow) and descending aorta (red arrow). The coronal scan on the right of Figure 7.63b shows the ascending aorta with both true and false lumens. The false lumen is opacified by the contrast as there is flow in that; intramural hematoma does not become opacified by the contrast. Type B (DeBakey type III) involves the descending aorta only and type I involves only the ascending aorta. Transesophageal echocardiography, CT, and MRI are equally sensitive and specific for the diagnosis of aortic dissection.

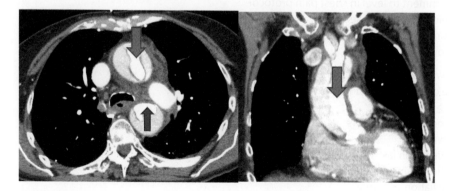

**Figure 7.63b**

**7.64.** D. Coronary angiogram followed by possible coronary reimplantation. The image shows origin of the left main coronary artery from the right coronary sinus with an anterior interarterial course between the aorta and pulmonary artery. This is associated with a high risk of sudden death and warrants surgical correction. RCA = Right coronary artery, LM = Left main coronary artery.

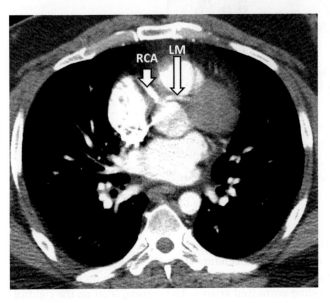

**Figure 7.64**

---

**Box 7.1     Suggested Chest Pain Triaging in ER and Role of Coronary CTA**

**Suggested steps in chest pain triaging in the ER (at discretion of ER physician)**

1. Obtain details on prognostic variables
2. Assignment to level in chest pain protocol
3. Choice of testing based on the level
4. Incorporation of coronary CTA test results and disposition
5. Follow-up plan

*1. Obtain details on prognostic variables*
- Type of chest pain (angina, atypical, noncardiac)
- Age ≥65
- ≥3 coronary risk factors
- Known CAD
- Aspirin use in last seven days
- ≥2 chest pain episodes in 24 hours
- ST deviation ≥0.5 mm
- Elevated cardiac enzymes
- TIMI score (1 point each for age >65, >3 coronary risk factors, known CAD, aspirin use in last 7 days, >2 chest pain episodes in 24 hours, ST deviation >0.5 mm, elevated cardiac enzymes)

*2. and 3. Assignment to level in chest pain protocol and appropriate testing*

See Figure B7.1.

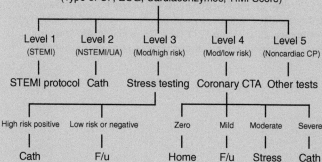

### ER Chest Pain Triage Protocol
Obtain Details on Prognostic Variables
(Type of CP, ECG, Cardiacenzymes, TIMI Score)

| Level 1 | Level 2 | Level 3 | Level 4 | Level 5 |
|---|---|---|---|---|
| (STEMI) | (NSTEMI/UA) | (Mod/high risk) | (Mod/low risk) | (Noncardiac CP) |
| STEMI protocol | Cath | Stress testing | Coronary CTA | Other tests |

High risk positive   Low risk or negative   Zero   Mild   Moderate   Severe
Cath                 F/u                    Home   F/u    Stress     Cath

**Figure B7.1**

- Level 1: ST-elevation myocardial infarction (STEMI) → STEMI protocol
- Level 2: non-STEMI, unstable angina → cardiac catheterization
- Level 3: TIMI score >2, typical angina, moderate ACS risk → stress testing
- Level 4: low to intermediate risk of ACS, TIMI score ≤2 → coronary CTA
- Level 5: noncardiac chest pain → look for noncardiac causes based on presentation

*4 and 5. Incorporation of coronary CTA test results and disposition*
- Zero: no stenosis → discharge home
- Mild: 1–49% → discharge home with follow-up within a week
- Moderate: 50–69% → noninvasive testing (stress test)
- Severe: ≥70% → admit and catheterization

### Choice of Stress Test

- If a patient can walk and ECG is normal → exercise stress ECG
- If a patient can walk and ECG is abnormal (not LBBB or RV paced rhythm) → exercise stress with imaging (echo or nuclear perfusion)
- If LBBB or paced rhythm → Lexiscan nuclear perfusion preferable (exercise perfusion results in false-positive perfusion defects). Dobutamine or exercise stress echo are also acceptable
- If a patient cannot walk → pharmacological stress test (dobutamine echocardiogram), vasodilator (Lexiscan) nuclear stress, vasodilator (Lexiscan) cardiac MRI when available

## Further Reading

Raff, G.L., Chinnaiyan, K.M., Cury, R.C. et al. (2014). SCCT guidelines on the use of coronary computed tomographic angiography for patients presenting with acute chest pain to the emergency department: a report of the Society of Cardiovascular Computed Tomography

Chapter 7

Guidelines Committee. *Journal of Cardiovascular Computed Tomography* 8 (4): 254–271. (An excellent review for chest pain triaging and appropriate use of cardiac CT in this situation.).

Taylor, A.J., Cerqueira, M., Hodgson, J.M. et al. (2010). ACCF/SCCT/ACR/AHA/ASE/ASNC/ NASCI/SCAI/SCMR 2010 appropriate use criteria for cardiac computed tomography. A report of the American College of Cardiology Foundation Appropriate Use Criteria Task Force, the Society of Cardiovascular Computed Tomography, the American College of Radiology, the American Heart Association, the American Society of Echocardiography, the American Society of Nuclear Cardiology, the North American Society for Cardiovascular Imaging, the Society for Cardiovascular Angiography and Interventions, and the Society for Cardiovascular Magnetic Resonance. *Circulation* 122 (21): e525–e555. https://doi.org/ 10.1161/CIR.0b013e3181fcae66. (A very useful resource that goes over appropriateness criteria for cardiac CT.).

# Cardiac Catheterization

# 8

**8.1.** Which of the images A, B, or C in Figure 8.1 depict the correct anatomic placement of the Kelly to identify the site of sheath entry for transfemoral access?

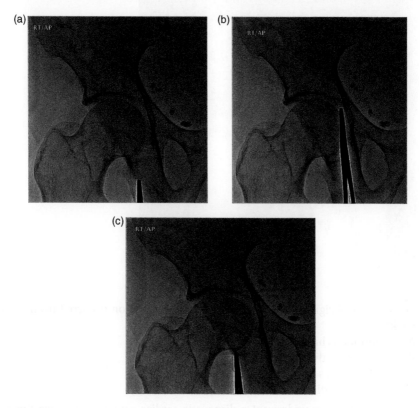

**Figure 8.1**

**8.2.** Where should the ideal location be of sheath entry in transfemoral access during cardiac catheterization?

    **A.** Above the inferior epigastric artery to stay as far away from the common femoral bifurcation as possible

    **B.** In the mid-common femoral artery above the bifurcation

    **C.** In the proximal profunda femoris

    **D.** In the superficial femoral artery

*Cardiology Board Review*, Second Edition. Ramdas G. Pai and Padmini Varadarajan.
© 2023 John Wiley & Sons Ltd. Published 2023 by John Wiley & Sons Ltd.

**8.3.** What are the possible complications associated with the access depicted in Figure 8.3?
  **A.** No complications as the access appears appropriate
  **B.** Pseudoaneurysm and arteriovenous malformations
  **C.** Retroperitoneal hemorrhage
  **D.** Intracranial hemorrhage

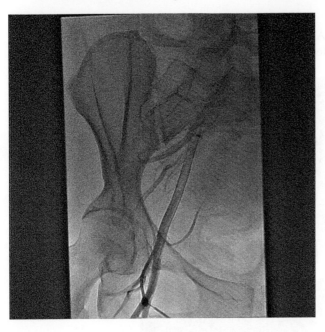

Figure 8.3

**8.4.** What physical sign would be expected if a complication occurred from a "low" stick?
  **A.** A continuous bruit over the access site
  **B.** Bruising over the skin
  **C.** A sudden and severe drop in blood pressure
  **D.** Angina chest discomfort

**8.5.** A 70-year-old man underwent a diagnostic cardiac catheterization via the right transfemoral approach prior to aortic valve replacement. Approximately one hour later, the nurse reports to you that he appears agitated and is complaining of lower abdominal discomfort. His systolic blood pressure is now 90 mmHg. The blood pressure prior to the procedure was 150 mmHg systolic. What is the next best step?
  **A.** Immediately start intravenous fluid and blood transfusion and obtain a non-contrast computed tomography (CT) of the abdomen and pelvis.
  **B.** Immediately start intravenous fluid and monitor blood pressure response
  **C.** Reassure the nurse that this is likely a vagal response and request that she monitor the blood pressure closely
  **D.** Immediately take the patient back to the catheterization laboratory to reevaluate his femoral anatomy.

**8.6.** Which of the femoral angiograms A or B in Figure 8.6 is most likely to be associated with the patient in Question 8.5?

(a)
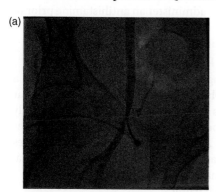

(b)
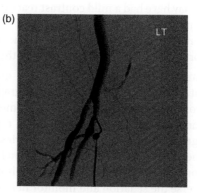

**Figure 8.6**

**8.7.** A 68-year-old man underwent an uncomplicated percutaneous coronary intervention of the mid-left anterior descending (LAD) artery. You are called about 30 minutes after the procedure as there is a large hematoma over the femoral access site. Manual pressure is applied for 40 minutes but the hematoma quickly reforms. What is the next best step?

A. Immediately start intravenous fluid and blood transfusion and obtain a non-contrast CT of the abdomen and pelvis

B. Immediately start intravenous fluid, apply a clamp for compression, and monitor blood pressure response

C. Reassure the nurse that this is likely a vagal response and request that she monitor the blood pressure closely

D. Immediately take the patient back to the catheterization laboratory to reevaluate his femoral anatomy

**8.8.** A 56-year-old man presents to the emergency department complaining of discomfort in the right groin. He underwent a diagnostic cardiac catheterization about three days previously. Examination reveals a loud, continuous bruit over the femoral artery. What test should be ordered next?

A. A complete lower extremity angiogram, as this patient likely has concomitant peripheral vascular disease

B. CT scan of the pelvis

C. Ultrasound evaluation of the right groin

D. No work-up is needed as he likely has chronic peripheral vascular disease and the discomfort is normal in this timeframe

**8.9.** A patient is being evaluated and consented prior to an outpatient cardiac catheterization. He reports that he had a CT angiogram about two years previously. After the procedure he developed hives and pruritus. His physician prescribed a medication for one week at that time, the name of which he cannot recall. How should he be managed?

A. Given that the procedure was remote, this is likely an idiosyncratic reaction; proceed with the planned procedure without additional evaluation or medication

B. He may have had a mild contrast reaction, which is unlikely to recur; proceed as planned without additional evaluation or medication

C. He may have had a mild contrast reaction; administer an antihistamine prior to the planned procedure

D. He may have had a mild contrast reaction; administer an antihistamine and a short course of oral steroids prior to the procedure

8.10. You are in the midst of completing a diagnostic cardiac catheterization on a patient. His coronary anatomy is angiographically normal and the left ventricular function is normal. He suddenly becomes profoundly hypotensive. He is fully alert and able to answer questions. A repeat angiography again demonstrates angiographically normal coronary arteries. A stat echocardiogram demonstrates that the left ventricular function is normal and there is no evidence of pericardial effusion. What is the next best step in his management?

A. Reverse the sedation and monitor hemodynamics

B. Administer a bolus of normal saline and monitor hemodynamic response

C. Start intravenous normal saline bolus followed by continued infusion and administer intravenous glucocorticoids

D. Start dopamine infusion immediately and admit to the intensive care unit. Consult cardiothoracic surgery

8.11. Which of the following statements is correct regarding sedation during transradial access?

A. No sedation is required as this is a minimal painful, quick access

B. Moderate sedation to achieve a completely comfortable response

C. Deep sedation, making sure the airway is protected but no response to painful stimuli

D. General anesthesia, as multiple sticks are often required and significant pain may occur

8.12. The right radial artery is successfully accessed for coronary angiography in a 55-year-old woman. The sheath is advanced without difficulty. What is the immediate next step?

A. Proceed with diagnostic catheter advanced under fluoroscopic guidance immediately as access may spasm

B. Administer a pharmacological cocktail containing heparin only before beginning catheterization

C. Administer a pharmacological cocktail containing heparin and a vasodilator before beginning catheterization

D. Administer a pharmacological cocktail containing only a vasodilator before beginning catheterization

8.13. The cardiac catheterization is successfully completed in the patient in Question 8.12. As the sheath is being removed, there is significant tension noted and the patient suddenly complains about pain in the forearm? How should you proceed?

A. This is a normal response; continue to steady negative tension and withdraw the sheath

B. Stop immediately, as the sheath is entrapped by arterial spasm; consult vascular surgery immediately

C. Administer a repeat bolus of the pharmacological cocktail containing vasodilator and heparin; reattempt retraction gently

D. Repeat sedation only and reattempt when the patient is sedated and able to tolerate the discomfort

8.14. A 6-French JL-4 is used to engage the left main coronary artery for coronary angiography. The pressure waveform in Figure 8.14 is recorded. What should you do next?

A. Proceed as usual with coronary angiogram

B. Retract the catheter and reposition the engagement; if the same waveform is present, proceed as usual

C. Retract the catheter and reposition the engagement; if the same waveform is detected then give a small gentle puff of contrast to visualize the anatomy

D. Abandon the procedure, as there may be severe left main stenosis; consult cardiothoracic surgery

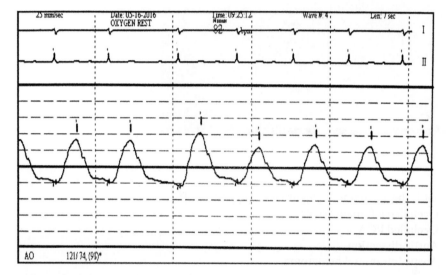

Figure 8.14

8.15. Coronary angiography is performed on a patient. What is depicted in the angiogram shown in Figure 8.15a?

A. Artifact from streaming of the contrast

B. A spiral dissection

C. Injection into the conus branch

D. Occluded right coronary artery

8.16. What should be the next step in treating the patient in Question 8.12?

A. Give a more brisk contrast injection to more forcefully displace the blood with contrast and better image the vessel

B. Advance a wire carefully to the distal vessel followed by a small-caliber over-the-wire balloon to verify intraluminal position

C. Proceed with angiography of the right coronary system, as no treatment is required for vessel tortuosity

D. Advance a floppy wire and treat the individual stenosis with stent implantation

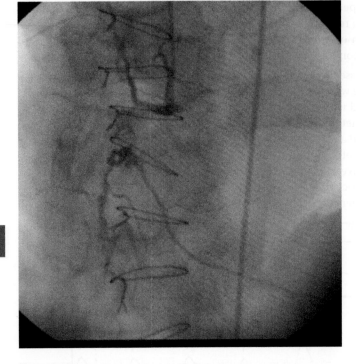

Figure 8.15a

8.17. What is the aortogram in Figure 8.17 suggestive of?
   A. Occluded left main artery
   B. Occluded RCA
   C. Aortic dissection
   D. Aortic intramural hematoma

8.18. The patient in Figure 8.18 presented with cardiogenic shock. What does the image show?
   A. Impella, RCA stent
   B. Intra-aortic balloon pump
   C. RCA stent and tandem heart catheter
   D. None of the above

8.19. What does the coronary angiogram in Figure 8.19 show?
   A. Significant distal left main coronary artery lesion
   B. LAD stenosis
   C. Severe circumflex lesion
   D. None of the above

8.20. What has the patient in Figure 8.20 likely presented with?
   A. Acute anterior ST-elevation myocardial infarction (STEMI)
   B. Acute inferior STEMI
   C. Chronic stable angina
   D. None of the above

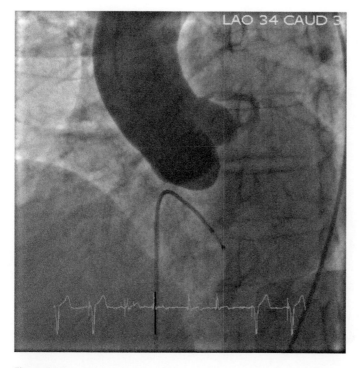

Figure 8.17

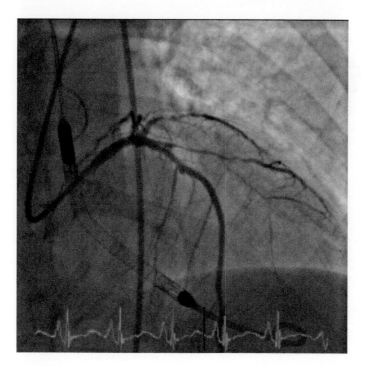

Figure 8.18

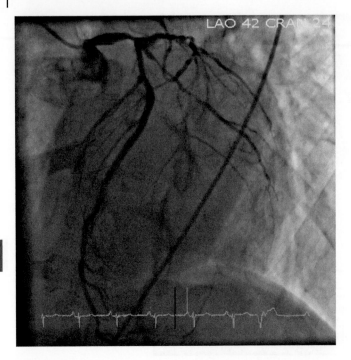

Figure 8.19

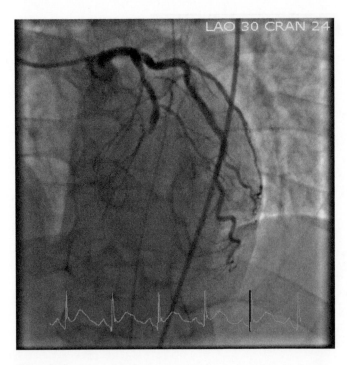

Figure 8.20

8.21. A 62-year-old Caucasian woman with a history of hypertension presented with sudden onset, sharp, squeezing discomfort in the center of her chest, radiating to her back and left shoulder. ECG showed diffuse T inversions in V1–V6 with a troponin I of 6 ng/ml. She underwent coronary angiography. Based on the coronary angiographic images in Figure 8.21, what is the most likely diagnosis for this patient?
   A. Severe coronary artery disease of the left anterior descending (LAD) artery
   B. Severe coronary artery disease of the left circumflex artery
   C. Severe coronary spasm of the LAD from catheter engagement
   D. Spontaneous coronary artery dissection involving the LAD

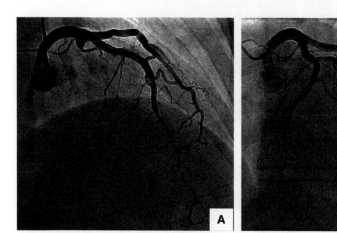

Figure 8.21

8.22. A 57-year-old Asian man presents to clinic with a history of gradually worsening dyspnea on exertion. Outpatient exercise treadmill stress test showed runs of non-sustained ventricular tachycardia (VT) at peak stress. Transthoracic echocardiography showed LVEF of 80% with mid to distal hypertrophy of the LV walls. Cardiac MRI confirmed the diagnosis of hypertrophic cardiomyopathy (HCM) with LV septal wall thickness of 35 mm and LV mid-cavity obliteration. Coronary angiography findings are as shown in Figure 8.22. A and B represent diastolic and systolic angiographic frames respectively. What is the diagnosis?
   A. Coronary spasm involving the LAD
   B. Myocardial bridge (intra-myocardial course) of the mid LAD
   C. Severe atherosclerosis of the LAD
   D. Spontaneous coronary artery dissection of the LAD

8.23. A 55-year-old woman with a history of diabetes type II and chronic tobacco use has been having class II angina not improving with anti-anginal therapy. She had a prior stress echocardiogram which demonstrated normal ejection fraction (EF) at rest and but she developed severe hypokinesis of the anterolateral wall with peak stress. She arrives for elective coronary angiogram. What is the diagnosis based on angiography in Figure 8.23?

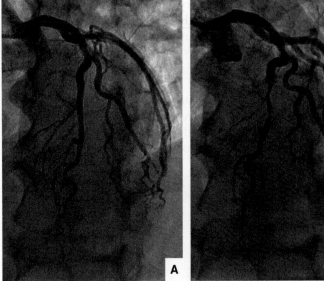

Figure 8.22

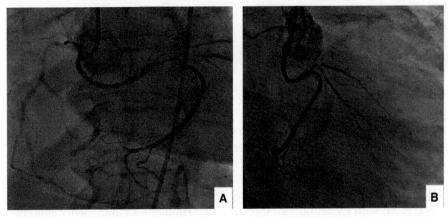

Figure 8.23

    A. RCA vessel visualized with significant stenosis at the mid-segment
    B. Anomalous left main artery with significant stenosis at the mid LAD
    C. Anomalous left circumflex artery with significant stenosis at the mid-segment
    D. Normal origin of left circumflex artery with significant stenosis at the mid-segment

8.24. A 55-year-old patient with a history of hypertension and type II diabetes presents with recurrent angina refractory to guideline-directed medical therapy. Coronary angiogram is done. What is the most significant findings in this angiogram?
    A. Severe stenosis of mid LAD with occluded left circumflex artery
    B. Severe stenosis of mid LCX with occluded LAD artery
    C. Absent left main artery with severe stenosis of the mid LAD
    D. Severe stenosis in the mid segment of both LAD and LCX

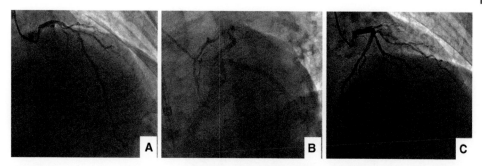

Figure 8.24

**8.25.** A 68-year-old male with a history of atrial fibrillation is being referred to an electrophysiologist for ablation. He has chronic angina, well controlled on guideline directed medical therapy. Prior coronary angiogram is shown below. What is the most significant finding?

A. Proximal ectasia of the RCA secondary to atherosclerotic disease
B. Anomalous conus branch origin from the posterolateral (PL) branch of RCA
C. Anomalous atrioventricular (AV) nodal branch origin from the PL branch of RCA
D. Anomalous origin of the left atrial branch from the PL branch of RCA

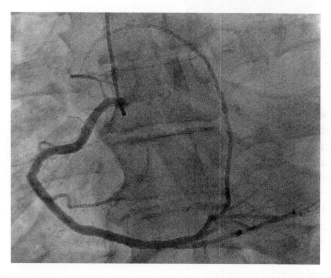

Figure 8.25

**8.26.** A 55-year-old man with a past medical history of hypertension, dyslipidemia and chronic tobacco use comes to the emergency room with chest pain that started 10 hours prior to presentation. ECG showed ST elevations in the inferior leads. Based on the angiographic finding in Figure 8.26, which of the following statements is false?

A. There is overall poor prognosis with a high risk for early and long-term adverse cardiac events
B. There is high-risk for distal embolization with coronary no-reflow phenomenon and risk for stent thrombosis after percutaneous intervention

C. Aspiration thrombectomy prior to stenting in this setting is associated with good long-term outcomes

D. Aspiration thrombectomy prior to stenting improves myocardial blush grade and rates of ST segment elevation resolution on ECG

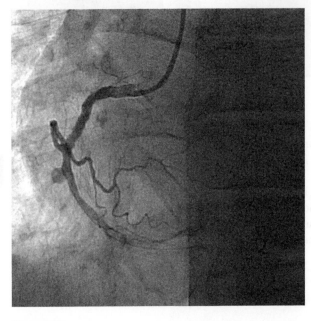

Figure 8.26

8.27. A 40-year-old woman with obesity and no other cardiac risk factors, presented to the clinic with complaints of lifestyle limiting angina brought on with minimal physical activity. Exercise treadmill stress test was non-diagnostic due to poor effort tolerance. Coronary angiography of the left system was normal, and angiography of the right system in the LAO (Panel A) and AP/Cranial (Panel B) projection is shown in Figure 8.27. What is the next best course of action?

A. Perform a coronary CT angiography

B. Start beta blockers and manage in a conservative fashion

C. Refer for cardiothoracic surgery evaluation as there is high risk for sudden death

D. Perform a sub-maximal exercise stress test

8.28. A 75-year-old man presented with left-sided chest pain moving to his left arm when he was lifting and moving boxes around his house. He has a history of peripheral vascular disease and had a stent placed in his left common iliac artery. He also has history of coronary artery disease and had a three-vessel bypass surgery 10 years previously. Nuclear stress test done as an outpatient showed extensive reversible ischemia involving the anterior wall with an ejection fraction of 25%. Coronary angiography showed severe native coronary artery disease with patent venous grafts to the left circumflex artery and to the right posterior descending artery and a patent left internal mammary artery graft. Based on the angiography shown in Figure 8.28, which of the following statements are true?

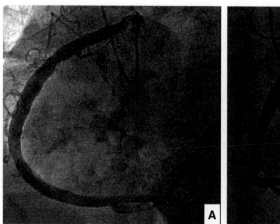 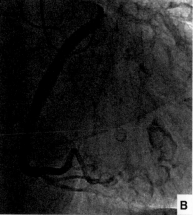

Figure 8.27

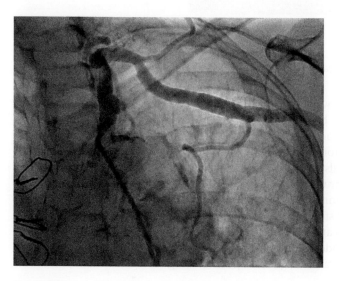

Figure 8.28

    A. Most common etiology is atherosclerosis
    B. Patient can also present with vertebrobasilar symptoms
    C. Endovascular revascularization is the preferred first approach
    D. All of the above

8.29. A 48-year-old woman with rheumatoid arthritis, diabetes mellitus and chronic active tobacco use is admitted from the emergency room with non-ST elevation MI. Coronary angiographic images are shown. What is the most common etiology of the condition demonstrated in this angiography?
    A. Vasculitis
    B. Connective-tissue disorder

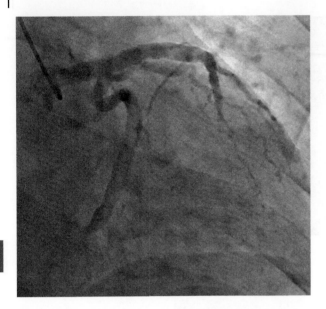

Figure 8.29

C. Atherosclerotic disease

D. Cocaine use

8.30. A 55-year-old woman with a history of coronary artery disease underwent three-vessel coronary artery bypass graft surgery the previous year. She presents with exertional angina to your outpatient clinic. Stress myocardial perfusion imaging with Sestamibi is performed and this shows mild reversible ischemia in the mid-to-distal anterior walls with no drop in ejection fraction from rest to stress. Coronary angiography was performed, and the venous grafts are noted to be patent. Left internal mammary artery (LIMA) angiography is shown in Figure 8.30. What is the next best step in her management?

A. Start beta blockers and long-acting nitrate therapy with close follow-up

B. Occlude thoracic side branch coming off the LIMA by coil-embolization

C. Refer to cardiothoracic surgeon to perform surgical ligation of the thoracic side branch

D. Perform revascularization of the proximal LAD by percutaneous intervention

8.31. A 65-year-old man with recurrent angina presents as an outpatient for elective coronary angiography. The left main is engaged with a 5 French diagnostic catheter and the following angiographic image is obtained (Figure 8.31). Shortly after, the patient starts complaining of chest pain and is noted to be hypotensive with systolic blood pressure of 80 mmHg. ST elevations were noted in the anterior leads on the monitor. What is the next immediate step?

A. Perform balloon angioplasty and stent implantation of the left anterior descending artery

B. Start 100% oxygen via a high-flow nasal cannula

C. Perform mechanical thrombectomy of the mid LAD

D. Prepare for emergency pericardiocentesis.

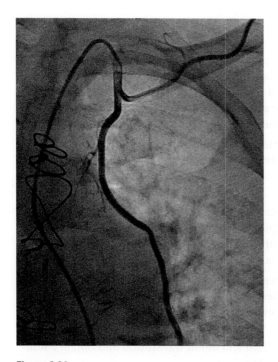

Figure 8.30

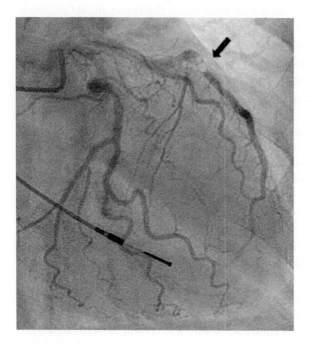

Figure 8.31

## Answers

8.1. C. An instrument such as a Kelly is placed over the patient skin to fluoroscopically identify the inferomedial femoral head. This is the ideal location for the needle to enter the skin at such an angle as to facilitate entry into the common femoral artery below the inferior epigastric artery and above the common femoral bifurcation. Entry at this location minimizes vascular complications.

8.2. B. In the mid-common femoral artery above the bifurcation.

The ideal location for sheath entry into the common femoral artery is below the inferior epigastric artery and above the bifurcation to minimize vascular complications.

8.3. B. Pseudoaneurysm and arteriovenous malformations.

This sheath has entered the superficial femoral artery and is considered a low stick. Low sticks are associated with arteriovenous fistulas and pseudoaneurysms as potential vascular complications.

8.4. A. A continuous bruit over the access site.

A low stick could result in an arteriovenous fistula or pseudoaneurysm. Physical examination would reveal a continuous murmur on auscultation over the arteriotomy site.

8.5. A. Immediately start intravenous fluid and blood transfusion and obtain a non-contrast CT of the abdomen and pelvis.

This patient most likely has a retroperitoneal hemorrhage. The sudden drop in blood pressure and the abdominal discomfort are big clues to this diagnosis. He should be immediately resuscitated with intravenous fluids and should receive a blood transfusion. A noncontrast CT scan of the abdomen and pelvis should be ordered when he is hemodynamically stable to confirm the diagnosis.

8.6. A. The first angiogram demonstrates a "high" stick just at the inferior epigastric artery. A high stick is associated with a retroperitoneal hemorrhage.

8.7. D. Immediately take the patient back to the catheterization laboratory to reevaluate his femoral anatomy.

A hematoma over the arteriotomy may develop from inadequate manual compression, failure of closure device, or vessel trauma. In a patient with a hematoma that is refractory to prolonged attempts at hemostasis with manual compression, the appropriate step would be to reevaluate the femoral anatomy. This allows for efficient decision making in the management of any potential vascular complication.

8.8. C. An ultrasound evaluation of the right groin.

An ultrasound is the test with the highest initial yield in this patient. It will identify potential local vascular complications such as a pseudoaneurysm, which is the most likely diagnosis.

8.9. C. The patient may have had a mild contrast reaction; administer an antihistamine prior to the planned procedure.

This patient likely had a mild contrast reaction and should be pretreated with antihistamines such as diphenhydramine 50 mg about one hour before the procedure.

**8.10.** C. Start intravenous normal saline bolus followed by continued infusion and administer intravenous glucocorticoids.

This patient is most likely having an immediate adverse contrast reaction. The angiography should be immediately stopped and he should be resuscitated with intravenous fluids. Glucocorticoids may be administered to suppress the immune response but will not be effective immediately. Epinephrine injection may be needed. In refractory or severe cases, vasopressor infusion may be needed to temporize the situation.

**8.11.** B. Moderate sedation to achieve a completely comfortable response.

Adequate moderate sedation is essential in transradial access as pain and anxiety may lead to more arterial spasm.

**8.12.** C. Administer a pharmacological cocktail containing heparin and a vasodilator before beginning catheterization.

The radial artery is small in caliber and prone to spasm; therefore, after radial access, it is generally recommended to administer a pharmacological cocktail of heparin and a vasodilator. Different regimens and dosages have been recommended. One such option is 5000 units of heparin, 200 μg of nitroglycerine, and 2.5 mg of verapamil.

**8.13.** C. Administer a repeat bolus of the pharmacological cocktail containing vasodilator and heparin; reattempt retraction gently.

If there is resistance while maneuvering catheters via the transradial approach, vasospasm should immediately be suspected. Aggressively removing the catheter may result in evulsion of the artery. Therefore, repeating the pharmacological cocktail of heparin and vasodilators is the most prudent course of action. Sedating the patient is appropriate, though not as a stand-alone therapy.

**8.14.** C. Retract the catheter and reposition the engagement; if the same waveform is detected then give a small gentle puff of contrast to visualize the anatomy.

The example shown is of a ventricularized arterial waveform. This is recognized as a slight decrease in systolic pressure but a large decrease in diastolic pressure. There is also a loss of, or significant smoothing out of, the dicrotic notch. It is commonly encountered when the angiography catheter passes through or is against a significant coronary stenosis. Readjusting the catheter to verify positioning is important before continuing on with the angiography. If the same waveform is verified, then a gentle "puff" of injection can be performed to visualize the anatomy and the potential cause of the waveform.

**8.15.** D. Occluded right coronary artery.

The arrow in Figure 8.15b points to the occluded proximal right coronary artery with bridging collaterals. The patient had prior coronary artery bypass surgery.

**8.16.** B. Advance a wire carefully to the distal vessel followed by a small-caliber over-the-wire balloon to verify intraluminal position.

A common technique in treating a coronary dissection is to leave the first wire in place within the dissection plane. An attempt is then made to advance a second wire into the true lumen. The first wire may act both as a guide as to the location of the dissection plane and also may deflect the second wire. Once the wire is advanced successfully, a small balloon may be advanced and dye injection performed to confirm intraluminal position.

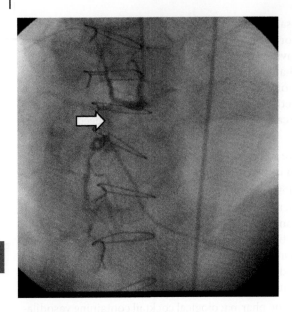

**Figure 8.15b**

**8.17.** **B.** Occluded RCA.

The RCA is also calcified. The ascending aorta is normal. Note a temporary right ventricular pacer and intermittent pacing.

**8.18.** **A.** Impella, RCA stent.

**8.19.** **A.** Significant distal left main coronary artery lesion.

**8.20.** **A.** Acute anterior ST-elevation myocardial infarction (STEMI).

Note the thrombotic occlusion of the mid LAD artery.

**8.21.** **D.** Spontaneous coronary artery dissection involving the LAD.

This case depicts a typical presentation of spontaneous coronary artery dissection (SCAD). SCAD is more common in women and unlike coronary artery disease (CAD), patients have a few or no CAD risk factors. SCAD is the most common cause of pregnancy-associated MI. Note the abrupt transition in lumen size of the LAD and a long segment of narrowing on angiography. This is typical for type II SCAD (long, diffuse and smooth narrowing). Catheter-induced spasm may occur in the proximal vessel if engaged deeply by the catheter. This is less likely to explain narrowing in the mid-distal LAD.

**8.22.** **B.** Myocardial bridge (intra-myocardial course) of the mid LAD.

Myocardial bridge is a congenital coronary anomaly in which the epicardial artery takes on an intramyocardial course resulting in compression of the tunneled artery during systole. This is demonstrated as "milking" of the mid LAD during systole (Figure 8.23 Panel A) followed by partial or complete decompression in diastole (Figure 8.23 Panel B) as demonstrated in the angiographic images. The LAD is the most common vessel involved, though any of the three epicardial coronary arteries can be affected. There is a strong association with myocardial bridging and hypertrophic cardiomyopathy (HCM) and can be seen in up to one third of patients with HCM. Most cases are benign, however myocardial bridge has been associated with objective evidence of ischemia on noninvasive testing as well as altered intracoronary hemodynamics. The first line of therapy are beta-blockers and calcium channel blockers. Percutaneous coronary intervention with stents are generally not recommended due to the high rate of target lesion failure. In cases refractory to medical therapy, surgical myotomy or coronary artery bypass surgery are suitable options.

8.23. C. Anomalous left circumflex artery with significant stenosis at the mid-segment.

Knowledge of normal coronary anatomy is important especially in the setting of anomalous aortic origin of coronary artery from inappropriate sinus of Valsalva. In this angiogram, we can see the anomalous left circumflex artery arising from the right coronary cusp with a separate ostia and taking course along the AV groove to reach the lateral wall. The RCA can be seen to the left of the vessel with faint contrast filling in Figure 8.23. This is a common coronary anomaly with incidence of 0.4–0.5% in the general population. Furthermore, one can appreciate the 80% stenosis in the mid-course of the artery that was responsible for her symptoms. This was successfully intervened upon with a stent.

8.24. C. Absent left main with severe stenosis of the mid LAD

The angiographic finding in Figure 8.24 is congenital absence of left main coronary artery (LMCA) and origin of left anterior descending artery (LAD) and left circumflex artery (LCX) with separate ostia from left sinus of Valsalva. This is best appreciated in panel B of the figure which is a LAO/Caudal ("spider") view that shows separate ostia of the LAD and LCX. Panel A shows the LAD and Panel C shows the LCX respectively, engaged and imaged in a selective manner. This finding is also a fairly common coronary artery anomaly with an incidence rate of 0.5%.

8.25. D. Anomalous origin of left atrial branch from the PL branch of RCA.

Typically, the left atrial (LA) branch comes off early from the left circumflex artery. In cases where the left circumflex is diminutive and RCA is super-dominant, the LA branch may come off the PL branch of the RCA. Knowledge of this unusual anatomy is important, especially during catheter ablation for atrial fibrillation. This course of the artery tends to cross ablation lines and is therefore at risk for thermal injury during ablation. Additionally, protected myocardium around the arterial branches may cause failure of ablation therapy and recurrence of atrial fibrillation.

8.26. C. Aspiration thrombectomy prior to stenting in this setting is associated with good long-term outcomes.

Angiogram shows heavy intracoronary thrombosis in the mid RCA which is a consequence of plaque rupture causing complete occlusion of the right coronary artery. This is the basic pathophysiological event in acute ST-elevation myocardial infarction. Presence of angiographically visible thrombus burden is a poor prognostic factor and is associated with high in-hospital and long-term adverse cardiac events. Additionally, distal embolization with coronary no-reflow phenomenon and risk for stent thrombosis are high in such cases. Aspiration thrombectomy prior to stenting is associated with improvement in myocardial blush grades and ST-elevation resolution on ECG, but there is no evidence that this intervention improves long-term outcomes. Routine aspiration thrombectomy in STEMI prior to PCI received a Class III recommendation (no benefit) in the latest ACC 2021 guidelines on myocardial revascularization.

**8.27.** A. Perform a coronary CT angiography.

The angiography demonstrates anomalous aortic origin of the right coronary artery (RCA) from the left coronary cusp. The patient has symptoms suggestive of angina but first she will need a CT coronary angiography to identify high-risk features that increase her risk for sudden cardiac death. These include slit-like orifice, acute angle take-off, inter-arterial/intramural course, and hypoplasia of the proximal coronary artery. In the presence of high-risk features, the next step would be to demonstrate objective evidence for ischemia in the RCA territory with a highly sensitive test such as a nuclear stress test prior to pursuing surgical evaluation. If no high-risk features are present, conservative management would be appropriate.

**8.28.** D. All of the above.

The diagnosis here is subclavian artery stenosis causing coronary subclavian steal syndrome from reduced blood flow in the LIMA graft and subsequent ischemia in the LAD territory. Patients usually present with anginal symptoms with use of the left upper extremity. They can also have vertebrobasilar symptoms (such as dizziness or syncope) due to retrograde flow in the ipsilateral vertebral artery. A gradient of >15 mmHg across the lesion is necessary for the stenosis to become hemodynamically significant. The most common cause is atherosclerosis and patients may have prior peripheral vascular disease as seen in this patient. The preferred first-line treatment is endovascular revascularization with a bare metal stent.

**8.29.** C. Atherosclerosis.

Angiography shows diffuse ectasia of the left coronary system with Thrombolysis in Myocardial Infarction (TIMI)-2 flow and no focal aneurysmal dilatations are noted. Coronary artery ectasia are rare findings and have an incidence of <1% based on data from cath registries. The underlying etiology depends upon the age of the patient at presentation. The common cause of coronary ectasia/aneurysm in children and young adults is vasculitis, particularly Kawasaki's disease. In adults, the most common etiology is atherosclerosis.

**8.30.** A. Start beta blockers and long-acting nitrate therapy with close follow-up.

The angiography of LIMA graft shows a large thoracic side branch coming off the LIMA graft proximally. This is suggestive of LIMA steal phenomenon in which an un-ligated branch vessel of the LIMA graft "steals" blood away from the LIMA. This may explain the patient's ischemic findings on stress testing localizing to the LAD territory. There is lack of consensus in the interventional community whether this phenomenon truly exists. Almost one-third of LIMA grafts can have an unligated side-branch on angiographic follow-up post CABG. Clinical benefit with surgical or percutaneous occlusion of the side branch have been reported in several case reports in the literature. However, physiological studies show that the blood flow in the LIMA graft is predominantly diastolic while flow in the thoracic side branch is predominantly systolic making it less likely to cause hemodynamically significant steal. Nevertheless, the first step in this patient with post-CABG angina should be intensification of antianginal therapy in the absence of high-risk findings on nuclear stress test.

**8.31.** B. Start 100% oxygen via high-flow nasal cannula.

Coronary artery air embolism is a rare complication (0.1–0.3%) of coronary angiography and most cases are iatrogenic from introduction of air in the contrast injection system or from inadequate de-aeration of the diagnostic catheter prior to use. The clinical consequence depends on the amount of air that enters the coronary arteries and the size of the parent vessel. Most cases are transient and respond to prompt institution of 100% oxygen therapy. This causes diffusion of nitrogen from the air bubble into the nitrogen-poor but oxygen-rich blood/tissues resulting in shrinkage of the bubble and eventual resolution.

Chapter 8

# Acute Coronary Syndromes

# 9

9.1. Of the following statements regarding a patient with multiple cardiac risk factors and angina-like chest pain lasting 30 minutes, which is the incorrect one?
   A. A normal echocardiogram (ECG) in the emergency room (ER) rules out myocardial infarction (MI)
   B. Ischemia in the circumflex area is more often electrically silent
   C. A negative first set of cardiac markers does not rule out MI
   D. ECG changes could be dynamic, and it is useful to repeat every 15 minutes in the first hour of chest pain or when chest pain recurs

9.2. The components of thrombolysis in MI (TIMI) risk score on initial patient evaluation for suspected acute coronary syndrome (ACS) include which of the following?
   A. Age >65 years
   B. More than three coronary artery disease (CAD) risk factors
   C. Prior CAD with >50% lesion
   D. More than two anginal events in 24 hours
   E. Use of aspirin in the previous seven days
   F. ST deviation on ECG
   G. Elevated cardiac markers
   H. All of the above
   I. Some of the above

9.3. Which of the following types of chest pain rule out ACS?
   A. Sharp stabbing chest pain
   B. Pleuritic chest pain
   C. Chest pain reproduced by palpation
   D. None of the above

9.4. Guideline recommendation for ECG for patients presenting with chest pain to the ER is the performance of ECG within how much time of arrival?
   A. 5 minutes
   B. 10 minutes
   C. 30 minutes
   D. 60 minutes

9.5. The GRACE risk model predicts in-hospital mortality in ACS patients and includes Killip class, systolic blood pressure (BP), heart rate, age, and serum creatinine level. Which one of the following may be negatively correlated with mortality?
   A. Heart rate
   B. Systolic BP

*Cardiology Board Review*, Second Edition. Ramdas G. Pai and Padmini Varadarajan.
© 2023 John Wiley & Sons Ltd. Published 2023 by John Wiley & Sons Ltd.

C. Killip class

D. None of the above

9.6. Which of the following are contraindications for nitroglycerin (NTG) in patients with ACS and continuing chest pain?

A. Systolic BP <90 mmHg

B. Inferior MI with positive Kussmaul

C. Sildenafil or vardenafil within 24 hours

D. Tadalafil within 48 hours

E. All of the above

F. None of the above

9.7. Regarding use of traditional nonsteroidal anti-inflammatory drugs (NSAIDs) and cyclooxygenase-2 (COX-2) inhibitors in the setting of ACS, which of the following statements is correct?

A. Traditional NSAIDs, but not COX-2 inhibitors can be used

B. Traditional NSAIDs should be used, but COX-2 inhibitors can be used

C. Neither traditional NSAIDs nor COX-2 inhibitors should be used

D. Either can be used with no risk of harm

9.8. Which calcium channel blockers are contraindicated in ACS?

A. Diltiazem

B. Verapamil

C. Short-acting nifedipine without a beta blocker

D. None of the above

9.9. The first dose and route of aspirin use in suspected ACS is which of the following?

A. 162 or 325 mg enteric coated

B. 162 or 325 mg nonenteric coated chewed

C. 81 mg orally

D. None of the above

9.10. Aspirin in suspected ACS is avoided in which of the following patients?

A. Aspirin allergy

B. Recent gastrointestinal (GI) bleed

C. Neither A nor B

D. Both A and B

9.11. For patients with ACS, what is the recommended duration of double antiplatelet therapy (DAPT)?

A. One month

B. Six months

C. One year

D. Forever, unless at high risk of bleeding

9.12. After NSTEMI, in addition to ASA, Plavix, beta blockers, and high-intensity statin therapy, which other agents are recommended for those with ejection fraction (EF) <40%?

A. Angiotensin-converting enzyme inhibitors (ACEIs), or angiotensin receptor blockers (ARBs) in those who are ACEI intolerant

B. Aldosterone blocking agent, provided creatinine is <2 mg/dl and K is <5 meq/l

Chapter 9

C. Diltiazem to prevent reinfarction
D. A and B
E. A and C

9.13. In a patient with non-ST elevation ACS, early coronary angiography is appropriate in which of the following situations?
A. TIMI score of 5
B. Continuing chest pain
C. EF <40%
D. Anterior wall motion abnormality
E. Dynamic mitral regurgitation (MR) murmur
F. All of the above

9.14. Based on current data, which of the following statements are correct in the setting of ACS?
A. In the setting of ST elevation MI (STEMI), nonculprit vessels should not be stented
B. In the setting of NSTEMI, it is also reasonable to perform percutaneous coronary intervention (PCI) on critically stenosed nonculprit vessels
C. Both A and B are correct
D. Neither A or B are correct

9.15. Which of the following statements are correct regarding prasugrel use?
A. It is used 10 mg once a day.
B. It reduces risk of stent thrombosis compared with clopidogrel
C. It has a higher risk of bleeding in those above 75 years of age or weight <60 kg
D. It is contraindicated in those with prior stroke or transient ischemic attack (TIA)
E. All of the above
F. None of the above

9.16. Which of the following should not be used as the sole anticoagulant during PCI?
A. Fondaparinux
B. Enoxaparin
C. Bivalirudin
D. None of the above

9.17. Which of the following statements are accurate regarding the duration of stoppage of antiplatelet drugs before elective coronary artery bypass grafting?
A. Clopidogrel for five days
B. Prasugrel for seven days
C. Eptifibatide and tirofiban for two to four hours
D. Abciximab for 12 hours
E. All of the above

9.18. Before coronary artery bypass grafting, which of the following statements is correct?
A. Aspirin should be stopped one week earlier
B. Aspirin should not be stopped
C. Aspirin should be stopped 24 hours before
D. None of the above

**9.19.** Which of the following statements are accurate regarding triple antithrombotic therapy after MI?

A. The duration should be minimized

B. Concomitant proton pump inhibitors should be used

C. Triple therapy should not be used

D. A and B are correct

**9.20.** Which of the following agents are useful for secondary prevention post MI?

A. Vitamin E

B. Folic acid

C. Beta carotene

D. Fish oil

E. None of the above

**9.21.** Which of the following statements are true for older patients with non-ST elevation ACS?

A. They may have atypical symptoms

B. Benefit with medical and catheter-based therapies is similar to younger patients

C. They receive less guideline-directed medical therapy

D. None of the above

E. All of the above

**9.22.** Compared with men, women presenting with ACS have which of the following?

A. More atypical symptoms

B. Greater chance of getting discharge from the ER

C. Higher risk of long-term complications such as heart failure (HF), shock, renal failure, stroke, readmission

D. All of the above

E. None of the above

**9.23.** Compared with men, women presenting with ACS have which of the following?

A. Greater incidence of normal coronary arteries

B. Higher percentage of normal EF

C. Fewer high-risk lesions

D. Same benefit with medicines

E. All of the above

F. None of the above

**9.24.** In ACS due to cocaine use, it is preferable to avoid which of these agents?

A. Heparin

B. Beta blocker

C. ACEI

D. None of the above

**9.25.** Which of the following are true regarding use of early glycoprotein (GP) IIb/IIIa inhibitor in the setting of acute STEMI receiving DAPT?

A. There is no clear benefit in terms of MI or death during follow-up

B. No clear evidence for a decrease in target vessel revascularization

C. There is evidence for rapidity of ST segment resolution, but not for improvement in TIMI grade 3 flow

D. All of the above

9.26. Adjunctive GP IIb/IIIa inhibitors are recommended in addition to DAPT and heparin in acute STEMI setting in which of the following situations?

A. At time of primary PCI

B. Routinely in the ER

C. Those with large thrombus burden

D. All of the above

E. At time of primary PCI or those with large thrombus burden

9.27. For a patient presenting with STEMI to a non-PCI facility, which of the following factors support immediate thrombolytic therapy?

A. Presentation within four hours of chest pain

B. Low-risk STEMI

C. Low bleeding risk with thrombolysis

D. PCI facility is far away

E. All of the above

F. There is no indication for thrombolysis; transfer to PCI facility

9.28. A 68-year-old man presents to a non-PCI facility with anterior STEMI with ST elevation from V2 to V5. He is short of breath with bilateral rales. Chest pain started four hours earlier. He had a TIA six weeks earlier and is on clopidogrel and statin. Estimated transport time to nearest catheterization laboratory is 75 minutes. After giving $O_2$, nitroglycerin (NTG), ASA, and heparin, what is the best next strategy?

A. Immediate transfer to the PCI facility

B. Give half-dose thrombolytic and then transfer

C. Patient is too high risk to transfer; give full-dose thrombolytic

D. None of the above

9.29. A 64-year-old man presents to a non-PCI facility with anterior STEMI with ST elevation from V2 to V4. He is short of breath with bilateral rales. Chest pain started three hours earlier. He is on aspirin and statin. Estimated transport time to the nearest catheterization laboratory is 4 H. There are no contraindications for thrombolytic therapy. After giving $O_2$, nitroglycerin (NTG), ASA chewed, and heparin, what is the best next strategy?

A. Full-dose thrombolytic and transfer to PCI facility

B. Half-dose thrombolytic and transfer to PCI facility

C. Immediately transfer to PCI facility

D. Treat medically as the patient is high risk to transfer

9.30. In patients presenting with acute MI, which of the following plasma glucose targets are desirable?

A. Tight control with glucose <110 mg/dl

B. Liberal control with glucose <300 mg/dl

C. Glucose <180 mg/dl

D. None of the above

9.31. A 65-year-old patient with diabetes mellitus and hypertension had an acute anterior MI treated within four hours of chest pain with drug-eluting stent (DES) in the left anterior descending (LAD) artery. He is stable. Serum creatinine is 1.3 mg/dl; creatine clearance 60 ml/minute. His home medications include aspirin, glybenclamide, metformin, and lisinopril. What would the appropriate actions be?

A. Start on insulin infusion 1 unit per hour and titrate to blood glucose <180 mg/dl
B. Continue current medications
C. Discontinue metformin
D. Discontinue lisinopril

9.32. Which of the following statements regarding thrombus aspiration are accurate in patients with acute MI undergoing PCI?

A. It is reasonable to perform in those presenting early and have large thrombus burden
B. It may not be useful in those presenting late
C. It is not useful in side branches subtending small myocardial territories
D. All of the above
E. None of the above

9.33. A 52-year-old man with no prior cardiac history presented with chest pain of four hours and was found to have acute anterior STEMI. He lost his job and medical insurance recently. He was on lisinopril and simvastatin. After administering aspirin and nitroglycerin (NTG), an immediate coronary angiography revealed a 90% lesion in the mid LAD artery with a reference diameter of 4 mm. The lesion length was 6 mm and type B. Other vessels were angiographically normal. What would the most appropriate therapy be?

A. A DES
B. A bare-metal stent (BMS)
C. Either
D. Immediate single-vessel bypass using left internal mammary artery on beating heart

9.34. In acute STEMI qualifying for reperfusion therapy, which of the following options is correct?

A. Desired door-to-needle is <30 minutes and door-to-balloon time is <90 minutes
B. Desired door-to-needle and door-to-balloon times are <90 minutes
C. There is no indication for thrombolysis
D. None of the above

9.35. Which of the following strategies may reduce time to reperfusion therapy in acute STEMI?

A. Media campaign to educate patients on signs of MI
B. Prehospital ECG
C. Use of 9-1-1 rather than being driven to the ER by a family member
D. An ER MI protocol
E. All of the above

9.36. In acute STEMI, fibrinolysis is preferred over primary PCI in which of the following situations?

A. Early presentation, <3 hours
B. Catheterization laboratory is not available or expert operator is not available
C. Predicted (door-to-balloon)-(door-to-needle) time is greater than 60 minutes
D. Medical contact to balloon or door-to-balloon time is likely to be >90 minutes
E. All of the above

Chapter 9

**9.37.** In acute STEMI, primary PCI is preferred over fibrinolysis in which of the following situations?
A. Late presentation, >3 hours of chest pain
B. Heart failure or cardiogenic shock
C. Contraindication to thrombolytics
D. Diagnosis of STEMI is in doubt
E. All of the above

**9.38.** Absolute contraindications for thrombolytics include which of the following?
A. Prior intracranial hemorrhage
B. Ischemic stroke within three months (except acute stroke <3 hours)
C. Closed head or facial trauma in last three months
D. Cerebral arteriovenous malformation, berry aneurysm, or neoplasms
E. All of the above
F. Above are only relative contraindications and decision depends upon risk/benefit ratio

**9.39.** Relative contraindication for thrombolytics include which of the following?
A. Systolic BP >180 mmHg or diastolic BP >110 mmHg
B. Prolonged cardiopulmonary resuscitation or major surgery in <3 weeks
C. Pregnancy
D. Current anticoagulant use
E. Noncompressible vascular punctures
F. All of the above
G. Some of the above

**9.40.** Which of the following statements about tissue plasminogen activator (tPA) are true?
A. It acts more rapidly than streptokinase
B. It acts better in the presence of fibrin; in its absence it is a weak plasminogen activator
C. It is a surface-active agent
D. Generally, dose for STEMI is 15 mg bolus + 50 mg over 30 minutes + 35 minutes over 60 minutes
E. All of the above
F. Some of the above

**9.41.** GUSTO-1 was a landmark trial that compared front-loaded alteplase with streptokinase in acute STEMI within 6 hours. What were the findings?
A. Reduced death with alteplase
B. Reduced myocardial reinfarction with alteplase
C. Trend to increased intracranial bleed with streptokinase
D. All of the above

**9.42.** A 48-year-old man with acute inferior MI has a heart rate of 74 bpm, BP of 90/60 mmHg. There are no murmurs. The jugular venous pressure (JVP) is 16 cm $H_2O$ and the column seems to rise during quiet breathing. The lungs are clear. What would the appropriate treatment for low BP include?
A. Intravenous bolus of normal saline
B. Normal saline and dobutamine infusion if BP is still low
C. Intravenous Lasix
D. Infusion of norepinephrine

**9.43.** A 52-year-old man with reperfused (with PCI with DES) acute anterior MI suffered recurrent chest pain, more on breathing, associated with an increase in ST elevation leads V2 to V5 on Day 3. What may this indicate?
A. Stent thrombosis
B. Dressler's syndrome
C. Chemical pericarditis
D. Potential for myocardial rupture

**9.44.** Left ventricle free wall rupture in the presence of acute MI is more common in which of the following?
A. The elderly
B. Women
C. Those without prior infarcts
D. Large infarcts
E. Reperfusion with lytics rather than PCI
F. All of the above
G. Some of the above

**9.45.** Which of the following are true about left ventricle free wall rupture?
A. It tends to occur at the junction of infarct and normal muscle
B. Generally occurs after one to four days of infarct, but can occur as late as three weeks
C. Usually occurs in left ventricle, but may involve right ventricle or atria
D. All of the above

**9.46.** A 46-year-old patient with inferior STEMI, post-primary PCI, became suddenly short of breath, rapidly evolving into pulmonary edema needing endotracheal intubation. On examination, his heart rate was 130 bpm, BP 80/50 mmHg, bilateral rales, and high jugular venous pressure. Cardiac sounds were soft, and there were no murmurs. The ECG showed sinus tachycardia with normal ST segments. What is the most likely diagnosis?
A. Coronary stent thrombosis
B. Acute pulmonary embolism
C. Papillary muscle rupture
D. Large RV infarct

**9.47.** Which of the following statements are true regarding papillary muscle rupture?
A. It can occur with small subendocardial infarcts affecting tip of papillary muscle
B. More commonly involves posteromedial papillary muscle
C. Anterolateral papillary muscle may derive dual blood supply from LAD and circumflex arteries and is less prone to rupture
D. All of the above

**9.48.** In the setting of acute MI, prophylactic lidocaine is recommended in which of the following situations?
A. Large anterior MI
B. Routinely in prehospital phase
C. Routinely on arrival to the ER
D. None of the above
E. All of the above

9.49. Patients with acute inferior MI may suffer which of the following types of atrio-ventricular (AV) conduction problems?
   A. Generally, first degree or Mobitz type I, but sometimes worse
   B. Generally intranodal problem due to ischemia or increased vagal tone
   C. May respond to atropine
   D. Rarely needs permanent pacemaker
   E. All of the above

9.50. Patients with acute MI, may get which of the following types of AV conduction problems?
   A. Generally, Mobitz type II or complete heart block
   B. Generally due to extensive myocardial ischemia
   C. In Mobitz type II AV block, atropine can make it worse by dropping the ventricular rate by increasing atrial rate
   D. Generally needs permanent pacemaker
   E. All of the above

9.51. A 62-year-old patient presents 3 weeks after an acute MI with fever and pleuritic chest pain. There was no cough, and chest X-ray showed blunting of costophrenic angles. ECG showed inferior Q waves with no ST elevation. The white cell count was 20 000 with neutrophilia; erythrocyte sedimentation rate (ESR) was 100 mm at the end of first hour. What would the best treatment be?
   A. Azithromycin
   B. Aspirin 650 mg q six hours
   C. NSAIDs
   D. Prednisone 40 mg/day
   E. None of the above

9.52. In a patient with acute anterior MI, post-primary PCI, and an EF of 30%, which of the following may reduce the risk of death in the ensuing three months?
   A. Beta blocker             C. rf-Sotalol
   B. Amiodarone               D. Flecainide

9.53. Which of the following statements about depression post MI are true?
   A. It is common
   B. It is associated with an increase in mortality
   C. It is associated with poor medication compliance
   D. Selective serotonin reuptake inhibitors improve survival
   E. All of the above
   F. B and D only are correct.

9.54. Which of the following statements are true about DAPT after an acute MI?
   A. DAPT reduces mortality only during the first year
   B. DAPT may reduce mortality beyond one year post MI
   C. DAPT reduces mortality beyond one year in only those with DES
   D. None of the above.

9.55. The results of the DAPT trial support the use of DAPT post MI even after 12 months. Which of the following were additional observations with use of DAPT?
   A. The rate of stent thrombosis was reduced beyond 12 months
   B. Risk of MI in nonstented areas was reduced
   C. There was a higher risk of bleeding
   D. All of the above

9.56. The PLATO trial (comparing clopidogrel with ticagrelor after ACS) showed which of the following?
  A. Ticagrelor was associated with reduced major adverse cardiac and cerebrovascular events (MACCEs) after ACS compared with clopidogrel
  B. Risk of major bleeding was similar for both agents overall
  C. Risk of intracranial bleeding was higher with ticagrelor
  D. Risk of MI was lower with ticagrelor, but stroke risk was similar
  E. All of the above

9.57. The TOTAL trial randomized patients undergoing primary PCI for STEMI to thrombectomy versus no thrombectomy. What were the findings?
  A. Thrombectomy did not reduce the primary end point of death, MI, stroke, and class IV HF
  B. Stroke risk was increased in thrombectomy patients
  C. No benefit of thrombectomy in the subset with high thrombus burden
  D. Bailout thrombectomy needed in 8% of non-thrombectomy group
  E. All of the above.

9.58. The MATRIX-ACCESS trial shows which of the following?
  A. The rate of major adverse cardiac events was similar between radial and femoral access approaches
  B. Net adverse cardiac events were lower in radial approach strategy
  C. Risk of bleeding was lower with a radial approach
  D. Major bleeding was associated with higher mortality
  E. All of the above are accurate

9.59. The DANAMI 3 trial tested the hypothesis that performing PCI on non-infarct-related artery (IRA) during primary PCI for STEMI may improve outcome. Which of the following were the results?
  A. The primary end point (death, MI, subsequent revascularization) was reduced by about 50% by performing PCI on non-IRA
  B. Only MI was reduced by performing PCI on non-IRA
  C. Only angina and repeat revascularization was reduced by performing PCI on non-IRA
  D. There was no difference in outcome by performing PCI on non-IRA

9.60. Based on the After Eighty trial, primary PCI for STEMI in the elderly,
  A. Increased stroke risk
  B. Reduced MACCEs
  C. Did not affect outcomes
  D. None of the above

9.61. Which of the following mechanical complications, after acute myocardial infarction, presents as sudden cardiac death?
  A. Papillary muscle rupture
  B. Pseudoaneurysm
  C. Left ventricular free wall rupture
  D. Ventricular septal defect

9.62. Which of the following cardiac biomarkers is the first to rise in acute myocardial infarction?
A. Creatinine kinase
B. Myoglobin
C. Troponin
D. ESR

9.63. Which of the following medications does not require activation through the CYP2C19 pathway?
A. Ticagrelor
B. Prasugrel
C. Clopidogrel

9.64. A 64-year-old man with history of CAD presents to the ER with NSTEMI. He undergoes coronary angiography and receives a DES to the mid LAD. He was previously on prasugrel, but it has been decided to switch him to ticagrelor. Which of the following is the most appropriate dose?
A. 180 mg immediately after the procedure, followed by 90 mg BID
B. No loading dose, start 90 mg BID
C. 180 mg immediately after the procedure, followed by 90 mg daily
D. Start 90 mg daily

9.65. A 72-year-old female presents to your office for pre-operative evaluation prior to a hernia repair. She had an MI six years previously which required placement of a drug-eluting stent. She has been on clopidogrel ever since. Which of the following is the correct mechanism of action of clopidogrel?
A. Inhibition of platelet aggregation through the reversible binding of its active metabolite to the P2Y12 class of ADP receptors
B. Inhibition of platelet aggregation through the irreversible binding of its active metabolite to the P2Y12 class of ADP receptors
C. Inhibition of platelet aggregation through the reversible binding of its inactive metabolite to the P2Y12 class of ADP receptors
D. Inhibition of platelet aggregation through the irreversible binding of its inactive metabolite to the P2Y12 class of ADP receptors

9.66. A 54-year-old man presents with 10 out of 10 pressure-like chest pain. His ECG shows ST elevations in leads II, III, and AVF. Soon after his presentation, he develops an intermittent high-grade AV block. What is the etiology of this rhythm?
A. Diffuse myocardial ischemia
B. Decreased perfusion of the AV node
C. Vasovagal response
D. Cardiogenic shock

9.67. A 77-year-old female presents 7 days after NSTEMI with acute shortness of breath. She has chest pain. Her oxygen saturation is 78%. Echocardiogram shows severe mitral regurgitation. Which artery was likely involved in her myocardial infarction?
A. Left anterior descending
B. Left circumflex artery
C. Diagonal
D. Posterior descending

**9.68.** Which of the following WOULD NOT result in an elevated troponin level?
A. Spontaneous coronary artery dissection
B. Coronary vasospasm
C. Pericarditis
D. Coronary embolus

**9.69.** A 97-year-old male presents with urosepsis. He is on several vasopressors. A troponin level is checked and is 1.95 (normal <0.005). Which of the following would describe this troponin elevation?
A. Type 1 MI
B. Type 2 MI
C. Type 3 MI
D. Type 4 MI
E. Type 5 MI

**9.70.** Which of the following DOES NOT meet criteria for ST-segment elevation myocardial infarction?
A. New ST-segment elevation of 0.1 mV in V4, V5, and V6.
B. In a patient with LBBB, ST-segment depression of 2 mm in leads V1, V2, or V3
C. New ST-segment elevation of 0.1 mV in leads V2 and V3
D. In a patient with LBBB, ST-segment elevation of 2 mm that is discordant with the QRS complex

**9.71.** A 57-year-old male with history of hypertension, hyperlipidemia and TIA presents with NSTEMI. He undergoes coronary angiography and receives a drug-eluting stent to the mid-RCA. Which anti-platelet therapy is contraindicated in this patient?
A. Ticagrelor
B. Aspirin
C. Prasugrel
D. Clopidogrel

**9.72.** Which of the following is not included in the TIMI scoring system?
A. Age greater than 65 years
B. History of hypertension, hyperlipidemia, tobacco use
C. Beta blocker use in the last seven days
D. Positive cardiac markers

**9.73.** What does the TIMI risk score assess?
A. 30-day mortality for patients with unstable angina or non-ST elevation MI
B. 15-day in-hospital mortality for patients with non-ST elevation MI
C. 30-day mortality for patients with ST-elevation MI
D. 15-day in-hospital mortality for patients with ST elevation MI

**9.74.** In the TIMI risk score, one point is given for how many episodes of severe angina over a 24-hour period?
A. Greater than one
B. Greater than two
C. Greater than three
D. Greater than four

9.75. Which of the following is NOT true regarding ST-elevation MI and non-ST-elevation MI?

A. ST-elevation MI results from complete and prolonged occlusion of an epicardial coronary artery

B. STEMI and NSTEMI cam both present with similar symptoms

C. Only STEMI patients must undergo coronary angiography emergently

D. NSTEMI is the result of severe coronary artery narrowing or transient occlusion.

9.76. Acute coronary syndrome is increasingly common in the female gender.

A. True

B. False

9.77. A 56-year-old male presents with chest pain not relieved by rest. He has a 5-year history of controlled stable angina. He has no ischemic changes on ECG. His cardiac troponin is elevated. Which of the following is the best diagnosis?

A. STEMI

B. NSTEMI

C. Unstable angina

D. Stable angina

9.78. Which of the following is contraindicated in Prinzmetal angina?

A. Calcium antagonists

B. Nitrates

C. Beta blockers

D. ACE inhibitors

9.79. A 67-year-old female presents with recurrent typical angina. She undergoes coronary angiography, which shows a 30% narrowing of the proximal LAD and a myocardial blush grade of 2. What is the most appropriate treatment for this patient?

A. Reassurance

B. Coronary artery bypass grafting

C. Prophylactic PCI of the proximal LAD

D. Treatment with ASA, clopidogrel, as well as antianginal therapy

9.80. Which of the following cardiac enzymes remain in the circulation the longest after myocardial infarction?

A. CK-MB

B. Myoglobin

C. Total CK

D. Troponin

9.81. After a large myocardial infarction, when does the troponin level peak?

A. 24–36 hours

B. 3–4 days

C. 2–4 hours

D. 6–7 days

9.82. Which of the following is NOT an indication for emergent coronary angiography?

A. A 44-year-old male with chest pain and new LBBB

B. A 67-year-old female with chest pain, hypotension, and T-wave inversions in anterolateral leads

C. A 34-year-old male with chest pain accompanied by troponin elevation. The chest pain is relieved by learning forward

D. A 44-year-old male with chest pain, hypotension, and new ST changes in inferior leads

9.83. Which of the following is NOT included in the original Sgarbossa criteria?

A. Concordant ST elevation >1 mm in leads with a positive QRS complex

B. Concordant ST elevation >1 mm in V4–V6

C. Concordant ST depression >1 mm in V1–V3

D. Excessively discordant ST elevation >5 mm in leads with a negative QRS complex

9.84. When is a bare metal stent preferred in patients?

A. Left main disease

B. History of diabetes

C. High risk of bleeding

D. In-stent restenosis

E. None of the above.

9.85. Which of the following is NOT typically a clinical presentation of acute coronary syndrome?

A. Diaphoresis

B. Shortness of breath

C. Headache

D. Diarrhea

## Answers

9.1. A. A normal echocardiogram (ECG) in the emergency room (ER) rules out myocardial infarction (MI).

This statement is wrong, as about 10% of acute non-ST-elevation MI (NSTEMI) may have a normal ECG. ECG changes could be dynamic, where even ST elevation can come and go.

9.2. H. All of the above.

Each has a score of 1 and the maximum total score is 7. The higher the score, the higher the 14-day event rate, progressively increasing from 4.7 to 40.9%. Note that ACS despite acetylsalicylic acid (ASA), ST deviation and positive cardiac markers portend high risk (Antman et al. 2000).

9.3. D. None of the above.

In a multicenter chest pain study, ACS was present in 22, 13, and 7%, respectively for choices A, B, and C.

9.4. B. 10 minutes.

9.5. B. Systolic BP.

The higher the systolic BP, the lower the risk. For others, higher numbers correlate with higher mortality (Granger et al. 2003).

9.6. E. All of the above.

This is because of risk of serious hypotension. Clinical scenario in B is indicative of right ventricular (RV) infarct.

9.7. C. Neither traditional NSAIDs nor COX-2 inhibitors should be used.
This is because of potential risk of platelet aggregation. Also, these may be associated with higher risk of gastrointestinal (GI) bleeding.

9.8. C. Short-acting nifedipine without a beta blocker.
This is because of the risk of reflex tachycardia.

9.9. B. 162 or 325 mg nonenteric coated chewed.

9.10. D. Both A and B.

9.11. C. One year.

9.12. D. A and B.
That is, ACEIs or ARBs in those who are ACEI intolerant, and aldosterone blocking agent provided creatinine is <2 mg/dl and K is <5 meq/l. Diltiazem reduced the reinfarction rate in NSTEMI in the diltiazem reinfarction trial when EF was >40%. Also, in this trial, a beta blocker was not used and this was before the days of statin therapy.

9.13. F. All of the above.
These are all high-risk markers.

9.14. C. Both A and B are correct.

9.15. E. All of the above.

9.16. A. Fondaparinux.
This is because of risk of catheter thrombosis.

9.17. E. All of the above.

9.18. B. Aspirin should not be stopped.
Should continue 81–324 mg/day.

9.19. D. A and B are correct.

9.20. E. None of the above.

9.21. E. All of the above.

9.22. D. All of the above.

9.23. E. All of the above.

9.24. B. Beta blocker.
This is because of possible risk of unopposed alpha action of cocaine on the coronary artery worsening spasm. The same principle also holds for amphetamine-induced ACS.

9.25. D. All of the above.
See discussions on BRAVE-3, ON-TIME 2 and Horizons-AMI trials in Box 9.1.

9.26. E. At the time of primary PCI or those with large thrombus burden.

9.27. E. All of the above.
The low-risk patients presenting early are suitable candidates. These patients may even be treated medically and noninvasively risk stratified unless there are high-risk features during hospital stay.

9.28. A. Immediate transfer to the PCI facility.
This is a high-risk patient and rapid PCI is in order. Also, the history of TIA poses a contraindication for thrombolytic therapy.

9.29. A. Full-dose thrombolytic and transfer to PCI facility.

This is a high-risk patient with anterior MI, pulmonary edema, and ACS, despite aspirin. In view of the considerable delay in transfer to a PCI facility and presentation within four hours of chest pain, administering thrombolytic with immediate arrangement to transfer to a PCI facility is appropriate as there are no contraindications for thrombolytics. See discussion on TRANSFER-AMI trial in Box 9.1. Early presentation, delay in transfer, and lack of contraindications for thrombolytics support thrombolytic therapy followed by PCI as soon as possible.

9.30. C. Glucose <180 mg/dl.

The 2009 guidelines recommend this conventional target rather than a tight control of normal glucose recommended in the 2004 guidelines. There are no trials comparing these two strategies in acute MI, but a large, randomized trial in intensive care unit patients (NICE-SUGAR) indicated higher mortality in the intensive glucose control arm.

9.31. C. Discontinue metformin.

Discontinue metformin in view of radiocontrast agent administration to reduce risk of lactic acidosis. Insulin infusion is no longer recommended for tight glycemic control in acute MI any more as per 2009 guidelines.

9.32. D. All of the above.

The choices are self-explanatory. Benefit is seen in those who present early, have a large thrombus burden, and large territory is jeopardized. The EXPIRA trial, which randomized 175 patients, showed greater myocardial blush, greater 90-minutes ST segment resolution, and smaller infarct size at 3 months in those undergoing thrombus aspiration.

9.33. B. A bare-metal stent (BMS).

This is in view of the fact that the patient may not be able to reliably take clopidogrel for one year (uninsured) and the fact that the stent size is 4 mm and short with low-risk of restenois. A DES is superior to a BMS in diabetics in those with long lesions and small vessels (<3 mm). There was no difference in outcomes between BMS and DES except rates of later ischemia-driven target vessel revascularization (HORIZONS-AMI trial).

9.34. A. Desired door-to-needle is <30 minutes and door-to-balloon time is <90 minutes.

9.35. E. All of the above.

All of these may speed up time to reperfusion.

9.36. E. All of the above.

The first trials to show the benefit of thrombolytics over placebo in STEMI included the British ISIS-2 trial and Italian GISSI trial.

9.37. E. All of the above.

This is provided a catheterization laboratory is available with expert operator and door or contact-to-balloon time is likely to be <90 minutes.

9.38. E. All of the above.

In view of a high risk of bleeding into brain. In addition, suspected aortic dissection or active bleeding (menses is not) are contraindications.

Chapter 9

9.39. F. All of the above.

9.40. E. All of the above.

In addition, there is a risk of allergy with streptokinase and should not be repeated in the next 6–12 months.

9.41. A. Reduced death with alteplase.

There was no difference in reinfarction rates. There was a trend to increased intracranial hemorrhage with alteplase.

9.42. B. Normal saline and dobutamine infusion if BP is still low.

The patient has classical RV infarct with raised jugular venous pressure, Kussmaul's sign, and clear lungs in the setting of inferior MI. Other signs may include ST elevation in right chest leads. Intravenous fluids help improve RV output, and dobutamine will recruit noninfarcted RV myocardium to increase its performance. BP may plummet with diuresis and NTG.

9.43. D. Potential for myocardial rupture.

The focal pericarditis causing recurrent ST elevation may be due to slow seepage of blood through a softened myocardium and is a marker of high risk of rupture. Dressler's syndrome occurs after two to three weeks. An echocardiogram would be valuable, and this may show intramural hematoma, pericardial fluid, or strands, which are risk factors for threatened myocardial rupture.

9.44. F. All of the above.

All are recognized risk factors for myomalacia cordis. In addition, being on steroids or NSAIDs and hypertension may predispose to it. The rupture could be acute or blowout (which results in immediate death), subacute (causing tamponade), or chronic (causing a pseudoaneurysm).

9.45. D. All of the above.

The rupture does not generally occur in the center of infarct. Adjacent hyperkinesis near a dyskinetic segment may promote rupture.

9.46. C. Papillary muscle rupture.

In view of flash pulmonary edema and hypotension. Hypotension combined with high left atrial pressure and large regurgitant orifice may not result in an MR murmur because of low driving pressure and lack of turbulence in the MR jet. Acute stent thrombosis is unlikely in view of the lack of ST elevation. Acute pulmonary embolism and RV infarct do cause pulmonary edema.

9.47. D. All of the above.

Posteromedial papillary muscle has blood supply from right coronary artery only and is more likely to rupture.

9.48. D. None of the above.

There is no benefit for prophylactic lidocaine. The Lown grading of ventricular arrhythmias as a basis for prophylactic lidocaine has not been supported by randomized trials.

9.49. E. All of the above.

9.50. E. All of the above.

9.51. B. Aspirin 650 mg q six hours.

This is classic Dressler's syndrome, which is thought to be autoimmune, occurring in about 1% of MIs. NSAIDs and steroids are best avoided as they may impair the left ventricle healing process and may promote rupture.

9.52. A. Beta blocker.

See details on CAST, SWORD, CAMIAT, and EMIAT in Box 9.1.

9.53. E. All of the above.

9.54. B. DAPT may reduce mortality beyond one year post MI.

Please see results of DAPT and TIMI-54 trials in Box 9.1.

9.55. D. All of the above.

See DAPT trial details in Box 9.1.

9.56. E. All of the above.

See details of PLATO trial in Box 9.1.

9.57. E. All of the above.

See Box 9.1.

9.58. E. All of the above are accurate.

Please see Box 9.1.

9.59. A. The primary end point (death, MI, subsequent revascularization) was reduced by about 50% by performing PCI on non-IRA.

See Box 9.1.

9.60. B. Reduced MACCEs.

See Box 9.1.

9.61. C. Left ventricular free wall rupture

LV free wall rupture often presents with sudden cardiac arrest. It is a dreaded complication which presents as hypotension and can quickly progress to PEA.

9.62. B. Myoglobin

Though rarely tested for in modern times, myoglobin is the first measurable protein in the blood after an acute myocardial infarction.

9.63. A. Ticagrelor

Ticagrelor is an orally administered PY12 receptor antagonist which reversibly and non-competitively binds to the P2Y12 receptor at a site distinct from ADP. Unlike prasugrel and clopidogrel, it does not require activation through the CYP2C19 pathway.

9.64. A. 180 mg immediately after the procedure, followed by 90 mg BID

This patient was previously on prasugrel and the decision has now been made to switch him to ticagrelor. A loading dose must be used when switching patients between antiplatelet medications. Ticagrelor has a loading dose of 180 mg following by 90 mg every 12 hours.

9.65. B. Inhibition of platelet aggregation through the irreversible binding of its active metabolite to the P2Y12 class of ADP receptors

Clopidogrel is a medication which works by inhibiting platelet activation by binding of its active metabolite to the P2Y12 class of ADP receptors

**9.66.** B. Decreased perfusion of the atrioventricular node

The atrioventricular node has a dual supply from the LAD and RCA, so the block is transient.

**9.67.** D. Posterior descending artery

The posterior descending artery is the only supply of the posteromedial muscle. A PDA infarct can thus cause severe mitral regurgitation as a late complication. The anterolateral papillary muscle has a dual blood supply, both from the LAD and LCX.

**9.68.** C. Pericarditis

Pericarditis does not involve the myocardium and, thus, does not present with a troponin elevation.

**9.69.** B. Type 2 MI

This patient is experiencing a Type 2 MI which occurs when there is a supply-demand mismatch. The patient is hypotensive due to sepsis, causing decreased perfusion to the coronary arteries.

**9.70.** C. New ST-segment elevation of 0.1 mV in leads V2 and V3

To qualify as a STEMI, the ST-segment in V2 and V3 must be 0.2 mV or greater, for men >40 and 0.25 mm for men <40 and >0.15 mm for women.

**9.71.** C. Prasugrel

Prasugrel should be avoided in patients with prior history of stroke or TIA. This was established in the TRITON-TIMI trial in 2007.

**9.72.** C. Beta blocker use in the last seven days

Aspirin use in the last seven days is included in the TIMI scoring system, not beta blocker use.

**9.73.** A. 30-day mortality for patients with unstable angina or non-ST elevation MI

The TIMI risk score is a well-established system to assess the 30-day mortality of patients how are presenting with unstable angina or NSTEMI

**9.74.** B. Greater than two

In the TIMI risk scoring system, one point is given for greater than two episodes of angina over a 24-hour period.

**9.75.** C. Only STEMI patients must undergo coronary angiography emergently

NSTEMI patients who are hemodynamically unstable or have refractory chest pain also qualify for emergent coronary evaluation. By the guidelines, these patients should undergo angiography within two hours. NSTEMI with hemodynamic instability carries with it a 50% in-hospital mortality.

**9.76.** A. True

Over the course of the last 20 years, women have seen an increased incidence of ACS. This is attributed to the rise in hypertension, diabetes, and obesity.

**9.77.** B. NSTEMI

This patient with a history of unstable angina now has a troponin elevation. This qualifies as an NSTEMI. If the patient had relentless chest pain without ECG changes or a troponin elevation, this would be unstable angina.

**9.78.** C. Beta blockers

Beta blockers, especially those with non-selective adrenoreceptor blocking effects, are contraindicated in patients with Prinzmetal angina as they can sometimes cause increased spasm leading to increased anginal symptoms.

**9.79.** D. Treatment with ASA, clopidogrel, as well as antianginal therapy

Microvascular angina is more common in women than men. It is treated the same way as classic coronary artery disease. WISE trial.

**9.80.** D. Troponin

Troponin levels can remain elevated for 7–14 days after myocardial infarction.

**9.81.** A. 24–36 hours

Troponin levels peak 24–36 hours after acute myocardial infarction and remain in the circulation for up to 7–14 days.

**9.82.** C. A 34-year-old male with chest pain accompanied by troponin elevation. The chest pain is relieved by learning forward.

A young patient without significant risk factors who presents with chest pain while leaning forward is suspicious for pericarditis. An elevated troponin indicates this may be myopericarditis.

**9.83.** B. Concordant ST elevation >1 mm in V4–V6

Sgarbossa criteria is used to identify STEMI in a patient with a left bundle branch block. This includes concordant ST elevation >1 mm in leads with a positive QRS complex, concordant ST depression >1 mm in V1–V3, and excessively discordant ST elevation >5 mm in leads with a negative QRS complex.

**9.84.** E. Current trials Onyx ONE clear study and POEM both showed noninferiority of 1 month DAPT vs 6–12-month DAPT.

**9.85.** D. Diarrhea

Acute coronary syndrome can present with a diverse array of symptoms including typical anginal chest pain, shortness of breath, dizziness, lightheadedness, diaphoresis, headache, anxiety, and nausea. However, diarrhea is not a known symptom of acute coronary syndrome.

---

**Box 9.1  Key Trials**

---

- CAST (The Cardiac Arrhythmia Suppression Trial (CAST) Investigators 1989): Cardiac Arrhythmia Suppression Trial based on premature ventricular complexes killer hypothesis. Strong type I antiarrhythmics (flecainide, encainide, and moricizine) were tested against placebo after acute MI. The study was prematurely stopped as these antiarrhythmics tripled the mortality through their proarrhythmic effects on ischemic substrate.
- SWORD trial (Waldo et al. 1996): d-Sotalol versus placebo in acute MI with EF <40%. Trial was prematurely stopped because of increased mortality with d-sotalol.
- CAMIAT (Cairns et al. 1997): Canadian trial testing amiodarone after acute MI. No reduction in mortality.
- EMIAT (Julian et al. 1997): European trial testing amiodarone after acute MI. No reduction in mortality.

- ISIS-1 trial (ISIS-1 (First International Study of Infarct Survival) Collaborative Group 1986): The First International Study of Infarct Survival. A placebo-controlled trial of the beta-blocker atenolol. It recruited 16 027 patients and was completed in 1985. Atenolol reduced mortality.
- ISIS-2 trial (ISIS-2 (Second International Study of Infarct Survival) Collaborative Group 1988): The Second International Study of Infarct Survival. A 2×2 factorial placebo-controlled trial of aspirin and the thrombolytic drug streptokinase. It recruited 17 187 patients. Aspirin and streptokinase reduced all-cause mortality.
- ISIS-3 trial (ISIS-3 (Third International Study of Infarct Survival) Collaborative Group 1992): The Third International Study of Infarct Survival. A 3×2 factorial trial that compared the three thrombolytic drugs streptokinase, tPA, and anistreplase with each other, and also compared the anticoagulant heparin with no heparin. All patients were also given aspirin. It recruited 41 299 patients. No significant difference in six-month survival was apparent overall or in the subset. Streptokinase versus tPA: tPA was associated with significantly fewer reports of allergy causing persistent symptoms and of hypotension requiring drug treatment, and with significantly more reports of non-cerebral bleeds, but not of transfused bleeds. There was a significant excess of strokes with tPA and being attributed to cerebral hemorrhage. Fewer reinfarctions were observed with tPA. There was no significant mortality difference during days 0 and 35 either among all randomized patients, and no difference in six-month survival was apparent.
- GISSI-1 trial (Gruppo Italiano per lo Studio della Streptochinasi nell'Infarto Miocardico (GISSI) 1 1986): 17 000 patients with acute MI randomized. Thrombolytic treatment with streptokinase significantly reduced mortality compared with placebo 10.7% SK versus 13% controls, for an 18% reduction ($p = 0.0002$, relative risk (RR) 0.81, 95% confidence interval (CI) 0.72–0.90).
- GUSTO trial (The GUSTO Investigators 1993): 41 021 patients with evolving MI were randomly assigned to four different thrombolytic strategies, consisting of the use of streptokinase and subcutaneous heparin, streptokinase and intravenous heparin, accelerated tPA and intravenous heparin, or a combination of streptokinase plus tPA with intravenous heparin. Accelerated tPA, given with intravenous heparin, provides a survival benefit over previous standard thrombolytic regimens.
- PAMI trial (The Global Use of Strategies to Open Occluded Coronary Arteries in Acute Coronary Syndromes (GUSTO IIb) Angioplasty Substudy Investigators 1997): 1138 patients with acute STEMI within 12 hours randomized to tPA versus primary angioplasty. Angioplasty was superior for primary study end point, which was a composite outcome of death, nonfatal reinfarction, and nonfatal disabling stroke at 30 days
- VANQWISH trial (Boden et al. 1998): In NSTEMI, early conservative and early invasive strategies were equivalent.
- FRISC-II trial (Lagerqvist et al. 2006): In 2500 NSTEMI patients, early invasive therapy showed superiority over early conservative therapy and the benefit persisted at five years.
- SHOCK trial (Hochman et al. 1999): 152 patients in cardiogenic shock post MI randomized. Emergency revascularization did not significantly reduce overall mortality at 30 days. However, after six months, there was a significant survival benefit.

Early revascularization should be strongly considered for patients with acute MI complicated by cardiogenic shock.

- PURSUIT trial (The PURSUIT Trial Investigators 1998): 11 000 patients with ACS with ST depression or raised cardiac markers randomized. Inhibition of platelet aggregation with eptifibatide reduced the incidence of the composite end point of death or nonfatal MI in patients with acute coronary syndromes who did not have persistent ST-segment elevation.
- PRISM-PLUS (Platelet Receptor Inhibition in Ischemic Syndrome Management in Patients Limited by Unstable Signs and Symptoms (PRISM-PLUS) Study Investigators 1998): 1915 patients with ACS randomized. When administered with heparin and aspirin, the platelet GP IIb/IIIa receptor inhibitor tirofiban was associated with a lower incidence of ischemic events in patients with ACSs than in patients who received only heparin and aspirin.
- BRAVE-3 trial (Mehilli et al. 2009): 800 patients with STEMI receiving DAPT were randomized to abciximab versus placebo. At 30 days, there was no difference in composites of death, recurrent MI, stroke, or urgent revascularization of infarct-related arteries (5% abciximab, 3.3% placebo).
- ON-TIME 2 trial (Van't Hof et al. 2008): 984 patients with acute STEMI randomized to tirofiban in addition to DAPT. Tirofiban treatment was associated with more rapid ST segment resolution, but no improvement in TIMI3 flow. No difference in 30-day mortality, MI, or urgent target vessel revascularization.
- Horizons-AMI trial (Stone et al. 2008). 3322 patients with acute STEMI receiving DAPT randomized to UFH plus GP IIb/IIIa inhibitor versus bivalirudin alone. At 30 days, total major bleeds and adverse events were lower in the bivalirudin arm.
- TRITON-TIMI 38 trial (Wiviott et al. 2007): 13 608 patients with moderate- or high-risk ACS were randomized to clopidogrel (300 mg loading followed by 75 mg/day) versus prasugrel (60 mg loading followed by 10 mg/day). Average follow up is 14.5 months. Prasugrel was associated with significant reduction in composite end points of death due to cardiovascular causes, nonfatal MI, nonfatal stroke (9.9% versus 12.1%). The difference was largely due to reduction in nonfatal MI. Prasugrel was associated with higher rates of major bleeds. The US Food and Drug Administration (FDA) cautions against use of prasugrel in those aged >75 years or weigh <60 kg. In those weighing <60 kg, the suggested dose by FDA is 5 mg/day. Prasugrel, as a part of DAPT, is contraindicated in those with prior stroke or TIA because of a higher risk of intracranial bleeds. ASSENT-4 trial (Assessment of the Safety and Efficacy of a New Treatment Strategy with Percutaneous Coronary Intervention (ASSENT-4 PCI) Investigators 2006): facilitated the PCI trial in STEMI. Fibrinolytic treatment before PCI was associated with higher risk of in-hospital death (6% versus 3%). This study is criticized for not using heparin infusion after bolus, lack of an upfront loading dose of clopidogrel, and prohibition of the use of GP IIb/IIIa during PCI.
- FINESSE trial (Ellis et al. 2004): No difference in outcomes of use of abciximab plus reteplase versus abciximab alone before PCI for STEMI.
- TRANSFER-AMI trial (Cantor et al. 2009): High-risk STEMI presenting to non-PCI facility were randomized to pharmacoinvasive arm (tenectaplace, ASA, heparin, clopidogrel,

and immediate transfer for PCI) versus standard treatment arm (same medical treatment, but rescue PCI only). Pharmacoinvasive arm was superior (events 11% versus 17%). DAPT trial (Mauri et al. 2014): clopidogrel or prasugrel added to ASA post MI versus ASA alone between 12 and 30 months post MI in 9961 patients. DAPT reduced stent thrombosis (0.4% versus 1.4%) and MACCEs (even MI in nonstented area) compared with ASA alone. DAPT was associated with higher risk of bleeding.

- TIMI-54 trial (Bonaca et al. 2015): 21 000 patients post MI 1 year randomized to ASA alone, ASA plus ticagrelor 90 mg BID or ASA plus ticagrelor 60 mg BID. MACCEs 9% in ASA alone group versus 7.8% in DAPT group at three years with no increase in intracranial bleed. "In patients with a myocardial infarction more than one year previously, treatment with ticagrelor significantly reduced the risk of cardiovascular death, myocardial infarction, or stroke and increased the risk of major bleeding."

- PLATO (Wallentin et al. 2009): 18 000 patients with ACS randomized to clopidogrel versus ticagrelor after loading. "At 12 months, the primary end point – a composite of death from vascular causes, myocardial infarction, or stroke – had occurred in 9.8% of patients receiving ticagrelor as compared with 11.7% of those receiving clopidogrel (hazard ratio, 0.84; 95% confidence interval [CI], 0.77 to 0.92; $P < 0.001$)"

- TOTAL trial (Jolly et al. 2015): A global trial enrolled 10 732 patients undergoing primary PCI for STEMI. Randomized to aspiration thrombectomy versus no thrombectomy. There was no difference in the primary end point of cardiovascular death, MI, shock, and HF class IV. Bail out thrombectomy in 8% of no thrombectomy group. Thrombectomy was associated with higher rates of stroke.

- MATRIX-Access trial (Valgimigli et al. 2015): 8404 patients with acute coronary syndrome, with or without ST-segment elevation, were randomly assigned "to radial (4197) or femoral (4207) access for coronary angiography and percutaneous coronary intervention. 369 (8.8%) patients with radial access had major adverse cardiovascular events, compared with 429 (10.3%) patients with femoral access (rate ratio [RR] 0.85, 95% CI 0.74–0.99; $p = 0.0307$), non-significant at $a$ of 0.025. 410 (9.8%) patients with radial access had net adverse clinical events compared with 486 (11.7%) patients with femoral access (0.83, 95% CI 0.73–0.96; $p = 0.0092$). The difference was driven by BARC [Bleeding Academic Research Consortium] major bleeding unrelated to coronary artery bypass graft surgery (1.6% vs 2.3%, RR 0.67, 95% CI 0.49–0.92; $p = 0.013$) and all-cause mortality (1.6% vs 2.2%, RR 0.72, 95% CI 0.53–0.99; $p = 0.045$)."

- DANAMI 3 (Engstrom et al. 2015): Danish trial testing the hypothesis that PCI of significant lesion in non-IRA (>50% and FFR <0.8 or >90% lesion) during primary PCI for STEMI improves outcomes; 627 patients randomized. Primary end point of death, MI subsequent to revascularization, was 13% in non-IRA PCI arm compared with 22% in IRA-only PCI arm ($p = 0.0004$).

- After Eighty trial (Tegn et al. 2016): 457 patients with STEMI in patients >80 years randomized to primary PCI versus medical treatment. 50% reduction of mortality in primary PCI arm.

# References

Antman, E.M., Cohen, M., Bernink, P.J. et al. (2000). The TIMI risk score for unstable angina/ non-ST elevation MI: a method for prognostication and therapeutic decision making. *JAMA* 284 (7): 835–842.

Assessment of the Safety and Efficacy of a New Treatment Strategy with Percutaneous Coronary Intervention (ASSENT-4 PCI) Investigators (2006). Primary versus tenecteplase-facilitated percutaneous coronary intervention in patients with ST-segment elevation acute myocardial infarction (ASSENT-4 PCI): randomised trial. *Lancet* 367 (9510): 569–578.

Boden, W.E., O'Rourke, R.A., Crawford, M.H. et al. (1998). Outcomes in patients with acute non-Q-wave myocardial infarction randomly assigned to an invasive as compared with a conservative management strategy. *The New England Journal of Medicine* 338: 1785–1792.

Bonaca, M.P., Bhatt, D.L., Cohen, M. et al. (2015). Long-term use of ticagrelor in patients with prior myocardial infarction. *The New England Journal of Medicine* 372 (19): 1791–1800. https://doi.org/10.1056/NEJMoa1500857.

Cairns, J.A., Connolly, S.J., Roberts, R., and Gent, M. (1997). Randomised trial of outcome after myocardial infarction in patients with frequent or repetitive ventricular premature depolari-sations: CAMIAT. *Lancet* 349 (9053): 675–682. [Erratum: *Lancet* (1997) 349(9067): 1776].

Cantor, W.J., Fitchett, D., Borgundvaag, B. et al. (2009). Routine early angioplasty after fibrinoly-sis for acute myocardial infarction. *The New England Journal of Medicine* 360 (26): 2705–2718. https://doi.org/10.1056/NEJMoa0808276.

Ellis, S.G., Armstrong, P., Betriu, A. et al. (2004). Facilitated percutaneous coronary intervention versus primary percutaneous coronary intervention: design and rationale of the Facilitated Intervention with Enhanced Reperfusion Speed to Stop Events (FINESSE) trial. *American Heart Journal* 147 (4): E16.

Engstrom, T., Kelbak, H., Helqvist, S. et al. (2015). Complete revascularisation versus treatment of the culprit lesion only in patients with ST-segment elevation myocardial infarction and multivessel disease (DANAMI-3—PRIMULTI): an open-label, randomised controlled trial. *Lancet* 386 (9994): 665–671.

Granger, C.B., Goldber, R.J., Dabbous, O. et al. (2003). Predictors of hospital mortality in the global registry of acute coronary events. *Archives of Internal Medicine* 163 (19): 2345–2353.

Gruppo Italiano per lo Studio della Streptochinasi nell'Infarto Miocardico (GISSI) 1 (1986). Effectiveness of intravenous thrombolytic treatment in acute myocardial infarction. *Lancet* 327 (8478): 397–402.

Hochman, J.S., Sleeper, L.A., Webb, J.G. et al. (1999). Early revascularization in acute myocar-dial infarction complicated by cardiogenic shock. *The New England Journal of Medicine* 1341 (9): 625–634.

ISIS-1 (First International Study of Infarct Survival) Collaborative Group (1986). Randomised trial of intravenous atenolol among 16,027 cases of suspected acute myocardial infarction: ISIS-1. *Lancet* 328 (8498): 57–66.

ISIS-2 (Second International Study of Infarct Survival) Collaborative Group (1988). Randomised trial of intravenous streptokinase, oral aspirin, both, or neither among 17,187 cases of suspected acute myocardial infarction: ISIS-2. *Lancet* 332 (8607): 349–360.

ISIS-3 (Third International Study of Infarct Survival) Collaborative Group (1992). ISIS-3: a randomised comparison of streptokinase vs tissue plasminogen activator vs anistreplase and of aspirin plus heparin vs aspirin alone among 41,299 cases of suspected acute myocardial infarction. *Lancet* 339 (8796): 753–770.

Chapter 9

Jolly, S.S., Cairns, J.A., Yusuf, S. et al. (2015). Randomized trial of primary PCI with or without routine manual thrombectomy. *The New England Journal of Medicine* 372: 1389–1398.

Julian, D.G., Camm, A.J., Frangin, G. et al. (1997). Randomised trial of effect of amiodarone on mortality in patients with left-ventricular dysfunction after recent myocardial infarction: EMIAT. *Lancet* 349 (9053): 667–674. [Errata: *Lancet* (1997) 349(9067): 1776; Lancet (1997) 349(9059): 1180].

Lagerqvist, B., Husted, S., Kontny, F. et al. (2006). 5-year outcomes in the FRISC-II randomised trial of an invasive versus a non-invasive strategy in non-ST-elevation acute coronary syndrome: a follow-up study. *Lancet* 368 (9540): 998–1004.

Mauri, L., Kereiakes, D.J., Yeh, R.W. et al. (2014). Twelve or 30 months of dual antiplatelet therapy after drug-eluting stents. *The New England Journal of Medicine* 371 (23): 2155–2166. https://doi.org/10.1056/NEJMoa1409312.

Mehilli, J., Kastrati, A., Schulz, S. et al. (2009). Abciximab in patients with acute ST-segment-elevation myocardial infarction undergoing primary percutaneous coronary intervention after clopidogrel loading: a randomized double-blind trial. *Circulation* 119 (14): 1933–1940.

Platelet Receptor Inhibition in Ischemic Syndrome Management in Patients Limited by Unstable Signs and Symptoms (PRISM-PLUS) Study Investigators (1998). Inhibition of the platelet glycoprotein IIb/IIIa receptor with tirofiban in unstable angina and non-Q-wave myocardial infarction. *The New England Journal of Medicine* 338 (21): 1488–1497. [Erratum: *The New England Journal of Medicine* (1998) 339(6): 415].

Stone, G.W., Witzenbichler, B., Guagliumi, G. et al. (2008). Bivalirudin during primary PCI in acute myocardial infarction. *The New England Journal of Medicine* 358 (21): 2218–2230. https://doi.org/10.1056/NEJMoa0708191.

Tegn, N., Abdelnoor, M., Aaberge, L. et al. (2016). Invasive versus conservative strategy in patients aged 80 years or older with non-ST-elevation myocardial infarction or unstable angina pectoris (after eighty study): an open-label randomised controlled trial. *Lancet* 387 (10023): 1057–1065.

The Cardiac Arrhythmia Suppression Trial (CAST) Investigators (1989). Preliminary report: effect of encainide and flecainide on mortality in a randomized trial of arrhythmia suppression after myocardial infarction. *The New England Journal of Medicine* 321 (6): 406–412.

The Global Use of Strategies to Open Occluded Coronary Arteries in Acute Coronary Syndromes (GUSTO IIb) Angioplasty Substudy Investigators (1997). A clinical trial comparing primary coronary angioplasty with tissue plasminogen activator for acute myocardial infarction. *The New England Journal of Medicine* 336: 1621–1628.

The GUSTO Investigators (1993). An international randomized trial comparing four thrombolytic strategies for acute myocardial infarction. *The New England Journal of Medicine* 329 (10): 673–682.

The PURSUIT Trial Investigators (1998). Inhibition of platelet glycoprotein IIb/IIIa with eptifibatide in patients with acute coronary syndromes. *The New England Journal of Medicine* 339 (7): 436–443.

Valgimigli, M., Gagnor, A., Calabro, P. et al. (2015). Radial versus femoral access in patients with acute coronary syndromes undergoing invasive management: a randomised multicentre trial. *Lancet* 385 (9986): 2465–2476. https://doi.org/10.1016/S0140-6736(15)60292-6.

Van't Hof, A.W., Ten Berg, J., Heestermans, T. et al. (2008). Prehospital initiation of tirofiban in patients with ST-elevation myocardial infarction undergoing primary angioplasty (On-TIME 2): a multicentre, double-blind, randomised controlled trial. *Lancet* 372 (9638): 537–546. https://doi.org/10.1016/S0140-6736(08)61235-0.

Chapter 9

Waldo, A.L., Camm, A.J., deRuyter, H. et al. (1996). Effect of d-sotalol on mortality in patients with left ventricular dysfunction after recent and remote myocardial infarction. *Lancet* 348 (9019): 7–12.

Wallentin, L., Becker, R.C., Budaj, A. et al. (2009). Ticagrelor versus clopidogrel in patients with acute coronary syndromes. *The New England Journal of Medicine* 361 (11): 1045–1057.

Wiviott, S.D., Braunwald, E., McCabe, C.H. et al. (2007). Prasugrel versus clopidogrel in patients with acute coronary syndromes. *The New England Journal of Medicine* 357 (20): 2001–2015.

# Chronic Coronary Artery Disease

# 10

10.1. The resting electrocardiogram (ECG) is normal in what percentage of patients with stable coronary artery disease (CAD)?
   A. About 10%
   B. About 50%
   C. About 75%
   D. 100%

10.2. The occurrence of conduction disturbances such as left bundle branch block (LBBB) and left anterior fascicular block (LAFB) are associated with which of the following?
   A. Good prognosis
   B. Poor prognosis
   C. Does not dictate prognosis
   D. None of the above

10.3. The presence of LV hypertrophy on the resting ECG in a patient with stable CAD may be suggestive of which of the following?
   A. Underlying hypertension
   B. Aortic stenosis
   C. Hypertrophic cardiomyopathy
   D. All of the above
   E. None of the above

10.4. In what percentage of patients does the resting ECG become abnormal in patients with stable CAD during an episode of angina?
   A. 100%
   B. 50%
   C. 75%
   D. 25%

10.5. What is the most common finding on the ECG in stable CAD patients during an episode of angina?
   A. ST segment depression
   B. ST segment elevation
   C. Normalization of previous ST abnormalities (pseudonormalization)
   D. None of the above

*Cardiology Board Review*, Second Edition. Ramdas G. Pai and Padmini Varadarajan.
© 2023 John Wiley & Sons Ltd. Published 2023 by John Wiley & Sons Ltd.

10.6. In a patient with chest pain and moderate probability of CAD and a normal resting ECG, what is the best test to order to evaluate for ischemia?
   A. Exercise stress ECG
   B. Exercise echo
   C. Dobutamine stress echo
   D. Stress nuclear

10.7. What is true of a negative stress ECG for a patient receiving anti-anginal medications when evaluating for ischemia?
   A. Reduces the sensitivity as a screening tool
   B. Does not have any effect on the test
   C. Increases the sensitivity as a screening tool
   D. None of the above

10.8. A stress nuclear test is helpful in which of the following situations?
   A. Abnormal resting ECG changes      C. LV hypertrophy
   B. LBBB                               D. All of the above

10.9. A pharmacological stress test can be ordered to evaluate for CAD in which of the following situations?
   A. Patients unable to exercise and achieve an adequate workload
   B. Peripheral vascular disease
   C. Patients with pulmonary disease
   D. All of the above

Chapter 10

10.10. Exercise testing in asymptomatic patients without known CAD may be appropriate in which situation?
   A. Patients with diabetes mellitus
   B. Severe coronary calcifications on electron beam computed tomography (CT)
   C. Evidence of ischemia on ambulatory ECG
   D. All of the above
   E. None of the above

10.11. Which of the following is a true statement?
   A. Stress test in females is associated with higher false-positive results compared with males
   B. Stress test in females is associated with a low rate of false-positive results compared with males
   C. Stress test in females is associated with higher rates of false-negative results compared with males
   D. Stress test in females is associated with low rates of false-negative results compared with males
   E. The results are similar in both men and women when stratified appropriately

10.12. In a patient with angina, with an intermediate to high pretest probability, with LBBB on ECG and with moderate ability for physical exercise, what is a reasonable diagnostic test to perform?
   A. Exercise stress ECG
   B. Exercise stress echo
   C. Coronary angiogram
   D. Adenosine stress cardiovascular magnetic resonance (CMR)

10.13. In a patient with angina, with intermediate pretest probability and able to perform moderate ability to function physically, what would be a reasonable test to perform?

A. Coronary angiography

B. Exercise stress ECG

C. Exercise stress echo

D. Coronary CT angiography (CCTA)

10.14. In a patient with an intermediate to high pretest probability for CAD and who is incapable of at least moderate exertion, what are the recommended tests for the diagnosis of CAD?

A. Dobutamine stress echo

B. Adenosine stress single-photon emission CT (SPECT)

C. Dobutamine stress SPECT

D. None of the above

E. All of the above

10.15. A 40-year-old woman is referred for evaluation of angina. Her physical examination is normal. Based on her history, she is at low pretest likelihood. She has severe knee pain and is unable to perform moderate physical activity. What is the best recommended diagnostic test to evaluate her angina?

A. Coronary angiogram

B. Adenosine stress CMR

C. CCTA

D. Dobutamine stress echo

E. B, C, and D

10.16. A 55-year-old male with a history of hypertension, diabetes, smoking, and family history of CAD is referred to you for evaluation of chest pain. He is unable to walk on the treadmill due to back pain. What is a reasonable diagnostic test to perform?

A. Coronary angiogram

B. Dipyridamole stress echo

C. Stress CMR

D. CCTA

10.17. A 65-year-old male is referred for evaluation of exercise-induced angina. He has a history of hypertension, diabetes mellitus, and hypercholesterolemia. He used to smoke one pack of cigarettes a day for 20 years and has quit recently. His father was diagnosed with CAD and underwent coronary artery bypass grafting (CABG) at age 68. He is on aspirin, amlodipine 10 mg daily, lisinopril 20 mg daily and Lipitor 40 mg qd. On examination, his heart rate is 60 bpm, BP 120/75 mmHg, and is otherwise unremarkable. He used to walk 2 miles a day. He now has intractable angina and is not able to perform low-intensity exercise. His primary care physician had started him on long-acting nitrates without relief. What is the best test to evaluate this patient's symptoms?

A. Exercise stress ECG

B. Exercise stress SPECT

C. Coronary angiogram

D. Dobutamine stress echo

10.18. A 63-year-old male with a history of hypertension, diabetes mellitus, hypercholesterolemia, and a past history of smoking has complaints of angina. His primary
care physician has optimized him on guideline-directed medical therapy and has
referred him to you for further evaluation. An echocardiogram is ordered and resting LV ejection fraction (EF) is 30%. What is the best test to evaluate this patient?
A. Exercise SPECT
B. Adenosine SPECT
C. Coronary angiogram
D. Exercise treadmill

10.19. A 60-year-old female with cardiac risk factors is being evaluated for ischemic heart
disease (IHD). She has complaints of new-onset angina. She is on optimal medical
therapy for hypertension, hypercholesterolemia and diabetes mellitus. She is unable to walk due to orthopedic limitations. She then has a dobutamine stress
echocardiogram, wherein she achieves 70% of her age-predicted maximum heart
rate at peak stress. What is the best approach in further evaluation of this patient?
A. Adenosine stress SPECT
B. Coronary angiogram
C. No further testing
D. Intensify medical therapy

10.20. A 69-year-old male has a history of hypertension, diabetes mellitus controlled on
long-acting insulin therapy, hypercholesterolemia, and a past history of smoking.
He is on optimal medical therapy. He has new onset of exercise-induced angina
of one month's duration. His primary care physician ordered a stress test. His
stress test was interpreted as negative. He is now referred to you for further eval-
uation. What is the best test to order?
A. No further testing
B. Stress nuclear imaging
C. Coronary angiogram
D. Adenosine stress CMR

10.21. A 59-year-old male patient with multiple cardiac risk factors and intractable
angina was referred for a coronary angiogram. His coronary angiogram revealed
a 60% stenosis in the mid LAD artery. What is the best approach in the treatment
of this patient?
A. Percutaneous coronary intervention (PCI) of the 60% stenosis with a bare-
metal stent
B. Fractional flow reserve (FFR)-guided PCI of the 60% stenosis
C. No further evaluation
D. PCI with a drug-eluting stent (DES)

10.22. A 71-year-old male underwent coronary angiogram to evaluate suspected IHD. His
angiogram revealed a 30% lesion in his mid-right coronary artery (RCA), a 40%
lesion in left circumflex artery, and a 60% stenosis of his proximal LAD artery. FFR of
the LAD artery lesion was 0.85. What is the best approach in managing this patient?
A. PCI with a DES to his proximal LAD stenosis
B. Intensify medical therapy
C. PCI of left circumflex and LAD stenosis
D. No further therapy

10.23. What is the US annual mortality rate in a middle-aged man with CAD?

A. 1.7–3%

B. 5–10%

C. 10–15%

D. None of the above

10.24. What is the US occurrence of major ischemic events in a middle-aged person with CAD?

A. 5–10%

B. 1.4–2.4%

C. 15–25%

D. None of the above

10.25. What is the five-year survival in a patient with triple-vessel disease with an LVEF of 30% and on medical therapy?

A. 70%

B. 60%

C. 40%

D. 25%

10.26. There is an increased gradient of risk based on angiographic extent of disease. Which of the following options best describes this statement?

A. True

B. False

C. Not enough information is provided

D. None of the above

10.27. In a patient with symptomatic CAD, with three-vessel CAD on coronary angiography and an EF of 40%, what would the best approach be?

A. Multivessel PCI with DES

B. Multivessel PCI with bare metal stents

C. Coronary artery bypass grafting (CABG) including left internal mammary artery (LIMA) to LAD artery

D. Medical therapy only

10.28. According to the SYNTAX trial, what was a low SYNTAX score?

A. 23 – 32

B. ≤22

C. ≥33

D. 50

10.29. In the SYNTAX trial, the combined end point of death, myocardial infarction (MI), and stroke for CABG was described as what compared with DES at five-year follow-up?

A. Equal

B. Lower

C. Higher

D. None of the above

10.30. In the SYNTAX trial, MI and repeat revascularization were described as what in the DES group compared with the CABG group?

A. Lower

B. Higher

C. Equal

D. None of the above

10.31. In the SYNTAX trial at five-year follow-up, the occurrence of major adverse cardiac and cerebrovascular events (MACCEs) was described as what in the PCI group compared with the CABG group?

A. Equal

B. Lower

C. Higher

D. Do not know

10.32. What is the best approach for revascularization in a patient with 70% distal left main coronary disease?
 A. PCI with DES
 B. CABG
 C. Medical therapy
 D. Medical therapy plus CABG

10.33. A 65-year-old male patient has complaints of severe angina. His coronary angiogram reveals a 50% mid RCA stenosis, FFR of 0.85, and a 30% left circumflex lesion. What is the best approach in treating this patient?
 A. DES to RCA stenosis only
 B. DES to RCA and left circumflex arteries
 C. CABG
 D. Guideline-directed medical therapy

10.34. In the COURAGE trial, is it true or false that PCI with optimal medical therapy reduced the risk of death or MI compared with optimal medical therapy alone?
 A. True
 B. False

10.35. A 69-year-old male with hypertension and diabetes mellitus had a coronary angiogram for symptoms of angina. His resting echocardiogram showed an EF of 35%. He underwent PCI with a DES to the mid LAD artery. He is on aspirin, clopidogrel, metoprolol, and high-intensity atorvastatin. Prior to discharge, what other medication is indicated?
 A. Hydrochlorothiazide
 B. Angiotensin-converting inhibitor
 C. Diltiazem
 D. Angiotensin receptor blocker

10.36. In the patient mentioned in Question 10.35, what is the optimal duration of dual antiplatelet therapy?
 A. 3 months
 B. 6 months
 C. 12 months
 D. 6–12 months

10.37. A 54-year-old male with CAD has complained of angina which occurs two or three times per week. He is on aspirin, long-acting metoprolol, and atorvastatin. What is the next best step to add?
 A. Nifedipine
 B. Switch metoprolol to atenolol
 C. Ranolazine
 D. Long-acting nitrates

10.38. The patient in Question 10.37 is started on a long-acting nitrate. He comes back to your office for a follow-up. He indicates that his angina is not completely resolved. He also says that his BP at home is elevated at 150/95 mmHg. What is the best course of action to take next?
 A. Add nicardipine
 B. Start ranolazine
 C. No need to add anything at this time
 D. Switch metoprolol to atenolol

10.39. By how much does ranolazine increase the plasma concentration of simvastatin?
  A. Threefold
  B. Twofold
  C. Fourfold
  D. Does not change the plasma concentration

10.40. How is the absorption rate of ranolazine affected by verapamil?
  A. Increased
  B. Decreased
  C. No change

10.41. How is the plasma concentration of ranolazine affected by ketoconazole?
  A. Decreased
  B. Increased
  C. It is not affected

10.42. Cocaine causes MI due to its effect on what?
  A. Alpha adrenergic stimulation
  B. Beta adrenergic stimulation
  C. Alpha and beta adrenergic stimulation
  D. Dopaminergic receptors

10.43. A 65-year-old man was admitted to the emergency room with acute anterior ST elevation MI. He underwent uneventful stenting of the proximal LAD artery within four hours of chest pain onset. He had mild congestive heart failure, and EF on echo was 30%. In addition to beta blocker, angiotensin-converting-enzyme inhibitor, high-dose statin, aspirin, and clopidogrel, what else is likely to improve his outcome, if done before discharge?
  A. Implantation of an implantable cardioverter-defibrillator
  B. Eplerenone 25 mg daily
  C. Amiodarone 200 mg daily to reduce risk for VT/Vfib
  D. Warfarin to get an INR to 2–3 to prevent LV thrombus

10.44. A 38-year-old athletic, very muscular individual is evaluated for numbness in the left arm during exercise and weightlifting. No other medical problems. Examination is normal, as is the resting ECG. He is 68 inches tall, weighs 180 lbs, and has a short muscular neck. On stress test using a ramp protocol, he attained 95% of age-predicted heart rate at 16 METs, there was no chest pain, but had 1 mm of upsloping ST depression in inferior leads resolving within 20 seconds. What will you recommend?
  A. Coronary angiogram
  B. Stress nuclear test or stress echo.
  C. Adson's test
  D. Magnetic resonance imaging of C spine.

## Answers

10.1. B. About 50%.
    The resting ECG can be normal in about 50% of patients with stable CAD. Nonspecific ST-T changes are most commonly found on the resting ECG in stable CAD patients.

10.2. B. Poor prognosis.

The presence or development of conduction disturbances in stable CAD patients is associated with a poor prognosis. This may be suggestive of reduced left ventricular (LV) function and or multivessel disease (Finh et al. 2014).

10.3. D. All of the above.

When LV hypertrophy is evident on the resting ECG, further evaluation is needed. Such patients should undergo an echocardiogram to evaluate LV function, wall motion, wall thickness and valve function.

10.4. B. 50%.

The resting ECG becomes abnormal in 50% of patients during an episode of angina in patients with stable CAD.

10.5. A. ST segment depression.

The most common finding on a resting ECG during an episode of angina is ST depression. The most common finding is ST segment depression.

10.6. A. Exercise stress ECG.

An exercise stress ECG is probably the best test to order in this situation. The stress ECG will be very useful to evaluate for ischemia especially when the resting ECG is normal and the patient is able to exercise and achieve a good workload (Finh et al. 2014).

10.7. A. Reduces the sensitivity as a screening tool.

In the presence of anti-anginal therapy, the sensitivity of a stress ECG is reduced and a negative stress test cannot be used to rule out significant CAD. Long-acting nitrates and beta blockers need to be stopped two to three days prior to the test.

10.8. D. All of the above.

A stress nuclear test will be helpful in the evaluation of ischemia in the presence of resting ECG changes, LBBB, LV hypertrophy, and in those receiving digoxin. In these patients, ST segments cannot be interpreted accurately during stress. An exercise stress nuclear test is relatively expensive (about three times) compared with a regular stress ECG test. Hence, a stress nuclear test should not be used as a screening tool especially in a patient with low probability of CAD. In patients with chest pain and a normal resting ECG, an exercise stress ECG should be used to screen for CAD. In patients with LBBB, pharmacological stress is preferable as exercise stress may result in false-positive septal perfusion defects.

10.9. D. All of the above.

A pharmacological stress nuclear test can be used to evaluate for ischemia in all of the situations A–C. Though pharmacological stress testing provides diagnostic accuracy comparable to an exercise stress nuclear test, exercise testing should be preferred as the exercise portion of the test provides additional information, such as heart rate and blood pressure (BP) response, amount of exercise and workload achieved, symptoms, and stress ECG abnormalities. Hence, whenever a patient can exercise and has a normal resting ECG, an exercise stress test is preferable (Finh et al. 2014).

10.10. D. All of the above.

10.11. A. A Stress test in females is associated with higher false-positive results compared with males.

Exercise stress ECG was associated with a higher rate of false-positive rates based on earlier studies. But when men and women are appropriately categorized based on their pretest probability, the results of stress test are similar in both men and women, though the specificity may be slightly lower (Finh et al. 2014).

10.12. D. Adenosine stress CMR.

In a person with angina and moderate physical limitation, a pharmacological stress is recommended. According to the 2012 ACC/AHA guidelines (Finh et al. 2012), pharmacological stress CMR is useful in the diagnosis of CAD (class IIa) recommendation (Nandalur et al. 2007; Hamon et al. 2010; Schuetz et al. 2010).

10.13. D. Coronary CT angiography (CCTA).

In a person with an intermediate pretest probability of CAD, with an ability to exercise moderately, a CCTA can be useful to diagnose CAD (class IIb) recommendation according to the 2012 ACC/AHA guidelines (Budoff et al. 2008; Schuetz et al. 2010; Finh et al. 2012).

10.14. E. All of the above.

In a patient with intermediate to high pretest likelihood of CAD and who is unable to perform to at least moderate exertion, then pharmacological stress with either echo or nuclear imaging is recommended (class 1) according to the 2012 ACC/AHA guidelines (Finh et al. 2012).

10.15. E. B, C, and D.

In a patient with low pretest likelihood and an inability to exercise, pharmacological stress or CCTA are reasonable diagnostic tests (class IIa, level of evidence C) (Finh et al. 2012).

10.16. C. Stress CMR.

In a patient with intermediate to high pretest likelihood and an inability to exercise, stress CMR is reasonable to perform for evaluation of angina (class IIa, level of evidence B). CCTA is reasonable to perform in a patient with low to intermediate likelihood of IHD, who is incapable of at least moderate physical activity (class IIa, level of evidence B) (Finh et al. 2012).

10.17. C. Coronary angiogram.

This patient has a high pretest likelihood of IHD and has intractable symptoms. Coronary angiogram is the best test to evaluate for CAD (class I, level of evidence C) as he is on optimal guideline-directed medical therapy and may be amenable for coronary revascularization (2014 ACC/AHA guideline update) (Finh et al. 2014).

10.18. C. Coronary angiogram.

This patient has a high probability of multivessel disease based on risk factors, angina, and low EF. His LV EF is 30%, which poses a high risk in the presence of IHD. Patients with a high likelihood of IHD, based on noninvasive testing, will benefit from a coronary angiogram provided they are amenable to revascularization (class IIa, level of evidence C).

Features of high risk (>3% annual mortality rate) include: resting LV EF <35%, high-risk treadmill score ≤11, severe exercise-induced LV dysfunction (<35%), stress-induced perfusion defect, especially the anterior wall, multiple perfusion defects of moderate size on stress-induced imaging, large fixed perfusion defect on thallium-201 imaging along with LV dilatation or increased lung uptake, moderate perfusion defect on thallium-201 imaging associated with LV dilatation or increased lung uptake, wall motion abnormality developing in two segments at a low dose of dobutamine (<10 μg/[kg min]) or at a low heart rate <120 bpm, or extensive ischemia on a stress echocardiogram.

10.19. **B. Intensify medical therapy.**

This patient has risk factors for IHD. Her primary care physician ordered a dobutamine stress echo. The results of the noninvasive test are indeterminate as she did not achieve target heart rate. Owing to her symptoms, she should undergo coronary angiogram for further evaluation. According to the 2014 ACC/AHA guidelines (Finh et al. 2014), coronary angiography is reasonable in patients with suspected symptomatic IHD who cannot undergo diagnostic stress testing, or have indeterminate or nondiagnostic stress tests, when there is a high likelihood that the findings will result in important changes to therapy (class IIa, level of evidence C).

10.20. **C. Coronary angiogram.**

This patient probably has a false-negative stress test. Based on his risk factors and symptoms his pre- and post-test, the likelihood of IHD is high. Despite a negative stress test, coronary angiogram is warranted here as the findings on coronary angiogram may result in important changes to therapy. The 2014 update of ACC/AHA guidelines (Finh et al. 2014) state that "Coronary angiography might be considered in patients with stress test results of acceptable quality that do not suggest the presence of CAD when clinical suspicion of CAD remains high and there is a high likelihood that the findings will result in important changes to therapy" (class IIb, level of evidence C).

There are high-quality clinical data to base recommendations for performing coronary angiography in suspected IHD patients. All prior trials in this subset of patients have required angiography. Additionally, the incremental benefits of detecting CAD by coronary angiography need to be determined. The ISCHEMIA (International Study of Comparative Health Effectiveness with Medical and Invasive Approaches) trial is an ongoing trial randomizing patients with at least moderate ischemia on stress testing to a strategy of optimal medical treatment alone versus routine coronary angiogram along with medical therapy. Prior to randomization, patients with normal renal function will undergo CCTA to exclude left main or severe CAD.

10.21. **B. Fractional flow reserve (FFR)-guided PCI of the 60% stenosis.**

This patient with a 60% stenosis of his mid LAD artery should undergo FFR. If the FFR is <0.80 then that lesion should be intervened on. The FAME-2 trial (see Box 10.1) showed that, in patients with stable CAD and functionally significant stenosis, FFR-guided PCI, along with best medical therapy compared with best medical therapy alone, decreased the need for urgent revascularization (De Bruyne et al. 2012).

10.22. B. Intensify medical therapy.

This patient has a coronary stenosis that was shown to be not significant for ischemia based on FFR. In the FAME-2 trial, it was shown that the outcomes were favorable with best medical therapy when there was no demonstrable ischemia by FFR. Hence, medical therapy should be intensified in this patient. Please refer to discussion in Question 10.21.

10.23. A. 1.7–3%.

10.24. B. 1.4–2.4%.

Data from the Framingham study before the widespread use of aspirin and beta blockers have shown the annual mortality rate in patients with chronic stable angina was 4%. The use of aggressive medical therapy has improved the prognosis. In recent studies, the annual mortality rate in stable patients with CAD has been shown to be 1.7–3% and the occurrence of major ischemic events was around 1.4–2.4% (The PEACE Trial Investigators 2004).

10.25. C. 40%.

Data from the CASS study (see Box 10.1) have shown that five-year survival in medically treated patients with severe triple-vessel disease and an LVEF ≤34% was poor at 40% (Emond et al. 1994). If the LVEF was greater than 50% then the five-year survival was around 80%. As the stenosis severity increases and LV function is reduced below 34%, prognosis is adversely affected.

10.26. A. True.

Studies have shown there is an increased gradient of risk with increased angiographic extent of disease. It has been shown that, in medically treated symptomatic CAD patients, the annual mortality rate is 2% when there is a 50% stenosis in only one of the major epicardial coronary vessels. In patients with an obstructive lesion proximal to the first septal perforator, the 5-year survival rate is 90%, compared with 98% in patients with more distal LAD stenosis (Califf et al. 1996).

10.27. C. C3oronary artery bypass grafting (CABG) including left internal mammary artery (LIMA) to LAD artery.

In the 2014 ACC/AHA guidelines (Finh et al. 2014), CABG received a class 1 recommendation in patients with diabetes mellitus and multivessel CAD (three vessel or complex two vessel including proximal LAD artery provided a LIMA graft can be anastomosed to the LAD artery). See Box 10.1 regarding the FREEDOM trial (Faroukh et al. 2012), the SYNTAX trial (Kappatein et al. 2013), and the meta-analysis of eight trials, including the FREEDOM trial (Verma et al. 2013).

10.28. B. ≤22.

A low SYNTAX score was defined as ≤22 in the SYNTAX trial. This score was based on location, severity, and extent of stenosis, with a low score indicating less complicated anatomy. A score of 23–32 was defined as intermediate, and a score ≥33 was defined as a high-risk score.

10.29. B. Lower.

In the SYNTAX study (see Box 10.1) the occurrence of combined end point in the CABG group was lower compared with DES (16.7% versus 20.8%, $P = 0.03$ respectively) (Kappatein et al. 2013).

10.30. B. Higher.

In the SYNTAX trial (see Box 10.1), the MI rate and repeat revascularization were higher in the DES group when compared with the CABG group: MI 3.6% in the CABG versus 7.1% in the DES group; repeat revascularization 10.7% for CABG versus 19.7% for the DES group (Kappetein et al. 2011).

10.31. C. Higher.

In the SYNTAX trial (see Box 10.1), at 5-year follow-up, the occurrence of MACCEs was higher in the DES group compared with the CABG group: 37.3% versus 26.9% respectively, $p < 0.0001$ (Serruys et al. 2009).

10.32. D. Medical therapy plus CABG.

The best approach to revascularization in this patient is optimizing medical therapy and CABG (class 1, level of evidence B) (Finh et al. 2012).

10.33. D. Guideline-directed medical therapy.

CABG or PCI in this patient is class III (harm) according to the 2012 ACC/AHA guidelines (Finh et al. 2012). CABG or PCI should not be performed with the sole intent of improving survival in patients with stable IHD with one or more coronary stenoses not anatomically significant (<70% in non-left main a coronary artery or FFR >0.80), no or mild ischemia on noninvasive testing, stenosis involving only the RCA or left circumflex artery, or subtend only a small area of viable myocardium.

10.34. B. False.

See Box 10.1 about the COURAGE trial results.

10.35. B. Angiotensin-converting inhibitor.

Since his LVEF is <40%, he should be started on angiotensin-converting enzyme inhibitor.

10.36. C. 12 months.

According to current ACC/AHA guidelines (Finh et al. 2014), dual antiplatelet therapy with aspirin and clopidogrel or prasugrel should be continued uninterrupted for 12 months, though the benefits and risks of treatment beyond 1 year are uncertain. See Box 10.1 about the DAPT study.

10.37. D. Long-acting nitrates.

This patient should be started on long-acting nitrates to help control his angina.

10.38. A. Add nicardipine.

This patient has elevated BP and his angina is persistent despite being on a long-acting nitrate and a beta blocker. The next best medication to add would be nicardipine, as he has an elevated BP. The half-life of this drug is two to four hours, but appears to have greater vascular selectivity. For chronic stable angina, it is supposed to be as effective as verapamil or diltiazem, and when combined with a beta blocker, the efficacy is enhanced.

10.39. B. Twofold.

Ranalozine increases plasma concentration of simvastatin twofold.

10.40. A. Increased.

The absorption of ranolazine is increased by verapamil by inhibition of P-glycoprotein system.

10.41. **B. Increased.**

Ranolazine is metabolized by the cytochrome P450 system. Ketoconazole is a strong inhibitor of cytochrome P450 system. Hence, the concentration of ranolazine will be increased when co-administered with ketoconazole.

10.42. **A. Alpha adrenergic stimulation.**

Cocaine causes MI by its alpha-adrenergic stimulation, which causes coronary vasoconstriction and increased myocardial oxygen demand. Thus, when treating such patients, pure beta blockers are contraindicated and drugs such as labetolol, which block both alpha- and beta-adrenergic receptors, should be used.

10.43. **B. Eplerenone 25 mg daily.**

As the EF is <35%, there is no indication for an implantable cardioverter-defibrillator unless EF remains <35% after 40 days.

10.44. **C. Adson's test.**

The features are consistent with thoracic outlet syndrome. The stress test is negative at very high workload and there is no indication for further ischemic work-up.

10.45. **B.** Ranolazine works by inhibiting the late inward sodium channel. As a result, there is less intracellular sodium that can be exchanged for calcium via Na+/Ca2+ exchanger. This results in decreased calcium overload in the myocyte.

---

**Box 10.1  Clinical Trials**

- **FAME-2** (De Bruyne et al. 2012). Hypothesis was that FFR-guided PCI of functionally significant stenosis, along with best medical therapy would be superior to best medical therapy alone. A total of 1220 patients were enrolled, 880 were randomized and 332 enrolled in registry. Primary end point was a composite of death, MI, or urgent revascularization. The trial was halted prematurely because of a significant difference in the primary outcome between the two groups: 4.3% in the PCI group and 12.7% in the medical therapy group (hazard ratio with PCI 0.32, 95% confidence interval [CI] 0.19–0.53, $P < 0.001$). The difference was driven by a lower rate of urgent revascularization in the PCI group. In patients without ischemia, the outcome appeared to be favorable with best medical therapy alone.
- **CASS trial** (Emond et al. 1994). This study describes the impact of clinical, angiographic, and demographic characteristics on the long-term survival of Coronary Artery Surgery Study (CASS) patients while they were under medical treatment. All CASS patients who had not received heart surgery before enrollment (23 467 patients) were included in this survival analysis while they were under medical treatment or surveillance. Follow-up time ranged from 0 to 17 years (median: 12 years). Overall, 12-year survival for patients with zero-, one-, two-, and three-vessel disease is 88, 74, 59, and 40%, respectively. The 12-year survival for patients with at least one diseased vessel and EFs in the ranges 50–100%, 35–49%, and 0–34% is 73, 54, and 21%, respectively.
- **FREEDOM trial** (Faroukh et al. 2012). In this trial, 1900 patients were randomized to either PCI or CABG. The primary outcome in this trial was a composite of death, nonfatal MI, or nonfatal stroke. The 5-year rates were 18.7% in the CABG group versus 26.6%

in the DES group ($p = 0.005$). The benefit of CABG was driven by differences in rates of MI ($p < 0.001$) and death from any cause ($p = 0.049$). Stroke was more frequent in the CABG group, and 5-year survival rates were 5.2% in the CABG group compared with 2.4% in the DES group ($p = 0.03$).

- **SYNTAX trial.**
  - The 5-year update from the SYNTAX trial (Kappatein et al. 2013) did not show a significant survival advantage with CABG over DES in patients with diabetes mellitus (12.9% with CABG versus19.5% with DES, $p = 0.065$).
  - In the SYNTAX trial, the occurrence of MACCEs correlated with the SYNTAX score for DES patients but not for those who had undergone CABG. At 12-month follow-up, the primary end point was similar in the CABG and DES groups in patients with a low SYNTAX score. In contrast, MACCEs occurred more often in DES patients when the SYNTAX scores were intermediate or high (Serruys et al. 2009). This difference in MACCEs increased at five years between those treated with a DES compared with CABG.

- **Meta-analysis** (Verma et al. 2013). The best evidence supporting the use of CABG in patients with multivessel CAD and diabetes mellitus comes from a meta-analysis of eight trials, including the FREEDOM trial. The study had 3131 patients and at five years, patients with diabetes mellitus randomized to CABG had a lower all-cause mortality than those randomized to PCI either with a bare-metal stent or DES (relative risk 0.67, 95% CI 0.52–0.86, $P = 0.002$).

- **COURAGE trial** (Boden et al. 2007). This was a randomized study which enrolled 2287 patients who had objective evidence of MI and significant CAD. Between 1999 and 2004, 1149 patients were assigned to undergo PCI with optimal medical therapy (PCI group) and 1138 to receive optimal medical therapy alone (medical-therapy group). The primary outcome was death from any cause and nonfatal MI during a median follow-up of 4.6 years. Cumulative primary-event rates were 19.0% in the PCI group and 18.5% in the medical-therapy group (hazard ratio for the PCI group, 1.05; 95% CI 0.87–1.27, $P = 0.62$). There were no significant differences between the PCI group and the medical-therapy group in the composite of death, MI, and stroke (20.0% versus 19.5%; hazard ratio 1.05, 95% CI 0.87–1.27, $P = 0.62$), hospitalization for acute coronary syndrome (12.4% versus 11.8%; hazard ratio 1.07, 95% CI 0.84–1.37, $P = 0.56$), or myocardial infarction (13.2% versus 12.3%; hazard ratio 1.13, 95% CI 0.89–1.43, $P = 0.33$). The trial concluded that, as an initial management strategy in patients with stable CAD, PCI did not reduce the risk of death, MI, or other major cardiovascular events when added to optimal medical therapy.

- **DAPT trial.** This enrolled 9961 patients who were either assigned to stop thienopyridine therapy after 12 months or to continue for another 18 months. The co-primary efficacy end points were stent thrombosis and MACCEs (a composite of death, MI, or stroke) during the follow-up period from 12 to 30 months. The primary safety end point was moderate or severe bleeding in this trial. Continued treatment with thienopyridine beyond 12 months, compared with placebo, reduced the rates of stent thrombosis (0.4% versus 1.4%; hazard ratio 0.29, 95% CI 0.17–0.48, $P < 0.001$) and MACCEs (4.3% versus 5.9%; hazard ratio 0.71, 95% CI 0.59–0.85, $P < 0.001$). The rate of moderate or severe bleeding was increased with continued thienopyridine treatment (2.5% versus 1.6%, $P = 0.001$). An elevated risk of stent thrombosis and MI was observed in both groups during the three months after discontinuation of thienopyridine treatment.

## References

Boden, W.E., O'Rourke, R.A., Teo, K.K. et al. (2007). Optimal medical therapy with or without PCI for stable coronary disease. *The New England Journal of Medicine* **356**: 1503–1516.

Budoff, M.J., Dowe, D., Jollis, J.G. et al. (2008). Diagnostic performance of 64-slice multidetector row coronary computed tomographic angiography for evaluation of coronary artery disease results from the prospective multicenter ACCURACY (assessment by coronary computed tomographic angiography in individuals undergoing invasive coronary angiography) trial. *Journal of the American College of Cardiology* **52**: 1724–1732.

Califf, R.M., Armstrong, P.W., Carver, J.R. et al. (1996). Task Force 5. Stratification of patients into high, medium and low risk subgroups for purposes of risk factor management. *Journal of the American College of Cardiology* **27**: 1007–1119.

De Bruyne, B., Pijls, N.H.J., Kalesan, B. et al. (2012). Fractional flow reserve-guided PCI versus medical therapy in stable coronary disease. *The New England Journal of Medicine* **367**: 991–1001.

Emond, M., Mock, M.B., Davis, K.B. et al. (1994). Long-term survival of medically treated patients in the Coronary Artery Surgery Study (CASS) registry. *Circulation* **90**: 2645–2657.

Faroukh, M.E., Domanski, M., Sleeper, L.A. et al. (2012). Strategies for multivessel revascularization in patients with diabetes mellitus. *The New England Journal of Medicine* **367**: 2375–2384.

Finh, S.D., Gardin, J.M., Abrams, J. et al. (2012). 2012 ACC/AHA/AATS/PCNA/SCAI/STS guideline for the diagnosis and management of patients with stable ischemic heart disease: a report of the American College of Cardiology Foundation/American Heart Association Task Force on Practice Guidelines, and the American College of Physicians, American Association for Thoracic Surgery, Preventive Cardiovascular Nurses Association, Society for Cardiovascular Angiography and Interventions, and Society of Thoracic Surgeons. *Journal of the American College of Cardiology* **60**: e44–e164.

Finh, S.D., Blankenship, J.C., Alexander, K.P. et al. (2014). 2014 ACC/AHA/AATS/PCNA/SCAI/STS focused update of the guideline for the diagnosis and management of patients with stable ischemic heart disease. A report of the American College of Cardiology/American Heart Association Task Force on Practice Guidelines, and the American Association for Thoracic Surgery, Preventive Cardiovascular Nurses Association, Society for Cardiovascular Angiography and Interventions, and Society of Thoracic Surgeons. *Circulation* **130**: 1749–1767.

Hamon, M., Fau, G., Née, G. et al. (2010). Meta-analysis of the diagnostic performance of stress perfusion cardiovascular magnetic resonance for detection of coronary artery disease. *Journal of Cardiovascular Magnetic Resonance* **12**: 29.

Kappatein, A.P., Head, S.J., Morice, M.C. et al. (2013). Treatment of complex coronary artery disease in patients with diabetes mellitus: 5 year results comparing outcomes of bypass surgery with percutaneous coronary intervention in the SYNTAX trial. *European Journal of Cardiothoracic Surgery* **43**: 1006–1013.

Kappetein, A.P., Feldman, T.E., Mack, M.J. et al. (2011). Comparison of coronary bypass surgery with drug eluting stenting for the treatment of left main/or three vessel disease: 3 year follow up of the SYNTAX trial. *European Heart Journal* **32**: 2125–2134.

Nandalur, K.R., Dwamena, B.A., Choudhri, A.F. et al. (2007). Diagnostic performance of stress cardiac magnetic resonance imaging in the detection of coronary artery disease: a meta-analysis. *Journal of the American College of Cardiology* **50**: 1343–1353.

Schuetz, G.M., Zacharapoulou, N.M., Schlattman, P., and Dewey, M. (2010). Meta-analysis: noninvasive coronary angiography using computed tomography versus magnetic resonance imaging. *Annals of Internal Medicine* **152**: 167–177.

Serruys, P.W., Morice, M.C., Kappetein, A.P. et al. (2009). Percutaneous coronary intervention versus coronary artery bypass artery grafting for severe coronary artery disease. *The New England Journal of Medicine* **360**: 961–972.

The PEACE Trial Investigators (2004). Angiotensin-converting-enzyme inhibition in stable coronary artery disease. *The New England Journal of Medicine* **351**: 2058–2068.

Verma, S., Farkouh, M.E., Yanagawa, B. et al. (2013). Comparison of coronary artery bypass surgery and percutaneous coronary interventions in patients with diabetes: a meta-analysis of randomized controlled trials. *The Lancet Diabetes & Endocrinology* **1**: 317–328.

Chapter 1

# Heart Failure, Transplant, Left Ventricular Assist Devices, Pulmonary Hypertension

# 11

11.1. A 62-year-old man with smoking, hypertension, and diabetes mellitus complains of shortness of breath on exertion. He gets short of breath walking up a flight of stairs. There is no chest pain. On physical examination, heart rate is 72 bpm and regular; blood pressure 148/90 mmHg with body mass index (BMI) of 24. Jugular venous pressure (JVP) and heart sounds are normal. The electrocardiogram shows normal sinus rhythm. The echocardiogram shows mild left ventricular (LV) hypertrophy, normal wall motion, normal valvular function, mitral E/A velocity ratio of 0.7, E/E′ ratio of 7, pulmonary artery (PA) systolic pressure of 50 mmHg. What is the most productive next step?

A. Add calcium channel blocker (CCB) as a lusiotropic agent as it may reduce PA pressure

B. Computed tomography (CT) pulmonary angiography to rule out pulmonary embolism

C. Right heart catheterization (RHC) to evaluate for pulmonary vascular resistance and its response to $O_2$ and pulmonary vasodilators

D. Diuresis to reduce left atrial (LA) pressure as this may reduce PA pressure

11.2. Which of the following agents are shown to improve survival in heart failure with reduced ejection fraction (HFrEF)?

A. Carvedilol and metoprolol succinate

B. Angiotensin-converting-enzyme inhibitor (ACEI)

C. Spironolactone

D. All of the above

E. None of the above

11.3. Which of the following agents are shown to improve survival in heart failure with preserved ejection fraction (HFpEF)?

A. Carvedilol and metoprolol succinate

B. ACEI

C. Spironolactone

D. All of the above

E. None of the above

*Cardiology Board Review*, Second Edition. Ramdas G. Pai and Padmini Varadarajan.
© 2023 John Wiley & Sons Ltd. Published 2023 by John Wiley & Sons Ltd.

**11.4.** A 62-year-old asymptomatic hypertensive had an echocardiogram for a murmur. The rest of the physical examination was normal. Echocardiogram showed normal LV wall thickness and wall motion with ejection fraction (EF) of 65%. Valves were normal. Mitral E/A velocity ratio was 0.7. What does the patient have?
A. Stage A heart failure (HF)
B. Stage B HF
C. HFpEF
D. None of the above

**11.5.** Diagnosis of HF by Framingham criteria requires which of the following?
A. Two major or one major and two minor criteria
B. Four major criteria
C. Two major criteria and raised serum brain natriuretic peptide (BNP)
D. None of the above

**11.6.** The major Framingham criteria for HF include:
A. S3
B. Paroxysmal nocturnal dyspnea
C. Basal rales
D. All of the above

**11.7.** The minor Framingham criteria for HF include which of the following?
A. Shortness of breath
B. Edema
C. Nocturnal cough
D. All of the above

**11.8.** Which of the following are class I indications for echocardiography, based on American College of Cardiology Foundation and imaging societies' appropriateness criteria in subjects with HF?
A. Clinical HF
B. Family history of cardiomyopathy, but no clinical HF
C. Cardiotoxic chemotherapy
D. All of the above

**11.9.** In which patients with HFrEF is coronary angiography most appropriate and clearly indicated?
A. A 52-year-old patient with EF of 30%, diabetes, and angina on walking one block
B. A 63-year-old man with prior ST elevation myocardial infarction, scarred left anterior descending artery area on nuclear testing, no reversible ischemia, EF of 30%, but short of breath on exertion
C. A 22-year-old patient with HF, EF of 10%, severely dilated left ventricle
D. None of the above

**11.10.** Compared with atrial myocyte, ventricular myocyte is which of the following?
A. Longer
B. Broader
C. Has more T tubules
D. All of the above
E. None of the above.

11.11. Which of the following has absent T tubules?
   A. Ventricular myocyte
   B. Atrial myocyte
   C. Purkinje cells
   D. None of the above

11.12. Which of the following have the most abundant gap junctions?
   A. Ventricular myocyte
   B. Atrial myocyte
   C. Purkinje cells
   D. None of the above

11.13. What is the increase in myocardial contractile force with increase in preload called?
   A. Frank-Starling phenomenon
   B. Anrep phenomenon
   C. Bowditch phenomenon
   D. None of the above.

11.14. What is the increase in myocardial contractile force with acute increase in afterload called?
   A. Frank-Starling phenomenon
   B. Anrep phenomenon
   C. Bowditch phenomenon
   D. None of the above.

11.15. What is the increase in myocardial contractile force with increase in heart rate called?
   A. Frank-Starling phenomenon
   B. Anrep phenomenon
   C. Bowditch phenomenon
   D. None of the above.

11.16. An increase in LV end-systolic size would increase which of the following?
   A. LV preload
   B. LV afterload
   C. None
   D. Both

11.17. What would an acute increase in afterload result in?
   A. Reduction in LV EF
   B. Increase in LV end-systolic volume
   C. Increased LV contractility
   D. All of the above.

11.18. Which of the following does the LVEF depend upon?
   A. LV preload                 C. LV contractility
   B. LV afterload               D. All of the above

11.19. Which of the following factors affect LV diastolic function?
   A. LV relaxation process
   B. Modulus of chamber stiffness
   C. LV recoil
   D. All of the above

**11.20.** Submassive acute pulmonary embolism may cause all of the following except which option?
- **A.** Increase in intrapericardial pressure
- **B.** Increase in LV end-diastolic pressure
- **C.** Reduced LV filling
- **D.** Increase in stroke volume

**11.21.** Which of the following is not acceptable as a donor heart for heart transplant?
- **A.** Bicuspid aortic valve
- **B.** History of meth use with normal EF and absence of LV hypertrophy
- **C.** Atrial septal defect with normal right ventricle function
- **D.** History of alcohol abuse and EF of 35% on pressors

**11.22.** What is your recommendation for a donor heart that is normal except for 3+ functional tricuspid regurgitation (TR)?
- **A.** Reject the heart
- **B.** Assign the heart to alternate list
- **C.** Do DeVega annuloplasty on bench and use the heart
- **D.** Do tricuspid valve replacement and use the heart

**11.23.** What are the likely outcomes after heart transplant in a patient with preoperative moderate PH and increased pulmonary vascular resistance?
- **A.** Right ventricular (RV) dilation and failure
- **B.** Tricuspid regurgitation
- **C.** Low output state
- **D.** None of the above
- **E.** Options A–C

**11.24.** Which of the following reduces serum levels of cyclosporine, tacrolimus, and sirolimus?
- **A.** Phenytoin
- **B.** Phenobarbital
- **C.** Rifampicin
- **D.** All of the above

**11.25.** Which of the following increases serum levels of cyclosporine, tacrolimus, and sirolimus?
- **A.** Erythromycin
- **B.** Ketoconazole and fluconazole
- **C.** Diltiazem and verapamil
- **D.** Amiodarone
- **E.** All of the above

**11.26.** Which of the following are potential side effects of tacrolimus?
- **A.** Diabetes mellitus
- **B.** Tremor
- **C.** Anemia
- **D.** All of the above
- **E.** None of the above

**11.27.** Potential side effects of cyclosporine include which of the following?
- **A.** Hypertension
- **B.** Hypertriglyceridemia

Chapter 1

C. Hypercholesterolemia

D. Increase in creatinine

E. All of the above

11.28. Which of the following are treatment options for antibody-mediated graft rejection?

A. High-dose corticosteroid

B. Intravenous (IV) immunoglobulin

C. Daily plasmapheresis

D. IV rituximab

E. All of the above.

11.29. Which of the following drugs may retard cardiac allograft vasculopathy?

A. Sirolimus

B. Everolimus

C. Statins

D. Mycophenolate mofetil

E. All of the above.

11.30. In an adult patient with heart transplant beyond six months, which of the following surveillance regimens for rejection is appropriate?

A. Biannual endomyocardial biopsy for the first five years

B. Biannual endomyocardial biopsy for an indefinite period of time

C. Echocardiography in place of biopsy

D. Cardiac magnetic resonance imaging with delayed enhancement in place of biopsy

E. All of the above

11.31. Which of the following are not acceptable practices for cardiac allograft surveillance?

A. Monitoring of serum BNP trends

B. Monitoring of troponin I and C-reactive protein

C. Echocardiography in place of biopsy

D. Cardiac magnetic resonance imaging with delayed enhancement in place of biopsy

E. All of the above

11.32. In a patient with heart transplant, pregnancy should be discouraged under which of the following circumstances?

A. Within a year of transplant

B. Evidence of LV dysfunction

C. Evidence of coronary vasculopathy

D. All of the above

E. None of the above.

11.33. Which of the following statements are true in a heart transplant patient who gets pregnant?

A. Discontinue all antirejection medications in the first trimester because of teratogenicity

B. Discontinue all antirejection medications throughout pregnancy because of fetal growth retardation

C. Continue corticosteroids and calcineurin inhibitors (cyclosporine or tacrolimus)

D. Continue corticosteroids, tacrolimus and mycophenolate mofetil

**11.34.** Which of the following statements are true regarding coronary angiography after heart transplant?

A. Reasonable to perform coronary angiogram at six months after heart transplant

B. Reasonable to perform coronary angiogram at five years after heart transplant and then annually

C. Both A and B

D. Neither A nor B

**11.35.** Which of the following patients are reasonable candidates to evaluate for heart transplant?

A. Male, 60 years, EF of 10%, class IV HF, inotrope dependent

B. Female, 57 years, EF 35%, class IV angina, poor targets for percutaneous coronary intervention or coronary artery bypass grafting and refractory to medical therapy

C. Male, 67 years, class III symptoms, EF 20%, $V_{O2}$ max 8 ml/(kg min)

D. All of the above

E. None of the above.

**11.36.** Which of the following are absolute contraindications for heart transplant?

A. Prostatic carcinoma, status post treatment with persistently elevated prostate-specific antigen

B. AIDS with opportunistic infections

C. Fixed PH with PA systolic pressure >60 mmHg or pulmonary vascular resistance >6 Wood units or transpulmonary gradient >15 mmHg

D. All of the above.

E. None of the above

**11.37.** Which of the following patients are undesirable candidates for heart transplant for class IV HF?

A. Male, 75 years, with HFrEF and EF 10%

B. Patient on hemodialysis for heart transplant alone

C. Living alone with no social support

D. BMI >35 kg/m²

E. All of the above

**11.38.** Which of the following statements are true regarding an implantable left ventricular assist device (LVAD)?

A. In patients with severe class IV HFrEF ineligible for heart transplant, it prolongs survival

B. It may be used as a bridge to transplant

C. It may be used as a bridge to recovery

D. It may be used as destination therapy

E. All are correct.

**11.39.** In a patient considered for LVAD, which of the following findings may increase associated risk?

A. Highly trabeculated left ventricle

B. LV apical thrombus

C. LV end diastolic diameter <63 mm
D. All of the above

11.40. Which of the following are red-flag findings in patients undergoing LVAD?
A. LA appendage thrombus
B. Severe RV dysfunction
C. Patent foramen ovale (PFO)
D. Ventricular septal defect (VSD)
E. All of the above.

11.41. Which of the following valvular lesions may be problematic in patients undergoing LVAD?
A. Moderate or severe aortic regurgitation (AR)
B. Moderate or severe mitral stenosis
C. Moderate or severe TR
D. All of the above

11.42. Which of the following valve lesions may not significantly impede LVAD function?
A. Mitral regurgitation          C. Pulmonary regurgitation
B. Aortic stenosis               D. All of the above.

11.43. Which of the following prosthetic valves may need to be explanted before LVAD implant?
A. Mechanical aortic valve
B. Bioprosthetic aortic valve
C. Normally functioning mechanical mitral valve
D. Mechanical mitral valve with 3+ mitral regurgitation (MR)
E. All of the above.

11.44. Which of the following are preferred surgical options to be included for severe AR before LVAD implant?
A. Bioprosthesis
B. Complete sewing and closure
C. Park stitch (central suture)
D. All of the above
E. None of the above

11.45. What is sudden desaturation soon after LVAD implant likely due to?
A. Unmasked PFO               C. Unmasked RV dysfunction
B. AR                         D. Pulmonary embolism

11.46. Which of the following options is true about AR quantitation after LVAD?
A. Should be upgraded by one grade based on traditional criteria
B. Should be downgraded by one grade
C. Should be based on aortic flow reversal in diastole
D. None of the above
E. All of the above

11.47. What is a recommended approach if leftward septal shift, severe RV dysfunction, and severe TR occur soon after LVAD implant even at low speed?
A. Reduce the LV cannula size
B. Perform tricuspid valve repair

    **C.** Infuse fluid

    **D.** Change to biventricular mechanical circulatory support

**11.48.** Which of the following echo findings indicate normal LVAD function?

    **A.** Inflow (LV) cannula velocity of <1.5 m/s without turbulence

    **B.** Ouflow (aortic) cannula velocity of <2.0 m/s without turbulence

    **C.** Intermittent opening of aortic valve

    **D.** Ventricular septum in the middle

    **E.** All of the above

**11.49.** What might signs of LVAD malfunction include?

    **A.** Diastolic flow reversal in inflow and outflow cannula with pump arrest

    **B.** Reduced response to increase in pump speed

    **C.** LV dilation

    **D.** Low velocities in cannula

    **E.** All of the above

**11.50.** What might persistent aortic valve closure in a patient with LVAD result in?

    **A.** Aortic root thrombus    **C.** Both A and B

    **B.** AR    **D.** Neither A nor B

**11.51.** What should one not do when aortic root thrombus is seen in a patient with LVAD?

    **A.** Reduce pump speed

    **B.** Increase pump speed

    **C.** Neither

**11.52.** What might signs of an LV suction event include?

    **A.** LV end diastolic diameter <3 cm

    **B.** Obstruction to inflow cannula

    **C.** Leftward septal shit

    **D.** Increase in TR

    **E.** All of the above.

    **F.** None of the above.

**11.53.** A patient with an LVAD presents with heart failure. An echocardiogram shows an increase in LV size and greater opening of the aortic valve with each beat from 90 to 200 ms. What is the most likely cause?

    **A.** Thrombosis of the LVAD    **C.** Pulmonary embolism

    **B.** Hypertension    **D.** None of the above

**11.54.** With increase in pump speed, which of the following may occur?

    **A.** Reduced opening of aortic valve

    **B.** A diminution of systolic velocity and an increase in diastolic velocity in the aortic cannula

    **C.** A diminution in LV size

    **D.** Septal shift to left

    **E.** All of the above

**11.55.** Which statin has least interaction with immune suppressants?

    **A.** Simvastatin

    **B.** Pravastatin

    **C.** Atorvastatin

    **D.** Rosuvastatin

**11.56.** Which immunosuppressant may increase serum creatinine level?
  A. Sirolimus
  B. Cyclosporine
  C. Mycophenolate mofetil
  D. Corticosteroid

**11.57.** A 45-year-old man with heart transplant performed 6 years previously is admitted with shortness of breath and fever. He is on prednisone, tacrolimus, mycophenolate mofetil, diltiazem, and pravastatin. Chest X-ray is suggestive of pneumonia. The echocardiogram showed normal LV function, wall thickness, and filling pressures. The white cell count is 16 000, and serum creatinine is 3.2 mg/dl. In addition to treating with appropriate antibiotics, what would you do?
  A. Start dobutamine infusion
  B. Discontinue tacrolimus
  C. Treat with IV immunoglobulin
  D. Perform plasmapheresis

**11.58.** In a patient with systolic heart failure on optimal doses of carvedilol and spironolactone, which drug is likely to produce maximum mortality and HF admission benefit?
  A. ACEI
  B. Angiotensin receptor blocker
  C. Neprilysin inhibitor
  D. Diuretic

In Questions 11.59–11.66, match the question's clinical scenario to the indicated risk of PH, if any, and to the type of pulmonary arterial hypertension (PAH) based on the current classification system. See Box 11.1 on the classification of pulmonary hypertension at the end of this chapter. Each option may apply to more than one clinical situation or none at all.

**11.59.** A 62-year-old woman, with a history of hypertension and obesity (current BMI 31), presents with dyspnea. On echo, there is normal LV and valvular function, mitral E/e' ratio is 6, and PA systolic pressure is 60 mmHg. She has used the appetite-suppressant drug fen-phen for two years in the past. Based on the current classification system, which of the following options best describe this patient's condition?
  A. No PH
  B. Group 1 PH
  C. Group 2 PH
  D. Group 3 PH
  E. Group 4 PH
  F. Group 5 PH

**11.60.** A 27-year-old woman has idiopathic PH. Based on the current classification system, which of the following options best describe this patient's condition?
  A. No PH
  B. Group 1 PH
  C. Group 2 PH
  D. Group 3 PH
  E. Group 4 PH
  F. Group 5 PH

**11.61.** A patient has PH in systemic sclerosis. Based on the current classification system, which of the following options best describe this patient's condition?

A. No PH
B. Group 1 PH
C. Group 2 PH
D. Group 3 PH
E. Group 4 PH
F. Group 5 PH

**11.62.** The PA pressure in a patient being evaluated for liver transplant because of end-stage liver disease is 65/40 mmHg. Echo shows normal LV and is consistent with normal left and right atrial pressures. Based on the current classification system, which of the following options best describe this patient's condition?

A. No PH
B. Group 1 PH
C. Group 2 PH
D. Group 3 PH
E. Group 4 PH
F. Group 5 PH

**11.63.** A 10-year-old boy has severe PH. His mother had a history of severe depression and committed suicide 6 years previously. Based on the current classification system, which of the following options best describe this patient's condition?

A. No PH
B. Group 1 PH
C. Group 2 PH
D. Group 3 PH
E. Group 4 PH
F. Group 5 PH

**11.64.** The PA pressure in a 37-year-old patient who had VSD patch closure at the age of 15 years is 60/35 mmHg. Based on the current classification system, which of the following options best describe this patient's condition?

A. No PH
B. Group 1 PH
C. Group 2 PH
D. Group 3 PH
E. Group 4 PH
F. Group 5 PH

**11.65.** A 52-year-old woman with shortness of breath, echo shows EF of 60%, thickened mitral leaflets with diastolic doming, mitral valve pressure half-time of 270 ms, isovolumic relaxation time 30 ms, mild TR with a velocity of 3.9 m/s, dilated inferior vena cava. Based on the current classification system, which of the following options best describe this patient's condition?

A. No PH
B. Group 1 PH
C. Group 2 PH
D. Group 3 PH
E. Group 4 PH
F. Group 5 PH

**11.66.** A 42-year-old woman presents with protein C deficiency, recurrent deep-vein thromboses and pulmonary embolism. She is uninsured with intermittent compliance with anticoagulation and has increasing dyspnea and bilateral pedal edema. JVP is elevated, and P2 is loud and palpable at left sternal border. Based on the current classification system, which of the following options best describe this patient's condition?

A. No PH

B. Group 1 PH

C. Group 2 PH

D. Group 3 PH

E. Group 4 PH

F. Group 5 PH

**11.67.** What is the commonest cause of moderate to severe PH worldwide?

A. Idiopathic

B. Mitral stenosis

C. Schistosomiasis

D. Pulmonary embolism

**11.68.** Which of the following mutations is responsible for the majority of patients with familial PH?

A. *BMPR2* mutations           C. *SMAD9* mutation

B. *BMPR1B* mutation          D. None of the above

**11.69.** Which is the preferred modality to diagnose thromboembolic PH?

A. V/Q scan

B. CT pulmonary angiography

C. Gd-enhanced MR pulmonary angiography

D. Transesophageal echocardiography

**11.70.** Is RHC indicated in patients with PH?

A. Yes

B. No

C. Depends upon the situation

**11.71.** Which of the following statements are true regarding RHC in those with PH?

A. RHC is recommended to confirm the diagnosis of PAH (group 1) and to support treatment decisions

B. In patients with PH, it is recommended to perform RHC in expert centers as it is technically demanding and may be associated with serious complications

C. RHC is recommended in patients with congenital cardiac shunts to support decisions on correction

D. RHC is indicated in patients with CTEPH (group 4) to confirm the diagnosis and support treatment decisions

E. All of the above

F. None of the above.

**11.72.** Which of the following statements is untrue about vasoreactivity testing in PH?

A. Vasoreactivity testing is recommended in patients with idiopathic PAH, hereditary PAH, and PAH associated with drugs used to detect patients who can be treated with high doses of a CCB

B. A positive response to vasoreactivity testing is defined as a reduction of mean PA pressure >10 mmHg to reach an absolute value of mean PA pressure <40 mmHg with an increased or unchanged cardiac output

C. Nitric oxide is recommended for performing vasoreactivity testing. IV epoprostenol is recommended for performing vasoreactivity testing as an alternative

D. Adenosine should be considered for performing vasoreactivity testing as an alternative

E. The use of oral or IV CCBs in acute vasoreactivity testing is recommended

**11.73.** Which of the following are acceptable recommendations in those with PAH?
A. Avoid pregnancy
B. Use flu and pneumococcal vaccines
C. Supervise training program or cardiopulmonary rehab
D. Those needing anesthesia, use epidural rather than general
E. All of the above.

**11.74.** Which of the following are class I indications in PAH?
A. Diuretic treatment is recommended in PAH patients with signs of RV failure and fluid retention
B. Continuous long-term $O_2$ therapy is recommended in PAH patients when arterial blood $O_2$ pressure is consistently <8 kPa (60 mmHg)
C. High doses of CCBs are recommended in patients with idiopathic PAH, hereditary PAH, and drug-induced PAH who are responders to acute vasoreactivity testing
D. Pulmonary vasodilators are generally recommended for group 1 PH
E. All of the above
F. None of the above

**11.75.** Which of the following drugs have class I recommendations for treatment of World Health Organization group 1 PH functional class II and III, either alone or sequentially, or in combination?
A. Ambrisentan
B. Bosentan
C. Sildenafil
D. Tadalafil
E. All of the above
F. The above are recommended only in class IV

**11.76.** Which of the following statements are correct regarding CTEPH?
A. Life-long anticoagulation is recommended in all patients with CTEPH
B. It is recommended that in all patients with CTEPH the assessment of operability and decisions regarding other treatment strategies should be made by a multidisciplinary team of experts
C. Surgical pulmonary endarterectomy in deep hypothermia circulatory arrest is recommended for patients with CTEPH
D. Riociguat is recommended in symptomatic patients who have been classified as having persistent/recurrent CTEPH after surgical treatment or inoperable CTEPH by a CTEPH team, including at least one experienced pulmonary endarterectomy surgeon
E. All of the above

**11.77.** What does the patient in Figure 11.77 have?

A. LVAD

B. Impella device

C. Tandem heart device

D. None of the above

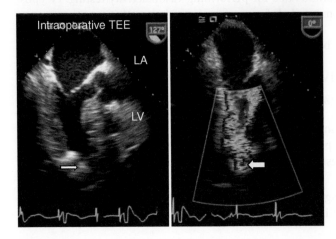

**Figure 11.77**

**11.78.** What does the patient in Figure 11.78 have?

A. LVAD

B. Impella device

C. Tandem heart device

D. None of the above

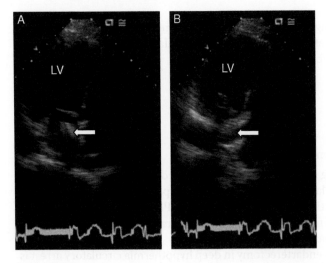

**Figure 11.78**

**11.79.** What does the patient in Figure 11.79 have?
   A. LVAD
   B. Impella device
   C. Tandem heart device
   D. None of the above

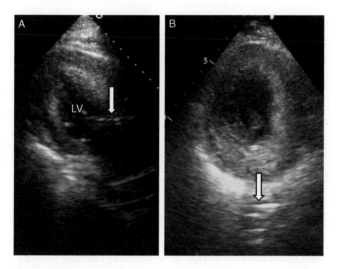

**Figure 11.79**

**11.80.** Which of the following is considered to be a diagnostic test for heart failure?
   A. Troponin
   B. NT-proBNP
   C. CXR
   D. Echo
   E. None of the above

**11.81.** What is the definition of "heart failure with reduced ejection fraction"?
   A. ≤30%
   B. ≤40%
   C. ≤45%
   D. ≤50%

**11.82.** What is the most common cause of heart failure with preserved ejection fraction?
   A. HTN
   B. Family history
   C. CAD
   D. DM2
   E. Atrial fibrillation

**11.83.** What is the considered to be the upper limit of normal mean pulmonary artery pressure?
   A. 15 mmHg
   B. 20 mmHg

C. 25 mmHg

D. 30 mmHg

11.84. Elevated mean pulmonary artery pressure in the 19–24 mmHg range is associated with which of the following?

A. RA enlargement

B. RV enlargement

C. Decreased RV systolic function

D. All of the above

11.85. The result of (mean pulmonary artery pressure – pulmonary artery wedge pressure)/cardiac output is?

A. Pulmonary vascular resistance

B. Cardiac index

C. RV end diastolic pressure

D. Pulmonary compliance

11.86. What is the threshold of pulmonary vascular resistance for diagnosing pulmonary arterial hypertension?

A. 2.0 woods units

B. 2.5 woods units

C. 3.0 woods units

D. 3.5 woods units

11.87. Measurements from a right heart catheterization show a mean pulmonary artery pressure of 24 mmHg, pulmonary vascular resistance of 1.9 woods units, and pulmonary artery wedge pressure of 28 mmHg. This patient will have which primary dysfunction?

A. Isolated pulmonary arterial hypertension

B. LV dysfunction

C. Chronic lung disease

D. Both A and B

11.88. Qp/Qs ratio of <1 signifies which direction of shunt?

A. Left-to-right shunt

B. Right-to-left shunt

11.89. The "a" wave on right atrial/central venous pressure waveform analysis represents which of the following?

A. Right atrial contraction

B. Tricuspid valve bulging into the right atrium

C. Right atrial relaxation

D. Rapid filling of the right atrium

E. Early rapid filling of the right ventricle

11.90. Which of the following are indications for CRT in heart failure patients?

A. LVEF ≤35%

B. Sinus rhythm

C. LBBB with QRS ≥150 ms

D. NYHA Class II, III, or IV symptoms on GDMT

E. A and C only

F. All the above.

**11.91.** How should one switch from ACE-I/ARB to an ARNI for a patient with HFrEF?
A. Stop ACE-I and start ARNI immediately
B. Stop ACE-I and start ARNI after 12 hours
C. Stop ACE-I and start ARNI after 36 hours
D. Stop ARB and start ARNI after 36 hours
E. Switch ACE-I/ARB to spironolactone and then start ARNI after 36 hours.

**11.92.** In which of the following heart failure patients would starting combination hydralazine and isosorbide dinitrate improve survival?
A. 50-year-old Caucasian male with HFrEF (NYHA IV) treated with ACE-I, BB, spironolactone
B. 64-year-old Black female with HFrEF (NYHA II) only on maximally tolerated BB
C. 72-year-old Hispanic female with HFrEF (NYHA II), CKD3 and treated with BB
D. 70-year-old Black male with HFrEF (NYHA III) treated with ARB, BB, and diuretics
E. 68-year-old Black male with HFpEF (NYHA II) treated with spironolactone

**11.93.** In patients with cardiogenic shock and a need for mechanical circulatory support, which of the following is not a contraindication for intra-aortic balloon pump (IABP)?
A. Severe aortic regurgitation
B. Severe mitral stenosis
C. Aortic dissection
D. Uncontrolled sepsis
E. Uncontrolled bleeding disorder

**11.94.** In patients undergoing cardiopulmonary stress testing (CPET), which of the following respiratory exchange ratio (RER) and peak oxygen consumption ($VO_2$) results would support listing for heart transplant?
A. RER of 0.95 and $VO_2$ 30
B. RER of 1.10 and $VO_2$ 8
C. RER of 1.10 and $VO_2$ 30
D. RER of 0.95 and $VO_2$ 8
E. None of the above

**11.95.** Which of the following is the least likely cause of death in the first year after heart transplantation?
A. Cardiac allograft vasculopathy
B. Graft failure
C. Infection
D. Acute rejection
E. Multiple organ failure

**11.96.** Which of the following is NOT an advantage of extracorporeal membrane oxygenation (ECMO) over percutaneous ventricular assist device (PVAD) for mechanical circulatory support?
A. Increased right ventricular unloading
B. Lower myocardial $O_2$ demand
C. Ability to oxygenate blood
D. Longer maximum implant duration

E. None of the above

**11.97.** In patients hospitalized with acute heart failure, which of the following conditions is an indication for pulmonary artery catheter placement?

A. Evidence of severe hypoperfusion or marked congestion at rest associated with acute ischemia, infarction, or renal failure

B. Fluid retention refractory to high-dose or combination diuretics

C. Hypoxemia with concomitant cardiac and pulmonary disease

D. Undifferentiated shock

E. All the above

**11.98.** In acute heart failure, patients who do not respond to initial IV diuresis regimen, which of the following is a reasonable therapeutic option?

A. Increase dose of diuretic

B. Initiate IV nitroprusside

C. Initiate IV dobutamine

D. Initiate Impella support

E. All the above.

**11.99.** Which of the following statements regarding inotropic therapy is true?

A. Dobutamine is not renally cleared

B. Dopamine has vasodilator effect at higher doses

C. Milrinone side effects include tachycardia, hypotension, and arrythmias

D. A and C only

E. All the above

**11.100.** Which of the following beta-blockers are indicated for HFrEF management in the US?

A. Labetalol

B. Bisoprolol

C. Carvedilol

D. Metoprolol succinate

E. A, C, and D only

F. B, C, and D only

G. All the above

## Answers

**11.1.** C. Right heart catheterization (RHC) to evaluate for pulmonary vascular resistance and its response to $O_2$ and pulmonary vasodilators.

Normal E/E' ratio indicates normal LA pressure and pulmonary hypertension (PH) being secondary to pulmonary vascular or parenchymal disease. Diuresis would not help. Shortness of breath is unlikely to be due to impaired LV relaxation as LA pressure is normal, and lusiotropic agents do not help hemodynamics in clinical settings apart from in patients with hypertrophic cardiomyopathy. A CT pulmonary angiogram is a poor test for chronic pulmonary emboli – a ventilation/perfusion (V/Q) scan would be better for this purpose.

**11.2.** D. All of the above.

Note that metoprolol tartrate, which is short acting, is not a good choice in HFrEF because of intermittent blockage of beta receptors, which may expose the patient to intermittent beta blocker withdrawal.

**11.3.** E. None of the above.

None of these have been shown to improve survival in HFpEF.

**11.4.** B. Stage B HF.

The pattern of impaired LV relaxation is consistent with stage B HF. He has no clinical HF and is not stage C. HFpEF needs clinical syndrome of HF, generally determined by Framingham criteria.

**11.5.** A. Two major or one major and two minor criteria.

For the Framingham study, see McKee et al. (1971) and Boxes 11.2 and 11.3.

**11.6.** D. All of the above.

Other major criteria include raised JVP, weight loss of 10 lb with diuresis.

**11.7.** D. All of the above.

**11.8.** D. All of the above.

**11.9.** A. A 52-year-old patient with EF of 30%, diabetes, and angina on walking one block.

In this patient with angina and diabetes, there is a high likelihood of having significant coronary artery disease (CAD) as the basis of LV dysfunction and constitutes class I indication. In scenario B, there is no ischemia or chest pain and coronary angiogram would be inappropriate. In C, the likelihood of CAD is very low.

**11.10.** D. All of the above.

That is, longer, broader, and more T tubules. Ventricular myocytes are about 60–140 p.m. in length, compared with 20 p.m. for atrial myocytes. The diameter of a ventricular myocyte is about 20 p.m., compared with 5 p.m. for an atrial myocyte Atrial myocytes are elliptical, and ventricular myocytes are branched tubules with plenty of mitochondria and sarcomeres.

**11.11.** C. Purkinje cells.

These have no T tubules as they do not contract and their function is mainly electrical conduction.

**11.12.** C. Purkinje cells.

To facilitate rapid electrical conduction, as their function is mainly electrical conduction.

**11.13.** A. Frank-Starling phenomenon.

**11.14.** B. Anrep phenomenon.

**11.15.** C. Bowditch phenomenon.

Otherwise known as the force–frequency relationship. Contractile force is maximal at a rate of about 150 bpm.

**11.16.** B. LV afterload.

LV end-systolic wall stress is a measure of LV afterload and is roughly proportional to blood pressure and LV end-systolic radius and is inversely proportional to LV wall thickness (Laplace equation).

**11.17.** D. All of the above.

An increase in afterload will increase contractility through the Bowditch effect, but this may not be enough to overcome the afterload and hence would cause an increase in LV end-systolic volume and a reduction in EF. Both EF and end-systolic volume are afterload dependent.

**11.18.** D. All of the above.

**11.19.** D. All of the above.

The relaxation process affects the early LV filling, chamber stiffness, the late filling, and recoil, which depends upon how well the left ventricle squeezes and then recoils, which affects early filling. In addition, LV filling is affected by pericardial restraint, intrathoracic pressure, and interactions with the right ventricle.

**11.20.** D. Increase in stroke volume.

Submassive pulmonary embolism may cause right ventricle distention and invoke pericardial restraint (due to noncompliant pericardium) through an acute increase in intrapericardial volume. This will increase intrapericardial pressure, reduced transmural LV diastolic pressure and hence a reduction in stroke volume in the face of reduced LV preload due to reduced transmural LV diastolic pressure.

**11.21.** D. History of alcohol abuse and EF of 35% on pressors.

The other options are acceptable. Minor defects can always be repaired on the bench.

**11.22.** C. Do DeVega annuloplasty on bench and use the heart.

**11.23.** E. Options A–C.

Because of acute afterload mismatch for right ventricle. May be treated with pulmonary vasodilators, diuresis, positive inotropes and, in rare instances, atrial septostomy to unload the right side and increase cardiac output.

**11.24.** D. All of the above.

**11.25.** E. All of the above.

**11.26.** D. All of the above.

**11.27.** E. All of the above.

**11.28.** E. All of the above.

**11.29.** E. All of the above.

**11.30.** A. Biannual endomyocardial biopsy for the first five years.

**11.31.** E. All of the above.

**11.32.** D. All of the above.

**11.33.** C. Continue corticosteroids and calcineurin inhibitors (cyclosporine or tacrolimus).

Mycophenolate mofetil is a class D drug. Use of azathioprine is controversial.

**11.34.** C. Both A and B.

**11.35.** D. All of the above.

**11.36.** D. All of the above.

**11.37.** E. All of the above.

**11.38.** E. All are correct.

**11.39.** D. All of the above.

The trabeculations may impede flow into inflow cannula and also predispose to thrombus formation. LV thrombus increases stroke risk. A small LV increases the risk of obstruction to inflow cannula.

**11.40.** E. All of the above.

LA thrombus increases the risk of thrombus as blood is sucked into the LVAD. Suction force also promotes right-to-left shunting through atrial septal defects or VSDs and systemic desaturation. The PFO should be closed before the LVAD and should also be checked for both before and after the LVAD, as it may open up with LA unloading. Patients with severe RV dilation and dysfunction may need a biventricular assist device as leftward shift of ventricular septum may aggravate RV dysfunction.

**11.41.** D. All of the above.

Post LVAD, AR occurs throughout the cardiac cycle and leads to a blind-loop type of circulation. Mitral stenosis impedes LV filling. The TR may worsen due to a leftward shift of the ventricular septum. Hence, all these lesions should be addressed before LVAD implant.

**11.42.** D. All of the above.

**11.43.** A. Mechanical aortic valve.

Due to the risk of thrombosis because of low/absent flow. Bioprosthetic aortic valve is not an issue. The mechanical mitral prosthesis with or without MR has a low risk of thrombosis with anticoagulation as flow through it is increased with the LVAD. However, stenotic mitral prosthesis would be a problem and may need to be replaced with a bioprosthesis.

**11.44.** D. All of the above.

It is important to eliminate AR.

**11.45.** A. Unmasked PFO.

LA unloading may open up the PFO which was not detected preoperatively even with "ventilator Valsalva" and may cause large right-to-left shunting and systemic desaturation.

**11.46.** A. Should be upgraded by one grade based on traditional criteria.

This is because the AR is both systolic and diastolic. In diastole, the aortic flow will all be forward because of LVAD flow and hence this sign is invalid. A vena contracta of >3 mm or jet height to LV outflow tract ratio of >46% is considered to indicate severe AR.

**11.47.** D. Change to biventricular mechanical circulatory support.

This is a sign of severe RV dysfunction.

**11.48.** E. All of the above.

**11.49.** E. All of the above.

**11.50.** C. Both A and B.

**11.51.** A. Reduce pump speed.

Reducing pump speed may open the aortic valve and dislodge the thrombus.

**11.52.** E. All of the above.

**11.53.** A. Thrombosis of the LVAD.

This would also result in reduced inflow velocity and reduced transpulmonary flow, as evidenced by reduced velocity–time integral of flow across pulmonary valve, which is very useful in monitoring total cardiac output.

**11.54.** A. Reduced opening of aortic valve.

As flow through the pump increases, there is less flow through aortic valve, greater LV unloading, and less pulsatility in aorta.

**11.55.** B. Pravastatin.

**11.56.** B. Cyclosporine.

**11.57.** B. Discontinue tacrolimus.

This is because it may be the cause of renal dysfunction. The patient has no signs of rejection, and so treatment for antibody-mediated rejection (C and D) is not indicated. You would need to increase corticosteroids to stress dose level.

**11.58.** C. Neprilysin inhibitor.

LCZ696 has shown a higher efficacy than enalpril in the PARADIGM-HF trial (see Box 11.3; McMurray et al. 2014; Simpson et al. 2015).

**11.59.** B. Group 1 PH.

PH is attributable to the banned appetite suppressant fen-phen, which causes pulmonary vascular disease. Use for >3 months is a risk factor. E/e' ratio <8 indicates probable normal LA pressure.

**11.60.** B. Group 1 PH.

**11.61.** B. Group 1 PH.

**11.62.** B. Group 1 PH.

Portopulmonary hypertension is group 1.

**11.63.** B. Group 1 PH.

This is likely due to *in utero* exposure to selective serotonin reuptake inhibitor, which causes PH in the child.

**11.64.** B. Group 1 PH.

It is residual PH after late VSD closure due to increased pulmonary vascular resistance.

**11.65.** C. Group 2 PH.

Clearly due to severe mitral stenosis. Pressure half-time of 270 ms indicates a mitral valve area of <0.7 cm² and isovolumic relaxation time of 30 ms indicates very high LA pressure.

**11.66.** E. Group 4 PH.

Due to pulmonary thromboembolism. Loud, palpable P2 indicates PH. In addition, this patient has features of right HF.

**11.67.** C. Schistosomiasis.

**11.68.** A. *BMPR2* mutations.

These account for 75% of the cases of familial type and 25% of cases of idiopathic type. *BMPR2* encodes a type 2 receptor for bone morphogenetic proteins involved in the control of vascular cell proliferation.

**11.69.** A. V/Q scan.

A V/Q lung scan should be performed in patients with PH to look for chronic thromboembolic PH (CTEPH). The V/Q scan has been the screening method of choice for CTEPH because of its higher sensitivity compared with CT pulmonary angiogram, especially in inexperienced centers. A normal- or low-probability V/Q scan effectively excludes CTEPH with a sensitivity of 90–100% and a specificity of 94–100%.

**11.70.** A. Yes.

All patients should have this to confirm the diagnosis and make treatment decisions.

**11.71.** E. All of the above.

**11.72.** E. The use of oral or IV CCBs in acute vasoreactivity testing is recommended.
All the other statements are accurate.

**11.73.** E. All of the above.

A and B are class I recommendations; C and D are class IIA recommendations.

**11.74.** E. All of the above.

The statements are self-explanatory.

**11.75.** E. All of the above.

Recommendation is for group 1 and functional class II or III, rather than too late or too early (i.e. class I recommendation). A and B are endothelin receptor antagonists, and C and D are phosphodiesterase type 5 inhibitors. Prostacyclin analogs epoprostenol (IV), iloprost (inhaled or IV) and treprostinil (subcutaneous or inhaled) also have class I recommendations in this patient category. When combination is used, use drugs from different categories.

**11.76.** E. All of the above.

These are based on 2015 European Society of Cardiology/European Respiratory Society guidelines (Galie et al. 2016). See Box 11.4.

**11.77.** A. LVAD.

Note the inlet cannula in the LV apex (arrow in Figure 11.77). The outflow cannula would be in ascending aorta (not shown).

**11.78.** C. Tandem heart device.

Note the inlet cannula in the left atrium.

**11.79.** B. Impella device.

Note the Impella catheter across the aortic valve in Figure 11.79a and in the descending thoracic aorta in Figure 11.79b– both pointed to by the arrow.

**11.80.** E. None of the above. There is no single diagnostic test for HF because it is largely a clinical diagnosis based on a careful history and physical examination.

**11.81.** B. Heart failure with reduced ejection fraction is defined as an EF ≤ 40%.

**11.82.** A. Hypertension remains the most common cause of heart failure with preserved ejection fraction with some studies estimated up to 60–89% of cases attributed to this etiology.

**11.83.** B. The upper limit of normal mean pulmonary artery pressure is considered to be 20 mmHg. Above this threshold, the mortality among patients with pulmonary hypertension increases up to 23% above the normal population.

**11.84.** D. All of the above were associated with even mildly elevated mean pulmonary artery pressure. This is why there is a greater emphasis in diagnosing and treating pulmonary hypertension in an earlier stage of the disease.

**11.85.** A. Pulmonary vascular resistance (in woods units) is calculated by taking the difference between pulmonary artery pressure and wedge pressure and dividing that quantity by the cardiac output. To convert this quantity to metric measurements (dynes/sec/cm$^3$), you must multiply by 80.

**11.86.** C. $\geq$3 woods units from data on right heart catheterization is diagnostic for pulmonary arterial hypertension.

**11.87.** B. A mean pulmonary artery pressure >20 mmHg, pulmonary vascular resistance <3 woods units, and pulmonary artery wedge pressure >15 mmHg signifies isolated LV dysfunction.

**11.88.** B. A right-to-left shunt will produce more flow in the systemic circulation compared to pulmonary circulation and cause the Qp/Qs to be <1.

**11.89.** A. The "a" wave represents right atrial contraction. Tricuspid valve bulging into the right atrium results in "c" wave. Right atrial relaxation results in "x" descent. Rapid filling of the right atrium results in "v" wave. Early right ventricular filling results in "y" wave.

**11.90.** F. CRT is indicated for patients who have LVEF $\leq$35%, sinus rhythm, LBBB with a QRS $\geq$150 ms, and NYHA class II (IA), III, or ambulatory IV symptoms on GDMT (I,B).

**11.91.** C. Ensure 36 hours off ACE-I before initiating sacubitril/valsartan (ARNI) (Guidelines). This delay is not required when switching from ARB to ARNI (Expert Consensus). Use of an aldosterone antagonist is not considered mandatory prior to changing a patient to ARNI (Expert Consensus).

**11.92.** D. A combination of hydralazine and isorbide dinitrate (BiDil) improves survival, incremental to the above drugs in black patients, as demonstrated in the A-HeFT Trial. Thus, in black patients with HFrEF NYHA III–IV already on ACEI/ARB and BB, starting hydralazine and nitrates combination therapy is a Class I indication.

**11.93.** B. Contraindications for IABP include severe aortic regurgitation, aortic dissection, uncontrolled sepsis, and uncontrolled bleeding disorders.

**11.94.** B. A maximal cardiopulmonary exercise test (CPET) is defined as one with a respirator exchange ratio (RER) >1.05 and achievement of an anaerobic threshold on optimal pharmacological therapy. If the above criteria are met, then a cutoff of peak VO$_2$ of $\leq$14 ml/kg/min should be used to guide listing. If the patient is on a beta blocker, then a cutoff of peak VO$_2$ $\leq$ 12 ml/kg/min should be used.

**11.95.** A. Graft failure, infection, and multiorgan dysfunction are the leading causes of death in the first year after heart transplantation. Acute rejection, though occurring in approximately 12.7% of patients over the first year post-transplant, accounts for <5% of deaths in that time period. After one year, cardiac allograft vasculopathy, malignancy, and renal failure are relatively more common causes of death.

**11.96.** B. Unlike PVADs such as Impella devices, ECMO enables RV decompression and offers the ability to oxygenate blood if needed. ECMO can also remain implanted for weeks, compared to seven days for PVAD. However, VA ECMO increases afterload due to oxygenated outflow being directed back into the arterial circulation. This, in turn, results in increased myocardial $O_2$ demand. PVADs decrease preload and LV distension/wall stress, thereby resulting in decreased myocardial $O_2$ demand.

**11.97.** E. Indications for pulmonary artery catheter placement include all of the above answers (hypoperfusion, refractory fluid retention, hypoxemia, undifferentiated shock) as well as patients undergoing evaluation or preoperative management for MCS/transplant, or patients with end-stage HF being considered for home inotropic support.

**11.98.** E. Other options for diuretic resistant patients include use of vasodilators (IV Nitroprusside or nitroglycerin or oral hydralazine/nitrates), positive inotropes (dobutamine, milrinone, dopamine), or temporary mechanical circulatory support (IABP, Impella, etc.). Vasodilators are preferred unless limited by hypotension. Positive inotropes may contribute to proarrhythmia and are associated with adverse outcomes.

**11.99.** D. Dobutamine is not cleared renally, unlike milrinone. Dopamine has vasopressor activity at higher doses, no vasodilator activity. Side effects of tachycardia, arrythmia and myocardial ischemia are common for all three inotropes. Milrinone typically leads to more hypotension than dobutamine.

**11.100.** F. Bisoprolol, metoprolol succinate, and carvedilol are the only beta-blockers indicated for guideline-directed medical therapy in patients with HFrEF.

**Box 11.1    Clinical Pearls, Facts, and Guidelines**

**Heart Failure Stages**

Stage A: risk factors for heart disease such as hypertension, diabetes, or CAD, but no functional or structural changes.
Stage B: structural or functional changes such as LV hypertrophy, low EF, abnormal LV diastolic function, or abnormal valve function, but no clinical HF.
Stage C: ambulatory clinical HF.
Stage D: HF with symptoms at rest.

### Framingham Criteria for Heart Failure

HF: two major or one major and two minor criteria.

Major criteria: jugular vein distension, hepatojugular reflux, S3, pulmonary edema, paroxysmal nocturnal dyspnea, 4.5 kg weight loss on diuresis, cardiomegaly on chest X-ray.

Minor criteria: dyspnea, nocturnal cough, bilateral edema, tachycardia >120 bpm, pleural effusions.

### Role of Brain Natriuretic Peptide in Heart Failure

1. BNP >400 pg/ml or N-terminal prohormone of BNP (NT-proBNP) >2000 pg/ml support diagnosis of HF.
2. If BNP <400 pg/ml or NT-proBNP <400 pg/ml in a patient with dyspnea, consider alternate diagnosis.
3. Persistently elevated levels predict poor prognosis and recurrent hospital admissions for HF.
4. Levels are also elevated with LV hypertrophy and atrial fibrillation.
5. May be false negative in obesity due to being metabolized by adipocytes.

### Treatment of Heart Failure with Reduced Ejection Fraction

1. Na restriction to <1–2 g/day.
2. Water restriction to <1 l/day in those with hyponatremia.
3. Treatment of underlying cause (e.g. alcohol or drug use, relief of ischemia).
4. Achieve euvolemic status: use JVP and daily weights to monitor.
5. Treatment of acute decompensation with IV diuresis.
6. Digoxin as an inotrope has neutral effect on mortality but may increase mortality in those with renal dysfunction, the aged, and women.
7. Beta blockers are important disease-modifying agents by blocking toxic effects of catecholamines on myocardium and upregulating beta receptors; carvedilol and metoprolol succinate have shown mortality benefit. Maximize doses.
8. ACEIs or angiotensin receptor blockers (ARBs) reduce mortality. Neprilysin inhibitor, LCZ696, was superior to enalapril in PARADIGM-HF trial (McMurray et al. 2014).
9. Spironalactone or eplerenone improve survival.
10. Combination of hydralazine and isorbide dinitrate (BiDil) improves survival incremental to above drugs in black patients.
11. Amiodarone has neutral effect on mortality. May be useful as a bridge to beta blockade in acute HF with rapid heart rates (Singh et al. 1995).
12. Inotropes increase mortality; they are used for palliative care and as a bridge to heart transplant.
13. An implantable cardioverter-defibrillator (ICD) for primary prevention of death is recommended in those with EF <35%.
14. Cardiac resynchronization therapy (CRT) with biventricular pacer or ICD is recommended for those with EF <35% and QRS duration >150 ms with left bundle branch block morphology.
15. Cardiac transplant improves outcome in end-stage HF patients who are candidates for heart transplant.

16. LVADs improve survival in selected patients with end-stage HF who are not transplant candidates.
17. Treatment of anemia with erythropoietin increased mortality.

## Treatment of Heart Failure with Preserved Ejection Fraction

1. Na restriction to <1–2 g/day.
2. Water restriction to <1 l/day in those with hyponatremia.
3. Treatment of underlying cause (e.g. hypertension, relief of ischemia).
4. Achieve euvolemic status: use JVP and daily weights to monitor.
5. Treatment of acute decompensation with IV diuresis.
6. Beta blockers have not shown a mortality benefit.
7. ACEIs and ARBs have not shown a mortality benefit, though ARBs may marginally reduce hospitalization.
8. Aldosterone blockade had no mortality benefit.
9. No role for ICD or CRT devices.
10. Exercise program improves exercise tolerance.

## Causes of Acute Heart Failure Decompensation

Keep these in mind.

1. Noncompliance with medical regimen.
2. Acute myocardial ischemia.
3. Uncorrected high blood pressure.
4. Atrial fibrillation and other arrhythmias.
5. Intake of negative inotropic agents (e.g. verapamil, diltiazem, sotalol, disopyramide).
6. Pulmonary embolism.
7. Use of nonsteroidal anti-inflammatory drugs causing fluid retention.
8. Excessive alcohol or illicit drug use.
9. Concurrent infections (e.g. pneumonia, viral illnesses).

**Chapter 11**

## Markers of Poor Prognosis in Heart Failure

1. Lower EF.
2. Higher functional class.
3. Hyponatremia.
4. Refractory symptoms.
5. Low blood pressure.
6. Tachycardia.
7. Intolerance to beta blockers and ACEIs.
8. Increasing creatinine.
9. Recurrent admissions.
10. Inotrope dependence.
11. Increasing QRS duration.
12. Higher BNP levels.
13. Anemia.

---

**Box 11.2  Updated Classification of Pulmonary Hypertension**

---

Adapted from Simonneau et al. (2013).

1. **PAH**
   - 1.1  Idiopathic PAH
   - 1.2  Heritable PAH
     - 1.2.1  *BMPR2*
     - 1.2.2  *ALK-1, ENG, SMAD9, CAV1, KCNK3*
     - 1.2.3  Unknown
   - 1.3  Drug and toxin induced
   - 1.4  Associated with:
     - 1.4.1  Connective tissue disease
     - 1.4.2  HIV infection
     - 1.4.3  Portal hypertension
     - 1.4.4  Congenital heart diseases
     - 1.4.5  Schistosomiasis
   - 1' Pulmonary veno-occlusive disease and/or pulmonary capillary hemangiomatosis
   - 1" Persistent PH of the newborn (PPHN)
2. **PH due to left heart disease**
   - 2.1  Left ventricular systolic dysfunction
   - 2.2  Left ventricular diastolic dysfunction
   - 2.3  Valvular disease
   - 2.4  Congenital/acquired left heart inflow/outflow tract obstruction and congenital cardiomyopathies
3. **PH due to lung diseases and/or hypoxia**
   - 3.1  Chronic obstructive pulmonary disease
   - 3.2  Interstitial lung disease
   - 3.3  Other pulmonary diseases with mixed restrictive and obstructive pattern
   - 3.4  Sleep-disordered breathing
   - 3.5  Alveolar hypoventilation disorders
   - 3.6  Chronic exposure to high altitude
   - 3.7  Developmental lung diseases
4. **CTEPH**
5. **PH with unclear multifactorial mechanisms**
   - 5.1  Hematologic disorders: chronic hemolytic anemia, myeloproliferative disorders, splenectomy
   - 5.2  Systemic disorders: sarcoidosis, pulmonary histiocytosis, lymphangioleiomy-omatosis
   - 5.3  Metabolic disorders: glycogen-storage disease, Gaucher disease, thyroid disorders
   - 5.4  Others: tumoral obstruction, fibrosing mediastinitis, chronic renal failure, segmental PH

---

**Box 11.3    Pulmonary Hypertension Take-home Points**

These take-home points are based on ESC/ERS 2015 recommendations. (Adapted from Galiè et al. 2016).

1. RHC is recommended to confirm the diagnosis of PAH (Group 1) and to support treatment decisions.
2. Vasoreactivity testing is recommended in patients with idiopathic PAH, hereditary PAH, and PAH induced by drugs used to detect patients who can be treated with high doses of a CCB.
3. It is recommended to avoid pregnancy in patients with PAH.
4. It is recommended for referral centers to provide care by a multi-professional team (cardiology and respiratory medicine physicians, clinical nurse specialist, radiologists, psychological and social work support, appropriate on-call expertise).
5. Initial approved drugs monotherapy is recommended in treatment-naive, low-, or intermediate-risk patients with PAH.
6. Initial approved oral drugs combination therapy is recommended in treatment-naive, low-, or intermediate-risk patients with PAH.
7. Sequential drug combination therapy is recommended in patients with inadequate treatment response to initial monotherapy or to initial double-combination therapy.
8. The use of PAH-approved therapies is not recommended in patients with PH due to left heart disease or lung diseases.
9. Surgical pulmonary endarterectomy in deep hypothermia circulatory arrest is recommended for patients with CTEPH and it is recommended that the assessment of operability and decisions regarding other treatment strategies (drugs therapy or balloon pulmonary angioplasty) be made by a multidisciplinary team of experts.

---

**Box 11.4    Summary of Pivotal Clinical Trials in Heart Failure**

- McKee et al. (1971) lists the Framingham criteria for HF that serves as the gold standard for its diagnosis
- The CONSENSUS trial (The CONSENSUS Trial Study Group 1987) is a large, randomized study that showed a large survival benefit with ACEIs in HFrEF which had been shown before a Veterans Administration randomized trial.
- Packer et al. (1996) was a randomized trial that clearly established the role for carvedilol in the treatment of HFrEF.
- The MERIT-HF Study Group (Hjalmarson et al. 2000) randomized trial showed mortality benefit with long-acting metoprolol in HFrEF. Note that short-acting metoprolol does not give the same benefit due to a lack of sustained beta blockade.
- Pitt et al. (1999) used aldosterone antagonist to improve survival incremental to beta blocker and ACEIs in HFrEF.
- The A-HeFT trial (Taylor et al. 2004) showed a mortality benefit with the combination of isosorbide dinitrate and hydralazine (BiDil) in African-American patients with HFrEF and this effect was incremental to beta blocker and ACEIs.

- The DIG trial (The Digitalis Investigation Group 1997) showed a neutral effect on mortality in HF. But subset analysis has shown a potential reduction in hospitalization in those with severe congestive HF and S3 and potential increased mortality in the elderly, women, and those with renal dysfunction, possibly as a result of digoxin toxicity in these subgroups with lower creatinine clearance rates.
- The CHF-STAT trial (Singh et al. 1995) showed that amiodarone had a neutral effect on mortality in HFrEF. It is possible that a slight reduction in mortality due to malignant ventricular arrhythmias was neutralized by an increase in bradycardic mortality.
- In the CHARM-Preserved Trial (Yusuf et al. 2003) the ARB candesartan did not reduce mortality in HFpEF, but there was a slight reduction in hospitalization.
- The SENIORS study (Flather et al. 2005) examined beta blockers. They did not reduce mortality in HFpEF.
- The Aldo-HF trial (Edelmann et al. 2013) examined spironolactone, which had a neutral mortality effect in HFpEF.
- In the Ex-DHF study (Edelmann et al. 2011), exercise training was found to improve exercise tolerance and LV filling dynamics in HFpEF.
- In the PARADIGM-HF trial (McMurray et al. 2014) the Angiotensin receptor-neprilysin inhibitor was superior to enalapril in addition to standard therapy in patients with systolic heart failure in terms of mortality and hospitalization. 8442 patients with class II, III, or IV HF and an EF of 40% or less were randomized.
- In the PARADIGM-HF trial (Simpson et al. 2015), MAGGIC (Meta-Analysis Global Group in Chronic Heart Failure) and EMPHASIS-HF (Eplerenone in Mild Patients Hospitalization and Survival Study in Heart Failure) risk scores are described and applied to the trial population. The benefit of LCZ696 was uniform across all risk groups based on these scores.
- The 2015 ESC/ERS Guidelines (Galie et al. 2016) is an excellent reference resource to understand the current classification, diagnostic approach, and treatment of patients with PH.

## References

Edelmann, F., Gelbrich, G., Dungen, H.-D. et al. (2011). Exercise training improves exercise capacity and diastolic function in patients with heart failure with preserved ejection fraction: results of the ex-DHF (exercise training in diastolic heart failure) pilot study. *Journal of the American College of Cardiology* 58 (17): 1780–1791.

Edelmann, F., Wachter, R., Schmidt, A.G. et al. (2013). Effect of spironolactone on diastolic function and exercise capacity in patients with heart failure with preserved ejection fraction: the Aldo-DHF randomized controlled trial. *Journal of the American Medical Association* 309 (8): 781–791.

Flather, M.D., Shibata, M.C., Coats, A.J.S. et al. (2005). Randomized trial to determine the effect of nebivolol on mortality and cardiovascular hospital admission in elderly patients with heart failure (SENIORS). *European Heart Journal* 26: 215–225.

Galie, N., Humbert, M., Vachiery, J.L. et al. (2016). 2015 ESC/ERS guidelines for the diagnosis and treatment of pulmonary hypertension: the joint task force for the diagnosis and treatment of pulmonary hypertension of the European Society of Cardiology (ESC) and the European Respiratory Society (ERS): endorsed by: Association for European Paediatric and Congenital

Cardiology (AEPC), International Society for Heart and Lung Transplantation (ISHLT). *European Heart Journal* 37 (1): 67–119. https://doi.org/10.1093/eurheartj/ehv317.

Hjalmarson, A., Goldstein, S., Fagerberg, B. et al. (2000). Effects of controlled release metoprolol on total mortality, hospitalizations, and well-being in patients with heart failure: the metoprolol CR/XL randomized intervention trial in congestive heart failure (MERIT-HF). MERIT-HF Study Group. *Journal of the American Medical Association* 283: 1295–1302.

McKee, P.A., Castelli, W.P., McNamara, P.M., and Kannel, W.B. (1971). The natural history of congestive heart failure: the Framingham study. *The New England Journal of Medicine* 285: 1441–1446.

McMurray, J.J., Packer, M., Desai, A.S. et al. (2014). Angiotensin-neprilysin inhibition versus enalapril in heart failure. *The New England Journal of Medicine* 371 (11): 993–1004.

Packer, M., Bristow, M.R., Cohn, J.N. et al. (1996). The effect of carvedilol on morbidity and mortality in patients with chronic heart failure. U.S. Carvedilol Heart Failure Study Group. *The New England Journal of Medicine* 334: 1349–1355.

Pitt, B., Zannad, F., Remme, W.J. et al. (1999). The effect of spironolactone on morbidity and mortality in patients with severe heart failure. Randomized Aldactone Evaluation Study Investigators. *The New England Journal of Medicine* 341: 709–717.

Simonneau, G., Gatzoulis, M.A., Adatia, I. et al. (2013). Updated clinical classification of pulmonary hypertension. *Journal of the American College of Cardiology* 62 (25 Suppl): D34–D41. https://doi.org/10.1016/j.jacc.2013.10.029 [Erratum: Journal of the American College of Cardiology (2014) 63(7): 746.].

Simpson, J., Jhund, P.S., Silva Cardoso, J. et al. (2015). Comparing LCZ696 with enalapril according to baseline risk using the MAGGIC and EMPHASIS-HF risk scores: an analysis of mortality and morbidity in PARADIGM-HF. *Journal of the American College of Cardiology* 66 (19): 2059–2071. https://doi.org/10.1016/j.jacc.2015.08.878.

Singh, S.N., Fletcher, R.D., Fisher, S.G. et al. (1995). Amiodarone in patients with congestive heart failure and asymptomatic ventricular arrhythmia. Survival trial of antiarrhythmic therapy in congestive heart failure. *The New England Journal of Medicine* 333: 77–82.

Taylor, A.L., Ziesche, S., Yancy, C. et al. (2004). Combination of isosorbide dinitrate and hydralazine in blacks with heart failure. *The New England Journal of Medicine* 351: 2049–2057.

The CONSENSUS Trial Study Group (1987). Effects of enalapril on mortality in severe congestive heart failure. Results of the Cooperative North Scandinavian Enalapril Survival Study (CONSENSUS). *The New England Journal of Medicine* 316: 1429–1435.

The Digitalis Investigation Group (1997). The effect of digoxin on mortality and morbidity in patients with heart failure. *The New England Journal of Medicine* 336: 525–533.

Yusuf, S., Pfeffer, M.A., Swedberg, K. et al. (2003). Effects of candesartan in patients with chronic heart failure and preserved left-ventricular ejection fraction: the CHARM-preserved trial. *Lancet* 362: 777–781.

Chapter 11

# Cardiomyopathies

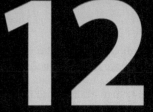

**12.1.** About 30% of dilated cardiomyopathies are inherited. What modes of transmission are included?
- **A.** Autosomal dominant
- **B.** Autosomal recessive
- **C.** X-linked
- **D.** Mitochondrial
- **E.** All of the above

**12.2.** What is the most common mode of inheritance in dilated cardiomyopathy (DCM)?
- **A.** Autosomal dominant
- **B.** X-linked
- **C.** Autosomal recessive
- **D.** Mitochondrial

**12.3.** A 19-year-old patient has DCM with an ejection fraction (EF) of 10%, complete heart block, junctional escape rhythm with left bundle branch block (LBBB), and muscle weakness. What is the likely mutation in?
- **A.** Lamin A/C gene
- **B.** Troponin T gene
- **C.** Desmin gene
- **D.** Titin gene

**12.4.** Which of the following gene mutations can cause DCM?
- **A.** Myosin heavy chain
- **B.** Cardiac actin
- **C.** Troponin T
- **D.** Titin
- **E.** Dystrophin
- **F.** All of the above

**12.5.** Which of the following is *not* a standard indication for anticoagulation in patients with dilated cardiomyopathy?
- **A.** Male, 30 years, DCM, EF of 10%
- **B.** Male, 30 years, DCM, EF of 25%, apical thrombus
- **C.** Male, 30 years, DCM, EF is 20%, multiple transient ischemic attacks (TIAs), no thrombus seen in left ventricle or left atrium, aorta is clear, no patent foramen ovale

*Cardiology Board Review*, Second Edition. Ramdas G. Pai and Padmini Varadarajan.
© 2023 John Wiley & Sons Ltd. Published 2023 by John Wiley & Sons Ltd.

   **D.** Male, 30 years, DCM, EF 35%, no left ventricular (LV) thrombus, no TIA or stroke, left ventricle is hypertrabeculated with noncompacted to compacted ratio of 2.5

**12.6.** Which of the following mutations may not cause hypertrophic cardiomyopathy (HCM)?
   **A.** Myosin heavy chain
   **B.** Myosin light chain
   **C.** Troponin T
   **D.** Desmin

**12.7.** Which of the following mutation can cause restrictive cardiomyopathy?
   **A.** Myosin heavy chain
   **B.** Cardiac actin
   **C.** Troponin T
   **D.** Troponin I

**12.8.** A 42-year-old man is diagnosed to have HCM with dynamic LV outflow tract (LVOT) obstruction. He has had two episodes of syncope, and maximum interventricular septal thickness is 30 mm. No genetic testing has been done. Which of the following statements is *not* accurate regarding screening?
   **A.** It is appropriate to screen first-degree relatives with an echocardiogram
   **B.** It is strongly recommended to screen first-degree relatives for high-risk genotypes
   **C.** It is appropriate to perform a physical examination and an electrocardiogram (ECG) in first-degree relatives
   **D.** It is appropriate to screen adult first-degree relatives every 5 years and children every 12–18 months.

**12.9.** Which of the following statements is inaccurate regarding genetic testing in HCM?
   **A.** Evaluation of familial inheritance and genetic counseling is recommended as part of the assessment of patients with HCM
   **B.** Patients who undergo genetic testing should also undergo counseling by someone knowledgeable in the genetics of cardiovascular disease so that results and their clinical significance can be appropriately reviewed with the patient
   **C.** Genetic testing is reasonable in the index patient to facilitate the identification of first-degree family members at risk for developing HCM
   **D.** Genetic testing is indicated in relatives when the index patient does not have a definitive pathogenic mutation as sporadic mutations may occur

**12.10.** A 45-year-old man has HCM and was found to have MHC gene mutation. The same mutation is found in one of his sons who is 20 years old. The son had a normal physical examination, ECG, and an echocardiogram. How frequently would you repeat an echocardiogram on this son?
   **A.** No need to repeat
   **B.** Every 12–18 months
   **C.** Every five years
   **D.** Only if symptoms occur or ECG becomes abnormal

Chapter 1

**12.11.** Which of the following statements are accurate regarding performance of a 24-hour Holter monitor in a patient with HCM?

**A.** Twenty-four-hour ambulatory (Holter) ECG monitoring is recommended in the initial evaluation of patients with HCM to detect ventricular tachycardia (VT) and identify patients who may be candidates for ICD therapy even if they have no palpitations or syncope

**B.** Twenty-four-hour ambulatory (Holter) ECG monitoring or event recording is recommended in patients with HCM who develop palpitations or lightheadedness

**C.** Twenty-four-hour ambulatory (Holter) ECG monitoring, repeated every 12 years, is reasonable in patients with HCM who have no previous evidence of VT to identify patients who may be candidates for implantable cardioverter-defibrillator (ICD) therapy

**D.** All of the above

**E.** None of the above

**12.12.** In a patient with known or suspected HCM, which of the following statements regarding echocardiography are accurate?

**A.** A transthoracic echocardiogram (TTE) is recommended in the initial evaluation of all patients with suspected HCM

**B.** A TTE is recommended as a component of the screening algorithm for family members of patients with HCM unless the family member is genotype negative in a family with known definitive mutations

**C.** Periodic (12–18 months) TTE screening is recommended for children of patients with HCM, starting by age 12 years or earlier if a growth spurt or signs of puberty are evident and/or when there are plans for engaging in intense competitive sports or there is a family history of sudden cardiac death (SCD)

**D.** All of the above

**12.13.** In a patient with known or suspected HCM, which of the following statements regarding cardiac magnetic resonance (CMR) imaging are accurate?

**A.** CMR imaging is indicated in patients with suspected HCM when echocardiography is inconclusive for diagnosis

**B.** CMR imaging is indicated in patients with known HCM when additional information that may have an impact on management or decision making regarding invasive management, such as magnitude and distribution of hypertrophy or anatomy of the mitral valve apparatus or papillary muscles, is not adequately defined with echocardiography

**C.** CMR imaging is reasonable in patients with HCM to define apical hypertrophy and/or aneurysm if echocardiography is inconclusive

**D.** In selected patients with known HCM, when SCD risk stratification is inconclusive after documentation of the conventional risk factors, CMR imaging with assessment of late gadolinium enhancement may be considered in resolving clinical decision making

**E.** All of the above

**12.14.** Which of the following drugs may prolong survival in an asymptomatic HCM patient?
A. Beta blocker
B. Verapamil
C. Amiodarone
D. None of the above

**12.15.** Which of the following therapies are indicated in asymptomatic HCM patients with no outflow obstruction?
A. Beta blocker to reduce atrial fibrillation risk
B. Calcium channel blocker as positive lusiotropic agents to improve cardiac performance
C. Amiodarone to reduce risk of sudden death
D. None of the above
E. All of the above

**12.16.** A patient with hypertrophic obstructive cardiomyopathy (HOCM) has a resting LVOT gradient of 80 mmHg despite verapamil of 480 mg/day. His heart rate is 58 bpm, blood pressure (BP) 125/70 mmHg and he is still in class III symptoms and short of breath on minimal exertion. Which of the following would you do?
A. Add nifedipine as a positive lusiotropic agent to improve LV diastolic function
B. Add small dose of frusemide to relieve pulmonary congestion
C. Consider dual-chamber pacer with short atrioventricular delay to cause asynchronous septal contraction and elimination of obstruction
D. Consider disopyramide as a negative inotropic agent

**12.17.** In a hypotensive patient with HOCM with high outflow gradient, in addition to intravenous fluids, which intravenous drug would be most useful?
A. Phenylephrine
B. Norepinephrine
C. Dopamine
D. Verapamil

**12.18.** Which of the following statements are accurate regarding septal reduction procedures in patients with HOCM?
A. Septal reduction therapy should be performed only by experienced operators in the context of a comprehensive HCM clinical program and only for the treatment of eligible patients with severe drug-refractory symptoms and LVOT obstruction
B. Surgical septal myectomy, when performed in experienced centers, can be beneficial and is the first consideration for the majority of eligible patients with HCM with severe drug-refractory symptoms and LVOT obstruction
C. When surgery is contraindicated or the risk is considered unacceptable because of serious comorbidities or advanced age, alcohol septal ablation, when performed in experienced centers, can be beneficial in eligible adult patients with HCM with LVOT obstruction and severe drug-refractory symptoms
D. All of the above

Chapter 12

**12.19.** Which of the following markers may be associated with elevated SCD risk in HCM patients?
   A. Family history of sudden death
   B. Syncope
   C. Nonsustained VT
   D. Hypotension on exercise
   E. LV wall thickness >30 mm
   F. All of the above

**12.20.** Which of the following markers may also be associated with elevated SCD risk in HCM patients?
   A. Delayed enhancement on CMR imaging
   B. Severe LVOT gradient
   C. Double and compound mutations
   D. All of the above
   E. None of the above

**12.21.** Which of the following statements are accurate regarding use of an ICD for primary prevention in a patient with HCM?
   A. An ICD can be useful in select patients with nonsustained VT (particularly those <30 years of age) in the presence of other SCD risk factors or modifiers
   B. An ICD can be useful in select patients with HCM with an abnormal blood pressure response with exercise in the presence of other SCD risk factors or modifiers
   C. It is reasonable to recommend an ICD for high-risk children with HCM, based on unexplained syncope, massive LV hypertrophy (LVH), or family history of SCD, after taking into account the relatively high complication rate of long-term ICD implantation
   D. All of the above

**12.22.** A 42-year-old man presents with shortness of breath, tingling of fingers, vague abdominal pains, and blurred vision. He is hypertensive, creatinine is 2.4 mg/dl, and has corneal opacities. He has reduced touch sensations in hands and feet. An echocardiogram shows moderate LVH with normal wall motion. What is the likely diagnosis?
   A. HCM
   B. Hypertensive heart disease
   C. Fabry disease
   D. Hemochromatosis

**12.23.** A 52-year-old man presented with anginal sounding chest pain. The ECG showed increased voltage and deep T-wave inversions V2 to V6. The cardiac enzymes were negative and the coronary angiogram was completely normal. What is the LV gram likely to show?
   A. Apical akinesis
   B. Severe LVH
   C. Dyskinesis distal 2/3 of left ventricle
   D. A spade-shaped left ventricle

**12.24.** A 42-year-old woman presented with abdominal pain, and an abdominal computed tomography scan showed possible LV apical pseudoaneurysm. A TTE was suboptimal. A transesophageal echocardiogram image is shown in Figure 12.24. What is the likely apical abnormality?

    **A.** LV apical aneurysm

    **B.** LV apical pseudoaneurysm

    **C.** LV apical diverticulum

    **D.** LV apex is normal

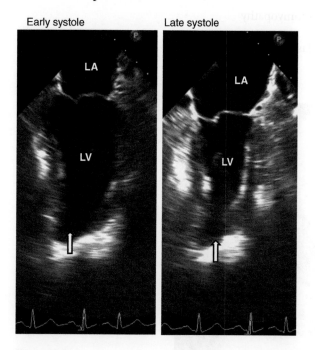

**Figure 12.24**

**12.25.** A 42-year-old man with a diagnosis of HOCM has shortness of breath on minimal exertion. He is on verapamil 240 mg BID and disopyramide 100 mg TID. His heart rate is 56 bpm, BP 120/70 mmHg, and examination shows a systolic murmur at the left sternal border increasing with Valsalva. The echocardiogram shows an EF of 75%, severe upper septal hypertrophy, severe systolic anterior motion (SAM) with a resting LVOT velocity of 4 m/s. The septal thickness at SAM-septal contact is 25 mm. What would the most appropriate treatment be?

    **A.** Referral to HCM center of excellence for surgical septal myectomy

    **B.** Alcohol septal ablation

    **C.** Mitral valve replacement

    **D.** Trial with dual-chamber pacemaker with short atrioventricular delay

**12.26.** A 22-year-old man is admitted with a history of syncope. He had a similar episode two months earlier. No other medical history. Family history is unremarkable. His resting ECG is normal and overnight monitoring shows frequent episodes of nonsustained VT of LBBB morphology. An echocardiogram, which is technically difficult, shows normal left ventricle and valvular function. The right ventricle

seems to be mildly dilated with a tricuspid annular plane systolic excursion of 15 mm. What would be the most useful test you could recommend at this time?
A. CMR imaging
B. Electrophysiology testing
C. Endomyocardial biopsy
D. A loop recorder

12.27. The 28-year-old patient in Figure 12.27 had syncope. What is the likely underlying cause?
A. LV noncompaction cardiomyopathy
B. HCM
C. Endomyocardial fibroelastosis
D. None of the above

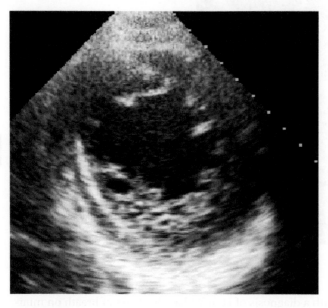

**Figure 12.27**

12.28. A 28-year-old man with no prior history presented with shortness of breath on minimal exertion. Images from a resting echocardiogram are shown in Figure 12.28. Which of the following may the shortness of breath respond to?
A. Aortic valve replacement
B. Frusemide
C. Beta blocker
D. Digoxin

12.29. What is auscultation of the patient's heart in Figure 12.29 likely to reveal?
A. Systolic murmur increased by Valsalva maneuver
B. Systolic murmur increased by hand grip
C. Systolic murmur with soft S1
D. Mid-diastolic murmur

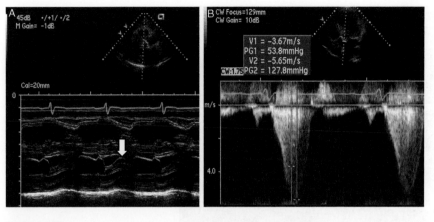

**Figure 12.28**

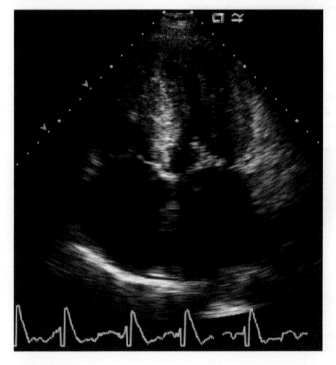

**Figure 12.29**

**12.30.** A 43-year-old woman with no prior medical history presented with a four month history of shortness of breath (see Figure 12.30). What could the likely explanation be?

**A.** Heart failure with reduced EF

**B.** Heart failure with preserved EF

**C.** Mitral stenosis

**D.** Mitral regurgitation

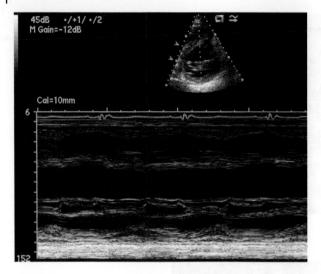

**Figure 12.30**

**12.31.** Which of the following is the patient in Figure 12.31 likely to have?
   **A.** HCM
   **B.** Restrictive cardiomyopathy
   **C.** Normal LV size and morphology
   **D.** LV noncompaction

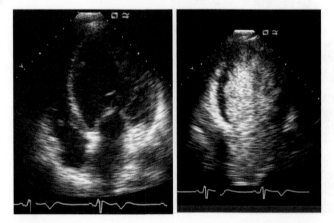

**Figure 12.31**

**12.32.** A 66-year-old patient presented with dyspnea and pedal edema. The ECG and an echo image are shown in Figure 12.32. The EF was about 25% and the left ventricle was globally hypokinetic. What is the possible diagnosis?
   **A.** Hypertensive heart disease
   **B.** HCM
   **C.** Cardiac amyloidosis
   **D.** None of the above

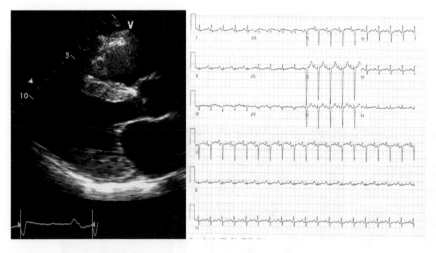

**Figure 12.32**

**12.33.** The 33-year-old woman shown in Figure 12.33 presented with shortness of breath and pedal edema of 4 weeks' duration. She also had low-grade fever, dry cough, and wheezing. There was no prior medical history, and she denied use of alcohol or recreational drugs. What does the possible diagnosis include?
**A.** Hypereosinophilic syndrome
**B.** Anterior myocardial infarction with large apical thrombus
**C.** Rib artifact in LV apex
**D.** Apical HCM

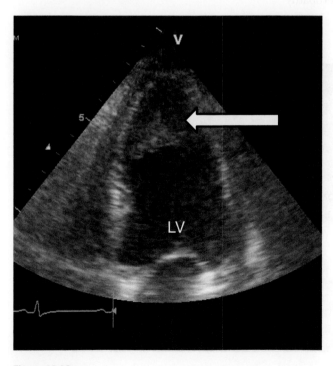

**Figure 12.33**

**12.34.** The 43-year-old African-American woman shown in Figure 12.34 (MDE: myocardial delayed enhancement) presented with syncope. What is the possible explanation?

A. LV diverticulum

B. Myocardial infarction

C. Cardiac sarcoid

D. None of the above

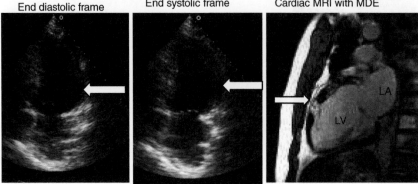

End diastolic frame     End systolic frame     Cardiac MRI with MDE

**Figure 12.34**

**12.35.** A 42-year-old woman presented with weight loss and diarrhea. A continuous-wave signal through the tricuspid valve is shown in Figure 12.35. What is the likely cause of her symptoms?

A. Hepatic congestion from severe tricuspid regurgitation

B. Protein-losing enteropathy

C. Carcinoid

D. None of the above

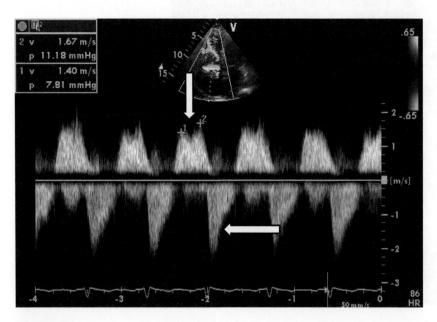

**Figure 12.35**

**12.36.** For the diagnosis of ARVD, which of the following criteria are required?
  A. Two major
  B. One major and two minor
  C. Four minor from different categories
  D. Any of the above

**12.37.** Which of the following are major criteria for ARVD diagnosis?
  A. On CMR imaging: RV regional wall dyskinesis plus RV EDV $\geq110\,ml/m^2$ in males/RV EDV $\geq 100\,ml/m^2$ in females or RV EF $\leq40\%$
  B. Epsilon wave (reproducible low-amplitude signals between end of QRS complex to onset of the T wave) in the right precordial leads (V1 to V3)
  C. Nonsustained or sustained VT of left bundle-branch morphology with superior axis (negative or indeterminate QRS in leads II, III, and aVF and positive in lead aVL)
  D. Arrhythmogenic RV cardiomyopathy (ARVC)/ARVD confirmed in a first-degree relative or identification of a pathogenic mutation categorized as associated or probably associated with ARVC/ARVD in the patient under evaluation
  E. All of the above

**12.38.** Which of the following facts are accurate regarding genetics of ARVD?
  A. Inheritance in familial cases is mostly autosomal dominant
  B. Mutations affect desmosomes with facilitate cell to cell connections
  C. Mutations have been found in plakoglobin *(JUP)*, desmoplakin *(DSP)*, plakophilin-2 *(PKP2)*, desmoglein-2 *(DSG2)*, desmocollin-2 *(DSC2)*, transforming growth factor beta-3 *(TGF3)*, and transmembrane protein 43 *(TMEM43)*.
  D. Mutations in *RYR2* coding the ryanodine receptor have been reported in ARVC/ARVD in patients with an arrhythmic presentation (stress-induced bidirectional VT) in the absence of significant electrocardiographic or structural abnormalities
  E. All of the above

Chapter 12

**12.39.** In the interventional management of HOCM, compared with surgical septal myectomy, alcohol septal ablation has a higher risk of all *except* which of the following?
  A. Right bundle branch block
  B. LBBB
  C. Complete heart block
  D. Sustained VT

**12.40.** What is the general approach for surgical myectomy?
  A. Transaortic
  B. Transatrial
  C. Through right ventricle
  D. None of the above

**12.41.** What is the risk of needing a permanent pacemaker with alcohol septal ablation?
  A. 2%
  B. 5%
  C. 20%
  D. 60%

**12.42.** Which of the following statements is most accurate regarding the amount of residual scar in the ventricular septum after surgical myectomy versus septal ablation?
A. Similar
B. More with surgical myectomy
C. More with alcohol septal ablation
D. None of the above

**12.43.** Following surgical septal myectomy or septal ablation with relief of obstruction, which of the following statements about LV mass regression are true at six months?
A. There is a reduction in septal LV mass only
B. There is a reduction in nonseptal LV mass only
C. There is reduction in both septal and nonseptal LV mass
D. There is no reduction in LV mass

**12.44.** Regarding residual outflow obstruction after surgical myectomy versus septal ablation, which of the following statements is most accurate?
A. Similar
B. More with surgical myectomy
C. More with alcohol septal ablation
D. None of the above

## Answers

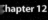

**12.1.** E. All of the above.

**12.2.** A. Autosomal dominant.

**12.3.** A. Lamin A/C gene.
The lamin A/C gene causes all these abnormalities.

**12.4.** F. All of the above.

**12.5.** A. Male, 30 years, DCM, EF of 10%.
This patient is least likely to benefit in the absence of LV thrombus, TIA, or atrial fibrillation. In option C, though there is no detectable LV thrombus, it is the likely cause of TIA. In D, patient has noncompaction and there is an indication for anticoagulation if EF is <40% even in the absence of TIA or thrombus as the deep LV crypts may promote thrombus formation and stroke.

**12.6.** D. Desmin.
Desmin mutation causes DCM. The other three cause HCM. Other mutations leading to HCM include troponin I, myosin-binding protein C, and titin. It is mostly the sarcomeric mutations that cause HCM. But DCM may be caused by mutations in sarcomeric proteins, cytosketetal proteins, as well as Z-disk associated protein.

**12.7.** D. Troponin I.

**12.8.** B. It is strongly recommended to screen first-degree relatives for high-risk genotypes.
In the absence of genotyping the index case, it is inappropriate to screen relatives for possible mutations. Genetic testing is not indicated in relatives when the index patient does not have a definitive pathogenic mutation.

**12.9.** D. Genetic testing is indicated in relatives when the index patient does not have a definitive pathogenic mutation as sporadic mutations may occur.

> The other statements are correct per ACC/AHA HCM guidelines.

**12.10.** C. Every five years.

> In adults every 5 years, and 12–18 months in children. As the genotype is positive, periodic screening for phenotype is indicated even in the absence of symptoms or physical signs as an echocardiogram is a lot more sensitive.

**12.11.** D. All of the above.

**12.12.** D. All of the above.

**12.13.** E. All of the above.

**12.14.** D. None of the above.

**12.15.** D. None of the above.

**12.16.** D. Consider disopyramide as a negative inotropic agent.

> This may reduce gradient without slowing heart rate further. As a matter of fact, its anticholinergic properties may increase the heart rate slightly. Diuretic and nifedepine as vasodilator will worsen the gradient by reducing the LV end-systolic volume. Despite initial enthusiasm, subsequent studies have not supported the use of a pacemaker to eliminate gradient.

**12.17.** A. Phenylephrine.

> This is a pure alpha stimulant. Dopamine, dobutamine, and norepinephrine have beta stimulant properties and would worsen outflow obstruction. Digoxin is contraindicated as well. Verapamil, through vasodilation, may drop the BP further.

**12.18.** D. All of the above.

**12.19.** F. All of the above.

**12.20.** D. All of the above.

**12.21.** D. All of the above.

**12.22.** C. Fabry disease.

> This is an X-linked recessive disease with manifest phenotype in males with wide variation in expressivity and penetrance. It is due to defective alpha glycosidase A deficiency, which leads to its deposition in nerves, vessels, intestines, cornea, heart, and kidneys. Hence, it may lead to cardiac hypertrophy, renal failure, hypertension, visual defects, and neuropathy. It is an orphan disease, and enzyme therapy is available at an annual cost of about $200 000.

**12.23.** D. A spade-shaped left ventricle.

> Indicates apical HCM. The presentation is typical. Option A is consistent with mid left anterior descending coronary artery lesion, and option C with Takatsubo syndrome.

**12.24.** C. LV apical diverticulum.

> The apical tip bulging does contract in systole, indicating it has muscular wall (muscular type of diverticulum). Neither the aneurysm nor pseudoaneurysm contract; aneurysm has a wide neck and pseudoaneurysm has a narrow neck.

**12.25.** A. Referral to HCM center of excellence for surgical septal myectomy.

> The patient, an otherwise healthy individual, has exhausted medical options. If the patient had multiple comorbidities and was of advanced age, alcohol septal

ablation would have been an option. Both should be done in experienced centers. Mitral valve replacement, though entertained as an option in the past, is not a recommended treatment. Despite some controversial data on the use of dual-chamber pacing in the 1990s, it is not considered an option in the current era.

**12.26.** A. CMR imaging.

The index of suspicion for right ventricular (RV) dysplasia is significant. CMR imaging would be helpful for assessment of RV volume and EF. An EF <40% or RV end-diastolic volume (EDV) >110 ml/m$^2$ would serve as a major criterion. VT is also a major criterion and a diagnosis of arrhythmogenic RV dysplasia (ARVD) can be established with two major criteria. Right ventricle biopsy may be negative due to sampling errors and can also be risky in a patient with thin right ventricle wall. Electrophysiology testing or loop recorder would not add much as the patient already has VT with LBBB morphology. ARVD major criteria are listed at the end of the chapter.

**12.27.** A. LV noncompaction cardiomyopathy.

Note the heavily trabeculated LV myocardium with noncompacted to compacted thickness ratio >2 in systole. CMR imaging and echo with contrast are other useful tools for the diagnosis. LV noncompaction results in cardiomyopathy, heart failure, ventricular arrhythmias, and formation of LV thrombus with embolization. Indications for anticoagulation include: LV thrombus, systemic embolism/stroke/TIA, atrial fibrillation, and EF <40% even without a thrombus. First-degree relatives should be screened as it is mostly transmitted in an autosomal dominant fashion.

**12.28.** C. Beta blocker.

The m-mode of the mitral valve in panel A shows SAM of the mitral valve (arrow). The continuous-wave Doppler signal in panel B is diagnostic of dynamic LVOT obstruction with a late-peaking signal. In valvular aortic stenosis, the signal would be more rounded as obstruction is present throughout the ejection period. Diuresis and digoxin are likely to worsen the dynamic obstruction. The other useful drugs are nondihydropyridine calcium channel blockers and disopy-ramide because of their negative inotropic properties.

**12.29.** A. Systolic murmur increased by Valsalva maneuver.

Note the SAM of the anterior mitral leaflet along with septal hypertrophy, suggesting HOCM.

**12.30.** A. Heart failure with reduced EF.

The m-mode examination of the left ventricle at the level of mitral leaflet tips shows dilated left ventricle with LV end-diastolic diameter of 62 mm, reduced contractile function, and increased mitral E wave-septal separation. Reduced mitral opening is due to reduced flow – the leaflets are not thickened and posterior leaflet does not move anteriorly during diastole with the anterior leaflet, as would occur with rheumatic mitral stenosis.

**12.31.** D. LV noncompaction.

Note the hypertrabeculated LV lateral wall. LV contrast is helpful. A noncompacted to compacted ratio of >2 is suggestive of noncompaction. Noncompaction can result in systolic heart failure, ventricular arrhythmias, sudden death, and LV thrombus formation with stroke. Anticoagulation is generally indicated when EF <40% or there is LV thrombus, systemic embolism, or atrial fibrillation.

**12.32.** C. Cardiac amyloidosis.

Note LVH on echo with low voltage in the limb leads of the ECG. Also note poor R wave progression V1 to V4 despite preserved septal wall thickness; that is, pseudo-anterior infarct pattern. These features are highly suggestive of cardiac amyloidosis.

**12.33.** A. Hypereosinophilic syndrome.

The patient has obliterative cardiomyopathy with filling of LV apex with fibrous tissue/thrombus. The patient had an eosinophilic count of 65% on the peripheral smear. Treatment with anticoagulation and prednisone resulted in marked improvement in the appearance of the LV apex and symptoms. In late stages, the patient may not respond and may need surgical resection of endocardial thickening or heart transplant.

**12.34.** C. Cardiac sarcoid.

The arrow points to a focal aneurysm in the mid anterior wall in both the echo and CMR images. The CMR image also shows patchy scarring of the anterior wall. The chest computed tomography scan was suggestive of pulmonary sarcoid. This patient is at high risk of sudden death in view of myocardial scarring and syncope, which may suggest VT. An ICD for primary prevention is indicated. These patients can get scarring in the right ventricle that mimics ARVD, which may cause focal aneurysms, causing severe LV dysfunction, typically in subtricuspid or other areas. They are also at risk for complete heart block. Diagnostic criteria from Heart Rhythm Society (HRS) expert panel are summarized in Box 12.1 at the end of this chapter.

**12.35.** C. Carcinoid.

Note that the patient has both severe tricuspid stenosis (mean diastolic gradient >5 mmHg) and severe tricuspid regurgitation with "V" wave cutoff sign (arrow). This is typical of carcinoid.

**12.36.** D. Any of the above.

See Box 12.2 at the end of this chapter for a summary from the 2010 criteria.

**12.37.** E. All of the above.

**12.38.** E. All of the above.

**12.39.** B. LBBB.

With septal ablation, there is higher risk of all except LBBB. Risk of LBBB is higher with surgical myectomy.

**12.40.** A. Transaortic.

Through the aortic valve.

**12.41.** C. 20%.

This is a lot higher than for surgical myectomy, where the risk is about 1–2%.

**12.42.** C. More with alcohol septal ablation.

This is because no muscle is removed and an uncontrolled infarction is produced. Hence, there is a concern for higher sudden death risk and there is a lower threshold to protect with an ICD. Overall survival and sudden death risk are lower with surgical myectomy. Survival of patients after surgical myectomy is fairly similar to the age-matched general population and much better than those with unoperated HOCM patients.

**12.43.** C. There is reduction in both septal and nonseptal LV mass.
Both regress by about 20%.

**12.44.** C. More with alcohol septal ablation.
Also, relief of obstruction takes several weeks.

---

**Box 12.1   Expert Consensus Recommendations on Criteria for the Diagnosis of Cardiac Sarcoid**

The diagnostic criteria for cardiac sarcoid are adapted from Birnie et al. (2014).
There are two pathways to a diagnosis of cardiac sarcoidosis.

1. *Histological diagnosis from myocardial tissue.* Cardiac sarcoid is diagnosed in the presence of non-caseating granuloma on histological examination of myocardial tissue with no alternative cause identified.
2. *Clinical diagnosis from invasive and noninvasive studies.* It is probable that there is cardiac sarcoid if (i) there is a histological diagnosis of extra-cardiac sarcoidosis and (ii) one or more of the following is present:
   - Steroid ± immunosuppressant-responsive cardiomyopathy or heart block
   - Unexplained reduced LV EF (<40%)
   - Unexplained sustained (spontaneous or induced) VT
   - Mobitz type II second-degree heart block or third-degree heart block
   - Patchy uptake on dedicated cardiac positron emission tomography (in a pattern consistent with cardiac sarcoid)
   - Late gadolinium enhancement on CMR imaging (in a pattern consistent with cardiac sarcoid)
   - Positive gallium uptake (in a pattern consistent with cardiac sarcoid)

---

**Box 12.2   Most Current and Comprehensive Summary and Guideline**

**Diagnostic Criteria for ARVD**

The following is summarized from adapted from Marcus et al. (2010).

**Diagnostic Terminology for Revised Criteria**

Definite diagnosis: two major or one major and two minor criteria or four minor from different categories.
Borderline: one major and one minor or three minor criteria from different categories.
Possible: one major or two minor criteria from different categories.

**Major Criteria for ARVD**

1. *Echo:* RV regional wall dyskinesis plus RV outflow tract end-diastolic (RVOTd) in long axis ≥32 mm or RVOTd in short axis ≥36 mm or RV fractional area change ≤33%.

2. *Magnetic resonance imaging:* RV regional wall dyskinesis plus RV EDV $\geq$110 ml/m$^2$ in males/RVEDV $\geq$100 ml/m$^2$ in females or RV EF <40% (note that RV scarring and fatty changes on CMR imaging have been removed as criteria).
3. *Histology:* Residual myocytes <60% by morphometric analysis (or <50% if estimated), with fibrous replacement of the RV free wall myocardium in $\geq$1 sample, with or without fatty replacement of tissue on endomyocardial biopsy.
4. *Repolarization abnormalities on ECG:* Inverted T waves in right precordial leads (V1, V2, and V3) or beyond in individuals >14 years of age (in the absence of complete right bundle-branch block QRS $\geq$120 ms).
5. *Depolarization abnormalities on ECG:* Epsilon wave (reproducible low-amplitude signals between end of QRS complex to onset of the T wave) in the right precordial leads (V1 to V3).
6. *Arrhythmias:* Nonsustained or sustained VT of left bundle-branch morphology with superior axis (negative or indeterminate QRS in leads II, III, and aVF and positive in lead aVL).
7. *Family history:* ARVC/ARVD confirmed in a first-degree relative.
8. *Genetic testing:* Identification of a pathogenic mutation categorized as associated or probably associated with ARVC/ARVD in the patient under evaluation.

**Minor Criteria for ARVD**

1. These are somewhat similar to major criteria, but less stringent or slightly more liberal.

Chapter 1

## References

Birnie, D.H., Sauer, W.H., Bogun, F. et al. (2014). HRS Expert Consensus Statement on the diagnosis and management of arrhythmias associated with cardiac sarcoidosis. *Heart Rhythm* 11: 1304–1323.

Marcus, F.I., McKenna, W.J., Sherrill, D. et al. (2010). Diagnosis of arrhythmogenic right ventricular cardiomyopathy/dysplasia: proposed modification of the task force criteria. *Circulation* 121: 1533–1541.

## Further Reading

Elliott, P.M., Anastasakis, A., Borger, M.A. et al. (2014). 2014 ESC guidelines on diagnosis and management of hypertrophic cardiomyopathy: the task force for the diagnosis and Management of Hypertrophic Cardiomyopathy of the European Society of Cardiology (ESC). *European Heart Journal* 35 (39): 2733–2779. http://dx.doi.org/10.1093/eurheartj/ehu284.

# Hypertension 13

13.1. A 61-year-old black gentleman is seen in your office. He denies any cardiac symptoms. He does not have a history of diabetes. His vitals show a heart rate of 75 bpm and blood pressure (BP) of 160/92 mmHg; examination otherwise is normal. You recommend lifestyle modification, including regular exercise and low-sodium diet. What is the initial drug of choice in managing his hypertension?
   A. Metoprolol
   B. Furosemide
   C. Amlodipine
   D. Lisinopril

13.2. A 25-year-old female patient comes to your office. She has a history of chronic kidney disease (CKD) stage 2. She denies any cardiac symptoms. Her vitals are heart rate 76 bpm, BP 170/98 mmHg, respiratory rate 14/min. Her physical examination is otherwise normal. She is on furosemide 40 mg daily. What would your add-on drug of choice in this patient be?
   A. Amlodipine
   B. Clonidine
   C. Lisinopril
   D. Hydralazine

13.3. A 49-year-old male comes to your office for an evaluation as part of his executive check-up. He reports feeling well. He denies previous history of diabetes or coronary artery disease. Physical examination is unremarkable except for his BP, which was measured at 165/98 mmHg. His BP rechecked after five minutes was 160/98 mmHg. What would your recommendation be to this patient?
   A. Reassurance
   B. Initiate drug therapy
   C. Come back for a follow up in three months
   D. Come back for a follow up after six months

13.4. A 50-year-old female is being evaluated in your office. She reports a history of diabetes mellitus and is taking metformin 500 mg BID. She reports no other history. She denies any cardiac symptoms. She exercises regularly. Her examination is unremarkable except for her high BP, which was measured on two occasions five minutes apart and was 170/92 mmHg. What is the initial drug of choice?
   A. Prazosin
   B. Clonidine

*Cardiology Board Review*, Second Edition. Ramdas G. Pai and Padmini Varadarajan.
© 2023 John Wiley & Sons Ltd. Published 2023 by John Wiley & Sons Ltd.

C. Atenolol

D. Lisinopril

**13.5.** A 40-year-old female is admitted to the hospital. On examination, she is found to have pulmonary edema. Her past history is only significant for hypertension. She is on a medical regimen consisting of a thiazide diuretic, amlodipine, losartan, and carvedilol. Her family also gave a history of recent uncontrolled high BP and one other episode of pulmonary edema two months ago. Her BP was 220/110 mmHg. The rest of her examination is unremarkable. What is the initial diagnosis?

A. Pseudohypertension

B. Primary hyperaldosteronism

C. Reno-vascular hypertension

D. Coarctation of aorta

**13.6.** What is the diagnostic test of choice for the patient in Question 13.5?

A. Captopril renogram

B. Intravenous pyelogram

C. Doppler ultrasound of the renal arteries

D. Magnetic resonance angiography (MRA)

E. Captopril-stimulated plasma renin activity (PRA)

**13.7.** A 60-year-old female is referred to you for uncontrolled hypertension. Her primary care physician was treating her for the previous five months. She denies any other history in the past. She drinks alcohol socially and is in the habit of chewing tobacco. On examination, she weighs 75 kg, BP is 200/100 mmHg. The rest of her examination is unremarkable except for trace pedal edema. Her lab values are as follows:

serum sodium 144 mEq/l

serum potassium 3 mEq/dl

serum chloride 100 mEq/l

serum bicarbonate 29 mEq/l

serum creatinine 0.9 mg/dl

blood urea nitrogen 20 mg/dl

PRA is 1.2 pg/(l h), plasma aldosterone (PA) level is 9.2 ng/l, and aldosterone excretion rate is 8 mg/day (normal is 5–10 mg/day). Urine test after salt loading yields creatinine 1 g, sodium 251 mEq, and potassium 130 mEq.

Which diagnostic test would you order next?

A. Computed tomography of adrenal glands

B. MRA of the renal $^{Cha}$

C. Serum cortisol and urinary free-cortisol measurement

D. Cosyntropin test

**13.8.** A 45-year-old male is referred to you for treatment of uncontrolled hypertension. He is on four different antihypertensives at maximal doses, including a thiazide-type diuretic. He denies any other medical history. He is active. His BP is 184/100 mmHg, sitting upright in a relaxed posture. His blood chemistry is unremarkable except for serum potassium of 2.9 mg/dl and a plasma renin level of <1 ng/(ml h). What is the cause of hypertension in this patient?

A. Reno-vascular hypertension

B. Primary aldosteronism

    C. Pheochromocytoma
    D. Renal parenchymal disease

13.9. What is the best screening test in evaluating the patient in Question 13.8?
    A. MRA of the renal arteries.
    B. Ratio of PA to PRA
    C. Urine metanephrine
    D. Intravenous pyelogram

13.10. You have been referred a 52-year-old male with refractory hypertension by a primary care physician. The patient gives a history of episodes of headache, sweating, and palpitations. On examination, his BP is 198/112 mmHg. Examination is otherwise unremarkable. What is the best screening test in evaluating this patient?
    A. Serum cortisol
    B. PA to PRA
    C. Plasma catecholamines and urinary metanephrines
    D. MRA of the abdomen

13.11. What is the BP goal for a 62-year-old patient according to the JNC 8 guidelines?
    A. <140/90 mmHg
    B. <150/90 mmHg
    C. <160/100 mmHg
    D. <160/90 mmHg

13.12. What is the BP goal for a 92-year-old patient according to the JNC 8 guidelines?
    A. <140/90 mmHg
    B. <150/90 mmHg
    C. <160/100 mmHg
    D. <160/90 mmHg

13.13. What is the BP goal for a 62-year-old patient with diabetes mellitus according to the JNC 8 guidelines?
    A. <140/90 mmHg
    B. <150/90 mmHg
    C. <160/100 mmHg
    D. <160/90 mmHg

13.14. What is the BP goal for a 42-year-old patient with diabetes mellitus according to the JNC 8 guidelines?
    A. <140/90 mmHg
    B. <150/90 mmHg
    C. <160/100 mmHg
    D. <160/90 mmHg

13.15. What is the BP goal for a 62-year-old patient with renal disease according to the JNC 8 guidelines?
    A. <140/90 mmHg
    B. <150/90 mmHg
    C. <160/100 mmHg
    D. <160/90 mmHg

13.16. What is the BP goal for a 42-year-old patient with diabetes mellitus according to the JNC 8 guidelines?
    A. <140/90 mmHg
    B. <150/90 mmHg

C. <160/100 mmHg

D. <160/90 mmHg

**13.17.** What is the drug of choice to treat hypertension in a black person with renal disease?

A. Diuretic

B. Calcium Channel Blockers (CCB)

C. Angiotensin-Converting Enzyme Inhibitors (ACEI) or Angiotensin Receptor Blockers (ARB)

D. Betablocker

**13.18.** What is the drug of choice to treat hypertension in a black person with diabetes mellitus?

A. Diuretic or Calcium Channel Blockers (CCB)

B. Angiotensin-Converting Enzyme Inhibitors (ACEI)

C. Angiotensin Receptor Blockers (ARB)

D. Any of the above

**13.19.** What is the drug of choice to treat hypertension in a nonblack person with diabetes mellitus?

A. Diuretic

B. Calcium Channel Blockers (CCB)

C. Angiotensin-Converting Enzyme Inhibitors (ACEI) or Angiotensin Receptor Blockers (ARB)

D. Any of the above

**13.20.** Which is the most preferred drug to treat hypertension in pregnancy according to the JNC 8 guidelines?

A. Labetalol

B. Methyldopa

C. Nifedipine

D. Angiotensin Enzyme Converting Inhibitors (ACEI)

**13.21.** Which is the most preferred drug to reduce the risk of recurrent stroke according to the JNC 8 guidelines?

A. Diuretic

B. Calcium Channel Blockers (CCB)

C. Clonidine

D. Betablocker

**13.22.** Which antihypertensive agent may reduce uric acid levels?

A. Diuretic

B. Calcium Channel Blockers (CCB)

C. Losartan

D. Candesartan

**13.23.** Which antihypertensive agent may reduce migraine attacks?

A. Diuretic

B. Calcium Channel Blockers (CCB)

C. Losartan

D. Candesartan

**13.24.** Which antihypertensive agent may result in gynecomastia?
A. Spironolactone
B. Calcium Channel Blockers (CCB)
C. Losartan
D. Candesartan

**13.25.** A 44-year-old man with hypertension received an escalating dose of lisinopril. At the clinic visit, his heart rate is 72 bpm and BP is 152/92 mmHg on lisinopril 40 mg/day. What will you recommend?
A. Ask to reduce Na intake to <1 g instead of <2 g/day
B. Add hydrochlorothiazide (HCTZ) 25 mg/day
C. Add losartan 50 mg/day
D. Add beta blocker

**13.26.** A 75-year-old man with hypertension is on lisinopril 40 mg/day and HCTZ 50 mg/day. His BP is 160/88 mmHg. Previously, he did not tolerate diltiazem because of edema. What would you do?
A. Start losartan 25 mg/day
B. Add amlodipine 5 mg/day
C. Add furosemide
D. Add carvedilol 6.25 mg BID

**13.27.** What is the recommended daily Na restriction in hypertension?
A. <2400 mg
B. <1200 mg
C. <500 mg
D. None of the above

**13.28.** What systolic BP (SBP) goal does the Systolic Blood Pressure Intervention Trial (SPRINT) support?
A. <120 mmHg
B. <130 mmHg
C. <140 mmHg
D. <150 mmHg

**13.29.** The Systolic Hypertension in the Elderly Program (SHEP) showed that, in elderly patients with isolated systolic hypertension, thiazide diuretic reduced which of the following?
A. SBP
B. Stroke risk
C. Cardiac events
D. All of the above

**13.30.** Which of the following statements are accurate about the results of the Antihypertensive and Lipid-Lowering Treatment to Prevent Heart Attack Trial (ALLHAT)?
A. The primary outcome was similar in the chlorthalidone, amlodipine, and lisinopril arms. Mortality was similar
B. The SBP was lower in the chlorthalidone group
C. The DBP was lower in the amlodipine group

    D. Stroke and cardiac events were higher in the lisinopril group compared with chlorthalidone

    E. All of the above

13.31. A 36-year-old woman presents for follow-up. She was recently admitted to hospital for three days due to headaches and dyspnea. Her blood pressure was 178/98 mmHg on presentation. She responded well to intravenous labetalol and was discharged on lisinopril. On examination, during the clinic visit, her blood pressure is 160/90 mmHg. She has a normal cardiovascular examination except for an abdominal bruit. Her blood tests are notable for a rise in creatinine from 0.8 to 1.8 mg/dl since hospital discharge. What is the most appropriate next step?

    A. 24-hour urinary-free cortisol

    B. Duplex ultrasonography of the renal arteries

    C. Coronary angiogram

    D. Urinary catecholamines

13.32. How do you measure BP correctly in the office?

    A. Using the same cuff size for all patients

    B. Taking the blood pressure in one arm with the patient standing

    C. Taking blood pressures in both arms, in the seated position

    D. Taking blood pressure in both legs and both arms

13.33. Which of the following does not cause hypokalemia as a side effect?

    A. Spironolactone

    B. Loop- diuretics

    C. Thiazides

    D. All of the above

13.34. You are seeing an otherwise healthy 65-year-old-woman for hypertension in clinic. She is on a thiazide diuretic; ACE inhibitor and her BP is 140/90 today. She has no complaints today. How should you manage her hypertension?

    A. No adjustments to medications

    B. Increase dose of thiazide

    C. Add clonidine

    D. Refer for renal angiography

Chapter 13

13.35. A 40-year-old man with no significant past medical history and who is asymptomatic has a BP of 140/90 mmHg in the clinic. Which of the following tests would be indicated at this time?

    A. He should return in one year for a routine physical examination

    B. He should have a repeat blood pressure measurement later during the visit and check his blood pressure at home if the repeat clinic BP is elevated

    C. Start patient on CCB immediately

    D. Check urine metanephrines

13.36. A 52-year-old woman currently taking hydrochlorothiazide 25 mg PO daily, comes to your clinic to establish care. She keeps a log of her home BP which shows her BP at home is always less than 140/80 mmHg, but in the clinic, it is always higher. What will you do next?

    A. Increase the dose of thiazide

    B. Stop her thiazide as she has white coat hypertension

    C. Addition of second antihypertensive medication

    D. Evaluate for secondary causes of hypertension

**13.37.** A 62-year-old man with hypertension, stage III chronic kidney disease (CKD), and diabetes is not yet at blood pressure goal on the following antihypertensives: lisinopril 40 mg, hydrochlorothiazide 25 mg, and metoprolol XL 150 mg. Which medication should not be added to his regimen?

    A. Amlodipine

    B. Hydrochlorothiazide

    C. Aliskiren

    D. Furosemide

**13.38.** A 58-year-old Caucasian man with diabetes presents for a follow-up visit after he was noted to have a blood pressure of 160/90 mmHg at his last visit. On repeat evaluation, his blood pressure is 155/95 mmHg. Which of the following is the least preferred therapy?

    A. Chlorthalidone 25 mg PO daily

    B. Lisinopril 10 mg PO daily

    C. Atenolol 25 mg PO daily

    D. Hydrochlorothiazide 25 mg PO daily

**13.39.** A 42-year-old woman with coronary artery disease, diabetes mellitus, and hypertension is currently taking clonidine. She is found to have a blood pressure of 170/90 mmHg after forgetting to take her medication for the last two days. What is the best next step?

    A. Restart clonidine

    B. Start esmolol

    C. Add thiazide diuretic

    D. Start nitroprusside

**13.40.** A 40-year-old woman is noted to have episodic high blood pressure of 180/110 mmHg. She undergoes screening for secondary causes of hypertension and is found to have a pheochromocytoma. What of the following medications is contraindicated as monotherapy?

    A. Metoprolol

    B. Lisinopril

    C. Phentolamine

    D. Hydrochlorothiazide

## Answers

**13.1.** C. Amlodipine.

    The 2014 hypertension guidelines clearly state that the initial drug of choice in black patients, including those with diabetes, is either a thiazide-type diuretic or a calcium channel blocker (CCB). This recommendation stems from a prespecified subgroup analysis of a single large trial (ALLHAT). In this study, a thiazide-type diuretic was shown to be more effective in improving stroke, heart failure (HF), and combined cardiovascular outcomes compared with an angiotensin converting-enzyme inhibitor (ACEI) in the black subgroup in both diabetic and nondiabetic subjects. Hence, the recommendation to choose a thiazide diuretic over an ACEI. Although a CCB was less effective than a thiazide diuretic in preventing HF in the black population, there were no differences in other outcomes; that is, cardiovascular, cerebrovascular, renal, or combined outcomes. Therefore, either a thiazide-type diuretic or a CCB is the initial drug of choice in black patients.

**13.2.** C. Lisinopril.

According to the 2014 hypertension guidelines, people aged 18 or older with CKD and hypertension, an initial or add-on medication should include either an ACEI or an angiotensin receptor blocker (ARB) to improve renal outcomes. This recommendation applies to those with and without proteinuria, as studies using an ACEI or an ARB showed improved renal outcomes in both groups. This recommendation is mainly based on kidney outcomes. The African American Study of Kidney Disease and Hypertension study showed benefit of ACEIs in black patients with CKD.

**13.3.** B. Initiate drug therapy.

The 2014 hypertension guidelines state that, in the general population younger than 60 years, to initiate pharmacological treatment to lower diastolic blood pressure (DBP) of 90 mmHg or higher to a goal of lower than 90 mmHg. For ages 30–59 years the recommendations are strong and for ages 18–29 years the recommendations are based on expert opinion. This recommendation is based on data from five DBP trials (Hypertension Detection and Follow-up Program, Hypertension-Stroke Cooperative Study, Medical Research Council trial, Australian National Blood Pressure Study, and VA Cooperative Study), which showed improvements in health outcomes in adults aged 30 through 59 with elevated BP. Initiating treatment at DBP 90 mmHg or higher and reducing the DBP to lower than 90 mmHg reduced cerebrovascular events, HF, and overall mortality. There was no benefit in treating patients to a goal of 80 or 85 mmHg based on the Hypertension Optimal Treatment trial. In patients younger than 30 years, there are no good or fair quality randomized control trails and hence the recommendation is to start treatment when DBP is 90 mmHg or higher to a goal of less than 90 mmHg.

**13.4.** D. Lisinopril.

The 2014 guidelines recommendation for initial treatment of the general population with diabetes is thiazide-type diuretic, CCB, ACEI, or ARB (moderate recommendation – grade B). Each of the four drug classes recommended by the panel yielded comparable effects on mortality and cardiovascular, cerebrovascular, and kidney outcomes, with one exception: HF. Initial treatment with thiazide-type diuretic was more effective than CCB or ACEI, and an ACEI was more effective than a CCB in improving HF outcomes. The panel did not recommend beta-blockers for the initial treatment of hypertension because, in one study, use of beta-blockers resulted in a higher rate of the primary composite outcome of cardiovascular death, myocardial infraction, or stroke compared with the use of an ARB. Alpha-blockers were not recommended as first-line therapy because, in one study, the initial treatment with an alpha-blocker resulted in worse cerebrovascular, HF, and combined cardiovascular outcomes than initial treatment with a diuretic.

**13.5.** C. Reno-vascular hypertension.

Clinical clues that point toward reno-vascular hypertension are: age greater than 55 years, accelerated or malignant hypertension, hypertension refractory to triple drug therapy, epigastric bruit, recurrent flash pulmonary edema, unexplained renal insufficiency, or ACEI-induced renal insufficiency.

**13.6.** D. Magnetic resonance angiography (MRA).

While renal arterial angiography is the gold standard, MRA is equally good. MRA has a sensitivity of 100% and specificity of 96% in diagnosing renal artery stenosis. Computed tomography angiogram has a sensitivity of 98% and a specificity of 94% and can be used if MRA is unavailable. Doppler ultrasound has a sensitivity ranging from 69% to 96% and a specificity of 86–90%. Intravenous pyelogram has a sensitivity of about 75% and a specificity of about 85%, while captopril renogram and captopril PRA have sensitivity of 70–93% and 75%, respectively and specificity of 95% and 89%, respectively.

**13.7.** C. Serum cortisol and urinary free-cortisol measurement.

This patient has uncontrolled hypertension, with metabolic alkalosis and hypokalemia. She also has a low normal level of PRA and urinary aldosterone. These are suggestive of mineralocorticoid excess. This can be due to her habit of chewing tobacco. Chewing tobacco can be adulterated with licorice – which contains glycyrrhizic acid. This inhibits the inactivation of cortisol by 11-beta-dehydrogenase. This results in increased activation of corticosteroid receptors by cortisol, more so for the renal mineralocorticoid receptors, which causes sodium retention and kaliuresis. Moderate elevation of serum cortisol and urinary level of free cortisol is diagnostic for licorice-induced hypertension.

**13.8.** B. Primary aldosteronism.

In a patient with refractory hypertension, hypokalemia and inappropriate kaliuresis (urine potassium >30 mEq/24 hours), primary aldosteronism should be considered. When serum potassium is <3.5 mg/dl despite ACEI or ARB therapy or potassium supplementation then one should suspect hyperaldosteronism.

**13.9.** B. Ratio of PA to PRA.

The best screening test for primary aldosteronism is the ratio between PA/PRA. All diuretics should be discontinued one week prior to obtaining the levels. Then an elevated PA/PRA alone does not establish the diagnosis. It is confirmed by demonstrating inappropriate aldosterone secretion. During salt loading, a nonsuppressed aldosterone excretion is diagnostic. A rate of >14 pg/24 hours following a salt load (24 ml/kg physiologic saline in four hours for three days or home oral salt load) distinguishes most of the cases.

**13.10.** C. Plasma catecholamines and urinary metanephrines.

The combination of plasma catecholamines (>2000 pg/ml) and urinary metanephrines (1.8 mg in 24 hours) has a diagnostic accuracy approaching 98% in diagnosing both sporadic and familial pheochromocytomas.

**13.11.** B. <150/90 mmHg.

See the JNC 8 recommendations in Box 13.1.

**13.12.** B. <150/90 mmHg.

See the JNC 8 recommendations in Box 13.1. Goals are divided depending upon whether the age is above or below 60 years – there is no other age threshold.

**13.13.** A. <140/90 mmHg.

See the JNC 8 recommendations in Box 13.1.

**13.14.** A. <140/90 mmHg.

See the JNC 8 recommendations in Box 13.1.

**13.15.** A. <140/90 mmHg.

See the JNC 8 recommendations in Box 13.1.

**13.16.** A. <140/90 mmHg.

See the JNC 8 recommendations in Box 13.1.

**13.17.** C. ACEI or ARB.

**13.18.** A. Diuretic or CCB.

According to the JNC 8 recommendations. See Box 13.1.

**13.19.** D. Any of the above.

**13.20.** A. Labetalol.

Nifedipine and methyldopa are acceptable. An ACEI is contraindicated.

**13.21.** A. Diuretic.

The other drug is an ACEI.

**13.22.** C. Losartan.

**13.23.** D. Candesartan.

**13.24.** A. Spironolactone.

**13.25.** B. Add hydrochlorothiazide (HCTZ) 25 mg/day.

That is, add a drug from a different class. Losartan belongs to the same class. Beta blocker is not a preferred drug according to the JNC 8 guidelines unless post-myocardial infarction (MI) or angina or has systolic HF. Further reducing Na intake is not a recommendation and is likely to be futile. CCB is also another option.

**13.26.** D. Add carvedilol 6.25 mg BID.

Losartan will not help as the patient is already on an ACEI. Amlodipine is likely to cause edema as he had on diltiazem. Furosemide is not recommended unless in HF or glomerular filtration rate is <40 ml/min. Carvedilol is the best choice.

**13.27.** A. <2400 mg.

**13.28.** A. <120 mmHg.

Please see the details for SPRINT in Box 13.2.

**13.29.** D. All of the above.

See Box 13.2 for details about SHEP.

**13.30.** E. All of the above.

**13.31.** B. Duplex ultrasonography of the renal arteries.

This young woman likely has hypertension secondary to renal artery stenosis which may be related to underlying fibromuscular dysplasia (FMD). A significant rise in creatinine after ACEI/ARB initiation and abdominal bruit may indicate the presence of renal artery stenosis. Duplex ultrasonography is a noninvasive investigation for diagnosis of renal artery stenosis. The classic "string-of-beads" appearance of the arteries may be seen on angiography in FMD.

24 hour urinary-free cortisol is required to diagnose Cushing syndrome. The patient usually has other symptoms of Cushing syndrome (Cushingoid facies, abdominal obesity, buffalo hump, easy bruising, abdominal stria, hyperglycemia, osteoporosis, etc.)

Urinary catecholamines are used to diagnose phaeochromocytoma which is a tumor of the adrenal medulla and causes paroxysmal episodic elevations in BP associated with flushing and sweating.

**13.32.** C. Taking BP in both arms with the patient seated.

Choosing an appropriate cuff size is required for accurate BP recording. A cuff that is too large will underestimate the blood pressure. The patient should be seated comfortably and, ideally, the blood pressure should be taken in both arms.

**13.33.** A. Spironolactone

Spironolactone reduces potassium excretion by the kidneys thereby causing hyperkalemia. It is used for treating primary aldosteronism. The most frequent adverse reaction to thiazides is hypokalemia, due to their effect on potassium excretion by the kidneys. Loop-diuretics are preferred over thiazides when renal function is impaired or in the presence of congestive heart failure. They also cause hypokalemia.

**13.34.** B. As per JNC 8 guidelines, in the general population (without diabetes and CKD) aged 60 years or more, antihypertensive treatment is initiated at systolic blood pressure (SBP) of 150 mmHg or diastolic blood pressure (DBP) 90 mmHg. In this age group, if pharmacological treatment results in lower achieved BP and treatment is well tolerated and without adverse effects on health or quality of life, treatment does not need to be adjusted.

**13.35.** B. The patient should have a repeat blood pressure measurement later during the visit and return in a few weeks to obtain repeat testing if that measurement is elevated. The JNC 7 guidelines suggest that the diagnosis of hypertension requires at least two separate blood-pressure measurements during a clinic visit. The patient should be resting in a chair for at least five minutes and should have his arm supported at heart level at the time of taking BP. Blood pressure measurements should be evaluated in the contralateral arm and while standing if there are complaints of dizziness/orthostatic hypotension. Ambulatory monitoring of blood pressure should be attempted.

**13.36.** B. Whitecoat hypertension is defined as a clinic blood pressure of >140/80 mmHg in at least three clinic settings, with blood pressure measurements of <140/80 mmHg in at least two non-clinic settings, and with the absence of end-organ damage. Patients with white coat hypertension should be monitored closely for the development of sustained hypertension, but do not need to be initiated on antihypertensive therapy.

**13.37.** C. Aliskiren is a direct renin inhibitor. The use of aliskiren, in combination with ACE inhibitors or angiotensin receptor blockers, is associated with a significantly increased risk of hyperkalemia compared with monotherapy using ACE inhibitors or angiotensin receptor blockers.

**13.38.** C. The least preferred therapy should be atenolol. The ALLHAT study showed that the use of thiazide diuretics as first-line therapy for the treatment of uncomplicated hypertension was as effective as, if not superior to, amlodipine and lisinopril. Initiating ACEI would be reasonable due to the patient's history of diabetes. β-Blockers would not be indicated as first-line therapy in this patient. Multiple meta-analyses comparing β-blockers with placebo or other antihypertensive agents have shown no statistically significant decreases in mortality, myocardial infarction, and stroke.

**13.39.** A. Restart clonidine. Rebound hypertension is a known complication of clonidine. Immediate treatment of clonidine withdrawal involves restarting of therapy with a slow taper.

**13.40.** A. Pheochromocytoma is a rare cause of hypertension. The use of β-blocker monotherapy is contraindicated because blockage of these peripheral β-receptors results in unopposed α-activation leading to peripheral vasoconstriction. This can result in severe hypertension. Typical medical management of pheochromocytomas involves the use of antihypertensives with α-blocking capability. For example, prazosin or phenoxybenzamine may be used. Only once α-blockade is established should the use of a β-blocker be used.

See Box 13.2 for details about ALLHAT.

---

**Box 13.1    JNC 8 Recommendations**

Chapter 1

There is a lot of controversy about the JNC 8 recommendations (James et al. 2014), which were not reviewed by the American College of Cardiology, the American Heart Association, or hypertension societies. The recommendations (nine of them) are as follows.

1. In the general population aged >60 years, initiate pharmacological treatment to lower BP at SBP >150 mmHg or DBP >90 mmHg and treat to an SBP goal of <150 mmHg and a DBP goal of <90 mmHg. (Strong recommendation – grade A.)
2. In the general population <60 years, initiate pharmacological treatment to lower BP at DBP >90 mmHg and treat to a DBP goal of <90 mmHg. (For ages 30–59 years.)
3. In the general population <60 years, initiate pharmacological treatment to lower BP at SBP >140 mmHg and treat to an SBP goal of <140 mmHg.
4. In the population aged >18 years with CKD, initiate pharmacological treatment to lower BP at SBP >140 mmHg or DBP >90 mmHg and treat to an SBP goal of <140 mmHg and a DBP goal of <90 mmHg.
5. In the population aged >18 years with diabetes, initiate pharmacological treatment to lower BP at SBP >140 mmHg or DBP >90 mmHg and treat to an SBP goal of <140 mmHg and a DBP goal of <90 mmHg.
6. In the general nonblack population, including those with diabetes, initial antihypertensive treatment should include a thiazide-type diuretic, CC, ACEI, or ARB. *Note that beta blocker is not a first-line drug.*
7. In the general black population, including those with diabetes, initial antihypertensive treatment should include a thiazide-type diuretic or CCB.

8. In the population aged >18 years with CKD, initial (or add-on) antihypertensive treatment should include an ACEI or ARB to improve kidney outcomes. This applies to all CKD patients with hypertension regardless, of race or diabetes status.

9. The main objective of hypertension treatment is to attain and maintain a BP goal. If the goal BP is not reached within one month of treatment, increase the dose of the initial drug or add a second drug from one of the classes in recommendation 6 (thiazide-type diuretic, CCB, ACEI, or ARB). The clinician should continue to assess BP and adjust the treatment regimen until the BP goal is reached. If the BP goal cannot be reached with two drugs, add and titrate a third drug from the list provided. Do not use an ACEI and an ARB together in the same patient. If the goal BP cannot be reached using only the drugs in recommendation 6 because of a contraindication or the need to use more than three drugs to reach the BP goal, antihypertensive drugs from other classes can be used. Referral to a hypertension specialist may be indicated for patients in whom a BP goal cannot be attained using the aforementioned strategy or for the management of complicated patients for whom additional clinical consultation is needed.

---

### Box 13.2    Clinical Trials

- **SPRINT** (The SPRINT Research Group 2015). About 9000 patients with hypertension and SBP >130 mmHg and at high cardiovascular risk (renal disease, heart disease, stroke), but not diabetes, were randomized to intensive BP control (SBP <120 mmHg) versus traditional control (SBP <140 mmHg). Both the cumulative events and deaths were about 25% lower than in the intensive treatment group.

- **Action to Control Cardiovascular Risk in Diabetes** (ACCORD) trial (Margolis et al. 2014). ACCORD enrolled 10 251 type 2 diabetes patients aged 40–79 years at high risk for cardiovascular disease (CVD) events. Participants were randomly assigned to hemoglobin A1c goals of <6.0% (<42 mmol/mol; intensive glycemia) or 7.0–7.9% (5363 mmol/mol; standard glycemia) and then randomized a second time to either (i) SBP goals of <120 mmHg (intensive BP) or <140 mmHg (standard BP) or (ii) simvastatin plus fenofibrate (intensive lipid) or simvastatin plus placebo (standard lipid). Proportional hazards models were used to assess combinations of treatment assignments on the composite primary (deaths due to CVD, nonfatal MI, and nonfatal stroke) and secondary outcomes. Compared with combined standard treatment, intensive BP or intensive glycemia treatment alone improved major CVD outcomes, without the additional benefit from combining the two.

- **ALLHAT** (ALLHAT Officers and Coordinators for the ALLHAT Collaborative Research Group 2002). A total of 33 357 participants aged 55 years or older with hypertension and at least one other coronary heart disease risk factor were randomly assigned to receive chlorthalidone, 12.5–25 mg/day (*n* = 15 255), amlodipine, 2.5–10 mg/day (*n* = 9048), or lisinopril, 10–40 mg/day (n = 9054) for planned follow-up of approximately four to eight years. Primary outcome was fatal coronary heart disease or nonfatal MI. Compared with chlorthalidone (six-year rate, 11.5%), the relative risks (RRs) were

0.98 (95% confidence interval [CI], 0.90–1.07) for amlodipine (six-year rate, 11.3%) and 0.99 (95% CI, 0.91–1.08) for lisinopril (six-year rate, 11.4%). The five-year SBPs were significantly higher in the amlodipine (0.8 mmHg, $P=$ 0.03) and lisinopril (2 mmHg, $P<$ 0.001) groups compared with chlorthalidone, and five-year DBP was significantly lower with amlodipine (0.8 mmHg, $P<$ 0.001). For amlodipine versus chlorthalidone, secondary outcomes were similar except for a higher six-year rate of HF with amlodipine (10.2% versus 7.7%; RR, 1.38; 95% CI, 1.25–1.52). For lisinopril versus chlorthalidone, lisinopril had higher six-year rates of combined CVD (33.3% versus 30.9%; RR, 1.10; 95% CI, 1.05–1.16), stroke (6.3% versus 5.6%; RR, 1.15; 95% CI, 1.02–1.30), and HF (8.7% versus 7.7%; RR, 1.19; 95% CI, 1.07–1.31). Thiazide-type diuretics are superior in preventing one or more major forms of CVD and are less expensive. They should be preferred for first-step antihypertensive therapy.

- **SHEP** (SHEP Cooperative Research Group 1991). 4736 persons aged 60 years and above were randomized (2365 to active treatment, 2371 to placebo). SBP ranged from 160 to 219 mmHg and DBP was less than 90 mmHg. The five-year incidence of total stroke was 5.2 per 100 participants for active treatment (HCTZ ± atenolol) and 8.2 per 100 for placebo. The RR by proportional hazards regression analysis was 0.64 ($P=$ 0.0003). For the secondary end point of clinical nonfatal MI plus coronary death, the RR was 0.73. Major cardiovascular events were reduced (RR 0.68). For deaths from all causes, the RR was 0.87.

## References

ALLHAT Officers and Coordinators for the ALLHAT Collaborative Research Group (2002). Major outcomes in high-risk hypertensive patients randomized to angiotensin-converting enzyme inhibitor or calcium channel blocker vs diuretic: the Antihypertensive and Lipid-Lowering Treatment to Prevent Heart Attack Trial (ALLHAT). *Journal of the American Medical Association* 288: 2981–2997.

James, P.A., Oparil, S., Carter, B.L. et al. (2014). 2014 evidence-based guideline for the management of high blood pressure in adults: report from the panel members appointed to the Eighth Joint National Committee (JNC 8). *Journal of the American Medical Association* 311 (5): 507–520.

Margolis, K.L., O'Connor, P.J., Morgan, T.M. et al. (2014). Outcomes of combined cardiovascular risk factor management strategies in type 2 diabetes: the ACCORD randomized trial. *Diabetes Care* 37: 1721–1728.

SHEP Cooperative Research Group (1991). Prevention of stroke by antihypertensive drug treatment in older persons with isolated systolic hypertension: final results of the Systolic Hypertension in the Elderly Program (SHEP). *Journal of the American Medical Association* 265: 3255–3264.

The SPRINT Research Group (2015). A randomized trial of intensive versus standard blood-pressure control. *The New England Journal of Medicine* 373: 2103–2116.

Chapter 13

# Diabetes Mellitus

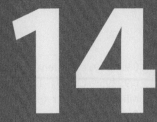

14.1. Which of the following criteria can be used to diagnose diabetes?
   A. Hemoglobin (Hb) A1C >6.5%
   B. Fasting glucose >126 mg/dl
   C. Two hours glucose >200 mg/dl
   D. All of the above
   E. None of the above

14.2. Which of the following criteria can be used to identify patients at increased risk for diabetes?
   A. Fasting glucose level of 100–125 mg/dl
   B. Two hours glucose of 140–199 mg/dl
   C. HbA1C of 5.7–6.4%
   D. None of the above
   E. All of the above

14.3. Studies have established a robust relationship between HbA1C and what conditions in initially nondiabetic patients?
   A. Future risk of diabetes mellitus
   B. Chronic kidney disease
   C. Coronary artery disease
   D. All-cause mortality
   E. All of the above
   F. None of the above

14.4. What type of exercise has been shown to be associated with lowering of HbA1C?
   A. Aerobic training
   B. Resistance training only
   C. Combined aerobic and resistance training
   D. None of the above

14.5. Which of the following is not a limitation to using HbA1C?
   A. Conditions interfering with interpretation, including hemoglobinopathies, alterations in red-cell turnover, such as hemolytic anemia, transfusion, pregnancy, blood loss
   B. Lack of standardization in many parts of the world
   C. Cost of the assay
   D. Less biological variability

*Cardiology Board Review*, Second Edition. Ramdas G. Pai and Padmini Varadarajan.
© 2023 John Wiley & Sons Ltd. Published 2023 by John Wiley & Sons Ltd.

**14.6.** Which of the following is false regarding hypertension control in diabetes mellitus?
A. For most individuals, the goal should be <130/80 mmHg; lower targets may be appropriate for younger patients
B. Therapy should include an angiotensin-converting-enzyme inhibitor (ACEI) or an angiotensin receptor blocker (ARB); if intolerant to one class, the other should be substituted
C. For patients with CKD, treatment should include ACEI or ARB
D. Beta blockers are the first drug of choice

**14.7.** Which of the following statements is not true regarding cholesterol management in diabetes mellitus?
A. Moderate-intensity therapy is recommended when low-density lipoprotein is between 70 and 189 mg/dl in patients aged 40–75 years of age
B. High-intensity therapy is recommended in patients aged 40–75 years when estimated risk for cardiovascular disease is >7.5%
C. Treat patients with fasting triglycerides greater than 500 mg/dl
D. Individualized therapy is recommended in patients <40 or >75 years of age
E. All of the above
F. None of the above

**14.8.** Which of the following statements is true about when bariatric surgery should be considered?
A. Body mass index (BMI) >40 kg/m² or >35 kg/m² with an obesity related comorbidity
B. BMI >35–40 kg/m²
C. BMI >40 kg/m² with no comorbidities or BMI >35 kg/m² with an obesity-related comorbidity with no response to behavioral or pharmacological treatment
D. None of the above

**14.9.** Which of the following drugs produce weight gain?
A. Thiazolidinediones
B. Sulfonylureas
C. Insulin
D. Glinides
E. All of the above
F. None of the above

**14.10.** Which of the following does not produce weight loss?
A. Metformin
B. Pramlintide
C. Exenatide
D. Liraglutide
E. Sodium-glucose cotransporter-2 inhibitors
F. Dipeptidyl peptidase-4 inhibitors

**14.11.** Which of the following is not true in diabetes mellitus?
A. Overweight and obese patients should be counseled to lose weight through exercise
B. Lifestyle changes can produce a 3–5% weight loss that can be sustained over time

C. For patients with a BMI >40 kg/m$^2$ or a BMI >35 kg/m$^2$ with an obesity-mediated comorbidity bariatric surgery may improve health when other methods have failed

D. Exercise and lifestyle changes have no benefit in the management of patients with diabetes mellitus

14.12. Which of the following is true regarding aspirin therapy in diabetes mellitus?

A. Low-dose aspirin (75–162 mg/day) is reasonable for those with a 10-year cardiovascular disease (CVD) risk of 10% without an increased risk of bleeding

B. Low-dose aspirin is reasonable in adults with diabetes mellitus with an intermediate risk (10-year CVD risk of 5–10%)

C. In the primary prevention population, aspirin is effective in preventing nonfatal myocardial infarction in men

D. In women, use of aspirin for primary prevention lessens the risk of stroke

E. All of the above

F. None of the above

14.13. Which of the following is true regarding management of hyperglycemia in type 2 diabetes patients?

A. In most patients, to reduce the incidence of microvascular disease, HbA1C should be lowered to <7.0%

B. Reducing HbA1C to <6.5% might be considered in some patients with short disease duration, long life expectancy, and no significant CVD, without causing significant hypoglycemia

C. HbA1c <8% is appropriate for patients with a history of hypoglycemia, limited life expectancy, advanced complications, and cognitive impairment

D. All of the above

E. None of the above

14.14. Which one of the following statements is false?

A. Type 2 diabetes mellitus is associated with a two- to fourfold increased risk of CVD, and event rates correlate with degree of hyperglycemia

B. In a large study, increase in fasting glucose was associated with 17% increased risk of future cardiovascular events or death

C. The correlation between hyperglycemia and microvascular disease is less strong than macrovascular disease with a 37% increased risk for retinopathy or renal failure with 1% increase in A1C

D. After adjustment for CVD risk factors, an increase in A1C of 1% is associated with an increased risk of CVD events, including 19% in myocardial infarction and 12–14% in all-cause mortality

14.15. Which of the following statements is not true regarding renal disease in diabetes?

A. Evidence suggests that the presence of diabetic kidney disease in type 2 diabetes is associated with an increased risk of mortality

B. Among adults with diabetes in the USA, the prevalence of diabetic kidney disease is 34.5%, 16.8% with albuminuria, 10.8% with impaired glomerular filtration rate (GFR) and 6.9% with both albuminuria and impaired GFR

C. It is recommended to screen yearly for diabetic kidney disease in all type 2 diabetes patients

D. Goals of care for patients with diabetic kidney disease include preventing progression to end-stage renal disease and reducing the risks of cardiovascular events and death

E. Among people with diabetes mellitus, albuminuria and impaired GFR are not associated with increased risks for acute kidney injury, cardiovascular events, and death.

14.16. Which of the following statements is not true regarding glycemic control in medical intensive care unit (ICU) patients?

A. Intensive glycemic control in the ICU targeting blood glucose <110 mg/dl is recommended

B. Intensive glycemic control is associated with excess 90-day mortality

C. Excess mortality was due to moderate to severe hypoglycemia

D. Guidelines suggest a target glucose of 140–180 mg/dl in ICU patients

14.17. Which of the following statements regarding type 1 diabetes mellitus and glycemic control is not true?

A. Strict glycemic control in type 1 diabetes patients can delay the onset of retinopathy, nephropathy, and neuropathy

B. Strict glycemic control can slow the progression of existing microvascular disease

C. The Diabetes Control and Complications Trial (DCCT) was able to demonstrate a reduction in cardiovascular events

D. Strict glycemic control is associated with higher (threefold) risk of hypoglycemia

14.18. Which of the following statements are true?

A. The FREEDOM trial showed that coronary artery bypass grafting (CABG) surgery is superior to percutaneous coronary intervention (PCI)

B. The benefit of CABG was due to lower rates of myocardial infarction and death from any cause

C. CABG was not associated with increased stroke rates

D. PCI was associated with higher strokes

14.19. Regarding sex differences and outcomes in diabetes, which of the following is not true?

A. Women with diabetes have a twofold excess risk for cardiovascular disease compared with men

B. Myocardial infarction usually occurs earlier and is associated with higher mortality in women with diabetes compared with men

C. Revascularization rates are similar in women when compared with men

D. Risk of occurrence of heart failure is higher in women with diabetes when compared to men

E. Long-term survival is less in women undergoing revascularization and also have higher post-surgical mortality when compared to men

F. Women with peripheral artery disease respond less well to exercise training when compared with men with and without diabetes

14.20. Which of the following statements is not true regarding the Bypass Angioplasty Revascularization Investigation 2 Diabetes (BARI 2D) trial?

A. This trial enrolled stable coronary artery disease patients with type 2 diabetes and compared PCI with CABG

Chapter 14

B. The majority of patients who underwent PCI had single-vessel interventions
C. There was a difference in survival in the PCI group compared with the CABG group
D. Subgroup analysis of the CABG group showed that those assigned to CABG and optimal medical therapy had more freedom from cardiovascular events compared with optimal medical therapy alone

14.21. Which of the following medications is considered to be a first-line treatment for diabetes mellitus?
A. Metformin
B. SGLT-2 inhibitors
C. Insulin
D. GLP-1 receptor antagonists

14.22. Which of the following social determinants of health are important when considering the treatment of diabetes?
A. Depression
B. Stress levels
C. Self-efficacy
D. Social support
E. All of the above

14.23. One daily serving of sweetened beverages raises the frequency of diabetes mellitus by how much?
A. 10%
B. 20%
C. 25%
D. 30%

14.24. What level of exercise has been shown to provide cardiovascular benefit to patients with type 2 diabetes?
A. 120 minutes per week of moderate intensity exercise
B. 150 minutes per week of moderate intensity exercise
C. 60 minutes per week of vigorous exercise
D. 75 minutes per week of vigorous exercise
E. Both A and C
F. Both B and D

14.25. What portion of adult Americans are pre-diabetic and are at risk for developing type 2 diabetes?
A. 1/5
B. 1/4
C. 1/3
D. 1/2

14.26. Which classes of diabetes medications have shown a benefit in cardiovascular risk reduction?
A. TZD
B. SGLT-2 inhibitors
C. Sulfonylureas
D. DPP-4 inhibitors

**14.27.** Which of the following is true when the BP goal for patients with diabetes was set to <120 mmHg?

A. It reduced the rate of composite outcome of fatal and nonfatal major adverse cardiac events

B. In secondary analysis, lowering the BP goal led to a reduction in stroke risk

C. A greater risk of adverse events was noted, such as self-reported hypotension and reduction in eGFR

D. Both B and C

E. All of the above

**14.28.** Which of the following statements are true regarding type 2 diabetes?

A. The higher the BMI, the greater the chance of developing type 2 diabetes

B. The larger the waist circumference, the greater the chance of developing type 2 diabetes.

C. The greater the hip circumference, the greater the chance of developing type 2 diabetes

D. Both A and C

E. All of the above

**14.29.** Sustained weight loss of 3–5% is likely to result in clinically meaningful benefits in which of the following factors?

A. Reduction in HbA1c

B. Increase in HDL

C. Prevention in developing type 2 diabetes

D. All of the above

**14.30.** Which of the following statements is false?

A. Approximately 1.5 million Americans are diagnosed with diabetes every year

B. Approximately 210 000 of Americans under the age of 20 have been diagnosed with diabetes

C. Diabetes is the seventh leading cause of death in the US

D. Average medical expenditures among people with diabetes were 2.3 times higher than those without diabetes

E. All of the above

F. None of the above

**14.31.** Patient A is a 60-year-old male with a history of diabetes, hypertension, hyperlipidemia, and BMI of 33.9 kg/m². Patient B is a 48-year-old male with diabetes over the previous 18 years who is recently diagnosed with hypertension. Patient C is a 45-year-old female with a history of diabetes over the previous seven years with no history of hyperlipidemia or hypertension. What cardiovascular risk class these patients be classified per 2019 ESC guidelines?

A. Patient A – high risk, Patient B – moderate risk, and Patient C – low risk

B. Patient A – very high risk, Patient B – high risk, and Patient C – moderate risk

C. Patient A – moderate risk, Patient B – moderate risk, and Patient C – low risk

D. Patient A – High risk, Patient B – High risk, and Patient C – moderate risk

**14.32.** What would be an ideal LDL target for the patients in above question?

A. Patient A LDL <55 mg/dl, Patient B LDL <70 mg/dl, and Patient C LDL <100 mg/dl

B. Patient A LDL <70 mg/dl, Patient B LDL <100 mg/dl, and Patient C LDL <140 mg/dl

Chapter 1

C. Patient A LDL <100 mg/dl, Patient B LDL <70 mg/dl, and Patient C LDL <55 mg/dl

D. Patient A LDL <100 mg/dl, Patient B LDL <140 mg/dl, and Patient C LDL <160 mg/dl

14.33. A 47-year-old-male with a history of diabetes has an atherosclerotic cardiovascular disease (ASCVD) risk of 4.5%. Which of the following should be done in regard to primary prevention of cardiovascular disease?

A. Exercise and dietary lifestyle changes. No cholesterol management
B. Moderate-intensity statin should be started
C. High-intensity statin should be started
D. Ezetimibe should be started

14.34. Ms. Brown came to your clinic for Cardiovascular screening. She is 45 years old and has a history of well-controlled type two diabetes (diagnosed six years previously), mild hypertension and psoriasis. Her ASCVD risk is 13%. What should the next best step for this patient be?

A. Moderate-intensity statin should be started
B. Exercise and dietary lifestyle changes. No cholesterol management
C. High-intensity statin should be started
D. PCSK 9 inhibitors should be started

14.35. Ms. Jones is a 60-year-old female with a history of non-obstructive coronary artery disease, diabetes, diabetic gastroparesis, hypertension, and osteoporosis. Her HBA1c is ~7. She is on aspirin, metformin, and lisinopril. What class of medications should be discussed in this patient?

A. High-dose statin and liraglutide
B. Moderate-intensity statin and liraglutide
C. Moderate-intensity statin and empagliflozin
D. High-intensity statin and empagliflozin

14.36. SGLT 2 inhibitors should be avoided or used with caution in which of the following?

A. Recurrent diabetic ketoacidosis
B. Patient with concomitant insulin use
C. History of genitourinary infections
D. A and C
E. A and B
F. All of the above

14.37. Diabetes increases atherosclerosis and cardiovascular mortality through which of the following mechanisms?

A. Reduced synthesis of nitric oxide (NO) from the endothelial cells
B. Phosphoinositide 3-kinase (PI3K) and nuclear factor kB mediated activation of adhesion molecule expression on endothelium
C. Overexpression of GP IIb/IIIa receptor causing increased platelet adhesion and activation.
D. A and C
E. B and C
F. All the above

14.38. Ms. Chandler is a 65-year-old female with a history of type 2 diabetes, obesity, hyperlipidemia, and non-obstructive coronary artery disease. She is on aspirin, metformin, and atorvastatin. Her family history is significant for multiple endocrine neoplasia. She is enquiring about drug therapy that can increase her life span. Which of the following would be ideal drug to start her on?
A. Linagliptin
B. Empagliflozin
C. Liraglutide
D. Insulin Therapy

14.39. Empagaliflozin is shown to reduce mortality in which group of patients?
A. HFrEF
B. HFmrEF
C. HFpEF
D. A & B
E. B & C
F. A, B, & C

14.40. A 69-year-old diabetic female is on maximal therapy for stable angina. Her symptoms are deemed well controlled. Her echocardiogram shows EF 55%, S1DD, and no major valvular abnormalities. HbA1c is 6.5 and his antidiabetic regimen includes metformin, glimepiride, and insulin. You decide to start the patient on SGLT2 inhibitor for mortality and heart failure hospitalization benefit. What should the next step be?
A. Consider reducing the total daily insulin dose by ~20% when starting therapy
B. Wean or stop sulfonylurea
C. Educate the patient to check blood glucose for the first four weeks of therapy.
D. Educate patients about symptoms of euglycemic diabetic ketoacidosis
E. None of the above
F. All of the above

## Answers

14.1. D. All of the above.

14.2. E. All of the above.

14.3. E. All of the above.

Studies have established a link between HbA1C and microvascular and macrovascular complications in initially nondiabetic persons using the new cut points put forth by the American Diabetic Association.

14.4. C. Combined aerobic and resistance training.

In a trial of 262 randomized patients, only combined aerobic and resistance training lowered Hb A1C (mean reduction, 0.34%, $P = 0.03$). The study by Church et al. (2010) highlights the importance of type of exercise in patients with type 2 diabetes mellitus to achieve better glycemic control.

14.5. D. Less biological variability.

The strength of using HbA1C is that it has less biological variability, eliminates the need for a fasting sample, and is a stronger predictor of complications compared with fasting blood glucose.

14.6. D. Beta blockers are the first drug of choice.

Beta blockers are not considered the drug of first choice in treating hypertension in patients with diabetes. An ACEI or an RB should be the first drug of choice.

14.7. E. All of the above.

14.8. C. BMI >40 kg/m$^2$ with no comorbidities or BMI >35 kg/m$^2$ with an obesity-related comorbidity with no response to behavioral or pharmacological treatment.

Bariatric surgery may be helpful in this case.

14.9. E. All of the above.

14.10. F. Dipeptidyl peptidase-4 inhibitors.

Dipeptidyl peptidase inhibitors are weight neutral, while the rest will result in weight loss when used to treat diabetes.

14.11. D. Exercise and lifestyle changes have no benefit in the management of patients with diabetes mellitus.

Exercise and lifestyle changes can produce a 3–5% rate of weight loss (American College of Cardiology (ACC)/American Heart Association (AHA) class 1 level of evidence A). For very obese patients who have not responded to behavioral treatment with or without pharmacological treatment, bariatric surgery may improve health (ACC/AHA, class II A, level of evidence A).

14.12. E. All of the above.

14.13. D. All of the above.

14.14. C. The correlation between hyperglycemia and microvascular disease is less strong than macrovascular disease with a 37% increased risk for retinopathy or renal failure with 1% increase in A1C.

All the other statements are true (Selvin et al. 2004).

14.15. E. Among people with diabetes mellitus, albuminuria and impaired GFR are not associated with increased risks for acute kidney injury, cardiovascular events, and death.

Albuminuria and impaired GFR portends an independent and additive risk for acute kidney injury, cardiovascular events, and death among people with diabetes mellitus.

14.16. A. Intensive glycemic control in the ICU targeting blood glucose <110 mg/dl is recommended.

Intensive glycemic control is no longer recommended in ICU patients. In the NICE-SUGAR trial (The NICE-SUGAR Study Investigators 2009), 6104 medical and surgical ICU patients were randomized to intensive glycemic control (blood glucose 81–108 mg/dl) versus conventional control (blood glucose <180 mg/dl). In this study, the intensive glycemic control arm was associated with a higher 90-day mortality. The authors followed up this initial study in 2012 and related the cause of excess mortality to moderate–severe hypoglycemia, especially in patients with distributive shock. Hence, intensive glycemic control is no longer recommended. Although there are no clear glucose targets, guidelines recommend a target glucose of 140–180 mg/dl in the ICU setting. This was true for both surgical and medical ICU patients.

14.17. C. The Diabetes Control and Complications Trial (DCCT) was able to demonstrate a reduction in cardiovascular events.

The DCCT was not able to show an education in cardiovascular events with strict glycemic control. This may be due to the study population being young (The Diabetes Control and Complications Trial Research Group 1993). However, studies have shown a reduction in cardiovascular events with strict glycemic control. All the other statements are true.

14.18. C. CABG was not associated with increased stroke rates.

The FREEDOM trial compared revascularization strategies in patients with advanced coronary artery disease and type 2 diabetes mellitus (Farkouh et al. 2012). The trial showed superiority of CABG over PCI. The primary outcome of all-cause mortality, non-fatal myocardial infarction, or non-fatal stroke occurred more frequently in the PCI group (26.6%) than in the CABG group (18.7%) at five years ($p = 0.005$). The benefit of CABG was due to less myocardial infarction ($p < 0.001$) and all-cause mortality (p = 0.049). Stroke was more frequent in the CABG group, with five-year rates of 2.4% in the PCI group versus 5.2% in the CABG group (p = 0.03).

14.19. C. Revascularization rates are similar in women when compared with men.

Revascularization rates (PCI, CABG) are found to be lower in women with diabetes compared with men (Regensteiner et al. 2015). All the other statements are true.

14.20. C. There was a difference in survival in the PCI group compared with the CABG group.

The BARI 2D trial showed no difference in survival or freedom from major cardiovascular events at five years between the PCI and CABG group (The BARI 2D Study Group 2009). All other statements are true.

14.21. A. Metformin is the first-line drug of choice for medication management of diabetes mellitus.

14.22. E. All of the above-mentioned factors play a crucial role in affecting the management of blood sugars in diabetes.

14.23. B. A 20% increase in frequency of diabetes mellitus was seen with one daily serving of sweetened beverages.

14.24. F. Adults with type 2 diabetes should perform at least 150 minutes per week of moderate-intensity physical activity or 75 minutes of vigorous-intensity physical activity to improve glycemic control, achieve weight loss if needed, and improve other ASCVD risk factors.

14.25. C. One-third of American adults are pre-diabetic and are at risk of developing type 2 diabetes.

14.26. B. The use of SGLT-2 inhibitors has demonstrated a significant improvement in control of heart failure as well as a reduction in ASCVD events.

14.27. D. In the ACCORD (Action to Control Cardiovascular Risk in Diabetes) trial (S4.4-51), lowering the BP target (SBP <120 mmHg) did not reduce the rate of the composite outcome of fatal and nonfatal major cardiovascular events and was associated with greater risk of adverse events, such as self-reported hypotension and a reduction in estimated glomerular filtration rate. Secondary analyses of the

Chapter 1

ACCORD trial demonstrated a significant outcome benefit of stroke risk reduction in the intensive BP/standard glycemic group.

14.28. E. All of the above statements have been demonstrated to be true.

14.29. D. All of the above benefits have been noted with a 3–5% reduction in weight through lifestyle modifications with or without the use of orlistat. Additionally, while some weight gain may occur in the subsequent years, the benefits achieved will continue to remain clinically significant.

14.30. F. None of the above. Each of the statements mentioned are true statistics as reported by the American Diabetes Association.

14.31. B. 2019 ESC guidelines classify patients with diabetes as follows
- **Very High Risk** – Patients with DM and CVD or DM with target organ damage (proteinuria or kidney failure [estimated glomerular filtration rate <30 ml/min/1.73 m$^2$], left ventricular hypertrophy, or retinopathy). Patients with DM with three or more major risk factors or with type 1 DM duration of >20 years.
- **High Risk** – Patients with DM duration of ≥10 years without target organ damage plus any other additional risk factor.
- **Moderate Risk** – Young patients (type 1DM aged <35 years or type 2DM aged <50 years) with DM duration of <10 years without other risk factors. Classification is important to make management decisions.

14.32. A. Per 2019 ESC guidelines, LDL-C targets have been lowered
- Moderate risk: LDL-C <2.6 mmol/l (<100 mg/dl)
- High risk: LDL-C <1.8 mmol/l (<70 mg/dl)
- Very high risk: LDL-C <1.4 mmol/l (<55 mg/dl)

14.33. B. Per ACC guidelines, in adults 40–75 years of age with diabetes, regardless of estimated 10-year ASCVD risk, moderate-intensity statin therapy is indicated (Class IA)

14.34. C. Per ACC guidelines, in adults 40–75 years of age with diabetes, ASCVD risk enhancer, and with intermediate risk 10-year ASCVD risk (7.5–20%), High-intensity statin should be started. Psoriasis is an ASCVD Risk enhancer (Class IIA).

Other risk enhancers include Family history of premature CAD, CKD, Metabolic Syndrome, Inflammatory diseases (RA, Psoriasis, HIV, etc.), South Asian ancestry, persistent elevated LDL >160 mg/dl, persistent elevated triglycerides greater than equal to 175 mg per deciliter. In selected individuals, high sensitivity CRP greater than 2.0 mg per liter, lipoprotein A levels greater than 50 mg per deciliter, apo lipoprotein B levels greater than 130 mg per deciliter, and or ankle brachial index ABI ∎.

Additionally, diabetes-specific risk enhancers are independent of other risk factors in diabetes mellitus.
- Long duration (≥10 years for T2DM or ≥20 years for type 1 diabetes mellitus)
- Albuminuria ≥30 mcg albumin/mg creatinine
- eGFR <60 ml/min/1.73 m$^2$
- Retinopathy
- Neuropathy
- ABI <0.9

14.35. D. High-intensity statin and empagliflozin

Patient has clinical ASCVD, thus, very high risk, necessitating use of high-intensity statin. Patient had clinical ASCVD (non-obstructive CAD) and would also benefit from sodium glucose cotransporter 2 inhibitors like empagliflozin. Liraglutide should be avoided in gastroparesis patient. Osteoporosis is a contraindication for canagliflozin.

14.36. F. There is increased hypoglycemia risk with insulin and insulin secretagogues (e.g. sulfonylureas). A lower dose of insulin or the insulin secretagogue may be required. There is increased risk of mycotic genital infections and should be used with extreme caution. There is increased risk of euglycemic ketoacidosis in vulnerable patients. SGLT 2 inhibitors should not be used in patients with ESRD or type 1 Diabetes.

14.37. F. Diabetes increases atherosclerosis and cardiovascular mortality through all of the following:
A. Reduced synthesis of nitric oxide (NO) from the endothelial cells
B. Phosphoinositide 3-kinase (PI3K) and nuclear factor kB mediated activation of adhesion molecule expression on endothelium
C. Overexpression of GP IIb/IIIa receptor causing increased platelet adhesion and activation.

14.38. C. Empagliflozin

Both empagliflozin and liraglutide can cause weight loss. However, liraglutide increased risk of medullary thyroid cancer and is contraindicated due to strong family history of MEN2a. Sulphonylureas and insulin increase weight. Sulphonylureas provide no cardiovascular mortality benefit.

14.39. F. SGLT 2 inhibitors are shown to reduce mortality and heart failure hospitalization in patients with all types of heart failure. The EMPEROR-preserved trial provided the first evidence of a cardio-protective effect of empagliflozin on the combined risk of HHF and CV death in subjects with HFpEF, an effect that is independent of the presence of diabetes. In other studies for empagliflozin, a lowered risk of CV death and HHF was also shown in the EMPA-REG OUTCOME trial in people with T2D and a history of CVD and in the EMPEROR-Reduced trial in people with HFrEF regardless of the presence of diabetes.

14.40. F. All of the above

When starting SGLT2i, consider reducing total daily insulin dose by ~20%, wean or stop sulfonylurea, especially in patients with well-controlled diabetes. Patients should be advised to check blood glucose for first four weeks of therapy and be cautious about nausea, vomiting, and diarrhea as symptoms of euglycemic diabetic ketoacidosis. Patients should also be educated about good genital hygiene.

## References

Church, T.S., Blair, S.N., Cocreham, S. et al. (2010). Effects of aerobic and resistance training on hemoglobin A1C levels in patients with type 2 diabetes: a randomized controlled trial. *Journal of the American Medical Association* 304: 2253–2262. [Erratum: *JAMA* (2011) 305: 892.].

Cosentino, F., Grant, P.J., Aboyans, V. et al. (2019, 2020). ESC guidelines on diabetes, pre-diabetes, and cardiovascular diseases developed in collaboration with the EASD. *European Heart Journal* 41 (2): 255–323. doi:10.1093/eurheartj/ehz486. Erratum in: Eur Heart J. 2020 Dec 1;41(45):4317. PMID: 31497854.

Das, S.R., Everett, B.M., Birtcher, K.K. et al. (2020). 2020 expert consensus decision pathway on novel therapies for cardiovascular risk reduction in patients with type 2 diabetes: a report of the American College of Cardiology Solution set Oversight Committee. *Journal of the American College of Cardiology* 76 (9): 1117–1145. https://doi.org/10.1016/j.jacc.2020.05.037. Epub 2020 Aug 5. PMID: 32771263; PMCID: PMC7545583.

Farkouh, M.E., Domanski, M., Sleeper, L.A. et al. (2012). Strategies for multivessel revascularization in patients with diabetes. *The New England Journal of Medicine* 367 (25): 2375–2384. https://doi.org/10.1056/NEJMoa1211585.

Löfvenborg, J.E., Andersson, T., Carlsson, P.-O. et al. (2016). Sweetened beverage intake and risk of latent autoimmune diabetes in adults (LADA) and type 2 diabetes. *European Journal of Endocrinology* 175: 605–614.

Margolis, K.L., O'Connor, P.J., Morgan, T.M. et al. (2014). Outcomes of combined cardiovascular risk factor management strategies in type 2 diabetes: the ACCORD randomized trial. *Diabetes Care* 37: 1721–1728.

Regensteiner, J.G., Golden, S., Huebschmann, A.G. et al. (2015). Sex differences in the cardiovascular consequences of diabetes mellitus: a scientific statement from the American Heart Association. *Circulation* 132: 2424–2447.

Selvin, E., Marinopoulos, S., Berkenbilt, G. et al. (2004). Meta-analysis: glysosylated hemoglobin and cardiovascular disease in diabetes mellitus. *Annals of Internal Medicine* 141: 421–431.

The BARI 2D Study Group (2009). A randomized trial of therapies for type 2 diabetes and coronary artery disease. *The New England Journal of Medicine* 360: 2503–2515.

The Diabetes Control and Complications Trial Research Group (1993). The effect of intensive treatment of diabetes on the development and progression of long-term complications in insulin-dependent diabetes mellitus. *The New England Journal of Medicine* 329: 977–986.

The NICE-SUGAR Study Investigators (2009). Intensive versus conventional glucose control in critically ill patients. *The New England Journal of Medicine* 360 (13): 1283–1297. https://doi.org/10.1056/NEJMoa0810625.

# Lipids

**15**

15.1. Which of the following are new categories for lipid management outlined in the 2013 American College of Cardiology (ACC)/American Heart Association (AHA) guidelines (see Box 15.1; Stone et al. 2013)?
   A. Individuals with clinical atherosclerotic coronary vascular disease (ASCVD)
   B. Individuals with primary elevations of low-density lipoprotein cholesterol (LDL-C) ≥190 mg/dl
   C. Individuals 40–75 years of age with diabetes with LDL-C 70–189 mg/dl
   D. Individuals without clinical ASCVD or diabetes who are 40–75 years of age with LDL-C 70–189 mg/dl and an estimated 10-year ASCVD risk of 7.5% or higher
   E. All of the above

15.2. What is the target goal low-density lipoprotein (LDL) recommendation (primary and secondary prevention) per the new ACC/AHA guidelines in patients with ASCVD?
   A. An LDL goal of <100 mg/dl if not diabetic
   B. An LDL goal of <70 mg/dl if diabetic
   C. No target goal recommendation
   D. None of the above

15.3. Which of the following is associated with microalbuminuria?
   A. Atorvastatin
   B. Metoprolol
   C. Amlodipine
   D. Lisinopril

15.4. The association of statin-induced microalbuminuria is increased with which of the following?
   A. Male gender
   B. Diabetes mellitus
   C. Coronary artery disease
   D. Smoking

15.5. According to the new ACC/AHA guidelines, what is the definition of high-intensity statin treatment?
   A. Daily statin dose reduces LDL-C by 30% to <50%
   B. Daily statin dose reduces LDL-C by >50%
   C. Daily statin dose reduces LDL-C by 80%
   D. Daily statin dose reduces LDL-C by 70%

*Cardiology Board Review*, Second Edition. Ramdas G. Pai and Padmini Varadarajan.
© 2023 John Wiley & Sons Ltd. Published 2023 by John Wiley & Sons Ltd.

15.6. According to the new ACC/AHA guidelines, what is the definition of moderate-intensity statin treatment?
   A. Daily statin dose reduces LDL-C by 30% to <50%
   B. Daily statin dose reduces LDL-C by >50%
   C. Daily statin dose reduces LDL-C by 80%
   D. Daily statin dose reduces LDL-C by 70%

15.7. A 67-year-old male with a known history of coronary artery disease (CAD) has an LDL-C of 180 mg/dl. Regarding statin treatment, what is the best course of action?
   A. No statin treatment
   B. High-intensity statin therapy
   C. Moderate-intensity statin therapy
   D. Low-intensity statin therapy

15.8. A 60-year-old male is referred to you for an evaluation. He has no known history of ASCVD, and his LDL-C is 160 mg/dl. What is the recommendation regarding statin therapy?
   A. No statin therapy
   B. Lifestyle modification
   C. Lifestyle modification and moderate-intensity statin therapy
   D. High-intensity statin therapy

15.9. A 45-year-old female has no known ASCVD. Her lab work-up reveals an LDL-C of 220 mg/dl. She has no other cardiac risk factors. What is the current recommendation for statin therapy?
   A. Lifestyle modification
   B. Lifestyle modification and reassess in six months
   C. High-intensity statin therapy
   D. Lifestyle modification and high-intensity statin therapy

15.10. A 60-year-old male is referred to you for an evaluation. He has no cardiovascular disease. On his lab work-up, triglycerides are 550 mg/dl. Which of the following is not a cause of elevated triglycerides?
   A. Oral estrogens
   B. Excessive alcohol intake
   C. Amiodarone
   D. Diabetes mellitus

15.11. Elevated LDL-C is associated with which of the following?
   A. Diuretics
   B. Cyclosporine
   C. Amiodarone
   D. Biliary obstruction
   E. All of the above
   F. None of the above

15.12. Regarding primary prevention, in a person with no diabetes, LDL-C between 70 and 189 mg/dl, and not receiving statin therapy, what is the current recommendation?
   A. Initiate statin therapy
   B. Estimate 10-year ASCVD risk every four to six years
   C. Estimate 10-year ASCVD risk every year
   D. None of the above

15.13. What is the current recommendation regarding primary prevention when the 10-year ASCVD risk is >7.5%?
A. No statin therapy
B. Moderate- or high-intensity statin therapy
C. Moderate-intensity statin therapy only
D. High-intensity statin therapy only
E. None of the above

15.14. What is the current recommendation regarding primary prevention when the 10-year ASCVD risk is 5–7.5%?
A. No statin therapy
B. Moderate- or high-intensity statin therapy
C. Moderate-intensity statin therapy
D. High-intensity statin therapy
E. None of the above

15.15. Dyslipidemia, consisting of an increase in LDL and triglycerides and a decrease in high-density lipoprotein (HDL), is not associated with which of the following?
A. Protease inhibitors
B. Non-nucleoside reverse transcriptase inhibitors
C. Nucleoside reverse transcriptase inhibitors
D. Fusion/entry inhibitors

15.16. A 45-year-old woman asks if she should take statins as her father had a myocardial infarction at the age of 60 and she smokes 10 cigarettes a day. She has no diabetes or hypertension and no cardiac history or symptoms and jogs 20 miles a week. Her body mass index (BMI) is 25 kg/m$^2$. What will be the LDL threshold for starting a statin based on the ACC/AHA guidelines for this patient?
A. >190 mg/dl
B. >160 mg/dl
C. >130 mg/dl
D. >100 mg/dl

15.17. A 45-year-old man post-renal transplant is referred for advice on lipid management. He is diabetic and hypertensive and is on aspirin, beta blocker, angiotensin converting-enzyme inhibitor, and cyclosporine. HDL-C is 30 mg/dl and LDL-C is 145 mg/dl; BMI is 25 kg/m$^2$. In addition to lifestyle changes, what else would you recommend?
A. Nothing else
B. Simvastatin 20 mg/day
C. Niacin
D. Pravastatin 40 mg/day

15.18. A 55-year-old man had an ST-elevation myocardial infarction and underwent a successful percutaneous coronary intervention. He has now returned for a follow-up visit after six weeks. He is doing well and is on atenolol 50 mg/day, aspirin 81 mg, clopidogrel 75 mg, atorvastatin 80 mg/day, and lisonopril 10 mg/day. His repeat HDL is 40 mg/dl; LDL is 78 mg/dl and triglycerides is 142 mg/dl. What would you recommend?
A. Switch to Crestor® 40 mg/day to achieve LDL of <70 mg/dl
B. Add ezetimibe

C. Add niacin

D. Stay on current therapy

15.19. A 42-year-old woman presents with hypertension and diabetes. Her weight is 320 lb (145 kg) and BMI is 43 kg/m². In addition to treating hypertension and diabetes, what are your other recommendations?

A. Moderate-dose statin therapy

B. Exercise, healthy diet, and target a net calorie deficit of 500–750 kcal/day

C. Lose 30 lb (~14 kg) of weight over next six months

D. All of the above

E. None of the above

15.20. According to 2013 obesity guidelines (Box 15.2), weight loss in recommended in which of the following?

A. Individuals with a BMI >30 kg/m² even without risk factors

B. Individuals with BMI 25–30 kg/m² with risk factors

C. Both A and B

D. Neither A nor B

15.21. Adding US Food and Drug Administration-approved pharmacotherapy as an adjunct to comprehensive lifestyle intervention is reasonable in which of the following conditions?

A. Those with a BMI >30 kg/m² who are motivated to lose weight

B. Those with a BMI >27 kg/m² with at least one obesity-associated comorbid condition who are motivated to lose weight

C. Both A and B

D. Neither A nor B

15.22. In the management of obesity, when is it appropriate to refer to an experienced bariatric surgeon for consultation and evaluation of patients who are motivated to lose weight and who have not responded to behavioral treatment (with or without pharmacotherapy)?

A. When BMI ≥40 kg/m²

B. When BMI ≥35 kg/m² with obesity-related comorbidities or complications

C. Both A and B

D. Neither A nor B

15.23. A 42-year-old man comes to see you to assess cardiovascular risk and recommendations. He is obese but has no other medical history and has started on an exercise and diet program. His height is 70", weight 220 lb (~100 kg), BMI 32 kg/m², heart rate 70 bpm, blood pressure 130/80 mmHg. His LDL is 135 mg/dl and HDL is 35 mg/dl, glucose is 88 mg/dl, hemoglobin A1C Jis 6.2%. His 10-year risk of a cardiovascular event is 3%. What will you recommend?

A. A stress test

B. Coronary computed tomography (CT) angiogram

C. Carotid intimal medial thickness with ultrasound

D. No further testing, continue current strategy

15.24. An 80-year-old man had a myocardial infarction seven years previously and is on atenolol 50 mg/day, aspirin 81 mg/day, and atorvastatin 20 mg/day. What is your recommendation for the statin as he is >75 years old?

A. Stop statin as he is above 75 years

B. Increase statin to 40 or 80 mg/day (high intensity)

C. Ask for patient preference in view of paucity of data in patients >75 years of age
D. Switch to ezetimibe

15.25. A 70-year-old Japanese woman received an left anterior descending coronary artery stent for ST-elevation myocardial infarction. She is doing well and is on atorvastatin 80 mg/day, atenolol 25 mg/day, aspirin 81 mg/day, and clopidogrel 75 mg/dl. Her LDL is 85 mg/dl. What would you recommend?
A. Reduce statin
B. Switch to rosuvastatin 40 mg/day
C. Add niacin
D. Add ezetimibe

15.26. Which of the following is a class I recommendation in assessing asymptomatic adults with no known CAD?
A. Genomic testing
B. Obtain global risk score (Framingham)
C. Assessment of lipoprotein and apolipoprotein
D. Measurements of natriuretic peptides

15.27. Which one of the following is a class I recommendation in assessing asymptomatic adults with no known CAD?
A. Genomic testing
B. Obtain family history
C. Assessment of lipoprotein and apolipoprotein
D. Coronary CT angiogram

15.28. Measurement of C reactive protein (CRP) is not recommended in which of the following?
A. In men over 50 years with an LDL of <130 mg/dl
B. In women over 60 years with an LDL <130 mg/dl not on hormone replacement therapy, and without diabetes or chronic kidney disease
C. In asymptomatic high-risk adults
D. In asymptomatic intermediate-risk men 50 years and younger or women 60 years and younger

15.29. Which of the following is not a class III recommendation in assessing low-risk asymptomatic adults with no known history of CAD?
A. Coronary CT angiogram
B. Magnetic resonance imaging (MRI) for plaque detection
C. Measurement of coronary calcium score
D. Resting electrocardiogram (ECG)

15.30. In patients with diabetes mellitus, which of the following is not recommended?
A. Stress echocardiogram
B. Stress myocardial perfusion imaging (MPI)
C. Coronary artery calcium (CAC) score measurement
D. Measurement of hemoglobin A1C

15.31. In asymptomatic women, which of the following is recommended?
A. Obtaining global risk score
B. Obtaining natriuretic peptides
C. MRI for plaque detection
D. Measurement of lipoprotein

**15.32.** Stress MPI is recommended in which of the following situations?
  A. In the assessment of a low-risk individual
  B. In the assessment of an intermediate-risk individual
  C. In an asymptomatic adult with diabetes mellitus
  D. None of the above

**15.33.** Which of the following is not true?
  A. Echocardiography is recommended to detect left ventricular hypertrophy in patients with hypertension
  B. Echocardiography is recommended in risk assessment of asymptomatic adults without hypertension
  C. A resting ECG is reasonable in asymptomatic adults with hypertension
  D. All of the above

**15.34.** Which of the following is a class III indication in the assessment of asymptomatic adults?
  A. Measurement of arterial stiffness
  B. Obtaining a resting ECG
  C. Obtaining an echocardiogram in a patient with hypertension
  D. Stress MPI in an individual with diabetes mellitus

**15.35.** Which of the following is not true regarding assessment of an asymptomatic adult with diabetes?
  A. Measurement of hemoglobin A1C
  B. Stress MPI
  C. Testing for microalbuminuria
  D. Coronary CT angiogram

**15.36.** Which of the following does not cause secondary dyslipidemia?
  A. Hyperthyroidism
  B. Obstructive liver disease
  C. Renal disorders including nephrotic syndrome and chronic renal failure
  D. Metabolic syndrome or diabetes mellitus (DM)

**15.37.** A 55-year-old woman presents to the clinic for follow-up after suffering a NSTEMI. She has hypertension, diabetes, has had two strokes. Her LDL-C was noted to be 120 mg/dl. She is on lisinopril 40 mg/dl, amlodipine 10 mg, metoprolol XL 25 mg, atorvastatin 80 mg, aspirin 81 mg, Plavix 75. What is the next best step?
  A. Add ezetimibe
  B. Add cilostazol
  C. Perform cardiac stress testing
  D. Increase atorvastatin to 100 mg

**15.38.** A 66-year-old male patient who is currently on lipitor 80 mg/day is being seen for follow-up. Which of the following is not considered a clinically significant adverse effect of statins?
  A. Myopathy
  B. Headache
  C. Renal insufficiency
  D. Diabetes

15.39. A 60-year-old woman was started on a statin one month previously and is here for a clinic follow-up. She has no muscle pain or weakness on examination. She denies the darkening of the urine. What is the next best step?

A. Measure CPK

B. Stop the statin

C. Perform muscle biopsy

D. Do nothing currently

15.40. You see a 48-year-old woman with diabetes, hypertension, current smoker with a brother with MI at age 54. Her LDL-C is 163 mg/dl, TG 275 mg/dl, and HDL-C 47 mg/dl. When first seen prior to initiation of any therapy, her lab revealed alanine transaminase (ALT)/aspartate transaminase (AST) of 102/96 (upper normal in the laboratory of 50/42 U/l). The patient is worried about taking statins due to concerns of liver failure. How should you proceed?

A. Statin therapy may lower the LFTs in patients with fatty liver infiltration

B. Elevations of LFTs greater than two times ULN is a contraindication to starting statins

C. Statin use has not been investigated in patients with baseline LFT abnormalities

## Answers

15.1. E. All of the above.

The statin randomized controlled trials (RCTs) provide the most extensive evidence for the greatest magnitude of ASCVD event reduction, with the best margin of safety (see Box 15.3). Four statin benefit groups – in which the potential for an ASCVD risk reduction benefit clearly exceeds the potential for adverse effects 15 in adults – have been identified in the new ACC/AHA guidelines. These include all of the scenarios listed in the question.

15.2. C. No target goal recommendation.

The panel makes no recommendations for or against specific LDL-C or non-high-density lipoprotein cholesterol (HDL-C) targets for primary or secondary prevention of ASCVD. Treating to a target LDL was the most widely used approach for the past 15 years. Three problems were identified in the ACC/AHA guidelines. First, current clinical trial data do not indicate what the target should be. Second, we do not know the magnitude of additional ASCVD risk reduction that would be achieved with one target lower than another. Third, it does not take into account potential adverse effects from multidrug therapy that might be needed to achieve a specific goal. Thus, in the absence of these data, this approach is less useful than it appears, and hence no target goal was set for treatment of LDL in patients with ASCVD (Stone et al. 2013).

15.3. A. Atorvastatin.

It has been shown that atorvastatin interferes with tubular reabsorption of albumin, which increases urinary albumin excretion. Robles et al. (2013) showed in their study that 27.1% of patients taking atorvastatin had microalbuminuria compared with 12.3% of patients taking simvastatin ($p = 0.012$). Statin-induced endothelial dysfunction of the glomerulus is the mechanism which induces microalbuminuria.

15.4. B. Diabetes mellitus.

Robles et al. (2013) used logistic regression analysis to show an independent relationship between statin treatment and microalbuminuria in diabetic patients.

15.5. B. Daily statin dose reduces LDL-C by >50%.

15.6. A. Daily statin dose reduces LDL-C by 30% to <50%.

15.7. B. High-intensity statin treatment.

According to the new ACC/AHA guidelines, if a person is >21 years and has clinical ASCVD and is aged <75 years, then high-intensity statin therapy should be initiated. Moderate-intensity statin therapy should be initiated in patients aged ≥75 years or if not a candidate for high-intensity statin therapy.

15.8. C. Lifestyle modification and moderate-intensity statin therapy.

In the situation given in the question, moderate-intensity statin therapy should be initiated. If the estimated 10-year ASCVD risk >7.5%, then high-intensity statin therapy should be initiated.

15.9. D. Lifestyle modification and high-intensity statin therapy.

The new ACC/AHA guidelines state that a person >21 years with no ASCVD and an LDL-C >190 mg/dl is a candidates for high-intensity statin therapy along with lifestyle modification.

15.10. D. Amiodarone.

All the options cause elevated triglycerides except for amiodarone. Excessive alcohol intake, refined carbohydrates, oral estrogens, glucocorticoids, bile acid sequestrants, protease inhibitors, retinoic acid, anabolic steroids, sirolimus, raloxifene, tamoxifen, beta blockers (except carvedilol), thiazides, nephrotic syndrome, chronic renal failure, lipodystrophies, poorly controlled diabetes mellitus, hypothyroidism, obesity, and pregnancy can all cause an increase triglycerides.

15.11. E. All of the above.

Saturated fats, anorexia nervosa, diuretics, cyclosporine, glucocorticoids, amiodarone, biliary obstruction, nephrotic syndrome, hypothyroidism, obesity, and pregnancy are all associated with elevated LDL-C.

15.12. B. Estimate 10-year ASCVD risk every four to six years.

15.13. B. Moderate- or high-intensity statin therapy.

If the 10-year risk for ASCVD is >7.5%, the current guideline recommendation is to initiate either moderate- or high-intensity statin therapy.

15.14. B. Moderate-intensity statin therapy.

If the 10-year ASCVD risk is between 5% and 7.5%, the current guideline recommendation is to initiate moderate-intensity statin therapy.

15.15. D. Fusion/entry inhibitors.

All of the options for medications except fusion/entry inhibitors, used in the treatment of HIV/AIDS, cause dyslipidemia, which can be atherogenic. Therefore, the ACC/AHA guideline recommendation is to treat these patients with statins at a higher dose.

15.16. A. >190 mg/dl.

As she has no CAD or diabetes mellitus and her 10-year risk is very low. Of course, she has to stop smoking.

15.17. D. Pravastatin 40 mg/day.

As simvastin metabolism is affected by cyclosporine and may lead to rhabdomyolysis. Niacin does not affect outcomes. As the patient is a diabetic, he should be on at least a modest dose of a statin.

15.18. D. Stay on current therapy.

Based on the ACC/AHA 2013 guidelines, the patient is already on high-intensity statin therapy and hence no further intervention is needed. Guidelines do not recommend "treat to target"

15.19. D. All of the above.

B and C are weight loss guidelines. The panel recommends as an initial goal the loss of 5–10% of baseline weight within six months.

15.20. C. Both A and B.

Risk factors include diabetes, prediabetes, hypertension, dyslipidemia, elevated waist circumference, and obesity-related complications.

15.21. C. Both A and B.

15.22. C. Both A and B.

15.23. D. No further testing, continue current strategy.

The risk is <5% over 10 years and hence no indication for statin either. In the absence of symptoms, A and B are inappropriate. C has not been shown to help risk stratify further.

15.24. C. Ask for patient preference in view of paucity of data in patients >75 years of age.

As per new lipid guidelines.

15.25. A. Reduce statin.

In view of the high risk of intracerebral hemorrhage with high-dose statins in Asians.

15.26. B. Obtain global risk score (Framingham).

Obtaining a global risk score in asymptomatic adults without a clinical history of CAD is a class I indication. These scores are helpful in combining individual risk factor measurements into a single quantitative estimate of risk that can be used in prevention strategies. It is not recommended to perform genomic testing or measure lipoprotein or natriuretic peptides in this population and is considered a class III indication (Greenland et al. 2010).

15.27. B. Obtain family history.

Obtaining a family history of ASCVD is recommended in the assessment of asymptomatic adults (Greenland et al. 2010).

15.28. C. In asymptomatic high-risk adults.

Measurement of CRP is not recommended in asymptomatic high-risk adults (class III). In men 50 years and older or women 60 years and older with an LDL of <130 mg/dl and not on lipid-lowering therapy, hormone replacement, or immunosuppressive therapy, and without clinical CAD, diabetes mellitus, chronic

Chapter 1

kidney disease, severe inflammatory conditions, or contraindications to statin therapy, CRP can be used to select patients for statin therapy (class IIa). It is also deemed reasonable to measure CRP in asymptomatic intermediate-risk men younger than 50 or women younger than 60 for assessment of CAD risk (class IIB) (Greenland et al. 2010).

15.29. D. Resting electrocardiogram (ECG).

A resting ECG may be reasonable in the assessment of asymptomatic adults with no history of hypertension or diabetes mellitus (class IIb). It is a class III indication to obtain a coronary CT angiogram, coronary calcium score, or MRI for plaque detection in low-risk asymptomatic individuals (Greenland et al. 2010).

15.30. A. Stress echocardiogram.

In asymptomatic adults with diabetes mellitus, it is reasonable to measure coronary calcium score (class IIa). It is also reasonable to measure hemoglobin A1C and stress MPI (class IIb). Stress MPI may be considered for patients with diabetes or when prior risk assessment suggests high risk, such as CAC of over 400 (Greenland et al. 2010).

15.31. A. Obtaining global risk score.

It is a class I indication to obtain a global risk score in all asymptomatic women.

15.32. C. In an asymptomatic adult with diabetes mellitus.

Stress MPI may be considered for advanced cardiovascular risk assessment in asymptomatic individuals with diabetes mellitus or in adults with a strong family history of CAD, or when there is prior risk assessment, such as a CAC score of over 400. Stress MPI is not recommended for assessment of low- or intermediate risk asymptomatic individuals (class III) (Greenland et al. 2010).

15.33. B. Echocardiography is recommended in risk assessment of asymptomatic adults without hypertension.

It is a class III indication to perform echocardiography in asymptomatic adults without hypertension. A resting ECG can be obtained in patients with hypertension or diabetes (class IIa) or obtain an echocardiogram in patients with hyper-l tension to detect left ventricular hypertrophy (class IIb) (Greenland et al. 2010).

15.34. A. Measurement of arterial stiffness.

This is a class III indication at the present time (Greenland et al. 2010).

15.35. D. Coronary CT angiogram.

It is a class III to obtain coronary CT angiogram in an asymptomatic adult with diabetes (Greenland et al. 2010).

15.36. A. Hyperthyroidism.

Identifying and treating secondary causes of dyslipidemia is important. Treating hypothyroidism and better control of diabetes may have a significant impact on correcting lipid abnormalities.

15.37. A. Add Ezetimibe

In very high-risk ASCVD, use an LDL-C threshold of 70 mg/dl to consider the addition of non-statins to statin therapy. Very high-risk ASCVD includes a history of multiple major ASCVD events or one major ASCVD event and multiple high-risk conditions. In very high-risk ASCVD patients, it is reasonable to add ezetimibe to maximally tolerated statin therapy when the LDL-C level remains

>70 mg/dl. In patients at very high risk whose LDL-C level remains >70 mg/dl on a maximally tolerated statin and ezetimibe therapy, adding a PCSK9 inhibitor is reasonable, although the long-term safety (>3 years) is uncertain.

15.38. C. Renal insufficiency.

Statins have not been shown to worsen renal function. In a meta-analysis by Naci et al. in 2013, comparing statins to placebo, the odds ratio for elevation in LFTs was 1.51, diabetes development 1.09, myalgia 1.07, CPK abnormality 1.13, and cancer 0.96, statistically significant only for liver test abnormalities and diabetes.

15.39. D. Do nothing

Routine measurement of CPK on statin therapy is not recommended but it is reasonable to obtain at baseline prior to therapy in individuals at higher risk for myopathy and if new symptoms develop on treatment. When a patient on statin presents with complaints of muscle pain, tenderness, stiffness, and weakness, the first approach should be to obtain CPK, creatinine, and urinalysis. It is important to exclude rhabdomyolysis, hypothyroidism, rheumatologic disorders, vitamin D deficiency, steroid use etc. If there are clinical signs of severe pain, new muscle weakness, CPK greater than 10 times ULN, or myoglobinuria, the statin should be stopped. If symptoms are mild to moderate and CPK is less than three times ULN it is reasonable to hold the statin until symptoms can be evaluated. If symptoms resolve, rechallenge with the same or lower dose of the statin to establish whether a causal relationship exists. If so, starting a low dose of a different statin is reasonably followed by slow titration. If CPK is greater than 10 times ULN, hold statin and evaluate for other causes for myopathies.

15.40. A. Statin therapy may lower LFTs in patients with fatty liver infiltration.

Unexplained ALT greater than three times ULN is a contraindication to statin therapy.

Chapter 15

---

Box 15.1    What's New in the 2013 ACC/AHA Guideline?

For the complete 2013 ACC/AHA guideline, see Stone et al. 2013.

1. Focus on ASCVD Risk Reduction: Four Statin Benefit Groups
   - Based on a comprehensive set of data from RCTs that identified four statin benefit groups which focus efforts on reducing ASCVD events in secondary and primary prevention.
   - Identifies high-intensity and moderate-intensity statin therapy for use in secondary and primary prevention.
2. New Perspective on LDL-C and/or Non-HDL-C Treatment Goals
   - The expert panel was unable to find RCT evidence to support continued use of specific LDL-C and/or non-HDL-C treatment targets.
   - The appropriate intensity of statin therapy should be used to reduce ASCVD risk in those most likely to benefit.
   - Non-statin therapies do not provide acceptable ASCVD risk-reduction benefits compared with their potential for adverse effects in the routine prevention of ASCVD.

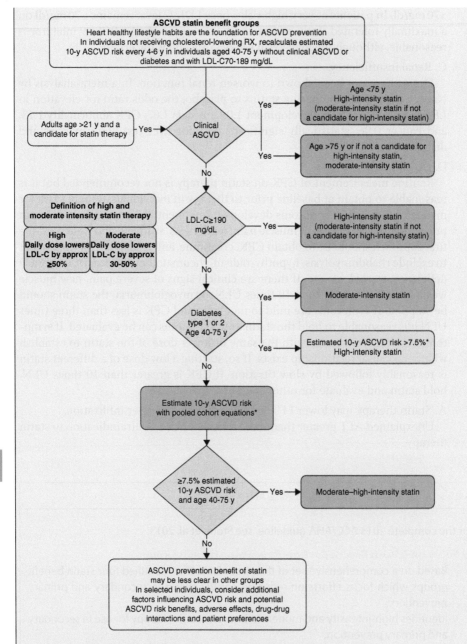

Figure 15.1 Major recommendations for statin therapy for ASCVD prevention.
*Source:* Adapted from Jensen et al. (2013).

## 3. Global Risk Assessment for Primary Prevention

- This guideline recommends use of the new pooled cohort equations to estimate 10-year ASCVD risk in both white and black men and women.
- By more accurately identifying higher risk individuals for statin therapy, the guideline focuses statin therapy on those most likely to benefit.

- It also indicates, based on RCT data, those high-risk groups that may not benefit.
- Before initiating statin therapy, this guideline recommends a discussion between clinician and patients.

### Patient Triaging for Statin Therapy

The flowchart in Figure 15.1 shows the decision process for statin therapy for ASCVD prevention.

---

### Box 15.2    Clinical Trials

- The Atherothrombosis Intervention in Metabolic Syndrome with Low HDL/High Triglycerides: Impact on Global Health Outcomes (AIM-HIGH) trial (AIM-HIGH Investigators 2011). A total of 3414 patients were randomly assigned to receive niacin (1718) or placebo (1696). All patients received simvastatin, 40–80 mg/day, plus ezetimibe, 10 mg/day, if needed, to maintain an LDL-C level of 40–80 mg/dl (1.03–2.07 mmol/l). The trial was stopped after a mean follow-up period of three years owing to a lack of efficacy.
- The Action to Control Cardiovascular Risk in Diabetes (ACCORD) study (ACCORD Study Group 2010). 5518 patients with type 2 diabetes who were being treated with open-label simvastatin were randomized to receive either masked fenofibrate or placebo. The primary outcome was the first occurrence of nonfatal myocardial infarction, nonfatal stroke, or death from cardiovascular causes. The combination of fenofibrate and simvastatin did not reduce the rate of fatal cardiovascular events, nonfatal myocardial infarction, or nonfatal stroke, compared with simvastatin alone.
- The PROspective Study of Pravastatin in the Elderly at Risk (PROSPER) (Shepherd et al. 2002). The aim was to test the benefits of pravastatin treatment in an elderly cohort of men and women with, or at high risk of developing, cardiovascular disease and stroke. Pravastatin given for three years reduced the risk of coronary disease in elderly individuals. PROSPER therefore extends to elderly individuals the treatment strategy currently used in middle-aged people.
- Cannon et al. (2004) enrolled 4162 patients who had been hospitalized for an acute coronary syndrome within the preceding 10 days to compare 40 mg of pravastatin daily (standard therapy) with 80 mg of atorvastatin daily (intensive therapy). An intensive lipid-lowering statin regimen provided greater protection against death or major cardiovascular events than a standard regimen did.
- Shepherd et al. (1995). This double-blind study was designed to determine whether the administration of pravastatin to men with hypercholesterolemia and no history of myocardial infarction reduced the combined incidence of nonfatal myocardial infarction and death from coronary heart disease. Treatment with pravastatin significantly reduced the incidence of myocardial infarction and death from cardiovascular causes without adversely affecting the risk of death from non-cardiovascular causes in men with moderate hypercholesterolemia and no history of myocardial infarction.

**Box 15.3    Primary Care of Overweight Patients with Obesity**

The flowchart in Figure 15.2 shows the chronic disease management model for primary care of overweight patients with obesity.

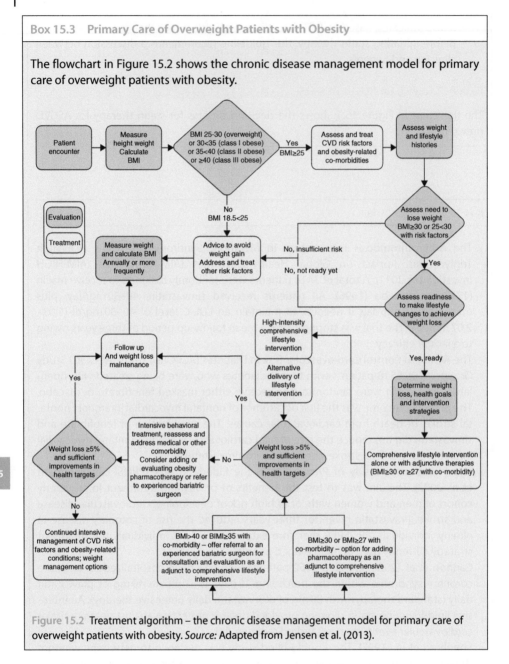

Figure 15.2 Treatment algorithm – the chronic disease management model for primary care of overweight patients with obesity. *Source:* Adapted from Jensen et al. (2013).

## References

AIM-HIGH Investigators (2011). Niacin in patients with low HDL cholesterol levels receiving intensive statin therapy. *The New England Journal of Medicine* 365: 2255–2267.

Cannon, C.P., Braunwald, E., McCabe, C.H. et al. (2004). Intensive versus moderate lipid lowering with statins after acute coronary syndromes. *The New England Journal of Medicine* 350: 1495–1504.

Greenland, P., Alpert, J.S., Beller, G.A. et al. (2010). 2010 ACCF/AHA guideline for assessment of cardiovascular risk in asymptomatic adults: executive summary. A report of the American College of Cardiology Foundation/American Heart Association task force on practice guidelines. *Circulation* 122: 2748–2764.

Jensen, M.D., Ryan, D.H., Apovian, C.M. et al. (2013). AHA/ACC/TOS guideline for the management of overweight and obesity in adults: a report of the American College of Cardiology/American Heart Association task force on practice guidelines and the Obesity Society. *Circulation* 129 (25 Suppl 2): S102–S138.

Robles, N.R., Velasco, J., Mena, C. et al. (2013). Increased frequency of microalbuminuria in patients receiving statins. *Clinical Lipidology* 8 (2): 257–262.

Shepherd, J., Cobbe, S.M., Ford, I. et al. (1995). Prevention of coronary heart disease with pravastatin in men with hypercholesterolemia. *The New England Journal of Medicine* 333: 1301–1307.

Shepherd, J., Blauw, G.J., Murphy, M.B. et al. (2002). Pravastatin in elderly individuals at risk of vascular disease (PROSPER): a randomised controlled trial. *Lancet* 360: 1623–1630.

Stone, N.J., Robinson, J., Lichtenstein, A.H. et al. (2013). 2013 ACC/AHA guideline on the treatment of blood cholesterol to reduce atherosclerotic cardiovascular risk in adults: a report of the American College of Cardiology/American Heart Association task force on practice guidelines. *Circulation* http://circ.ahajournals.org/lookup/suppl/doi:10.1161/01.cir.0000437738.63853.7a/-/DC1 (accessed March 26, 2017).

The ACCORD Study Group (2010). Effects of combination lipid therapy in type 2 diabetes mellitus. *The New England Journal of Medicine* 362: 1563–1574.

# Valvular Heart Disease

# 16

**16.1.** For a 62-year-old patient with mild aortic stenosis (AS; V2 2–3 m/s) who is asymptomatic, what is the recommendation for follow-up echocardiogram?
- **A.** Only when symptoms develop
- **B.** Every 3–5 years
- **C.** Every 1–2 years
- **D.** Every 6–12 months

**16.2.** For a 72-year-old patient with AS with V2 of 4.2 m/s, aortic valve area (AVA) 0.8 cm², ejection fraction (EF) of 65% and normal pulmonary artery (PA) pressure and no symptoms, what would be your recommendation based on current guidelines?
- **A.** Aortic valve replacement (AVR) as patient is likely to become symptomatic soon
- **B.** Follow-up clinic and echo every 1–2 years
- **C.** Follow-up clinic and echo every 6–12 months
- **D.** No follow up till symptoms develop

**16.3.** A 22-year-old Asian woman presents with shortness of breath and has mitral stenosis. What will you do about rheumatic fever prophylaxis?
- **A.** Prophylaxis for the next 10 years
- **B.** Prophylaxis till she turns 40 years
- **C.** No prophylaxis as she is >21 years old
- **D.** Prophylaxis for the next 5 years

**16.4.** Which of the following are acceptable for rheumatic heart disease prophylaxis?
- **A.** Penicillin G benzathine 1.2 million units intramuscularly every four weeks
- **B.** Penicillin V potassium 250 mg orally BID
- **C.** Sulfadiazine 1 g orally once daily
- **D.** Any of the above

**16.5.** Prophylaxis against infective endocarditis (IE) is reasonable for which of the following patients at highest risk for adverse outcomes from IE before dental procedures that involve manipulation of gingival tissue, manipulation of the periapical region of teeth, or perforation of the oral mucosa?
- **A.** Patients with prosthetic cardiac valves
- **B.** Patients with previous IE
- **C.** Cardiac transplant recipients with valve regurgitation due to a structurally abnormal valve

*Cardiology Board Review*, Second Edition. Ramdas G. Pai and Padmini Varadarajan.
© 2023 John Wiley & Sons Ltd. Published 2023 by John Wiley & Sons Ltd.

D. Patients with congenital heart disease with: (i) unrepaired cyanotic congenital heart disease, including palliative shunts and conduits; (ii) completely repaired congenital heart defect repaired with prosthetic material or device, whether placed by surgery or catheter intervention, during the first six months after the procedure; or (iii) repaired congenital heart disease with residual defects at the site or adjacent to the site of a prosthetic patch or prosthetic device.

E. All of the above

**16.6.** Prophylaxis against IE is indicated in a patient with a prosthetic mitral valve (MV) undergoing which of the following procedures in the absence of local infection in the instrumented area?

A. Transesophageal echocardiogram (TEE)

B. Esophagogastroduodenoscopy

C. Colonoscopy

D. Cystoscopy

E. All of the above

F. None of the above

**16.7.** Definition of severe AS includes which of the following?

A. Aortic valve area <1.0 cm$^2$

B. Transaortic velocity >4 m/s on echo

C. Transvalvular mean gradient >40 mmHg

D. Any of the above

E. Need all of the above

**16.8.** A 75-year-old man with no symptoms has severe aortic valve calcification, aortic valve velocity of 4.5 m/s and EF of 65%. What stage is he in?

A. Stage B

B. Stage C1

C. Stage C2

D. Stage D

**16.9.** A 72-year-old woman is found to have severe aortic stenosis (AS) with V2 of 4.6 m/s and mean gradient of 47 mmHg. The EF is 60% and pulmonary artery systolic pressure is normal by echo. She claims she has no symptoms, but the daughter thinks she has slowed down. It is reasonable to do which of the following?

A. An exercise stress test to confirm the asymptomatic status

B. Dobutamine echo to evaluate LV response to stress

C. Refer for cardiac catheterization and AVR

D. Follow up every 6–12 months

**16.10.** Aortic valve replacement (AVR) is recommended in which of the following situations of severe AS?

A. For symptomatic patients with severe high-gradient AS who have symptoms (chest pain, shortness of breath, or syncope) by history or on exercise testing

B. For asymptomatic patients with severe AS (stage C2) and LVEF <50%

C. For patients with severe AS (stage C or D) when undergoing other cardiac surgery

D. All of the above

**16.11.** AVR is reasonable in which of the following situations of severe AS?

A. Asymptomatic patients with very severe AS (stage C1, aortic velocity >5.0 m/s) and low surgical risk

**B.** Asymptomatic patients (stage C1) with severe AS and decreased exercise tolerance or an exercise fall in blood pressure

**C.** Symptomatic patients with low-flow/low-gradient severe AS with reduced LVEF (stage D2) with a low-dose dobutamine stress study that shows an aortic velocity >4.0 m/s (or mean pressure gradient >40 mmHg) with a valve area >1.0 cm² at any dobutamine dose

**D.** Patients with moderate AS (stage B) (aortic velocity 3.0–3.9 m/s) who are undergoing other cardiac surgery

**E.** Symptomatic patients who have low-flow/low-gradient severe AS (stage D3) who are normotensive and have an LVEF >50% if clinical, hemodynamic, and anatomic data support valve obstruction as the most likely cause of symptoms

**F.** All of the above

**16.12.** Transcatheter AVR (TAVR) is reasonable in which of the following situations?
**A.** Severe AS patients who meet an indication for AVR who have a prohibitive surgical risk and a predicted post-TAVR survival >12 months
**B.** As an alternative to surgical AVR in patients who meet an indication for AVR and who have high surgical risk
**C.** Neither A nor B
**D.** Both A and B

**16.13.** Which of the following statements is not true about balloon aortic valvuloplasty?
**A.** It is a good treatment for many forms of congenital AS
**B.** It is a good definitive treatment for calcific AS of the elderly
**C.** Percutaneous aortic balloon dilation may be considered as a bridge to surgical AVR or TAVR in severely symptomatic patients with severe AS
**D.** It is helpful to predilate the aortic valve just before TAVR

**16.14.** A 65-year-old woman with no prior cardiac history is short of breath on walking a flight of stairs and doing her daily activities for the previous 6 months and is getting worse. Echocardiogram showed an EF of 65%, probable bicuspid aortic valve with V2 of 3.5 m/s, aortic mean gradient of 30 mmHg, V1 0.8 m/s, and LV outflow tract diameter (LVOTd) of 20 mm. She walked 4 Mets and ramp II protocol on the treadmill. A TEE confirmed bicuspid aortic valve with a planimetered AVA of 0.7 cm² both on 2D and 3D. Normal coronaries on coronary angiography. PA pressure was normal. PFTs were normal. Hemoglobin 13.8 g/dl. What would be your recommendation?
**A.** Monitor the patient and repeat echo in six months
**B.** Do a dobutamine stress echo (DSE)
**C.** Enroll in an exercise program
**D.** Refer for AVR

**16.15.** A 72-year-old man with history of hypertension and diabetes is short of breath on walking a flight of stairs and doing his daily activities for the previous 6 months and is getting worse. Echocardiogram showed an EF of 30%, calcific AS with V2 of 3.5 m/s, aortic mean gradient of 30 mmHg, V1 0.8 m/s, stroke volume index 32 ml/m², and LVOTd of 20 mm. Normal coronaries on coronary angiography. What would be your recommendation?
**A.** AS is not severe; treat with beta blockers and angiotensin-converting-enzyme inhibitor
**B.** Low dose dobutamine echo for contractile reserve and hemodynamics

C. Refer for balloon valvotomy to see if the patient improves
D. Refer for TAVR

16.16. In the patient in Question 16.15, what is the approximate AVA by the continuity equation?
A. 0.7 cm$^2$
B. 0.9 cm$^2$
C. 1.2 cm$^2$
D. Cannot calculate with the data given

16.17. In a patient with suspected AR, which is the preferred diagnostic modality?
A. Echocardiography
B. Contrast aortography
C. Cardiac magnetic resonance imaging
D. Radionuclide angiography

16.18. Severe AR is suggested by which of the following echocardiographic measures?
A. Doppler jet width ≥65% of LVOT
B. Vena contracta >0.6 cm
C. Holodiastolic flow reversal in the proximal abdominal aorta
D. Regurgitant volume ≥60 ml/beat, or regurgitant fraction ≥50%, or effective regurgitant orifice (ERO) area ≥0.3 cm$^2$
E. All of the above

16.19. In a patient with chronic severe AR, which of the following constitute a definite indication for AVR?
A. Symptomatic patients with severe AR regardless of LV systolic function, even if EF is <30%
B. Asymptomatic patients with chronic severe AR and LV systolic dysfunction (LVEF <50%)
C. Patients with severe AR (stage C or D) while undergoing cardiac surgery for other indications
D. All of the above

16.20. In a patient with chronic severe AR, which of the following constitute a reasonable indication for AVR?
A. Asymptomatic patients with severe AR with normal LV systolic function (LVEF <50%) but with severe LV dilation (LV end-systolic dimension [LVESD] >50 mm, stage C2)
B. Moderate AR (stage B) patients who are undergoing other cardiac surgery
C. Asymptomatic patients with severe AR and normal LV systolic function (LVEF >50%, stage C1) but with progressive severe LV dilation (LV end-diastolic dimension [LVEDD] >65 mm) if surgical risk is low
D. All of the above

16.21. According to the AHA/ACC 2014 valve guidelines (Nishimura et al. 2014), when is MS considered severe?
A. MV area (MVA) <1.0 cm$^2$ and mean gradient >10 mmHg
B. MVA <1.0 cm$^2$
C. MVA <1.5 cm$^2$
D. MVA <1.5 cm$^2$ and mean gradient >10 mmHg

**16.22.** A 42-year-old patient is being followed up in the valve clinic for rheumatic MS. She is asymptomatic and has no other comorbidities. Her echocardiogram shows an EF of 65%, severe left atrial enlargement, and a calculated MVA of 0.7 cm². PA systolic pressure is 40 mmHg, and Wilkins score is 6 out of 16 without commissural calcification. There was no MR. What would you recommend?
**A.** Follow up in six months
**B.** Refer for mitral balloon valvotomy
**C.** Refer for MV replacement and appendage ligation
**D.** Perform an exercise tolerance test

**16.23.** A 52-year-old man with rheumatic MS has been having progressive shortness of breath. His LVEF is normal, mean mitral gradient is 8 mmHg at a heart rate of 65 bpm, mitral pressure half-time is 180 ms. There is also moderate MR and the Wilkins score is 7. What would you recommend?
**A.** Continue to follow up as MS is not severe
**B.** Refer for mitral balloon valvotomy after coronary angiogram
**C.** Refer for MV replacement after coronary angiogram
**D.** Refer for MV repair after coronary angiogram

**16.24.** What are the echocardiographic indices of severe MR?
**A.** Central jet with the jet occupying >40% LA area
**B.** Holosystolic eccentric MR jet, which is wall hugging reaching posterior LA wall
**C.** Vena contracta >0.7 cm, or regurgitant volume > 60 ml, or regurgitant fraction >50%
**D.** ERO area >0.40 cm²
**E.** Systolic flow reversal in pulmonary vein or veins
**F.** Any of the above

**16.25.** Which of the following are clear indications for surgical repair of primary severe MR?
**A.** Symptomatic patients with chronic severe primary MR (stage D) and LVEF >30%
**B.** Asymptomatic patients with chronic severe primary MR and LV dysfunction (LVEF 30–60% and/or LVESD >40 mm, stage C2)
**C.** Patients with chronic severe primary MR undergoing cardiac surgery for other indications
**D.** All of the above

**16.26.** In a patient undergoing MV surgery for severe MR, which type of anatomy is most suitable for successful repair?
**A.** Flail P2                    **C.** Bileaflet MV prolapse
**B.** Flail A2                    **D.** Barlow's disease

**16.27.** A 62-year-old man with previous anterior myocardial infarction has an EF of 30%, LV dilation, and bileaflet tethering causing MR. The MR jet area is 4 cm², vena contracta 5 mm, and the ERO area is 0.25 cm². Which of the following describes the state of MR?
**A.** Mild                    **C.** Severe
**B.** Moderate               **D.** Need more data

**16.28.** Criteria for severe tricuspid regurgitation (TR) include which of the following?
   A. Central jet area >10 cm$^2$
   B. Vena contracta width >0.70 cm
   C. Continuous wave (CW) jet density and contour: dense, triangular with early peak
   D. Hepatic vein flow: systolic reversal
   E. All of the above

**16.29.** Reasonable indications for tricuspid valve (TV) surgery include which of the following?
   A. Patients with severe TR (stages C and D) undergoing left-sided valve surgery
   B. Patients with symptoms due to severe primary TR unresponsive to medical therapy
   C. Asymptomatic or minimally symptomatic patients with severe primary TR (stage C) and progressive degrees of moderate or greater right ventricle dilation and/or systolic dysfunction
   D. All of the above

**16.30.** Indicators of severe tricuspid stenosis include which of the following?
   A. Mean diastolic gradient >5 mmHg
   B. PHT >190 ms
   C. Valve area by continuity equation <1.0 cm$^2$
   D. All of the above

**16.31.** Indicators of severe pulmonary stenosis include which of the following?
   A. Transvalvular velocity >4 m/s
   B. Peak gradient >40 mmHg
   C. V2 > 5 m/s
   D. None of the above

**16.32.** For a 52-year-old man with bileaflet mitral mechanical valve without atrial fibrillation, LV dysfunction, prior thromboemboli, or hypercoagulable state, what is the preferred anticoagulation regimen?
   A. Warfarin to an international normalized ratio (INR) goal of 3.0 and aspirin 81 mg daily
   B. Warfarin to an INR goal of 3.0 only
   C. Warfarin to an INR goal of 3.5
   D. Warfarin to an INR goal of 2.5 and aspirin 81 mg

**16.33.** For a 52-year-old man with bileaflet aortic mechanical valve without atrial fibrillation, LV dysfunction, prior thromboemboli, or hypercoagulable state, what is the preferred anticoagulation regimen?
   A. Warfarin to an INR goal of 3.0 and aspirin 81 mg daily
   B. Warfarin to an INR goal of 3.0 only
   C. Warfarin to an INR goal of 3.5
   D. Warfarin to an INR goal of 2.5 and aspirin 81 mg daily

**16.34.** For a 52-year-old man with bileaflet aortic mechanical valve with one of the risk factors such as atrial fibrillation, LV dysfunction, prior thromboemboli,or hypercoagulable state, what is the preferred anticoagulation regimen?
   A. Warfarin to an INR goal of 3.0 and aspirin 81 mg daily
   B. Warfarin to an INR goal of 3.0 only
   C. Warfarin to an INR goal of 3.5
   D. Warfarin to an INR goal of 2.5 and aspirin 81 mg daily

**16.35.** For a patient with mechanical MV undergoing noncardiac surgery needing interruption of anticoagulation, what would you recommend?
A. Minimize nonanticoagulated period; bridge with heparin or LMWH
B. No bridging needed
C. Bridge with novel anticoagulant
D. Use fresh frozen plasma to cover surgery

**16.36.** For a patient with mechanical aortic valve undergoing noncardiac surgery needing interruption of anticoagulation, what would you recommend? Patient has no risk factors for higher embolic risk.
A. Minimize nonanticoagulated period; bridge with heparin or LMWH
B. Minimize nonanticoagulated period; no bridging needed
C. Bridge with novel anticoagulant
D. Use fresh frozen plasma to cover surgery

**16.37.** In patients with risk factors for IE presenting with fever of >48 hours duration, which of the following guidelines for blood cultures are recommended?
A. At least two sets of blood cultures should be obtained, which may give positive culture rate of about 90%
B. In patients with a chronic (or subacute) presentation, three sets of blood cultures should be drawn >6 hours apart at peripheral sites before initiation of antimicrobial therapy
C. If option B is not feasible or safe in patients with severe sepsis or septic shock, two or more cultures at separate times are acceptable
D. All of the above

**16.38.** Based on the Duke criteria, a diagnosis of IE can definitely be made with which of the following present?
A. Two major criteria
B. One major and three minor criteria
C. Five major criteria
D. All of the above

**16.39.** In a patient with risk factors for IE presenting with persistent fever, a TEE would be appropriate in which of the following situations after obtaining blood cultures B and a transthoracic echocardiogram (TTE)?
A. Nondiagnostic TTE
B. IE complication is suspected
C. Presence of intracardiac lead
D. All of the above

**16.40.** In a patient with proven endocarditis who also has a pacemaker device, device and lead removal is indicated or reasonable under which of the following situations?
A. Infection of lead or device pocket
B. Needs valve surgery for IE, but leads and pocket look normal
C. IE due to resistant organism such as *Staphylococcus aureus* or fungi
D. All of the above

**16.41.** In a pregnant patient with mechanical valve prosthesis, which of the following anticoagulation regimens are acceptable during the first trimester of pregnancy?
A. Warfarin if therapeutic INR can be achieved with a dose of 5 mg or less
B. Intravenous (IV) UFH to achieve partial thromboplastin time (PTT) twice the control
C. LMWH twice a day to achieve anti-Xa level 0.8–1.2 units/ml four to six hours after the dose
D. All of the above

16.42. A 52-year-old woman has a history of abdominal bloating and diarrhea of six months' duration. The echocardiogram of the TV is shown in Figure 16.42. What is the likely diagnosis?

A. Carcinoid syndrome  C. Flail TV

B. Rheumatic heart disease  D. None of the above

End-diastole  Systole

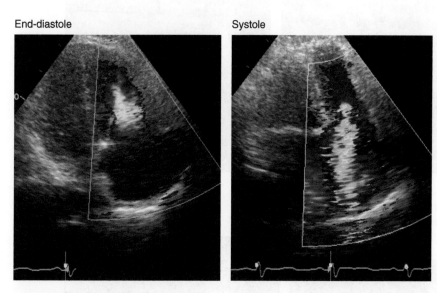

Figure 16.42

16.43. The flow across the mitral bioprosthesis in the patient in Figure 16.43 is indicative of what? (the MV PHT was 120 ms)?

A. Normal function

B. Mild stenosis

C. Moderate stenosis

D. Severe stenosis

16.44. Figure 16.44 is of a patient with a prior bioprosthetic valve. What is the likely cause of dyspnea in the patient?

A. Severe paravalvular AR

B. Severe prosthetic valve stenosis

C. Severe MR

D. None of the above

16.45. What is the m-mode in the patient in Figure 16.45 suggestive of?

A. MS

B. Low cardiac output state

C. Severe AR

D. None of the above

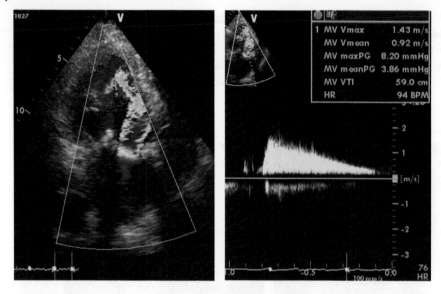

**Figure 16.43**

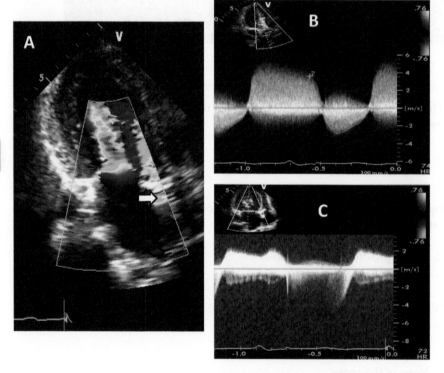

**Figure 16.44**

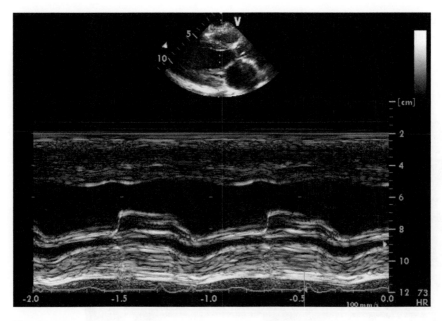

Figure 16.45

16.46. What is the TR velocity profile in the patient in Figure 16.46 with corrected tetralogy of Fallot and pulmonary valve replacement with an V2 of 2.4 m/s suggestive of?
A. Pulmonary hypertension
B. First-degree atrioventricular (AV) block or long AV delay on pacemaker
C. Severe pulmonary regurgitation (PR)
D. None of the above

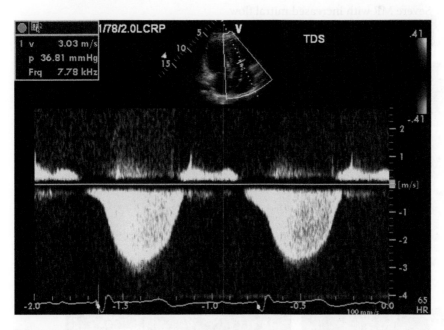

Figure 16.46

**16.47.** Figure 16.47 shows a CW signal across a bioprosthetic pulmonary valve. What is it suggestive of?

A. Pulmonary valve stenosis

B. Mild PR

C. Moderate PR

D. Severe PR

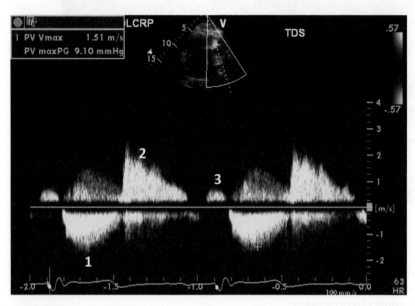

**Figure 16.47**

**16.48.** What is the mitral flow in Figure 16.48 suggestive of?

A. Normal flow

B. Severe MR with increased mitral flow

C. MS

D. Severe AR impeding mitral flow

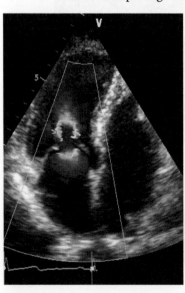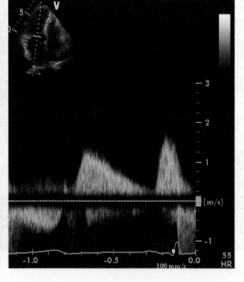

**Figure 16.48**

**16.49.** What does the patient in Figure 16.49 have?
A. Acute severe AR
B. Chronic severe AR
C. MS
D. None of the above

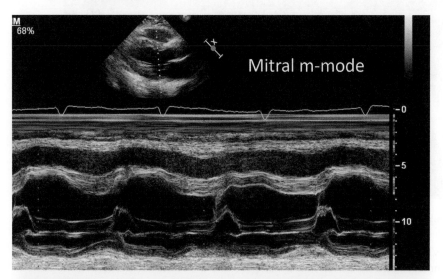

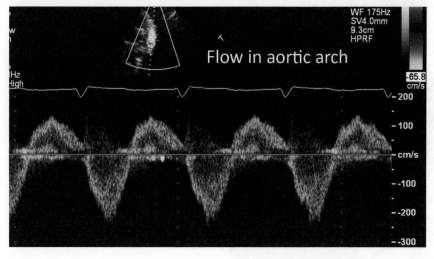

**Figure 16.49**

**16.50.** In a patient with suspected endocarditis, what is the Doppler signal in Figure 16.50 diagnostic of?
A. Acute severe AR
B. MS
C. AS
D. None of the above

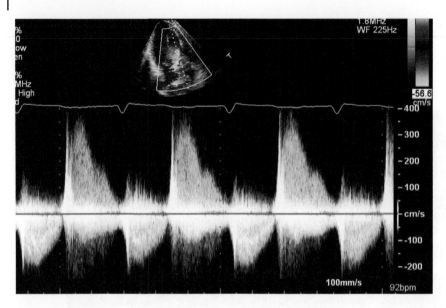

Figure 16.50

16.51. What is the image of the patient with a prosthetic MV and dyspnea in Figure 16.51 indicative of?
   A. Severe paravalvular MR
   B. MS
   C. AR
   D. AS

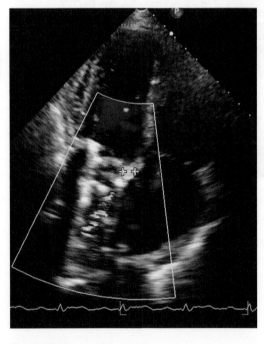

Figure 16.51

**16.52.** Figure 16.52 shows a 48-year-old man who presented with acute severe short-ness of breath. What would be the most optimal treatment?
A. MV repair
B. MVR
C. AVR
D. Prolonged antibiotic therapy

Systole                                    Diastole

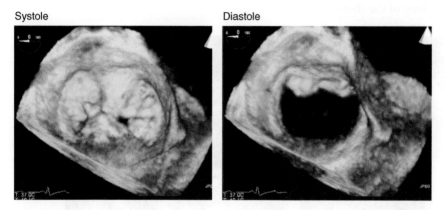

**Figure 16.52**

**16.53.** A patient with heart transplant presented with pedal edema and abdominal bloating. Figure 16.53 is of the TV. What is this suggestive of?
A. Severe TR
B. Moderate TR
C. Tricuspid stenosis
D. Normal function of TV in a transplanted patient

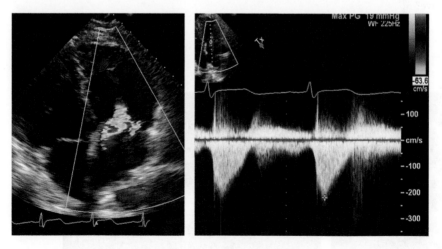

**Figure 16.53**

16.54. An 88-year-old man with multiple comorbidities and Society of Thoracic Surgeons score of 12 is scheduled for TAVR. Aortic valve images are shown in Figure 16.54. There was no fever, and blood cultures were negative. What would a prudent step be?

A. Proceed with TAVR

B. Proceed with TAVR using carotid protection

C. Cancel TAVR and treat with antibiotic for six weeks and repeat TEE

D. None of the above

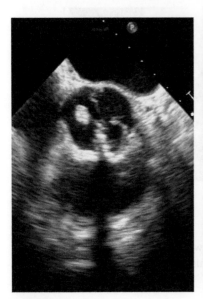 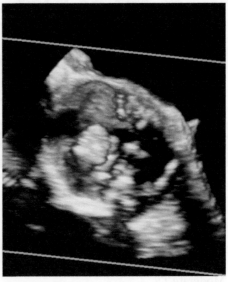

Figure 16.54

16.55. What condition does the patient in Figure 16.55 with a St Jude mechanical MV have?

A. Severe stenosis

B. Mild stenosis

C. Severe MR

D. None of the above

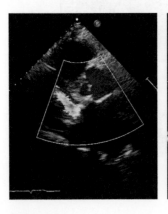 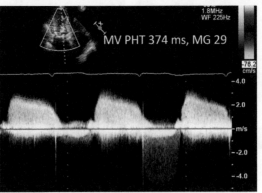

Figure 16.55

**16.56.** Figure 16.56 shows a patient who presented with shortness of breath. What condition does the patient have?
  **A.** Severe subvalvular AS
  **B.** Severe valvular AS
  **C.** Hypertrophic obstructive cardiomyopathy (HOCM)
  **D.** None of the above

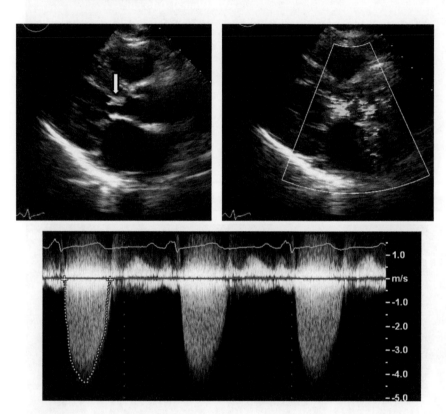

**Figure 16.56**

**16.57.** What is the Doppler signal in Figure 16.57 indicative of?
  **A.** Critical AS with high LA pressure
  **B.** Severe AS with atrial fibrillation
  **C.** Severe MR
  **D.** None of the above

**16.58.** A 19-year-old patient with a mechanical MV was admitted with shortness of breath. Within an hour of admission, she had to be intubated and ventilated for respiratory distress. The blood pressure dropped to 60/40 mmHg unresponsive to pressures. The TEE images are shown in Figure 16.58. What would the next logical step be?
  **A.** IV thrombolytic
  **B.** IV heparin only
  **C.** IV beta blocker to slow the heart rate
  **D.** Wait for the cardiac operating room to be ready, which may take two to three hours to finish the patient on the table

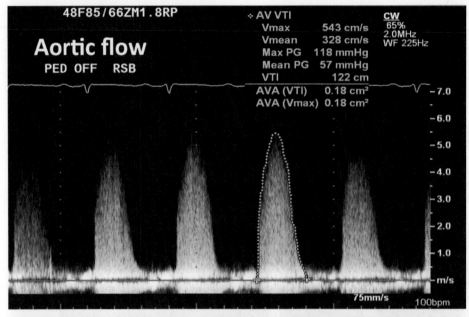

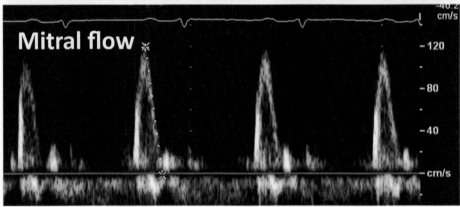

Figure 16.57

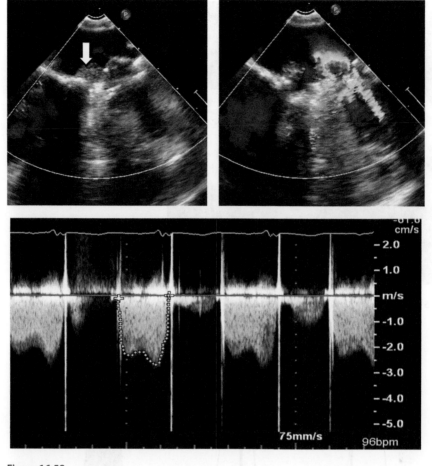

**Figure 16.58**

**16.59.** What is the arrow in Figure 16.59 pointing to?
   A. Thrombus or pannus on a bileaflet mechanical MV
   B. Sewing rim
   C. Artifact
   D. None of the above

**16.60.** Figure 16.60 is a pressure tracing of a patient with AS. Which of the following statements are true?
   A. A is the peak-to-peak gradient obtained by catheterization and is not physiological
   B. B is the peak instantaneous gradient obtained by Doppler peak velocity V2
   C. C is the mean gradient obtained by catheterization or Doppler echocardiography
   D. All of the above

**16.61.** What is the patient whose results are given in Figure 16.61 likely to have?
   A. Severe valvular AS
   B. Severe subvalvular AS
   C. HOCM
   D. No AS; has catheter entrapment

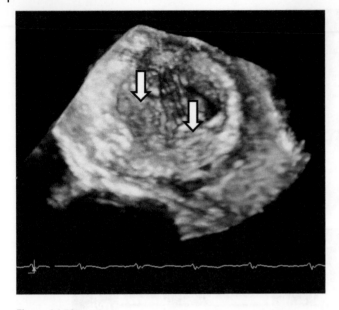

Figure 16.59

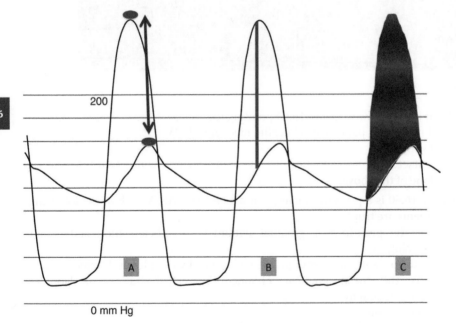

Figure 16.60

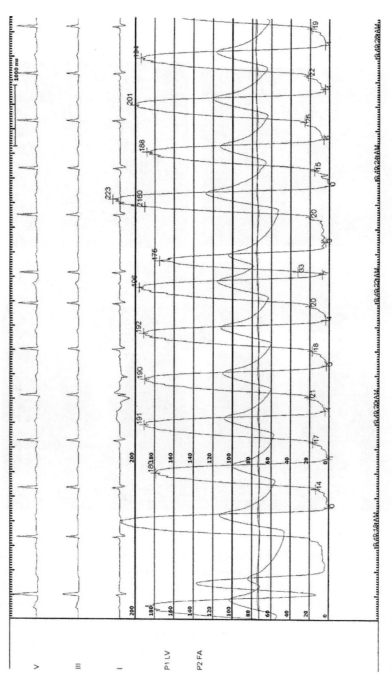

Figure 16.61

**16.62.** What does the patient (body surface area 1.8 m²) in Figure 16.62 have?
   A. Critical AS, high gradient despite low flow
   B. Low-flow, low gradient AS
   C. Normal flow, low gradient AS
   D. None of the above

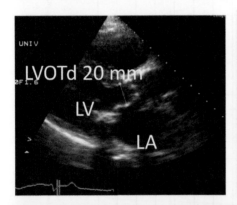
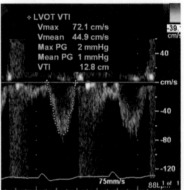

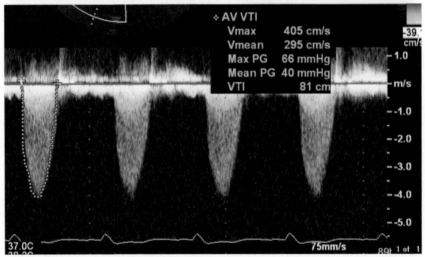

**Figure 16.62**

**16.63.** A 32-year-old man has had a history of murmur for several years. On examination, he has a 3/6 early diastolic murmur at the left sternal border. He is tall and has skeletal features of Marfan syndrome. He is on atenolol 50 mg/day, and his heart rate is 60 bpm and blood pressure 110/70 mmHg. His echocardiogram shows normal-sized LV with EF of 65%, mild AR, trileaflet aortic valve, and aortic sinus dimension of 51 mm and the ascending aorta 44 mm. What will you recommend?
   A. Close monitoring with echo every six months for ascending aortic dimensions
   B. Add losartan
   C. Refer for valve sparing root and ascending aortic replacement with coronary implantation
   D. None of the above

**16.64.** A 60-year-old male presents to your outpatient clinic for a murmur. His echocardiogram showed aortic stenosis with a $V_{max}$ of 4 m/s, aortic valve area 0.9 cm², and mean gradient 42 mmHg. He denies any functional limitation and walks more than one mile daily without shortness of breath. Which stage of valvular heart disease does this patient belong?

A. Stage A
B. Stage B
C. Stage C
D. Stage D

**16.65.** A 52-year-old male with a history of mild aortic stenosis presents for follow-up echocardiogram. His ECHO shows the aortic valve area is 1.5 cm², $V_{max}$ 3.2 m/s, mean gradient 31 mmHg. He denies exertional chest pain or shortness of breath. When should his subsequent echocardiogram be?

A. Every 3–5 years
B. Every five to 10 years
C. Every one to 2 years
D. Every 6–12 months
E. He should get a CT scan

**16.66.** A 29-year-old female who has recently immigrated from South America presents to your office for mitral regurgitation. She was diagnosed with rheumatic heart disease and had been taking antibiotics. For how long does this patient need to take antibiotics?

A. 10 years or until patient is 40 years of age (whichever is longer)
B. 10 years or until patient is 21 years of age (whichever is longer)
C. Five years or until 30 years of age (whichever is longer)
D. Until patient is 45 years of age.

**16.67.** Which of the following is not true regarding infective endocarditis prophylaxis?

A. Dental procedures in patients with prosthetic cardiac valves, including catheter implanted valves and homograft
B. Dental procedures in patients with prosthetic material used for cardiac valve repair, such as Angelo plastic rings, chords or clips
C. Previous infective endocarditis
D. Unrepaired cyanotic congenital heart disease or repaired congenital heart disease with residual shunts or valvular regurgitation
E. Cardiac transplant patients with valvular regurgitation attributable to a structurally abnormal valve
F. Recommended in patients with valvular heart disease who are at high risk of infective endocarditis and are undergoing colonoscopy or cystoscopy in the absence of active infection.

**16.68.** A 70-year-old male with a history of Aortic stenosis is seen in the outpatient clinic after transcatheter aortic valve replacement. How often should we do screening echocardiograms?

A. Baseline, 5 and 10 years after surgery, and then annually
B. Baseline and then annually
C. Baseline, one year, and then every two to three years
D. Baseline only

Chapter 1

**16.69.** A 67-year-old female is seen in your clinic for symptomatic aortic stenosis. Her echocardiogram shows LVEF 55%, severely reduced leaflet motion of aortic valve, indexed $AVA \leq 0.6\,cm^2/m^2$, aortic Vmax ~3.2 m/s, and mean gradient 34 mmHg. What are the requirements to diagnose this patient with paradoxical low-flow aortic stenosis?
   A. Dobutamine stress echocardiogram with $AVA \leq 1.0\,cm^2$ with $Vmax \geq 4\,m/s$
   B. Stroke volume index $< 35\,ml/m^2$
   C. $AVA \leq 1.0\,cm^2$, Vmax of $< 4\,m/s$, and mean gradient of $< 40\,mmHg$
   D. Measurements should be performed on a patient with systolic blood pressure $< 140\,mmHg$
   E. Both B and C
   F. A, B, and C

**16.70.** A 63-year-old male with history of hypertension, hyperlipidemia, and chronic aortic regurgitation presents with progressively worsening dyspnea on exertion. His echocardiogram shows aortic regurgitation with vena contracta >0.6, regurgitant volume 62 ml, EROA $0.34\,cm^2$, LVEF 54%, and no other abnormalities. As you discuss valve replacement, which of the following is not recommended?
   A. Patient should undergo surgical aortic valve replacement
   B. Patient can be considered for mechanical aortic valve based on shared decision making
   C. Patient can be considered for transcatheter aortic valve replacement
   D. BP control of less than $< 140\,mmHg$ with ACEi or ARBs
   E. Entresto can be initiated as per GDMT

**16.71.** You follow up on a patient with a bicuspid aortic valve (BAV). He was diagnosed during a screening echocardiogram after BAV and aortic dissection diagnosis in one of his first-degree cousins. Patient denies chest pain but complains of progressive shortness of breath during exertion. His echocardiogram shows an aortic sinus diameter of 5.0 cm, LVEF 50%, severe AS, and no AR. Which of the following is most appropriate?
   A. Aortic sinus and/or ascending aortic replacement is reasonable
   B. TAVR is recommended
   C. Surgery is not recommended as the aortic diameter is less than 5.5 cm
   D. SAVR and aortic sinus/ascending aortic replacement is reasonable
   E. Valve sparing aortic root replacement is indicated

**16.72.** A 42-year-old female with a history of mitral valve prolapse is following up for chronic mitral regurgitation. She denies chest pain, shortness of breath, leg swelling and is functionally active. Her latest echocardiogram shows mitral regurgitation with central jet >40% of LA, regurgitant fraction $\geq 50\%$, vena contracta $\geq 0.7\,cm$, EROA $\geq 0.4\,cm^2$, LVEF 55%, and LVESD 45 mm. Which of the following statements is most appropriate for the management of this patient?
   A. Patient should undergo mitral valve repair
   B. Surgery is not recommended as the patient is asymptomatic
   C. Patient should be followed up within 6–12 months before deciding about surgery
   D. Mitral valve replacement is recommended in preference to mitral valve repair
   E. PMBC is the treatment of choice

**16.73.** A 70-year-old male with a history of non-ischemic cardiomyopathy, congestive heart failure with LVEF 35% presents to your office with progressively worsening dyspnea on exertion, despite being on maximally tolerated goal-directed medical therapy. His transesophageal echocardiogram shows LVEF 30%, LVESD 60 mm, mitral regurgitation (A2, P2 segment) with regurgitant volume >60 ml, effective regurgitant orifice area of 0.5 cm², regurgitate fraction of 55%, and PASP of 65 mmHg. His recent coronary angiogram showed non-obstructive coronary artery disease. Which of the following is the most appropriate next step in the management?

A. Mitral valve replacement is indicated as it provides maximum benefit
B. Transcatheter edge-to-edge mitral valve repair
C. Medical management only as the patient has an elevated PASP
D. Mitral valve repair surgery

**16.74.** A 25-year-old male with a history of tetralogy of fallout repair presents to your office with gradually worsening exercise tolerance. His echocardiogram shows LVEF 55%, normal LV and LA size, RVEF 45%, severe PR. However, his cardiac stress test with Bruce protocol is unremarkable with 10 METS. Which of the following is the best next step in risk stratification of this patient?

A. Nuclear medicine perfusion stress testing
B. Left heart coronary angiography
C. Right heart coronary angiography
D. Cardiac magnetic resonance imaging
E. Gated CT cardiac

**16.75.** Cardiac MRI in the above patient showed MPA Distal 20 mm, Proximal RPA 12 mm, Distal RPA 15 mm, Proximal LPA 20 mm, Distal LPA 20 mm, LVEDVi 66 ml/m², LVESVi 31 ml/m², RVEF 40%, RV end-diastolic volume index of 160 ml/m², RV end-systolic volume index of 85 ml/m², and RV/LV EDV ratio of 2.5. What should be the next step in the management of this patient?

A. Brock valvuloplasty
B. Pulmonary valve replacement
C. Pulmonary conduit
D. Blalock Taussig shunt

Chapter 16

## Answers

**16.1.** B. Every three to five years.

According to American Heart Association (AHA)/American College of Cardiology (ACC) 2014 valve guidelines (Nishimura et al. 2014) – see Box 16.1. This is mild stage B disease. The same guidelines also apply to mild mitral stenosis (MS), mitral regurgitation (MR), and aortic regurgitation (AR).

**16.2.** B. Follow-up clinic and echo every one to two years.

According to the AHA/ACC 2014 valve guidelines (Nishimura et al. 2014). This is stage C disease. Evidence, based on natural history studies, is accumulating that option A may be true. Same principle applies to severe asymptomatic AR, MR, and MS.

**16.3.** B. Prophylaxis till she turns 40 years.

As per AHA/ACC 2014 valve guidelines. The recommendations are as follows. Rheumatic fever with carditis and residual heart disease (persistent valvular heart disease): 10 years or until patient is 40 years of age (whichever is longer). Rheumatic fever with carditis but no residual heart disease (no valvular disease): 10 years or until patient is 21 years of age (whichever is longer). Rheumatic fever without carditis: 5 years or until patient is 21 years of age (whichever is longer).

**16.4.** D. Any of the above.

**16.5.** E. All of the above.

**16.6.** F. None of the above.

**16.7.** D. Any of the above.

**16.8.** B. Stage C1.

As he has asymptomatic severe AS with normal left ventricular (LV) function. Stage C2 entails LV dysfunction. Stage D is symptomatic. Stage B is mild or moderate AS, and Stage A is at risk (i.e. calcified aortic valve with V2 < 2 m/s).

**16.9.** A. An exercise stress test to confirm the asymptomatic status.

As there is ambiguity about symptoms (class IIa indication). About 50% of patients who claim to be asymptomatic become symptomatic for the first time on a stress test as patients learn to live within symptoms. If a stress test confirms limitation of exercise tolerance, AVR would be indicated. If patient was clearly asymptomatic, option D would have been reasonable. Dobutamine echo is indicated in patients with low-gradient-severe AS to make sure that it is not pseudo AS and that there is contractile reserve.

**16.10.** D. All of the above.

These are class I indications for AVR in those with severe AS.

**16.11.** F. All of the above.

These are all class IIa recommendations for AVR.

**16.12.** D. Both A and B.

These conclusions are based on the PARTNER trial where, in nonsurgical patients, TAVR was superior to medical management alone and in high-risk patients, it was equivalent to surgical AVR.

**16.13.** B. It is a good definitive treatment for calcific AS of the elderly.

The results are only transient in calcific AS.

**16.14.** D. Refer for AVR.

This patient has an AVA of <1 cm² despite normal EF and low gradient and is symptomatic. In such patients, where symptoms are most likely due to AS, AVR is recommended as per current guidelines (Nishimura et al. 2014). As the EF is normal, a DSE has limited value. A recent meta-analysis has shown that low-gradient-severe AS patients have a survival advantage with AVR even if there no low flow (Dayan et al. 2015). Low flow is a stroke volume index of <35 ml/m².

**16.15.** B. Low-dose dobutamine echo for contractile reserve and hemodynamics.

Mostly to make sure that it is not pseudo AS; that is, valve opening more fully when the stroke volume is increased. In pseudo AS, with the increase in stroke volume, V2 will not increase proportionately resulting in an increase in V1/V2 velocity ratio or the dimensionless index. Generally, a dimensionless index of <0.25 indicates severe AS. Dobutamine also helps to evaluate the contractile reserve. Based on current valve guidelines, with a DSE, if AVA remains <1 cm² and V2 increases to >4 m/s, AVR is indicated (class IIa recommendation). Please see Figure 16.15 from the AHA/ACC 2014 valve guidelines (Nishimura et al. 2014). However, a large meta-analysis shows a benefit even in the absence of contractile reserve (Dayan et al. 2015) – see Box 16.2.

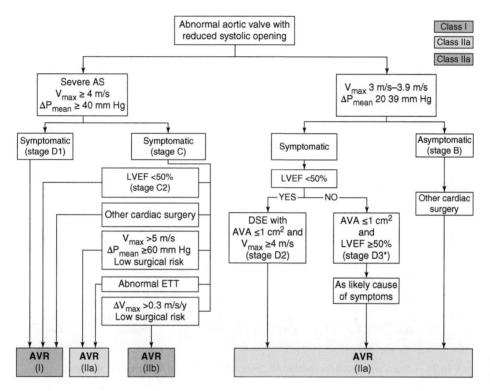

**Figure 16.15** Indications for AVR in patients with AS (ETT: exercise tolerance test). *Source:* adapted from Nishimura et al. (2014).

**16.16.** A. 0.7 cm².

By the continuity equation, A1 × V1 = A2 × V2 using peak velocities, where A1 is LV outflow tract (LVOT) area (3.14 cm² assuming circular geometry), V1 is LVOT velocity, V2 is transvalvular velocity, A2 is AVA. Plugging in the values: 3.14 × 0.8 = A2 × 3.5. Hence, A2 = 0.72 cm².

**16.17.** A. Echocardiography.

This has become the gold standard for assessment of all valvular disorders.

**16.18.** E. All of the above.

As per Nishimura et al. (2014). In addition, diagnosis of chronic severe AR requires evidence of LV dilation (in acute AR, LV does not dilate).

**16.19.** D. All of the above.

All are class I indications for AVR in severe AR.

**16.20.** D. All of the above.

Please refer to the flowchart in Figure 16.20 from the AHA/ACC 2014 valve guidelines (Nishimura et al. 2014).

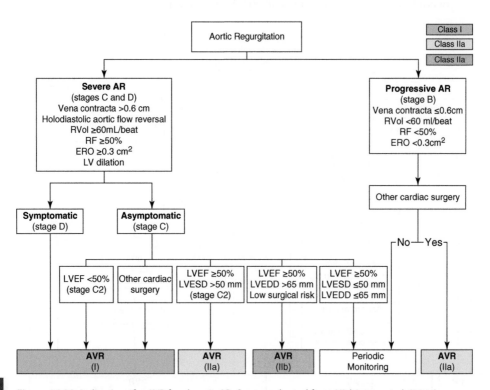

Figure 16.20 Indications for AVR for chronic AR. *Source:* adapted from Nishimura et al. (2014).

**16.21.** C. MVA <1.5 cm².

Or pressure half-time (PHT) >150 ms. MVA <1.0 cm² or PHT >220 ms is considered very severe.

**16.22.** B. Refer for mitral balloon valvotomy.

This patient has very severe MS and favorable anatomy for balloon valvotomy with a Wilkins score <8 and no commissural calcification and no MR. Exercise testing is reasonable, but there are no clear guidelines how to incorporate that data in decision making. Exercise limitation with an exercise-induced PA systolic pressure >60 mmHg are reasonable indications for intervention. Please see the flowchart in Figure 16.22 from the AHA/ACC 2014 valve guidelines (Nishimura et al. 2014).

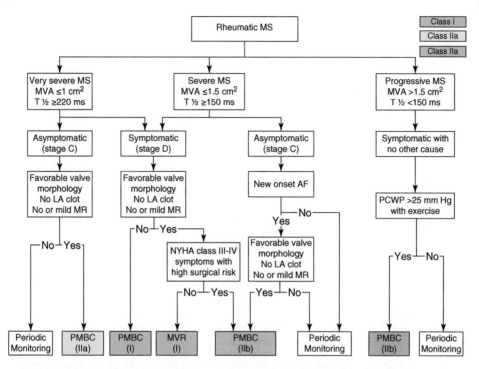

Figure 16.22 Indications for intervention for rheumatic MS (AF: atrial fibrillation; LA: left atrium; NYHA: New York Heart Association; PCWP: pulmonary capillary wedge pressure; PMBC: percutaneous mitral balloon commissurotomy). *Source:* adapted from Nishimura et al. (2014).

**16.23.** C. Refer for MV replacement after coronary angiogram.

Patient symptomatic and has severe MS (PHT >150 ms). As he has moderate MR, he is not an ideal candidate for balloon valvotomy, though the Wilkins score is low. Rheumatic valves are too scarred to give a good result with repair. Please see the flowchart in Figure 16.22.

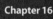

Chapter 16

**16.24.** F. Any of the above.

As per AHA/ACC 2014 valve guidelines (Nishimura et al. 2014).

**16.25.** D. All of the above.

Please see the flowchart in Figure 16.25 from the AHA/ACC 2014 valve guidelines (Nishimura et al. 2014).

**16.26.** A. Flail P2.

This is most suitable for repair, generally with resection of the segment and ring annuloplasty. Repair of anterior leaflet is more difficult. Barlow's disease will have extensive pathology of both leaflets, annulus, and the chords and the most difficult to repair, if at all, and durability may be compromised because of disease progression.

**16.27.** C. Severe.

For functional MR, ERO area >0.2 cm² or regurgitant volume >30 cm³ is deemed to be severe. MR due to valve leaflet tethering is functional as there is no leaflet pathology.

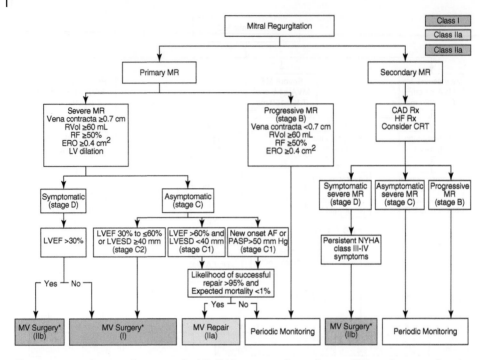

**Figure 16.25** Indications for surgery for MR (CAD: coronary heart disease; CRT: cardiac resynchronization therapy; HF: heart failure; Rx: treatment). *Source:* adapted from Nishimura et al. (2014).

**16.28.** E. All of the above.

**16.29.** D. All of the above.
  See the flowchart from the AHA/ACC 2014 valve guidelines in Figure 16.29.

**16.30.** D. All of the above.

**16.31.** A. Transvalvular velocity >4 m/s.
  Or peak gradient >64 mmHg.

**16.32.** A. Warfarin to an international normalized ratio (INR) goal of 3.0 and aspirin 81 mg daily.
  Based on AHA/ACC 2014 valve guidelines (Nishimura et al. 2014). Addition of aspirin further reduces embolic risk by 50–70%. See the flowchart in Figure 16.32.

**16.33.** D. Warfarin to an INR goal of 2.5 and aspirin 81 mg daily.
  Based on the AHA/ACC 2014 valve guidelines (Nishimura et al. 2014).

**16.34.** A. Warfarin to an INR goal of 3.0 and aspirin 81 mg daily.

**16.35.** A. Minimize nonanticoagulated period; bridge with heparin or LMWH.
  Novel anticoagulants are contraindicated for mechanical valves as they increase risk of thrombosis.

**16.36.** B. Minimize nonanticoagulated period; no bridging needed.

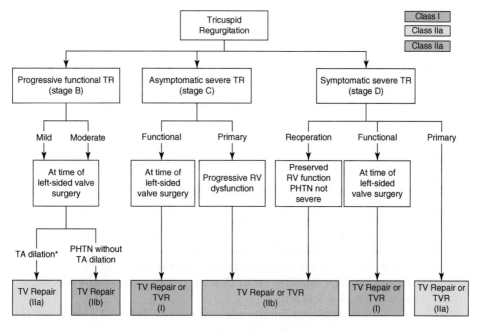

**Figure 16.29** Indications for surgery for TR (PHTN: pulmonary hypertension; RV: right ventricle; TA: tricuspid annular; TVR: TV replacement). *Source:* adapted from Nishimura et al. (2014).

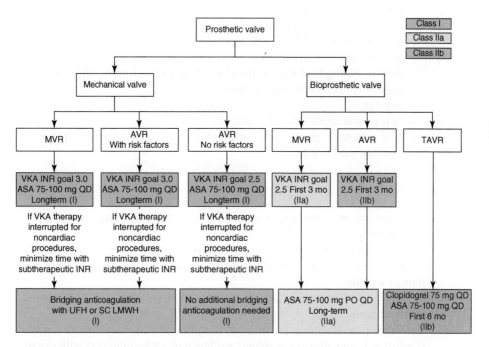

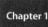

**Figure 16.32** Anticoagulation for prosthetic valves (ASA: aspirin; LMWH: low molecular weight heparin; MVR: mitral valve replacement; SC: subcutaneous; UFH: unfractionated heparin; VKA: vitamin Kantagonist). *Source:* adapted from Nishimura et al. (2014).

However, bridging is recommended for mechanical aortic valves when risk factors are present.

**16.37.** D. All of the above.

As per AHA/ACC 2014 valve guidelines (Nishimura et al. 2014).

**16.38.** D. All of the above.

The modified Duke criteria for the diagnosis of IE are as follows.

## Major Criteria

1. Blood culture positive for IE

Typical microorganisms consistent with IE from two separate blood cultures:
- viridans streptococci, *Streptococcus bovis*, HACEK group (Haemophilus spp., *Actinobacillus actinomycetemcomitans*, *Cardiobacterium hominis*, Eikenella spp., and *Kingella kingae*), *Staphylococcus aureus*; or community-acquired enterococci, in the absence of a primary focus; or
- microorganisms consistent with IE from persistently positive blood cultures, defined as follows:
  - at least two positive cultures of blood samples drawn 12 hours apart; or
  - all of three or a majority of four separate cultures of blood (with first and last samples drawn at least one hour apart)
  - single positive blood culture for *Coxiella burnetii* or antiphase I immunoglobulin G antibody titer >1 : 800.
2. Evidence of endocardial involvement
- Echocardiogram positive for IE defined as follows:
  - oscillating intracardiac mass on valve or supporting structures, in the path of regurgitant jets, or on implanted material in the absence of an alternative anatomic explanation;
  - abscess; or
  - new partial dehiscence of prosthetic valve
  - new valvular regurgitation (worsening or changing of preexisting murmur not sufficient).

## Minor Criteria

1. Predisposition, predisposing heart condition, or injection drug use.
2. Fever, temperature >38 °C (100.4 °F).
3. Vascular phenomena, major arterial emboli, septic pulmonary infarcts, mycotic aneurysm, intracranial hemorrhage, conjunctival hemorrhages, and Janeway lesions.
4. Immunologic phenomena: glomerulonephritis, Osier's nodes, Roth's spots, and rheumatoid factor.
5. Microbiological evidence: positive blood culture but does not meet a major criterion as noted above or serologic evidence of active infection with organism consistent with IE.

**16.39.** D. All of the above.

In addition, it is appropriate if a patient is undergoing valve surgery for IE, there is *S. aureus* bacteremia without a clear source, or there is prosthetic valve with persistent fever. See the flowchart in Figure 16.39 from the AHA/ACC 2014 valve guidelines (Nishimura et al. 2014).

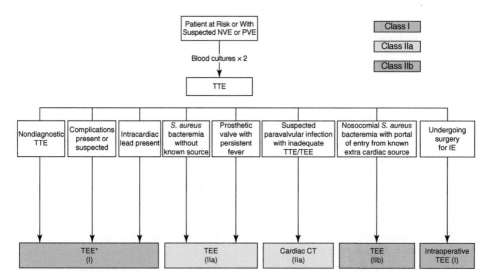

**Figure 16.39** Imaging studies in native valve endocarditis (NVE) and prosthetic valve endocarditis (PVE). *Source:* adapted from Nishimura et al. (2014).

**16.40.** D. All of the above.

Option A is a class I indication and other two are class IIa indications. See the flowchart in Figure 16.40.

**16.41.** D. All of the above.

With LMWH, monitoring is critical. See the flowchart in Figure 16.41.

**16.42.** A. Carcinoid syndrome.

Note the restricted opening of the TV during diastole suggesting tricuspid stenosis and severe TR. These are diagnostic of carcinoid in this clinical context.

**16.43.** B. Mild stenosis.

Note flow acceleration across the MV and a mean gradient of only 4 mmHg with pressure equilibration across the valve in end diastole. Normal PHT is generally about 60–80 ms.

**16.44.** A. Severe paravalvular AR.

Indicated by the arrow with a large proximal isovelocity surface area. The V2 across the aortic valve is about 2 m/s, and hence not stenotic. The MR signal on CW is faint, indicating that it is likely mild. The MS, however, seems to be significant and may be contributing to symptoms.

Chapter 16

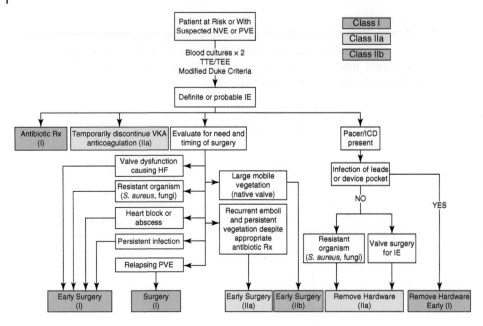

**Figure 16.40** Diagnosis and treatment of IE (ICD: implantable cardioverter defibrillator). *Source:* adapted from Nishimura et al. (2014).

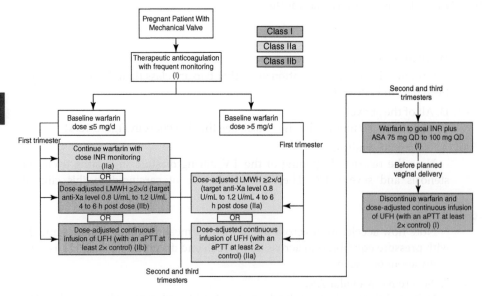

**Figure 16.41** Anticoagulation of pregnant patients with mechanical valves (aPTT: activated PTT). *Source:* adapted from Nishimura et al. (2014).

**16.45.** A. MS.

The m-mode of the MV shows slow EF slope and paradoxical anterior motion of posterior mitral leaflet indicating commissural fusion with posterior leaflet moving anteriorly with anterior leaflet during diastole. This is typical of MS – MS is likely to be severe as the EF slope is very flat and hence MV PHT is likely to be long.

**16.46.** B. First-degree atrioventricular (AV) block or long AV delay on pacemaker.

Note the diastolic TR indicating long AV delay. Also note the pacer lead.

**16.47.** C. Moderate PR.

The transvalvular velocity (i) is low, ruling out stenosis. The PR signal is quite dense, indicating that PR (ii) is either moderate or severe. However, there is still an end-diastolic PR signal (iii) after temporary interruption with right atrial systole. In severe PR, the signal generally ends in mid diastole due to PA/right ventricle diastolic pressure equilibration.

**16.48.** C. MS.

Note doming of the mitral leaflet and flow acceleration.

**16.49.** A. Acute severe AR.

Note the premature MV closure on MV m-mode and marked holodiastolic flow reversal in the aorta.

**16.50.** A. Acute severe AR.

Dense, rapidly decelerating AR signal indicates acute severe AR.

**16.51.** A. Severe paravalvular MR.

The measurement is of the MR vena contracta. Note that the MR jet reaches the posterior left atrial wall.

**16.52.** A. MV repair.

This is classical P2 flail, which is very amenable to repair.

**16.53.** A. Severe TR.

Note the vena contracta diameter of 15 mm and triangular TR signal indicating severe TR. Many times severe TR occurs because of flail TV due to damage to chords during endomyocardial biopsy or dilated tricuspid annulus.

**16.54.** B. Proceed with TAVR using carotid protection.

We did this. The mobile mass on the aortic valve did not embolize and was crushed against the aortic wall. The patient had no signs of endocarditis. Masses on aortic valve like this seem to embolize very rarely. We also avoided aortic valve predilatation to minimize embolic risk.

**16.55.** A. Severe stenosis.

Note a mean gradient of 29 mmHg and PHT of 374 ms.

**16.56.** A. Severe subvalvular AS.

The arrow points to the membrane in the LVOT. Note that the aortic valve opens well.

**16.57.** A. Critical AS with high LA pressure.

Note that V2 is >5 m/s and the calculated AVA is ^ 0.7 cm$^2$, indicating critical AS. The patient is in sinus rhythm but has no "A" wave and has very rapid E wave deceleration, indicating very high LA pressure.

**16.58.** A. IV thrombolytic.

As the operating room was not available and patient was worsening very rapidly, we took this approach. The patient had dramatic improvement within 30 minutes without any neurologic sequelae. The arrow points to a large thrombus on the valve, and Doppler signals are indicative of severe obstruction.

**16.59.** A. Thrombus or pannus on a bileaflet mechanical MV.

This is the LA side of the bileaflet mechanical MV with completely opened discs.

**16.60.** D. All of the above.

**16.61.** A. Severe valvular AS.

There is a peak-to-peak gradient of about 80 mmHg. In the post-premature atrial contraction beat (though not post-premature ventricular contraction), the gradient increases with an increase in aortic pulse pressure, suggesting it is not HOCM. In HOCM, the pulse pressure drops (Brockenbrough phenomenon). In subvalvular AS, as long as the distal catheter is still in the LV, the diastolic pressure would be same as main body of the LV.

**16.62.** A. Critical AS, high gradient despite low flow.

There is critical AS, as the AVA by the continuity equation is $0.5\,cm^2$ $(3.14 \times 12.8/81)$. The gradient is high as the peak gradient is >64 mmHg and the mean gradient is 40 mmHg. The stroke volume is low at $40\,cm^3$ $(3.14 \times 12.8)$ or $22\,cm^3/m^2$, but this has not lowered the gradient, suggesting the critical nature of AS. The gradient is proportional to the square of the flow following the Bernoulli equation. Low flow is defined as stroke volume index $<35\,cm^3/m^2$.

**16.63.** C. Refer for valve sparing root and ascending aortic replacement with coronary implantation.

Ascending aortic dimension >50 mm is an indication for surgery as the risk of rupture and dissection increases markedly at this point. If the aortic dimension was <50 mm, follow-up at six months for aortic growth rate would have been appropriate. He is well beta blocked.

**16.64.** C.

The patient belongs to stage C1-in symptomatic patients with severe valvular heart disease in whom the LV or RV remains compensated. There are four stages of valvular heart disease. Stage A includes at-risk patients with risk factors for the development of valvular heart disease. Stage B refers to progressive VHD where patients are asymptomatic and have mild to moderate severity. Stage C is sub-classified into stage C1 and stage C2. C1 patients are asymptomatic and have severe VHD but LV and RV remain compensated. Stage C2 refers to asymptomatic patients with severe VHD but with the LV or RV decompensation. Stage D refers to severe symptomatic patients with symptoms resulting from severe VHD.

**16.65.** C.

Per ACC 2020 valvular heart disease guidelines, patients with stage B Aortic stenosis with moderate severity (Vmax 3–3.9 m/s) should have a repeat echocardiogram done every one to two years. Patients with stages C&D should be given an echocardiogram every 6–12 months.

**16.66.** A.

As per 2020 ACC guidelines, the duration of secondary prophylaxis for rheumatic fever depends on carditis and residual heart disease. Patients with rheumatic fever with carditis and residual heart disease (persistent VHD) should take antibiotics for 10 years or until the patient is 40 years of age (whichever is longer). Patients with rheumatic fever with carditis but no residual heart disease (no valvular disease) should take antibiotics for 10 years or until the patient is 21 years of age (whichever is longer). Rheumatic fever without carditis should take antibiotics for 5 years or until 21 years of age (whichever is longer).

**16.67.** F.

As per 2020 ACC guidelines, in patients with valvular heart disease who are at high risk of infective endocarditis, antibiotic prophylaxis is not recommended for non-dental procedures (EGD, colonoscopy, or cystoscopy) in the absence of active infection.

**16.68.** B.

As per 2020 ACC guidelines, transcatheter bioprosthetic valve replacement needs periodic echocardiograms annually. A baseline echocardiogram should be done either one day before discharge or, more ideally, within one to three months after transcatheter valve replacement.

**16.69.** F.

AVA $\leq 1.0\,cm^2$ or indexed AVA $\leq 0.6\,cm^2/m^2$, Vmax of <4 m/s, and mean gradient of <40 mmHg in a patient with normal LVEF suggests the diagnosis of symptomatic severe low gradient aortic stenosis with normal LVEF or paradoxical low flow severe aortic stenosis. The next step is to measure the stroke volume index (<35 ml/$m^2$) when the patient's SBP is less than 140 mmHg.

**16.70.** C.

In patients with isolated severe AR who have indications for SAVR and are candidates for surgery, transcatheter aortic valve replacement should not be performed. TAVR for isolated chronic aortic regurgitation can be challenging because of the dilation of aortic root and lack of calcification to hold the valve in place. Significant complications include valve migration and paravalvular leak. Therefore, it should be considered only in patients with severe AR and heart failure symptoms who have prohibitive surgical risk. Even then, valvular calcification needs to be evaluated carefully.

**16.71.** D.

In patients with a bicuspid aortic valve and indications for surgical aortic valve replacement and a diameter of the aortic sinus/ascending aorta $\geq 4.5\,cm$, replacement of the aortic sinus/ascending aorta is reasonable if the surgery is performed at a comprehensive valve center (Class 2a). Moreover, this patient's family history of aortic dissection in a first-degree cousin makes him a high-risk candidate for dissection (Class 2a). The patient has severe aortic stenosis and should undergo surgical replacement with aortic sinus replacement and not just TAVR.

**16.72.** A.

Mitral valve surgery is recommended in patients with severe primary MR and evidence of left ventricular systolic dysfunction (LVEF ≤60% and LVESD ≥40 mm), regardless of the symptoms (Class 1B). Mitral valve repair is preferred over mitral valve replacement in patients with severe primary MR due to degenerative disease (Class 1B). PMBC is not the treatment of choice and is contraindicated in patients with MR.

**16.73. B.**

Based on the COAPT Trial, transcatheter edge-to-edge repair is recommended in patients with chronic severe secondary MR related to LV systolic dysfunction (EF <50%) who have NYHA class II-IV symptoms while being on optimal GDMT, with appropriate anatomy as defined on TEE and with LVEF between 20 and 50%, LVESD <70 mm, and pulmonary artery systolic pressure <70 mmHg. Mitral valve repair surgery would have been the best choice if the patient had obstructive coronary artery disease and was a candidate for coronary artery bypass grafting. Similarly, mitral replacement is not preferred for this patient.

**16.74. D.**

Cardiac MRI can help risk stratifying patients with pulmonary regurgitations and history of surgical repair of congenital heart disease. Cardiac MRI can show RV dysfunction and dilation that can be used in decision-making for pulmonary valve replacement. This patient had an unremarkable exercise stress test; therefore, left heart catheterization is unlikely to provide additional diagnostic information. Similarly, nuclear medicine perfusion stress testing is also not recommended. Right heart coronary angiography can be performed but will not offer end-systolic and diastolic volume indices and is an invasive procedure. Gated cardiac CT can provide information about indices but lacks cine resolution, especially in congenital heart disease repair cases.

**16.75. B.**

Severe PR in a symptomatic patient, or asymptomatic patient with severe PR and moderate to severe RV dilatation are Class 1 indications for pulmonary valve replacement. Progressive RV dysfunction (RVEF 40–45%) and large RV aneurysm are Class 2 indications for pulmonary valve replacement. This patient's RVEF 40%, RVEDVi of 160 ml/m$^2$, RVESVi of 85 ml/m$^2$, and RV/LV EDV ratio of 2.5 suggest severe RV dilatation and this patient should be sent for PVR. Patients can be evaluated for transcatheter versus surgical PVR at a tertiary care center (ACHD guidelines).

---

**Box 16.1  AHA/ACC 2014 Valve Guidelines**

Staging of valve disease (A–D) in Nishimura et al. (2014) is new compared with the 2008 guidelines. Generally, if the valve disease is severe and symptomatic, there is an indication for intervention; if the valve disease is severe, asymptomatic, and there is no damage to the heart, there is no indication for intervention; if the valve disease is severe, asymptomatic, and there is damage to the heart, then there is an indication for intervention; if the valve disease is severe, asymptomatic, there is no damage to the heart, but the patient is undergoing another heart surgery, there is an indication for intervention. In other words, in asymptomatic severe disease, there is indication for intervention or surgery, if there is damage to the heart or the patient is undergoing another heart surgery.

---

**Box 16.2    Meta-analysis of Aortic Valve Replacement**

The meta-analysis by Dayan et al. (2015) analyzed studies of mortality and survival impact of AVR in patients with low-gradient (LG) AS and preserved left ventricular EF, including paradoxical low flow (i.e. stroke volume index <35 ml/m$^2$), low-gradient (LF-LG) and normal-flow, low-gradient (NF-LG), and those with high-gradient (>40 mmHg) AS or moderate AS. Eighteen studies were included in the analysis. Patients with LF-LG AS have increased mortality compared with patients with moderate AS (hazard ratio (HR): 1.68; 95% confidence interval (CI): 1.31–2.17), NF-LG AS (HR: 1.80; 95% CI: 1.29–2.51), and high-gradient AS (HR: 1.67; 95% CI: 1.16–2.39). AVR was associated with reduced mortality in patients with LF-LG (HR: 0.44; 95% CI: 0.25–0.77). Similar benefit occurred with AVR in patients with NF-LG (HR: 0.48; 95% CI: 0.28–0.83). Compared with patients with high-gradient AS, those with LF-LG AS were less likely to be referred to AVR (odds ratio: 0.32; 95% CI: 0.21–0.49).

---

# References

Dayan, V., Vignolo, G., Magne, J. et al. (2015). Outcome and impact of aortic valve replacement in patients with preserved LVEF and low-gradient aortic stenosis. *Journal of the American College of Cardiology* 66 (23): 2594–2603.

Nishimura, R.A., Otto, C.M., Bonow, R.O. et al. (2014). 2014 AHA/ACC guideline for the management of patients with valvular heart disease: a report of the American College of Cardiology/American Heart Association Task Force on Practice Guidelines. *Journal of the American College of Cardiology* 63: e57–e185.

Chapter 1

# Adult Congenital Heart Disease

# 17

**17.1.** What are the most common lesions associated with Noonan syndrome?
  A. Pulmonary stenosis (PS) and atrial septal defect (ASD)
  B. Ventricular septal defect (VSD)
  C. Patent ductus arteriosus (PDA)
  D. Coarctation of aorta and aortic stenosis (AS)

**17.2.** What is the most common lesion associated with Williams syndrome?
  A. VSD
  B. Supravalvular AS
  C. Valvular AS
  D. ASD

**17.3.** What are the most common anomalies seen in DiGeorge syndrome (22q11)?
  A. VSD and arch anomalies
  B. Pulmonary valve stenosis
  C. ASD
  D. Supravalvular AS

**17.4.** What is the most common congenital heart lesion seen in Holt-Oram syndrome?
  A. Arch anomalies
  B. Coarctation of aorta
  C. ASD
  D. AS

**17.5.** What is the most common cardiac anomaly seen in Turner syndrome?
  A. Coarctation of aorta
  B. Tetralogy of Fallot (TOF)
  C. VSD
  D. Partial anomalous pulmonary venous drainage

**17.6.** Bicuspid aortic valves are seen in what percentage of the population?
  A. 4–6%
  B. 20%
  C. 1–2%
  D. 10%

**17.7.** Of the total number of congenital heart defects, simple shunts (ASD, VSD, PDA) are seen in what proportion of them?
  A. 75%
  B. 25%
  C. 50%
  D. 90%

**17.8.** Which of the following congenital cardiac lesions are seen in trisomy 21?
  A. VSD
  B. Atrioventricular (AV) canal defects
  C. ASD
  D. All of the above
  E. None of the above

**17.9.** Which of the following congenital cardiac defects are seen in trisomy 13?
    **A.** VSD
    **B.** PDA
    **C.** Dextrocardia
    **D.** All of the above
    **E.** None of the above

**17.10.** Which of the following congenital lesions are not seen in trisomy 18?
    **A.** VSD
    **B.** PDA
    **C.** PS
    **D.** AS

**17.11.** What is the chamber that dilates in a patient with a significant VSD?
    **A.** Right atrium
    **B.** Right ventricle
    **C.** Left atrium and left ventricle
    **D.** Left ventricle

**17.12.** What is the most common lesion associated with supracristal VSD?
    **A.** AS
    **B.** Aortic regurgitation
    **C.** Pulmonary regurgitation (PR)
    **D.** PS

**17.13.** A patient has a small restrictive perimembranous VSD. The velocity across the defect is 5 m/s. Blood pressure (BP) recorded at the time of the echocardiogram is 125/75 mmHg. What is the right ventricular (RV) systolic pressure?
    **A.** 40 mmHg
    **B.** 25 mmHg
    **C.** 100 mmHg
    **D.** 125 mmHg

**17.14.** A patient has a small perimembranous VSD. He is undergoing dental work. His dentist recommends that he sees you regarding endocarditis prophylaxis. What would your recommendation be?
    **A.** Amoxicillin 2 g prior to commencement of dental work
    **B.** Vancomycin 1 g IV prior to dental work
    **C.** Clindamycin 600 mg prior to dental work
    **D.** No antibiotic prophylaxis is indicated at this time

**17.15.** The short view of pulmonary artery (PA) branching and continuous-wave Doppler signal through the area of abnormal color flow in Figure 17.15 shows which of the following?
    **A.** ASD
    **B.** VSD
    **C.** PDA
    **D.** Coarctation of aorta

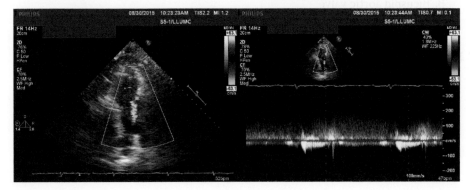

**Figure 17.15**

**17.16.** A 26-year-old patient is referred to you for a murmur. A transthoracic echocardio-gram (TTE) is performed which fails to show any valvular pathology or a shunt lesion. The TTE is remarkable for dilatation of right atrium and right ventricle. What would the next step be?
  A. Reassure the patient; no further test is needed
  B. Cardiac catheterization
  C. Transesophageal echocardiogram (TEE)
  D. Cardiac magnetic resonance imaging (MRI)

**17.17.** A sinus venosus ASD is commonly associated with which of the following?
  A. Cleft mitral valve
  B. Partial anomalous pulmonary venous drainage
  C. Persistent left superior vena cava (SVC)
  D. Goose-neck deformity

**17.18.** In the patient mentioned in Question 17.16, a TEE was performed which showed a sinus venosus ASD with a partial anomalous venous return of the right upper pulmonary vein. What is the next step in management?
  A. Cardiac catheterization to evaluate Qp/Qs
  B. Cardiac MRI
  C. Cardiac computed tomography (CT)
  D. Consultation with a CT surgeon
  E. Referral for percutaneous closure of the ASD

**17.19.** Secundum ASDs make up what proportion of ASDs?
  A. 90%                           C. 80%
  B. 25%                           D. 75%

**17.20.** A primum ASD is commonly associated with which of the following?
  A. Left axis deviation on surface electrocardiogram (ECG)
  B. Cleft of the anterior mitral leaflet
  C. Left axis deviation and cleft mitral leaflet
  D. Persistent left SVC

**17.21.** A patient with hypertension is diagnosed with coarctation of the aorta. What is the most common associated finding one should look for?
  A. Pulmonary valve stenosis
  B. Bicuspid aortic valve
  C. Cleft mitral valve
  D. Ebstein's anomaly

**17.22.** A patient is diagnosed with a PDA. The peak systolic gradient across the defect is 105 mmHg. No other abnormality is noted on the echocardiogram. The BP recorded at the time of the echocardiogram is 130/77 mmHg. Based on the data given, what does the patient have?
  A. Suprasystemic RV pressure
  B. Normal RV pressure
  C. Systemic RV pressure
  D. Cannot tell

**17.23.** Which of the following does TOF not include?

- **A.** Overriding of the aorta
- **B.** RV hypertrophy
- **C.** PS
- **D.** VSD
- **E.** ASD

**17.24.** Which of the following is an anomaly that should be sought out in a patient with TOF being referred for surgical repair?

- **A.** Anomalous origin of left anterior descending (LAD) artery from right coronary artery (RCA)
- **B.** Anomalous RCA from LAD
- **C.** Anomalous left circumflex artery from RCA
- **D.** None of the above

**17.25.** A patient with a history of repaired TOF is referred to you for complaints of fatigue and lack of exercise tolerance. Her echocardiogram shows moderate RV enlargement with mild hypokinesis. What is the probable cause of her right-sided enlargement?

- **A.** Severe tricuspid regurgitation (TR)
- **B.** Severe pulmonary valve regurgitation
- **C.** Severe mitral regurgitation
- **D.** Severe aortic regurgitation

**17.26.** What is the treatment of choice for the correction of dextro (D)-transposition of great arteries (TGA)?

- **A.** Senning procedure
- **B.** Mustard procedure
- **C.** Jatene arterial switch
- **D.** Rastelli procedure

**17.27.** What is the position of the aorta in D-TGA?

- **A.** Central
- **B.** Anterior and rightward
- **C.** Anterior and leftward
- **D.** Posterior

**17.28.** What is the position of the aorta in levo (L)-TGA?

- **A.** Anterior and rightward
- **B.** Anterior and to the left
- **C.** Central
- **D.** Posterior

**17.29.** In what percentage of patients with L-TGA is complete heart block seen?

- **A.** 90%
- **B.** 30%
- **C.** 50%
- **D.** 10%

**17.30.** Ebstein's anomaly can be seen in up to what proportion of patients with L-TGA?

- **A.** 100%
- **B.** 90%
- **C.** 80%
- **D.** 25%

**17.31.** The classic Blalock-Taussig shunt is a connection between which of the following?

- **A.** Ascending aorta to PA
- **B.** Subclavian artery to PA
- **C.** Descending aorta to left PA
- **D.** SVC to right PA

**17.32.** What is a Rastelli repair?

- **A.** Closure of VSD and placement of right ventricle-PA conduit
- **B.** Balloon atrial septostomy
- **C.** Repair of VSD
- **D.** Repair of ASD

Chapter 1

**17.33.** The Fontan operation is used to repair which of the following defects?

A. Hypoplastic left heart syndrome
B. Triscuspid or mitral atresia
C. Hypoplastic right heart syndrome
D. Double inlet single ventricle
E. None of the above
F. All of the above

**17.34.** Right aortic arch is associated with which of the following?

A. TOF
B. *Truncus* arteriosus
C. Pulmonary atresia
D. None of the above
E. All of the above

**17.35.** A patient with a history of a Fontan operation presents with complaints of edema. On examination, he has ascites, and his serum chemistry is significant for a low albumin level. What does this patient have?

A. Celiac disease
B. Pericardial constriction
C. Renal failure
D. Protein-losing enteropathy

**17.36.** Which of the following is/are a current class I indication regarding surgery for anomalous coronary arteries?

A. An anomalous left main coronary artery coursing between the aorta and PA
B. Ischemia caused by coronary compression (when coursing between the great arteries or has an intramural course)
C. An anomalous RCA between aorta and PA causing ischemia
D. All of the above
E. None of the above

**17.37.** Which of the following is not a class I indication regarding congenital heart disease in an adult >40 years of age?

A. Atrial level shunts with right ventricle enlargement and without pulmonary arterial hypertension (PAH) are recommended closure to prevent right ventricle failure, improve exercise capacity, and decrease atrial arrhythmia
B. Intervention is recommended for coarctation with obstruction for palliation of hypertension
C. Complex congenital heart disease with *de novo* presentation should receive comprehensive care at an adult congenital heart disease (ACHD) center with multidisciplinary input
D. In adults with a new presentation of a simple shunt or valve lesion and no hemodynamic compromise, evaluation by a general cardiologist in consultation with an ACHD cardiologist is reasonable
E. Patients with newly diagnosed coronary artery anomalies should be evaluated by an ACHD team with expertise in imaging, coronary artery disease management, intervention, and surgical revascularization

**17.38.** Regarding hypertension and coarctation of aorta, which of the following is the true statement?

A. The prevalence of hypertension is higher with later repair
B. The prevalence of hypertension is lower regardless of age of repair
C. The prevalence of hypertension is similar to people with no coarctation
D. Hypertension is not a problem after repair

**17.39.** Regarding the use of angiotensin-converting-enzyme (ACE) inhibitors in coarctation of the aorta, which of the following is the true statement?
  **A.** ACE inhibitors have no known side effect in patients with coarctation of aorta
  **B.** ACE inhibitors have been reported to precipitate acute renal failure in the setting of coarctation
  **C.** Neither A nor B
  **D.** Both A and B

**17.40.** Regarding screening for diabetes in ACHD, which of the following is the true statement?
  **A.** Screening for diabetes mellitus should be undertaken in patients >40 years, body mass index >25 kg/m² with or without risk factors
  **B.** Appropriate screening can include fasting glucose, hemoglobin A1C, or two-hours 75 g oral glucose tolerance test
  **C.** If tests are normal, repeat testing at three-year intervals
  **D.** All of the above
  **E.** None of the above

**17.41.** Regarding arrhythmias in ACHD, the following are true except:
  **A.** Wolff-Parkinson-White syndrome and accessory-pathway-mediated tachycardia are associated with Ebstein anomaly
  **B.** The most common arrhythmia facing older adults with congenital heart disease is intra-atrial reentrant tachycardia (IART)
  **C.** The highest incidence of IART is seen in those who have undergone Mustard or Senning repair for D-TGA or the Fontan procedure for single-ventricle physiology
  **D.** In the older adults, ventricular tachycardia (VT) is seen in patients with repaired TOF
  **E.** All of the above
  **F.** None of the above

**17.42.** Which of the following are true regarding pulmonary disease in ACHD?
  **A.** Clinicians should have a low threshold for assessing patents with ACHD for PAH, with echocardiogram and hemodynamic cardiac catheterization
  **B.** Patients with Eisenmenger's should be followed up closely by an ACHD specialist
  **C.** Treatment of PAH in the setting of ACHD with pulmonary vasodilator drugs can be useful and may lead to functional improvement
  **D.** It is reasonable to consider serial evaluations of lung function in all adults with CHD
  **E.** All of the above

**17.43.** Which of the following are true regarding recommendations for liver disease in ACHD?
  **A.** Serial evaluation of liver function should be performed in all patients with a previous history of Fontan palliation
  **B.** Patients with palliation for CHD prior to 1992 should be screened for hepatitis C
  **C.** Gallstones necessitating cholecystectomy are seen with increasing frequency in ACHD patients
  **D.** All of the above
  **E.** None of the above

**17.44.** Which of the following are not true regarding renal disease in ACHD?
A. Renal function should be routinely assessed in all patients with moderate to complex CHD
B. In the presence of renal dysfunction, all effort must be made to minimize additional renal injury
C. Novel biomarkers such as urinary interleukin 18 and neutrophil gelatinase-associated lipocalin may be predictive of acute kidney injury
D. Renal dysfunction is not a poor prognostic marker in patients with ACHD

**17.45.** Which of the following is not a class I recommendation regarding diagnostic testing in an ACHD patient?
A. Echocardiography in the ACHD patient should be interpreted by physicians with expertise in both acquired and congenital heart disease
B. Echocardiography reporting should include both anatomic diagnoses and quantitative assessment of chambers, valves, and great vessels in a format accessible to physicians caring for ACHD patients
C. Diagnostic cardiac catheterization in the older adult with CHD should use a team approach that includes interventionalists skilled in the evaluation of the physiology associated with CHD, as well as being skilled in selective coronary angiography.
D. Sixty-four detector row or higher CT angiography can be useful in lieu of invasive coronary angiography to exclude important coronary artery disease when the pretest probability is low to intermediate

**17.46.** TOF may be associated with which of the following genetic defects?
A. Point mutation in major histocompatibility complex gene
B. 22q11 deletion
C. 9–22 translocation
D. None of the above

**17.47.** In a patient who had complete repair of TOF, which of the following sequelae may exist?
A. PR or pulmonary stenosis
B. Branch PA stenosis
C. VSD
D. Aortic regurgitation
E. All of the above

**17.48.** In a 19-year-old patient with severe asymptomatic PR post TOF repair, what would be the best monitoring strategy in addition to symptoms and heart failure?
A. Serial TTE with monitoring of right ventricle diameter
B. Annual cardiac CT scan for right ventricle volume and ejection fraction (EF)
C. Annual cardiac MRI for right ventricle volume and EF
D. Clinical follow-up alone

**17.49.** What are the indications for redo surgery in a TOF patient with prior repair?
A. Severe symptomatic PR or severe PR with RV dysfunction
B. Valvular or subvalvular PS with a gradient of >50 mmHg or RVOT obstruction with RV dysfunction
C. Residual VSD with a shunt ratio of >1.5
D. Severe aortic regurgitation with LVEF <50%
E. All of the above
F. None of the above

**17.50.** The electrical abnormalities post TOF repair include which of the following?

A. VT and sudden death

B. Atrial flutter or fibrillation

C. Right bundle branch block

D. AV block

E. All of the above

F. None of the above

**17.51.** Which of the following are predictors of sudden death post TOF repair?

A. Severe PR

B. RV dilation or dysfunction

C. QRS duration of >180 ms

D. Nonsustained VT

E. Syncope

F. All of the above

**17.52.** An 18-year-old patient with prior Mustard procedure for TGA has developed facial swelling with suffusion. The jugular venous pressure is markedly raised. There is no edema, liver is normal sized, and there are no murmurs. What is the likely explanation?

A. Constrictive pericarditis

B. Failure of subpulmonic ventricle

C. Baffle obstruction

D. Systolic anterior motion (SAM) with dynamic subpulmonic obstruction

**17.53.** What is the frequency of baffle leaks post Mustard procedure?

A. 5%

B. 25%

C. 50%

D. 90%

**17.54.** What are the consequences of baffle leaks post Mustard procedure?

A. May be none

B. Systemic desaturation

C. Paradoxical embolization

D. All of the above

**17.55.** What do the potential consequences of atrial switch operation include?

A. Obstruction to systemic venous baffle

B. Baffle leak

C. Stenosis of pulmonary venous baffle

D. Failure of systemic ventricle and TR

E. Dynamic subpulmonic obstruction due to SAM

F. Atrial arrhythmias and AV conduction defects

G. All of the above

**17.56.** Potential complications after arterial switch operation for TGA include which of the following?

A. Stenosis of pulmonary arterial anastomosis site

B. Aortic aneurysm

C. Coronary artery stenosis

D. Neo-aortic regurgitation (native pulmonary valve)

E. All of the above

**17.57.** What percentage of patients with Ebstein's anomaly may have right-to-left shunt at atrial level?

A. 0%

B. 0%

C. 50%

D. 90%

**17.58.** Ebstein's anomaly may involve which of the following changes to the tricuspid valve?

A. Adherence of the tricuspid valve leaflets to the underlying myocardium or failure of delamination

Chapter 1

**B.** Apical displacement into the right ventricle of the septal and posterior leaflets of the tricuspid valve below the AV junction resulting in atrialization of right ventricle

**C.** Redundancy, tethering, and fenestrations of the anterior tricuspid valve leaflet

**D.** All of the above

**17.59.** The ECG changes in Ebstein's anomaly may include which of the following
  **A.** Pre-excitation due generally to a right-sided accessory pathway
  **B.** Giant P wave
  **C.** QR pattern in V1 to V4
  **D.** All of the above

**17.60.** The 19-year-old patient in Figure 17.60 presented with shortness of breath and large RV and RA, PA systolic pressure of 30 mmHg. What would the definitive treatment be?
  **A.** Annual follow-up
  **B.** Surgical repair
  **C.** Percutaneous closure
  **D.** None of the above

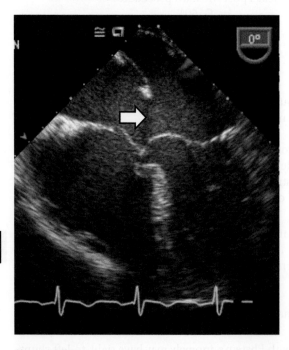

**Figure 17.60**

**17.61.** What type of ASD is shown in Figure 17.61?
  **A.** Secundum ASD
  **B.** Primum ASD
  **C.** Sinus venosus ASD of IVC type
  **D.** Sinus venosus ASD of SVC type

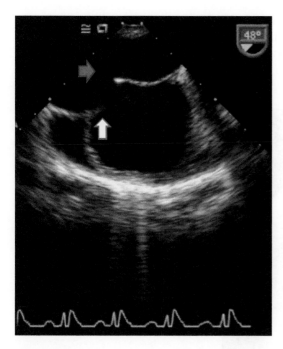

Figure 17.61

**17.62.** What condition does the patient in Figure 17.62 have?
  **A.** Sinus venosus ASD with anomalous drainage of right upper pulmonary vein
  **B.** Sinus venosus ASD with anomalous drainage of right lower pulmonary vein
  **C.** Secundum ASD
  **D.** None of the above

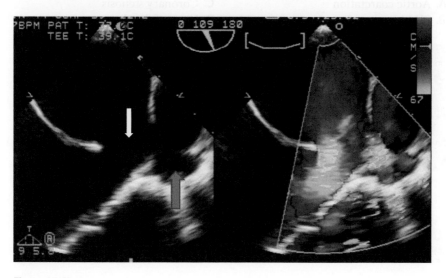

Figure 17.62

**17.63.** What procedure did the patient in Figure 17.63 have?
- **A.** Closure of secundum ASD with Amplatzer device
- **B.** Closure of patent foramen ovale (PFO) with Amplatzer device
- **C.** Surgical patch of ASD
- **D.** None of the above

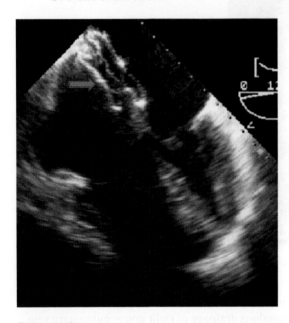

**Figure 17.63**

**17.64.** The CW Doppler signal in Figure 17.64 was obtained from a suprasternal window. What is it indicative of?
- **A.** Aortic coarctation
- **B.** PDA
- **C.** Coronary stenosis
- **D.** None of the above

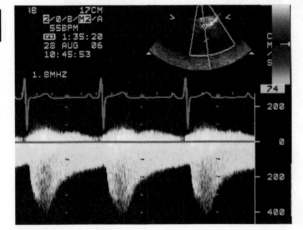

**Figure 17.64**

**17.65.** What does the patient in Figure 17.65 have? (DTA: descending thoracic aorta; MPA: main PA; RPA: right PA)

    **A.** PDA                     **C.** PS

    **B.** PR                      **D.** None of the above

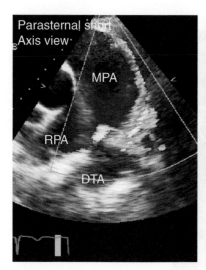
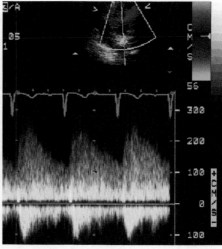

Figure 17.65

**17.66.** What does the patient in Figure 17.66 have?

    **A.** Congenitally corrected great arteries

    **B.** D-TGA

    **C.** Ebstein's anomaly

    **D.** None of the above

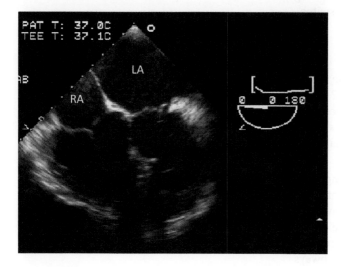

Figure 17.66

**17.67.** The TEE image in Figure 17.67a (LA: left atrium) is diagnostic of what?
  A. Congenitally corrected transposition of great arteries
  B. TGA, status post arterial switch
  C. Normal anatomy
  D. None of the above

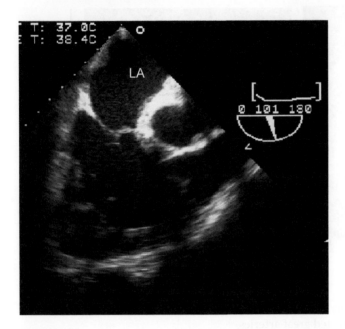

**Figure 17.67a**

**17.68.** The patient shown in Figure 17.68 (LA: left atrium; LV: left ventricle; MV: mitral valve; RA: right atrium; RV: right ventricle; TV: tricuspid valve) has what condition?
  A. D-TGA with atrial switch
  B. L-TGA
  C. Cor tiatriatum
  D. None of the above

**17.69.** What procedure is the patient in Figure 17.69 (LV: left ventricle; RV: right ventricle) likely to have had?
  A. Congenitally corrected TGA
  B. D-TGA with atrial switch
  C. D-TGA with arterial switch
  D. None of the above

**17.70.** Which of the following statements are true about the patient in Figure 17.70a? (LA: left atrium; LV: left ventricle; RA: right atrium; RV: right ventricle)
  A. The patient may have severe TR and heart failure
  B. The patient may be cyanotic
  C. The patient may present with atrial arrhythmias and reentrant arrhythmias due to accessory pathways
  D. All of the above

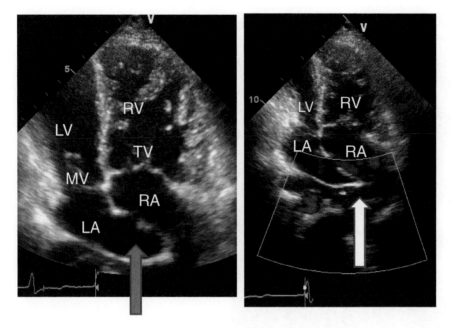

Figure 17.68

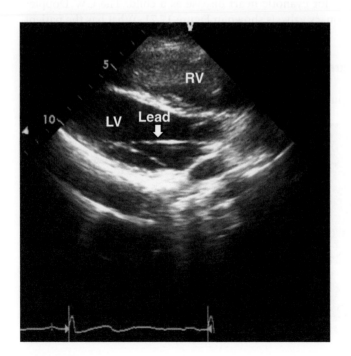

Figure 17.69

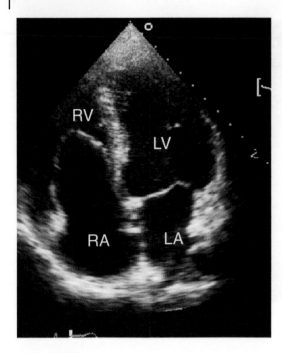

Figure 17.70a

17.71. A patient had surgery for cyanotic heart disease as a child. The CW Doppler signal from the pulmonary valve is shown in Figure 17.71. What has the patient most likely had?

A. TOF

B. Transposition of great vessels

C. Tricuspid atresia

D. Total anomalous pulmonary venous drainage

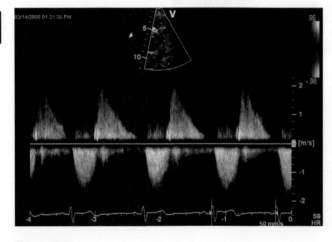

Figure 17.71

**17.72.** What is Figure 17.72 consistent with?
   **A.** Aortic coarctation
   **B.** Aortic interruption
   **C.** PDA
   **D.** A and B

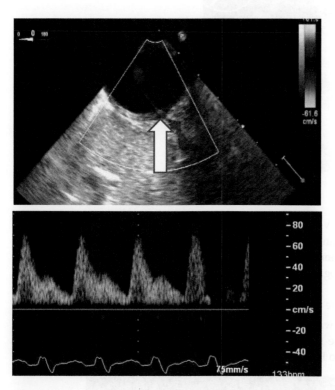

**Figure 17.72**

**17.73.** The TEE image in Figure 17.73 (Ao: aorta; LA: left atrium; LV: left ventricle) of the aortic annulus is suggestive of what?
   **A.** Normal aortic annulus
   **B.** Abscess
   **C.** Anomalous coronary artery with retroaortic course
   **D.** None of the above

**17.74.** A 30-year-old female undergoes an echocardiogram for evaluation of fatigue and dyspnea. ECG reveals normal sinus rhythm, incomplete right bundle branch block (IRBBB) with right axis deviation. Her blood pressure was measured at 118/70 mmHg, Echocardiogram shows 2 cm secundum atrial septal defect (ASD). Shunt is predominantly left to right. Both the right atrium and right ventricle are moderately dilated. Tricuspid jet velocity is 2.5 m/s and right atrial pressure is 5 mmHg. She undergoes a right heart catheterization which shows a

TEE T <37.0C

LA

Ao

0 125 1

LV

**Figure 17.73**

PASP of 31 mmHg, PVR 2 woods units. Calculated Qp : Qs was 2. What would be the best way to manage this patient?

**A.** Medical management with Bosentan

**B.** Repeat echocardiogram in six months to evaluate progression

**C.** Closure of ASD

**D.** Nothing to be done at this time

**17.75.** An 18-year-old male was being evaluated for symptoms of fatigue. Patient had an echocardiogram. The figure shows subcostal image. What condition does the patient have? Refer to Figure below.

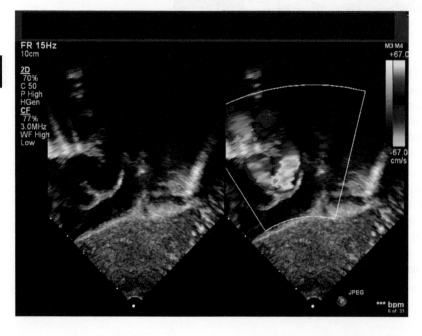

A. Ventricular septal defect
B. Atrial septal defect IVC type
C. Atrial septal defect, sinus venosus type
D. Patent ductus arteriosus

**17.76.** On further workup, the right ventricle was enlarged. Cardiac catheterization revealed normal pulmonary arterial pressures with a Qp : Qs of 2.4 : 1. What is the best way to manage this patient?
A. Percutaneous closure of the atrial septal defect
B. Nothing to do at this time
C. Surgical closure of the atrial septal defect
D. Medical management

**17.77.** A 22-year-old female patient presents to you to establish care. She gives you a history of repair for Tetralogy of Fallot when she was young. She has not followed up with a cardiologist for the previous five years. She complains of dyspnea on exertion with minimal activity. You perform an echocardiogram which is significant for normal left ventricular function, moderately dilated right ventricle with moderate hypokinesis. She is noted to have severe pulmonary regurgitation. Her ECG reveals right bundle branch block with rare premature ventricular beats. How would you classify her according to the new AP classification?
A. AIPA
B. AIIPA
C. AIIPC
D. AIIIPD

**17.78.** Endocarditis prophylaxis should be given to all patients with ACHD except?
A. Those with previous history of endocarditis
B. Patients with uncorrected cyanotic heart disease
C. Patients with prosthetic valves (surgical or transcatheter)
D. Patients within 12 months of placement of prosthetic material

**17.79.** Up to 5% of children born with congenital heart disease can be attributed to what syndrome?
A. Noonan syndrome
B. Down syndrome
C. Williams syndrome
D. DiGeorge syndrome

**17.80.** A 53-year-old patient comes to your office to establish care. He gives a history of Tetralogy of Fallot repair when he was five years of age. Which of the following should be part of his screening?
A. Hepatitis A
B. Hepatitis C
C. Hepatitis B
D. Hepatitis E

**17.81.** With regard to patients with congenital heart disease undergoing non cardiac surgery, all of these contribute to increased perioperative mortality and morbidity except:
A. Congestive heart failure
B. Older age of the patient
C. Cyanotic heart disease
D. Pulmonary hypertension

**17.82.** High maternal mortality and morbidity with pregnancy can be seen in all except:
A. Pulmonary hypertension
B. Severe systemic ventricular dysfunction, ejection fraction <30%, NYHA class III–IV symptoms
C. Secundum atrial septal defect with predominant left to right shunt
D. Severe aortic stenosis

**17.83.** Estrogen containing contraceptives are contraindicated in which of the following conditions?

**A.** Patient with Fontan repair
**B.** Mechanical aortic valve
**C.** Pulmonary hypertension
**D.** Cyanosis
**E.** All of the above

**17.84.** A 30-year-old female is referred to your clinic for evaluation of a murmur. She does not recall any past history but has symptoms of dyspnea on exertion. On examination, her heart rate was 80 /min, BP was 110/40 mmHg, oral mucosa was pink, with no chest wall deformities. Cardiac examination reveals a normal chest, both S1 and S2 were preserved, with a loud decrescendo diastolic murmur at the right second intercostal space. Lung examination was normal. ECG performed in the clinic showed normal sinus rhythm with no other abnormalities. Echocardiogram was performed in the clinic which showed mild dilatation of the left ventricle, with ejection fraction 60%. There was no mitral regurgitation. Aortic valve evaluation showed severe aortic regurgitation with prolapse of the right aortic cusp. Further evaluation also demonstrated a supracristal ventricular septal defect with a calculated Qp : Qs of 1.9 : 1. Cardiac catheterization did not reveal pulmonary hypertension and Qp : Q. The recommendations regarding management of this patient are:

**A.** Continued observation with another echocardiogram six months
**B.** Closure of supracristal VSD alone
**C.** Aortic valve repair
**D.** Closure of supracristal VSD and aortic valve repair or replacement

**17.85.** A 30-year-old male is referred to your clinic for a consult for evaluation of murmur. He gives a history of recent dyspnea on exertion. Examination reveals heart rate of 75/min, BP 129/76 mmHg, mildly elevated jugular venous pressure, systolic murmur at the second right intercostal space. He then undergoes an echocardiogram which reveals normal left ventricular size, severe concentric left ventricular hypertrophy with an ejection fraction of 60%. Mitral valve shows mild mitral and aortic regurgitation. What is the murmur due to? Please refer to the image below.

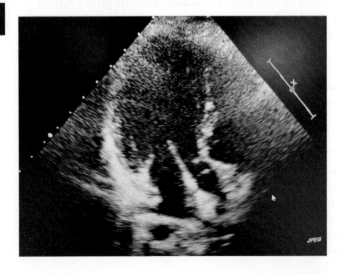

A. Mitral stenosis
B. Rheumatic aortic valve disease
C. Subaortic membrane
D. None of the above

**17.86.** Continuous wave Doppler in the patient in Question 17.85 is shown below. What is the next step?

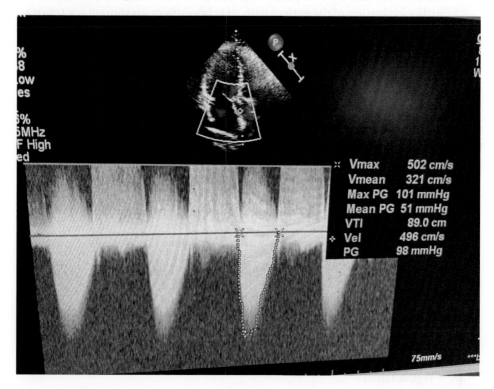

| | Vmax | 502 cm/s |
| --- | --- | --- |
| | Vmean | 321 cm/s |
| | Max PG | 101 mmHg |
| | Mean PG | 51 mmHg |
| | VTI | 89.0 cm |
| ÷ | Vel | 496 cm/s |
| | PG | 98 mmHg |

75mm/s

A. Observation
B. Repeat echocardiogram in six months
C. Surgical resection of the subaortic membrane
D. Low dobutamine stress echo

**17.87.** A 32-year-old male is referred to your clinic for evaluation of murmur. He gives a history of recent dyspnea on exertion. Examination reveals heart rate of 80/min, BP 121/70 mmHg, mildly elevated jugular venous pressure, systolic murmur at the second right intercostal space. He then undergoes an echocardiogram which reveals normal left ventricular size, severe concentric left ventricular hypertrophy with an ejection fraction of 45%. Aortic valve is trileaflet and opens well with no evidence of stenosis. Doppler evaluation shows flow acceleration below the aortic valve, Peak velocity is 3.7 m/s, Peak gradient of 55 mmHg. Careful evaluation then shows a discrete membrane just below the aortic valve. Mitral valve shows mild mitral and aortic regurgitation. What is the best management strategy in this patient?

A. Repeat echocardiogram in 3 months
B. Surgical resection of subaortic membrane
C. Medical management
D. Repeat echocardiogram in 6 months

**17.88.** A 22-year-old male is referred to your clinic with symptoms of dyspnea on exertion. One year ago, the patient was being evaluated for similar complaints. Further evaluation of the patient with an echocardiogram showed cor triatriatum sinister with a gradient of 10 mmHg. Patient was referred to surgery and had the membrane resected. Patient felt better soon after the surgery, but a few months later started noticing dyspnea. What would you suspect in this patient?

A. Recurrence of cor triatriatum
B. Pulmonary vein stenosis
C. Atrial septal defect
D. Mitral stenosis
E. None of the above

**17.89.** Which of the following is/are true in a patient with supravalvular aortic stenosis?

A. Commonly seen in Williams syndrome or homozygous familial hypercholesterolemia
B. Coronary imaging is recommended in patients with suspected ischemia
C. Impaired coronary perfusion can occur
D. Cardiac MRI or cardiac CT are superior to transthoracic echo in imaging supra valvular aortic stenosis
E. All of the above

**17.90.** Significant coarctation of aorta is defined as:

A. Upper extremity/lower extremity resting peak-to-peak gradient >20 mmHg or mean Doppler systolic gradient >20 mmHg
B. Upper extremity/lower extremity gradient >10 mmHg or mean Doppler gradient >10 mmHg in the presence of reduced left ventricular function or aortic regurgitation
C. Upper extremity/lower extremity gradient >10 mm Hg or mean Doppler gradient >10 mmHg in the presence of collateral flow
D. All of the above
E. None of the above

**17.91.** Which is true regarding coarctation of aorta?

A. About 2% have intracranial aneurysms
B. Patients with surgical patch repair are at high risk for aneurysm formation
C. About 25% will need reintervention
D. Bicuspid aortic valve is seen in 5% of patients

**17.92.** A 27-year-old male was referred for an echocardiogram. Based on the Figure 17.92 below, what does the patient have?

A. Trileaflet aortic valve
B. Bicuspid aortic valve
C. quadricuspid aortic valve
D. Unicuspid aortic valve

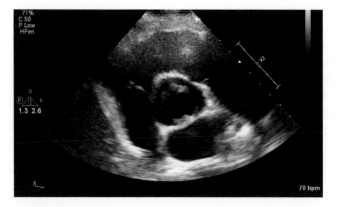

**Figure 17.92**

**17.93.** What does Figure 17.93 below show?

    **A.** Supravalvular mitral ring

    **B.** Cortriatriatum sinister

    **C.** Cortriatriatum dexter

    **D.** Left atrial cyst

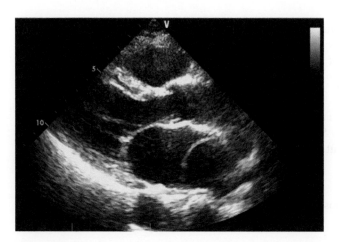

**Figure 17.93**

**Chapter 17**

**17.94.** A 27-year-old male is referred to your clinic with complains of chest pain. On further questioning, the patient complains of chest pain, characterized as a pressure-like feeling, exacerbated with exertion and relieved with rest. He does not have any significant past history or family history. On examination, vital signs are stable. Cardiac examination is within normal limits. He then undergoes an echocardiogram. His images are difficult. Since he was symptomatic, he undergoes coronary CT angiogram which shows anomalous origin of right coronary artery from the left coronary sinus. What is the next best step?

    **A.** Nothing to be done at this time

    **B.** Stress test

    **C.** Coronary angiogram

    **D.** Medical therapy

**17.95.** The patient in Question 17.94 had stress perfusion cardiac MRI, which did not reveal stress induced perfusion defects. He then underwent an event monitor which subsequently revealed several runs of non-sustained ventricular arrhythmia. What is the recommended best management strategy in this patient?
A. Continued observation
B. Coronary angiogram
C. Surgical intervention
D. Percutaneous intervention

## Answers

**17.1.** A. Pulmonary stenosis (PS) and atrial septal defect (ASD).

**17.2.** B. Supravalvular AS.
The second common associated defect is supravalvular PS.

**17.3.** A. VSD and arch anomalies.
The most common anomaly seen in DiGeorge syndrome is VSD, followed by arch anomalies. ASD and supravalvular AS are seen in this syndrome.

**17.4.** C. ASD.

**17.5.** A. Coarctation of aorta.
The most common congenital cardiac lesion associated with Turner syndrome (45X) is coarctation of aorta, followed by AS and then ASD.

**17.6.** C. 1–2%.

**17.7.** C. 50%.
Simple shunts, such as ASD, VSD, and PDA, are seen in about 50% of the congenital heart defects. Simple obstructions such as AS, PS, and coarctation of aorta are seen in about 20%, and complex lesions are seen in 30%.

**17.8.** D. All of the above.

**17.9.** D. All of the above.
In trisomy 13, most lesions seen are VSDs followed by PDAs and then dextrocardia.

**17.10.** D. AS.
AS does not form a part of syndromic lesions in trisomy 18. The most common lesion noted is VSD, followed by PDA, and then PS.

**17.11.** C. Left atrium and left ventricle.
A significant VSD will cause enlargement of the left atrium as well as the left ventricle. The blood goes across the shunt and is delivered to the lungs and then to the left atrium, which results in dilatation of this chamber.

**17.12.** B. Aortic regurgitation.
The most common associated finding seen in a supracristal VSD is aortic regurgitation, which occurs due to valve distortion.

**17.13.** B. 25 mmHg.
The left ventricle-right ventricle gradient across the VSD is $4 \times VSD^2$ that is, $4 \times 5 \times 5 = 100$ mmHg. The systolic BP is 125 mmHg. Right ventricular systolic pressure is then equivalent to 125–100 mmHg, which calculates to 25 mmHg.

**17.14.** D. No antibiotic prophylaxis is indicated at this time.

According to the new endocarditis prophylaxis guidelines, a simple shunt such as a VSD does not warrant endocarditis prophylaxis (Wilson et al., 2007).

**17.15.** C. PDA.

There is color flow in the PA and the accompanying Doppler shows continuous flow through systole and diastole, which is suggestive of a PDA.

**17.16.** C. Transesophageal echocardiogram (TEE).

The patient was referred for a murmur. The TTE is remarkable for dilatation of right-sided chambers. Though the TTE failed to show a shunt lesion, the TEE should be performed to look for sinus venosus ASD or partial anomalous pulmonary venous drainage that can be easily missed on a TTE. The cause of right-sided dilatation needs to be worked up further, and hence just reassuring the patient is not sufficient.

**17.17.** B. Partial anomalous pulmonary venous drainage.

Sinus venosus ASD is most commonly associated with partial anomalous venous return of the pulmonary veins. Usually, the right upper pulmonary vein drains anomalously into the right atrium.

**17.18.** D. Consultation with a CT surgeon.

This patient has a sinus venosus ASD associated with partial anomalous drainage of the right upper pulmonary vein and significant shunt as judged by right ventricle size. This person should be referred to a cardiothoracic surgeon for a complete repair. No need for coronary angiogram as the patient is young.

**17.19.** D. 75%.

Secundum ASDs are the most common form.

**17.20.** C. Left-axis deviation and cleft mitral leaflet.

A primum ASD is often associated with a left-axis deviation on the surface ECG. The most common associated anomaly seen on echocardiogram is a cleft of the anterior mitral leaflet. In this abnormality, the AV valves are at the same level and the left ventricular outflow tract is elongated and narrow, giving the characteristic "goose-neck" deformity. Primum ASDs constitute a partial AV canal defect.

**17.21.** B. Bicuspid aortic valve.

Bicuspid aortic valve is present in 50% of cases with coarctation of the aorta.

Chapter 1

**17.22.** B. Normal RV pressure.

The peak gradient across the PDA is 105 mmHg and systolic BP is 120 mmHg. Right ventricular systolic pressure is 130–105 which is 25 mmHg, which is in the normal range.

**17.23.** E. ASD.

TOF includes four components: VSD, RV hypertrophy, PS, and overriding of the aorta. ASD is not commonly seen in classic TOF, but when it is present it is called pentalogy of Fallot.

**17.24.** A. Anomalous origin of LAD artery from RCA.

Coronary artery anomalies are seen in 5% of TOF patients. The most common anomaly one should look out for is anomalous origin of the LAD artery from the

RCA. This has great clinical implication. When surgery is performed on the RV outflow tract (RVOT), if an anomalous coronary artery is not identified, the surgeon may inadvertently cut it, leading to catastrophe.

**17.25.** B. Severe pulmonary valve regurgitation.

Patients who have undergone repair of TOF, especially pulmonary valvotomy or removal of pulmonary valve, will go on to develop severe PR later on. When there is evidence of RV enlargement, severe PR should be sought out on echocardiogram. Owing to the severity of PR, color flow can be misleading, but continuous-wave Doppler can correctly help in identifying severe PR. When severe PR causes right-sided volume overload, pulmonary valve replacement is the treatment of choice.

**17.26.** C. Jatene arterial switch.

The procedure of choice to correct D-TGA is the Jatene arterial switch. The Senning and Mustard operations, which are atrial switch procedures, have largely been abandoned. The Rastelli procedure is usually done when there is associated pulmonary or subpulmonary stenosis, wherein a right ventricle-PA conduit is placed. This procedure may require conduit replacement and future operations.

**17.27.** B. Anterior and rightward.

Normally, the aorta is central and the PA wraps around it. In D-TGA, both the great arteries have a parallel course and the aorta is situated anterior and to the right of a centrally located PA.

**17.28.** B. Anterior and leftward.

Normally, the aorta is central and the PA wraps around it. In a levo-transposition, the great arteries have a parallel course. The aorta is anterior and to the left of a centrally located PA.

**17.29.** B. 30%.

Patients with L-TGA can have associated defects. One of them is rhythm abnormalities. The most common rhythm abnormality is complete heart block, which can be seen in 30% of the patients with L-TGA.

**17.30.** B. 90%.

Ebstein's anomaly of the systemic AV valve (morphologic tricuspid valve) can occur in up to 90% of patients with L-TGA. It is very important to recognize this anomaly as Ebstein's anomaly can result in severe valve regurgitation, which is less well tolerated and needs early aggressive intervention.

**17.31.** B. Subclavian artery to PA.

When a Gore-Tex™ interposition graft is used to anastomose the subclavian artery to the PA, it is called a modified Blalock-Taussig shunt. These two shunts are done to increase pulmonary blood flow in TOF patients. The ascending aorta to PA graft is called the central shunt. A descending aorta to left PA graft is called the Pott's shunt, while an ascending aorta to right PA graft is called a Waterston shunt. An SVC to right PA shunt is called a Glenn shunt, which is designed to provide flow to the PAs under lower pressure.

**17.32.** A. Closure of VSD and placement of a right ventricle-PA conduit. Usually, this is undertaken when there is a VSD and associated subpulmonic or pulmonic stenosis. Balloon atrial septostomy is called the Rashkind procedure.

**17.33.** F. All of the above.

The Fontan operation is used to repair all of the listed congenital heart defects. The goal of the Fontan operation is to separate systemic and pulmonary circulations and also to remove excess load on a single pumping chamber. In this operation, the systemic blood is directed to the lungs either by a modified Fontan-Kreutzer operation using the right atrium to direct blood to the PAs or by total cavo-pulmonary anastomosis, wherein the inferior vena cava (IVC) and SVC are joined directly through a tunnel in the right atrium to the PAs. There is no pumping chamber to the pulmonary circuit, and the single ventricle is then allowed to pump pulmonary venous blood to the body. The pulmonary flow is passive and depends upon venous pressure and will fail if there is an increase in pulmonary vascular resistance or left atrial pressure.

**17.34.** E. All of the above.

A right-sided aortic arch can be seen in 25% of cases with TOF and in about 40% of cases with pulmonary atresia.

**17.35.** D. Protein-losing enteropathy.

Patients with a history of Fontan surgery can present late in life with symptoms such as edema, ascites, and low albumin level, which is characteristic of protein losing enteropathy. This condition carries a high mortality when present.

**17.36.** D. All of the above.

All of the above are *class I indications* for surgical intervention in the face of anomalous coronary arteries.

**17.37.** D. In adults with a new presentation of a simple shunt or valve lesion and no hemodynamic compromise, evaluation by a general cardiologist in consultation with an ACHD cardiologist is reasonable.

Class IIa, level of evidence C. All the others are class I indications.

**17.38.** A. The prevalence of hypertension is higher especially with later repair.

All other statements are false (Webb 2005; Kenny and Hijazi 2011).

**17.39.** B. ACE inhibitors have been reported to precipitate acute renal failure in the setting of coarctation.

ACE inhibitors should be used with caution in patients with coarctation, especially if hemodynamically significant. This condition can mimic bilateral renal artery stenosis. ACE inhibitors have been known to precipitate acute renal failure because of already low flow to the renal arteries with significant coarctation (Woodmansey et al., 1994).

**17.40.** D. All of the above.

According to the current ACHD guidelines (Bhatt et al., 2015).

**17.41.** E. All of the above.

Association of accessory-pathway-mediated tachycardia is seen with Ebstein anomaly. Catheter ablation is curative in this setting, or intraoperative ablation can be performed when patients are undergoing surgery for valve repair/replacement. IART is the most common arrhythmia seen in older adults with coronary heart disease (CHD), which is a macroreentrant circuit within the atrial tissue that occurs due to patches, atriotomy incisions, and scars.

**Chapter 17**

Cavo-tricuspid-isthmus-dependent atrial flutter may be common, though unusual circuits are often present. Unlike the classic saw-tooth flutter waves occurring at 300 bpm, IART can be associated with varying P wave morphologies at 170–250 bpm, facilitating 1 : 1 conduction causing syncope, hypotension, and even death. Highest incidence of IART is seen post Mustard/Senning or Fontan procedure. Treatment could be elective electrical cardioversion after ruling out atrial thrombi with TEE and chronic AV nodal blockade. If accompanied by bradycardia, a pacemaker is helpful. VT is prototypically seen in patients with TOF. The classic presentation is a macroreentrant tachycardia seen as a late complication of ventriculotomy or VSD patch. These arrhythmias revolve around the RVOT. Most of the VTs are rapid, causing cardiac arrest. In older adults with repaired TOF, sudden cardiac death is the most common cause of late mortality, with an incidence of 2%/decade, reaching 10% by 35 years after surgery. Older age at the time of repair, advanced RV dilatation, presence of an RVOT patch, QRS interval ≥180 ms, and annual increase in QRS interval are independent risk factors for the development of VT.

**17.42.** E. All of the above.

A and B are class 1 indications, level of evidence C. Options C and D are class IIa, level of evidence B.

**17.43.** D. All of the above.

**17.44.** D. Renal dysfunction is not a poor prognostic marker in patients with ACHD.

Renal dysfunction is actually a marker of poor prognosis in patients with ACHD. Over six years, mortality risk was fivefold higher in those with moderate to severe renal impairment and twofold higher with mild impairment compared with those with normal function.

**17.45.** D. Sixty-four detector row or higher computed tomography angiography can be useful in lieu of invasive coronary angiography to exclude important coronary artery disease when the pretest probability is low to intermediate.

This is class IIa, level of evidence C. The first three options are class I recommendations, level of evidence C.

**17.46.** B. 22q11 deletion.

Screening for mutations should be offered to all patients with TOF, and all patients, especially those with a heritable mutation, should be offered genetic counseling before a planned pregnancy.

**17.47.** E. All of the above.

PR jet may be transient when severe and can be missed with color flow imaging. Continuous-wave (CW) signal may show rapid deceleration and equilibration of pressure in PA and right ventricle in mid-diastole.

**17.48.** C. Annual cardiac MRI for right ventricle volume and EF.

Even in asymptomatic individuals, moderate or severe right ventricle enlargement or dysfunction is an indication for repair. TTE is not reliable unless 3D echo is performed. Annual cardiac CT exposes the patient to lot of radiation as it has to be retrospectively gated for RV function analysis. In an asymptomatic patient with severe PR, any of the following two may constitute a reasonable indication for valve replacement: RV end-diastolic volume index EDVI >150 cm$^3$/m$^2$, RV end-systolic volume index >80 cm³/m², RV/LV end-diastolic volume index ratio >2, RVEF <47%, QRSd >140 ms, RVOT aneurysm, tachyarrhythmias.

**17.49.** E. All of the above.

For obvious reasons! TOF patients are also prone to ascending aortic aneurysms and need to be monitored for this.

**17.50.** E. All of the above.

Mechanical correlates of VT include PR and RV dilation; mechanical correlates of atrial arrhythmia include TR.

**17.51.** F. All of the above.

**17.52.** C. Baffle obstruction.

The presentation is typical for obstruction to the superior limb of the baffle. This is a lot more common than obstruction to the inferior limb. Constriction would cause hepatomegaly and ascites as well. A small subpulmonic left ventricle may be predisposed to SAM and dynamic outflow obstruction, but this patient does not have any murmurs to suggest this. In addition, the features are not suggestive of heart failure and more of SVC syndrome.

**17.53.** B. 25%.

**17.54.** D. All of the above.

The risk of paradoxical embolism is increased by atrial arrhythmias, endocardial pacer leads, and venous thrombosis.

**17.55.** G. All of the above.

Baffle leak is assessed with saline contrast echocardiography.

**17.56.** E. All of the above.

**17.57.** C. 50%.

**17.58.** D. All of the above.

**17.59.** D. All of the above.

**17.60.** B. Surgical repair.

The arrow in Figure 17.60 points to ostium primum ASD in the lower part of the septum. The patient has volume overload with normal PA pressure and has an indication for closure. This is not amenable to percutaneous closure, unlike a secundum ASD.

**17.61.** C. *Sinus* venosus ASD of IVC type.

In Figure 17.61, the blue arrow points to the defect and the white arrow to the Eustachian valve, and the IVC is to the left of that.

**17.62.** A. *Sinus* venosus ASD with anomalous drainage of right upper pulmonary vein.

The white arrow is pointing to the ASD and blue arrow to right upper pulmonary vein. This is not amenable to percutaneous closure either.

**17.63.** A. Closure of secundum ASD with Amplatzer device.

The arrow in Figure 17.63 points to the device. In the ASD device, the left disk is larger than the right, as in this case. In a PFO closure device, the right disk is larger.

**17.64.** A. Aortic coarctation.

Note that the systolic gradient is about 64 mmHg and there is a gradient throughout diastole. This is indicative of severe aortic coarctation.

**17.65.** A. PDA.

The color jet on the left panel coming from the arch-DTA junction into the PA is classic for PDA. Note that the flow is continuous, as shown on the CW Doppler signal on the right.

**17.66.** A. Congenitally corrected great arteries.

Note that the left AV valve is more apical, indicating that it is the tricuspid valve and the ventricle that goes with it is the right ventricle. Hence, the mitral valve and morphological LV are on the right side. There is AV discordance. This would, in addition, be associated with ventriculoarterial discordance (right ventricle to aorta and left ventricle to PA), with the two wrongs making a right, and the circulation would be normal except that the systemic ventricle is a morphologically right ventricle and systemic AV valve is a tricuspid valve. There is higher risk of TR and right ventricle (systemic ventricle) failure in these patients.

**17.67.** A. Congenitally corrected transposition of great arteries.

As shown in Figures 17.67b and 17.67c (AO: aorta; LA: left atrium; LV: left vent; RA: right atrium; RV: right ventricle), the left atrium is connected to the right ventricle and anterior aorta, and the right atrium is connected to the left ventricle and posterior PA. Also note a pacer lead in the right atrium.

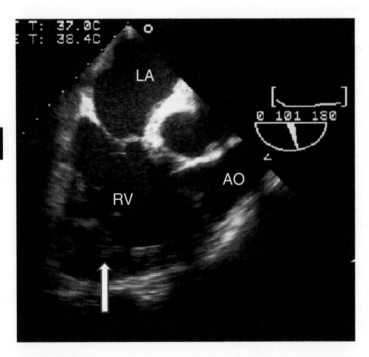

**Figure 17.67b**

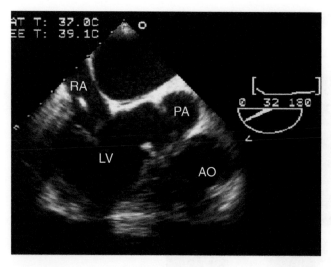

**Figure 17.67c**

**17.68.** A. D-TGA with atrial switch.

Note that the right atrium is connected to the right ventricle but gets pulmonary venous blood (white arrow in Figure 17.68) and left atrium is connected to smaller, smoother-walled left ventricle and receives vena caval blood (blue arrow in Figure 17.68). The nature's "wrong" is ventriculoarterial discordance; that is, right ventricle connected to aorta and left ventricle connected to PA. Atrial switch is "man-made wrong" and the two wrongs make one right. As the morphological right ventricle is the systemic ventricle, it is prone to dysfunction, and TR can occur as well.

**17.69.** B. D-TGA with atrial switch.

Note the pacer lead in the left ventricle (smooth walled), indicating that it pumps into the pulmonary circulation. This is indicative of atrial switch. In an arterial switch, the left ventricle would pump into the aorta. In L-TGA or congenitally corrected TGA, the posterior ventricle would be a morphological right ventricle, which pumps into the aorta.

**17.70.** D. All of the above.

This patient has Ebstein's anomaly with apical displacement of septal tricuspid leaflet and large sail-like anterior leaflet (arrow in Figure 17.70b). About 25% have accessory pathways, mostly right, and 50% have PFO or ASD, facilitating right-to-left shunting. See Figure 17.70b (LA: left atrium; LV: left ventricle; RA: right atrium; RV: right ventricle; RVa: atrialized right ventricle; TV: tricuspid valve). Note that a large portion of right ventricle is atrialized (RVa).

**17.71.** A. TOF.

Figure 17.71 shows severe PR, which is an important sequela of TOF repair.

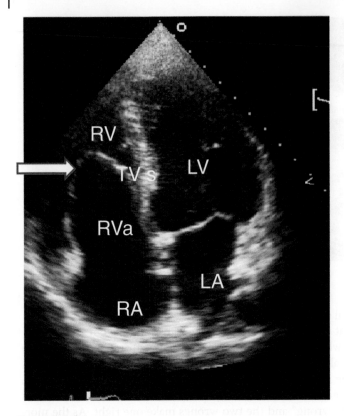

**Figure 17.70b**

**17.72.** D. A and B.

Note the retrograde flow (arrow in Figure 17.72) into descending thoracic aorta from intercostal arteries suggestive of collateral dependent flow in distal thoracic aorta. This is suggestive of severe aortic coarctation or aortic interruption. This patient had the latter.

**17.73.** C. Anomalous coronary artery with retroaortic course.

The arrow in Figure 17.73 points to a rounded structure. This was anomalous circumflex originating from the RCA with retroaortic course discovered incidentally during a TEE for suspected endocarditis.

**17.74.** C. This patient is symptomatic and has significant ASD with a Qp : Qs of 2. Her PASP is 31 mmHg and PVR is not elevated. She already has evidence of right-sided chamber enlargement. Hence, she would warrant closure of the secundum ASD either surgical or catheter based. According to the 2018 ACHD guidelines, please refer to the flow chart for appropriate management of symptomatic secundum ASD:

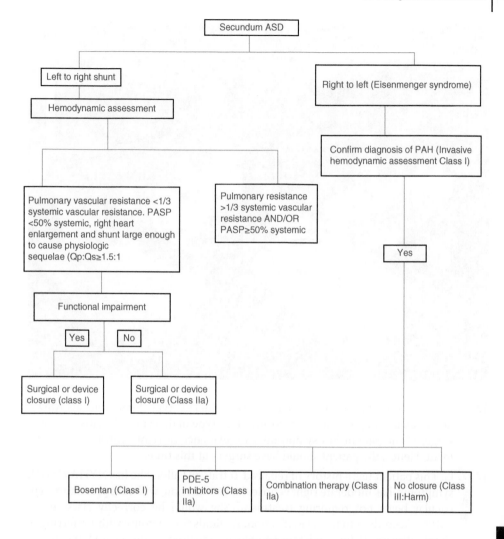

Patients who are left untreated with an ASD have been shown to have worse outcomes, including reduced functional capacity, being prone to atrial arrhythmias, and pulmonary hypertension. In patients with no impairment in functional capacity, the long-term benefit of ASD closure is less clear. Till further data is available, it is deemed reasonable to close a hemodynamically significant ASD without pulmonary arterial hypertension (Stout et al. 2018).

**17.75.** Atrial septal defect, IVC type. The image subcostal view. The left atrium is not seen well. The atrial septum is well depicted with a defect near the IVC. The color flow Doppler shows a shunt flow from left to right. (Blue arrow).

Chapter 1

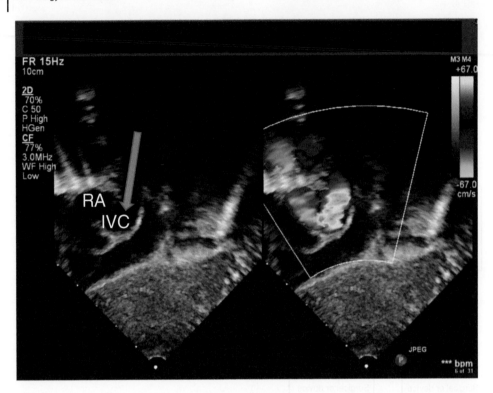

**17.76.** C. The patient has a sinus venosus ASD of the IVC type. Sinus venosus ASD is not amenable to percutaneous closure. This type of defect can be closed only by surgery. The patient has symptoms with evidence of right ventricular enlargement. Hence, the patient should have surgery at this time.

**17.77.** C. This patient has a history of repaired Tetralogy Fallot. She has NYHA class III symptoms, has moderate right ventricular dysfunction, with rare premature ventricular beats not requiring treatment. She would be correctly classified as AIIPC. According to this classification, A stands for anatomy with I referring to simple disease, II for moderate complexity repaired or unrepaired and III for complex congenital heart disease. Similarly P stands for Physiology with I relating to mild symptoms, no hemodynamic or anatomic sequelae, no arrhythmia, normal exercise capacity, B-mild symptoms, mild hemodynamic sequelae, mild valve disease, arrythmia not requiring treatment, C-NYHA class III symptoms, moderate or greater valve disease, moderate aortic enlargement, moderate or greater ventricular dysfunction, less than severe pulmonary dysfunction, end-organ dysfunction responsive to therapy, D-NYHA class IV symptoms, severe aortic enlargement, arrhythmias refractory to therapy, Eisenmenger syndrome, refractory end-organ dysfunction. Please refer to the ACHDAP classification table (Stout et al. 2018).

**17.78.** D. The current Infectious endocarditis guidelines recommend endocarditis prophylaxis in the following.
- Patients with a history of previous endocarditis
- Patients with prosthetic valves (biological, mechanical surgical, and transcatheter)
- Patients within six months of placement of prosthetic material
- Patients with residual shunts at the site of or adjacent to previous repair with prosthetic materials or devices
- Patients with uncorrected cyanotic heart disease

**17.79.** D. DiGeorge syndrome affects up to 5% of children born with congenital heart disease. It is autosomal dominant, associated with 22q11.2 deletion. Most common defects in this syndrome are conotruncal anomalies. Genetic testing for 22q11.2 deletion is reasonable in patients with conotruncal anomalies to evaluate for and manage comorbid conditions and risk of recurrence in offspring.

**17.80.** B. Patients with congenital heart disease are at very high risk for contracting hepatitis C due to exposure to blood during surgery. This is especially true for patients undergoing surgery prior to 1992 before universal screening for Hepatitis C was set. Our patient who is 53 years old had surgery when he was 5 years old, which puts his surgery prior to 1992. Hence, he should be screened for Hepatitis C.

**17.81.** B. Factors that lead to increased perioperative morbidity and mortality include: heart failure, cyanosis, pulmonary hypertension, poor general health, urgent or emergent procedures, respiratory or nervous system surgeries, complex congenital heart disease and younger age of the patient.

**17.82.** C. Patients with high risk for maternal mortality and severe morbidity include patients with severe systemic ventricular dysfunction, EF <30% or NYHA class III–IV symptoms, pulmonary hypertension, severe left-heart obstruction such as severe valve stenosis, severe native coarctation. If patients with any of the above become pregnant, option of termination of pregnancy should be discussed. Secundum atrial septal defect is not associated with maternal mortality or severe morbidity.

**17.83.** Prior thrombotic events, Fontan correction, pulmonary hypertension, mechanical valves, cyanosis are associated with high risk for thrombosis. Estrogen containing contraceptives are harmful in patients with the above listed conditions.

**17.84.** D. This patient has evidence of a significant supracristal VSD with a Qp : Qs of 1.9 : 1. Her echocardiogram and cardiac catheterization did not reveal evidence of pulmonary hypertension. She has evidence of severe aortic regurgitation due to prolapsing right coronary cusp. Both the VSD and aortic regurgitation should be addressed at the time of surgery. Please refer to the table below. (Stout et al. 2018).

Chapter 17

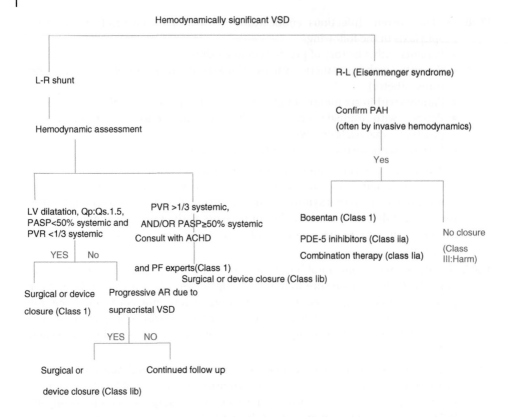

Hemodynamically significant VSD

L-R shunt

R-L (Eisenmenger syndrome)

Confirm PAH
(often by invasive hemodynamics)

Hemodynamic assessment

Yes

LV dilatation, Qp:Qs.1.5,
PASP<50% systemic and
PVR <1/3 systemic

PVR >1/3 systemic,
AND/OR PASP≥50% systemic
Consult with ACHD

Bosentan (Class 1)

No closure

PDE-5 inihibitors (Class IIa)

Combination therapy (class IIa)

(Class
III:Harm)

YES | No

and PF experts(Class 1)
Surgical or device closure (Class IIb)

Surgical or device
closure (Class 1)

Progressive AR due to
supracristal VSD

YES | NO

Surgical or
device closure (Class IIb)

Continued follow up

**17.85.** C. The echo cardiogram shows a subaortic membrane. The arrow in the image points to a structure below the aortic valve which is a subaortic membrane.

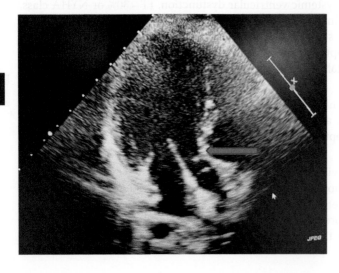

**17.86.** C. This patient has severe subaortic stenosis. This patient needs to undergo surgery to resect the membrane.

**17.87.** B. In patients with subaortic stenosis due to a membrane, surgical resection is recommended (class1 C-LD) when gradient is <50 mmHg, in the presence of heart failure, ischemic symptoms or left ventricular dysfunction. Patients with reduced left ventricular function and severe sub-aortic stenosis, may not manifest a gradient of ≥50 mmHg. In this subset of patients, decisions to cause relief of sub-aortic stenosis may be extrapolated form aortic stenosis data. In some patients with preserved systolic left ventricular function, compliance may be poor and result in heart failure symptoms and a resting maximum gradient of <50 mm. Surgical resection in these patients may be beneficial. Patients with resting or stress induced ischemia in the absence of obstructive coronary artery disease but with moderate sub-aortic stenosis (maximum gradient >30 and <50 mmHg) may benefit from surgical resection. This patient has left ventricular dysfunction with maximum sub-aortic gradient of 40 mmHg. Surgical resection of the membrane will be beneficial.

**17.88.** B. In patients who undergo surgery for cor triatriatum and with recurrence of symptoms, pulmonary vein stenosis can occur after surgery. Such patients should undergo evaluation for pulmonary vein stenosis. Pulmonary vein stenosis does not progress over time and has not been associated with pulmonary arterial hypertension.

**17.89.** E. Supra valvular aortic stenosis can be seen in Willaims syndrome or homozygous familial hypercholesterolemia. Transthoracic echo can be limited in assessment of supra-aortic stenosis. Cardiac MRI and CT are superior in imaging the narrowed part of the aorta. Unlike sub valvular or valvular aortic stenosis, coronary arteries are exposed to higher pressures generated by the supra valvular aortic stenosis. Surgical repair s recommended when symptoms occur or when left ventricular function is reduced secondary to the narrowing. Coronary perfusion can be impaired due to aortic valve leaflet adhesion to the narrowed segment or fibrotic thickening in the coronary ostia. Surgical revascularization is recommended in patients with coronary ischemia.

**17.90.** D.

**17.91.** B. Intracranial aneurysms are seen in about 10% of patients with coarctation. Eleven percent may need reintervention. Bicuspid aortic valve is seen in 50–70% of patients with coarctation. Patients with a history of surgical patch repair are at high risk for aneurysm formation.

**17.92.** D. The figure shows echocardiographic image of the aortic valve in short axis. It shows a single cusp with a circular opening. This is indicative of unicuspid aortic valve.

**17.93.** B. Cor triatriatum sinister.

Chapter 1

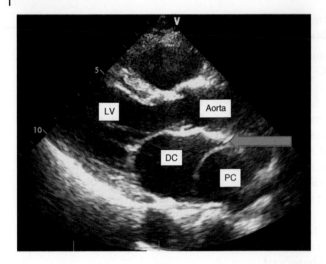

Blue arrow points to a membrane dividing the left atrium into a proximal chamber containing the pulmonary veins and a more distal chamber connected to the mitral valve.

**17.94.** B. Stress test in patients with anomalous coronary artery origin. Stress testing should be performed to elicit ischemia, which will dictate further management. Please see flow chart below (2018 ACHD guidelines).

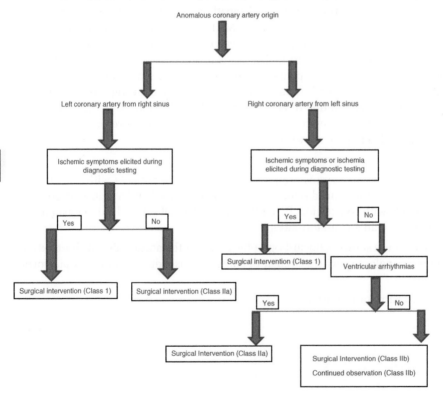

**17.95.** C. Surgical intervention. This patient has anomalous RCA origin. Stress testing did not show perfusion defects. As he is symptomatic, event monitoring was performed which revealed ventricular arrhythmias. This warrants surgical intervention (Class IIb) recommendation. Please refer to the flow chart in Answer 17.94.

## References

Bhatt, A.B., Foster, E., Kuehl, K. et al. (2015). Congenital heart disease in the older adult: a scientific statement from the American Heart Association. *Circulation* 131: 1884–1931.

Kenny, D. and Hijazi, Z.M. (2011). Coarctation of the aorta: from fetal life to adulthood. *Cardiology Journal* 18: 487–495.

Stout, Stout, K.K., Daniels, C.J., and Aboulhosn, J.A. (2018). AHA/ACC Guideline for the Management of Adults With Congenital Heart Disease: A Report of the American College of Cardiology/American Heart Association Task Force on Clinical Practice Guidelines. *Circulation* 2019: e698–e800.

Webb, G. (2005). Treatment of coarctation and late complications in the adult. *Seminars in Thoracic and Cardiovascular Surgery* 17: 139–142.

Wilson, W., Taubert, K.A., Gewitz, M. et al. (2007). Prevention of infective endocarditis. Guidelines from the American Heart Association: a guideline from the American Heart Association Rheumatic Fever, Endocarditis, and Kawasaki Disease Committee, Council on Cardiovascular Disease in the Young, and the Council on Clinical Cardiology, Council on Cardiovascular Surgery and Anesthesia, and the Quality of Care and Outcomes Research Interdisciplinary Working Group. *Circulation* 116: 1736–1754.

Woodmansey, P.A., Yeo, W.W., Jackson, P.R., and Ramsay, L.E. (1994). Acute renal failure with ACE inhibitors in aortic coarctation. *Postgraduate Medical Journal* 70: 927–929.

# Pericardial Diseases

# 18

**18.1.** What is the normal amount of pericardial fluid?

A. 0

B. 20–50 cm³

C. 50–100 cm³

D. 100–200 cm³

**18.2.** Which of the following statements about pericardial anatomy is incorrect?

A. Visceral layer is thin and has a single layer of mesothelial cells adherent to epicardial fat and reflected at the base onto the parietal pericardium

B. The parietal pericardium is tough and fibrous; it is flask-shaped and has attachments to the sternum and diaphragm

C. The visceral and parietal layers are adherent to each other

D. There are two pericardial sinuses

E. The parietal pericardium is continuous with adventitia of great vessels

**18.3.** Which of the following statements about pericardial sinuses are correct?

A. The transverse sinus is between the ascending aorta and pulmonary trunk anteriorly and superior vena cava posteriorly

B. The oblique sinus is posterior to the left atrium and lies between the left and right pulmonary veins

C. Both A and B are correct

D. Neither A nor B are correct

**18.4.** What is the normal intrapericardial pressure?

A. $0 \pm 3$ mmHg

B. $5 \pm 3$ mmHg

C. $10 \pm 3$ mmHg

D. $15 \pm 3$ mmHg

**18.5.** A 24-year-old man presents with a 5-day history of low-grade fever, malaise, cough and recent chest pain. He has a triphasic pericardial rub and concave-up ST elevation in most of the electrocardiogram (ECG) leads. Erythrocyte sedimentation rate (ESR) is 96 mm at the end of first hour, and complete blood count is normal. Serum troponin I level is 15 times the normal. What is the most likely cause of his pericarditis?

A. Idiopathic

B. Viral

C. Bacterial

D. Tubercular

**18.6.** What is the most common type of pericardial rub in acute pericarditis?

A. Triphasic

B. Biphasic

C. Monophasic

D. Quadriphasic

**18.7.** Some of the characteristics of pericardial rub include which of the following?

A. Scratchy or grating superficial sound that is heard close to the ears; best heard with diaphragm with pressure

*Cardiology Board Review*, Second Edition. Ramdas G. Pai and Padmini Varadarajan.
© 2023 John Wiley & Sons Ltd. Published 2023 by John Wiley & Sons Ltd.

    B. Best heard sitting up, leaning forward, in expiration

    C. May vary with position and heartbeats

    D. All of the above

    E. None of the above

**18.8.** What is the most common etiology of acute pericarditis?

    A. Idiopathic                         C. Bacterial

    B. Viral                               D. Autoimmune

**18.9.** Some of the acute ECG changes during acute pericarditis include which of the following?

    A. Concave-up ST elevation with upright T in most of the leads; ST depression in aortic valve replacement (aVR)

    B. PR segment depression in most of the leads

    C. PR segment elevation in aVR

    D. All of the above

**18.10.** Acute pericarditis can be differentiated from early repolarization by which of the following features?

    A. Progressive changes over days

    B. PR segment depression

    C. ST segment/T wave height ratio of $>0.25$

    D. All of the above

**18.11.** A 52-year-old man underwent successful left anterior descending artery stent placement for acute anterior ST-elevation myocardial infarction (MI). The next day, he complains of left-sided severe chest pain on inspiration and you hear a triphasic, grating sound at the low left sternal border. What is the explanation likely to be?

    A. Focal pericarditis due to transmural MI

    B. Dressler's syndrome

    C. Ventricular septal rupture

    D. Left anterior descending artery perforation

**18.12.** Which of the following would you suggest for the patient in Question 18.11?

    A. Increase the dose of aspirin         C. Start corticosteroid

    B. Start indomethacin               D. Start heparin

**18.13.** Three weeks after mitral valve repair, a 56-year-old patient presents with features of pericarditis, fever, and a normal complete blood count. He is on aspirin 81 mg/ day and warfarin for postoperative atrial fibrillation along with low-dose amiodarone. He is in sinus rhythm. What would you recommend?

    A. Start corticosteroids

    B. Stop warfarin and increase the dose of aspirin to 3 g/day with food, in divided doses for two weeks

    C. Start colchicine

    D. No change in treatment

**18.14.** A 30-year-old man with no other issues is admitted with a second episode of acute pericarditis in 2 months. The first episode was treated with a 10-day course of the nonsteroidal anti-inflammatory drug (NSAID) ibuprofen, 400 mg TID. His autoantibodies were negative. What is your recommendation?

Chapter 1

A. Start high-dose NSAID along with colchicine 0.6 mg BID

B. Start indomethacin because of ibuprofen failure

C. Start high-dose steroid with rapid taper

D. Start high-dose steroid with slow taper and low-dose maintenance for 36 months

18.15. In a patient with suspected tubercular pericarditis, which test is likely to give the highest diagnostic yield?

A. Acid-fast bacilli culture of pericardial fluid

B. Tuberculin test

C. Pericardial biopsy

D. Adenosine deaminase elevation in pericardial fluid

18.16. On pericardial biopsy, caseating granulomas are seen. What is the likely cause of pericarditis?

A. Tuberculosis

B. Sarcoid

C. Rheumatoid

D. Fungal

18.17. Which of these drugs can potentially result in pericarditis?

A. Hydralazine

B. Methyldopa

C. Penicillin

D. Sodium cromoglycate

E. All of the above

F. None of the above

18.18. What is the most common cause of malignant pericardial effusion with tamponade?

A. Lung cancer

B. Breast cancer

C. Lymphoma

D. Renal cancer

18.19. Indications for pericardiocentesis in a patient with pericarditis include which of the following?

A. Tamponade

B. Suspicion of pyogenic cause

C. Nonresolving, large effusion despite treatment

D. All of the above

18.20. What is the best approach for pericardiocentesis?

A. Subxiphoid with ECG monitoring of a lead connected to the needle

B. Echo guided

C. Magnetic resonance imaging (MRI) guided

D. Surgical

18.21. What is the normal pericardial thickness?

A. <3 mm on echo

B. <2 mm on computed tomography (CT)

C. <4 mm on MRI

D. All of the above

18.22. A 67-year-old patient presents with dyspnea and abdominal swelling. He had coronary artery bypass grafting procedure five years earlier. The physical examination reveals raised jugular venous pressure with Kussmaul's sign and ascites. The echocardiogram shows normal LV wall motion, ejection fraction of 60%, septal bounce, a severely dilated inferior vena cava, E/A ratio of 1.3, E/e' ratio of 10, septal e' velocity of 15 cm/s and lateral e' of 12 cm/s. Pericardium looked

normal. A gated contrast CT scan was performed and the pericardial thickness was <2 mm with no pericardial thickness. Grafts are patent, and invasive hemodynamics was inconclusive. What will you do?
- A. Treat for restrictive cardiomyopathy with diuretics
- B. Perform cardiac MRI
- C. Refer the patient for pericardiectomy
- D. None of the above

18.23. What are the indications for corticosteroids in pericarditis?
- A. Unresponsive to NSAID and colchicine
- B. Autoimmune etiology
- C. Recurrence despite colchicine
- D. All of the above
- E. None of the above

18.24. Pericardial calcification is best detected by which of the following?
- A. Fluoroscopy
- B. CT scan
- C. MRI
- D. Echocardiography

18.25. With which of the following is the risk of constriction the highest?
- A. Idiopathic pericarditis
- B. Tubercular pericarditis
- C. Uremic pericarditis
- D. Malignant pericarditis

18.26. Indications for pericardiectomy in pericarditis include which of the following?
- A. Multiple recurrences despite chronic NSAID and colchicine
- B. Steroid dependence
- C. Constriction
- D. Effusive-constrictive
- E. All of the above

18.27. Prednisone may be helpful to reduce the risk of constriction in which of the following etiologies of pericarditis, in addition to specific antimicrobial therapy?
- A. Tubercular
- B. Purulent
- C. Fungal
- D. All of the above

18.28. In a patient with malignant pericardial effusion, which of the following options may reduce recurrence?
- A. Intrapericardial tetracycline as a sclerosing agent
- B. Intrapericardial chemotherapy
- C. Pericardial window
- D. All of the above

18.29. A patient with end-stage renal disease (ESRD) on hemodialysis has moderate pericardial effusion. What is your recommendation?
- A. Intensify dialysis
- B. Switch to peritoneal dialysis
- C. Start NSAID
- D. Perform pericardiocentesis

18.30. The cause of pericardial effusion in ESRD patients on dialysis includes which of the following?
- A. Uremic pericarditis
- B. Volume excess
- C. Minoxidil
- D. Hydralazine
- E. All of the above

Chapter 18

18.31. Poor prognostic markers in pericarditis include which of the following?
   A. Fever >38 °C
   B. Subacute onset
   C. Large pericardial effusion or cardiac tamponade
   D. Lack of response to aspirin or NSAIDs after at least one week of therapy
   E. All of the above
   F. None of the above

18.32. A 27-year-old man with no cardiac symptoms was found to have heart entirely in left chest in left lateral decubitus X-ray and entirely on the right in right lateral decubitus X-ray. What is the patient likely to have?
   A. Mesocardia
   B. Dextrocardia
   C. Congenital absence of the pericardium
   D. It is normal

18.33. Which of the following has a higher risk of complications?
   A. Total absence of pericardium          C. They are similar
   B. Partial absence of pericardium         D. Both are benign

18.34. Which type of pericardial defect is least common?
   A. Partial left          C. Total
   B. Partial right         D. All are equally common

18.35. Some variants of constriction include which of the following?
   A. Annular variety with mitral stenosis
   B. Annular variety with tricuspid stenosis
   C. Pulmonary outflow stenosis
   D. All of the above
   E. None of the above

18.36. A 54-year-old asymptomatic man was found to have "fluid" around his right atrium on an echocardiogram. Images were difficult, and cardiac MRI was obtained. A FIESTA freeze frame is shown in Figure 18.36. What will you do next?

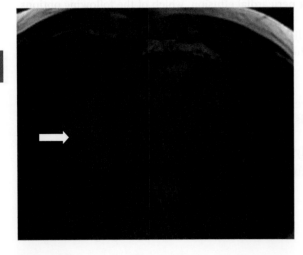

Figure 18.36

A. Reassure, do nothing, monitor for any symptoms
B. CT-guided needle aspiration
C. Surgical resection
D. Positron emission tomography (PET) scan

18.37. A 60-year-old man with systolic heart failure and atrial fibrillation presented with shortness of breath. He was on carvedilol, benazepril, amiodarone, and furosemide. Heart rate was 110 bpm. Blood pressure was 85/60 mmHg and jugular venous pressure was severely elevated. A CT scan image is shown in Figure 18.37. What will you do next?

A. Pericardiocentesis
B. Intravenous fluids
C. Intravenous diuresis
D. Refer to cardiothoracic surgery

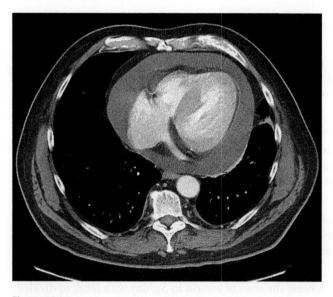

Figure 18.37

## Answers

18.1. B. 20–50 cm³.
It is an ultrafiltrate, acting as a lubricant. Accumulation of >100–150 cm³ may increase the pericardial pressure, depending upon the rapidity of accumulation.

18.2. C. The visceral and parietal layers are adherent to each other.
The visceral and parietal layers are not adherent to each other. The pericardial fluid lubricates the opposing surfaces such that the layers slide on each other. The other statements are correct.

18.3. C. Both A and B are correct.

18.4. A. 0 ± 3 mmHg.
It is atmospheric or the same as intrapleural pressure, being negative during inspiration and slightly positive during expiration.

**18.5.** B. Viral.

This is in view of substantial subepicardial myocardial involvement (ECG changes and positive troponin) which generally does not occur with idiopathic causes. Absence of high-grade fever with leukocytosis and a short history mitigate against choices C and D respectively.

**18.6.** A. Triphasic.

In 50–60% of cases when it is heard; the three phases are due to atrial systole, ventricular systole, and early left ventricular (LV) filling, and hence are presystolic, systolic, and early diastolic. Monophasic would be systolic and may be mistaken for a systolic murmur.

**18.7.** D. All of the above.

**18.8.** A. Idiopathic.

An etiology may not be discoverable in 60–80% of patients.

**18.9.** D. All of the above.

Changes in aVR are reciprocal to changes in all other leads. The ECG changes are progressive and progress to ST segment normalization with T wave flattening (stage 2), T wave inversion (stage 3, and normalization of ECG (stage 4).

**18.10.** D. All of the above.

These are features of pericarditis.

**18.11.** A. Focal pericarditis due to transmural MI.

This occurs in about 50% of ST-elevation MIs, though getting less frequent with acute revascularization therapies. Dressler's syndrome takes two to three weeks to develop.

**18.12.** A. Increase the dose of aspirin.

For both pain control and anti-inflammatory properties. Indomethacin and corticosteroids may increase the risk of LV rupture. Heparin may cause hemorrhagic pericarditis.

**18.13.** B. Stop warfarin and increase the dose of aspirin to 3 g/day with food, in divided doses for two weeks.

Anticoagulation may make the pericarditis hemorrhagic – as he is in sinus rhythm and has no mechanical valves, the risk of embolic event is rather low.

**18.14.** A. Start high-dose NSAID along with colchicine 0.6 mg BID.

Colchicine continued for six months may reduce pericarditis recurrence by 50% (Colchicine for Recurrent Pericarditis [CORP] trial – see Box 18.1). Use of steroids may increase the recurrence rates. No substantial difference in acute response to any of the NSAIDs used in high dose, though indomethacin is a classic time-honored drug; use of high dose of NSAID is important.

**18.15.** C. Pericardial biopsy.

The yield is nearly 100%. Yields with acid-fast bacilli cultures and adenosine deaminase test are about 50 and 80%, respectively. Tuberculin test could be either false positive or false negative.

**18.16.** A. Tuberculosis.

Caseation is typical of tuberculosis. The other options listed can result in granulomas.

**18.17.** E. All of the above.

Options A and B through systemic lupus erythematosus (SLE4) syndrome (also isoniazid), and options C and D through hypersensitivity reaction.

**18.18.** A. Lung cancer.

Followed by breast cancer and lymphoma.

**18.19.** D. All of the above.

**18.20.** B. Echo guided.

This is easy to perform, is bedside, and has the lowest risk. Most often, an apical window is suitable. Echo helps to choose the window, guide the needle, confirm its location in pericardium, and completeness of drainage. A sterile sleeve should be used on the echo probe.

**18.21.** D. All of the above.

These are approximate.

**18.22.** C. Refer the patient for pericardiectomy.

Given the clinical and echo features, the probability that he has constriction is >90% and no negative test can reduce it to zero. Hence, surgical exploration is appropriate. A higher septal e' compared with lateral e is called annulus paradoxus, which is reported in constriction and is attributed to tethered LV lateral wall by pericardium with compensatory increased medial annular motion in early diastole. An e' of >8 cm/s goes against a primary myocardial restrictive process. In about 25% of patients with constriction following heart surgery, pericardium has normal thickness.

**18.23.** D. All of the above.

**18.24.** B. CT scan.

This is the most sensitive. Calcium is not imaged or seen by MRI.

**18.25.** B. Tubercular pericarditis.

This is >50%. With viral or idiopathic pericarditis it is <1%. In malignancy, the risk is low because of short life span, though the effusion may be hemorrhagic.

**18.26.** E. All of the above.

**18.27.** D. All of the above.

**18.28.** D. All of the above.

**18.29.** A. Intensify dialysis.

This is likely to be uremic pericarditis. This should cause its resolution in 10–14 days. Both hemodialysis and peritoneal dialysis are equally efficacious. Peritoneal dialysis is not needed unless patient's blood pressure drops during hemodialysis.

**18.30.** E. All of the above.

These have to be kept in mind in an ESRD patient having pericardial effusion.

**18.31.** E. All of the above.

See Imazio et al. (2007).

**18.32.** C. Congenital absence of the pericardium.

Chapter 18

This is a typical presentation. It is mostly asymptomatic and benign, but excess mobility of the heart may predispose to cardiac contusion and aortic dissection with trauma. On a supine chest X-ray, the apex will be pointing posteriorly.

18.33. B. Partial absence of pericardium.

This is because of herniation of the heart through these defects, resulting in strangulation. Symptoms may include chest pain, shortness of breath, syncope, or sudden death. Surgical pericardioplasty with Dacron, Gore-Tex, or bovine pericardium is indicated in these situations.

18.34. C. Total.

Partial left-sided defect is the most common.

18.35. D. All of the above.

The other variants include left ventricle variety affecting mostly the left side, right ventricle variety, global variety, global variety with severe ventricular atrophy (where pericardiectomy is futile and contraindicated), and tubular variety, where both ventricles look like a tube because of constriction from both sides.

18.36. A. Reassure, do nothing, monitor for any symptoms.

Nothing to do as there are no symptoms. This is a typical pericardial cyst, which generally occurs at the right cardiophrenic angle. They have low intensity on T1W imaging and high intensity on T2W imaging. They do not enhance on perfusion imaging. When large or symptomatic, resection or percutaneous drainage is appropriate; recurrence rate with drainage is about 30%.

18.37. A. Pericardiocentesis.

Note the large pericardial effusion. The patient had tamponade, and $1200\,cm^3$ of fluid was drained with prompt relief of symptoms. The fluid was turbid with high protein content. The thyroid stimulating hormone was 80 mU, suggestive of severe amiodarone-induced hypothyroidism, which likely caused the effusion. The high Hounsfield unit of pericardial fluid was due to high protein content.

---

**Box 18.1   CORP Trial**

In the CORP trial (Imazio et al. 2011), 120 patients with a second episode of acute pericarditis were randomized to receive colchicine for six months versus placebo. There was about 50% reduction in risk of recurrent pericarditis.

---

# References

Imazio, M., Cecchi, E., Demichelis, B. et al. (2007). Indicators of poor prognosis of acute pericarditis. *Circulation* 115: 2739–2744.

Imazio, M., Brucato, A., Cemin, R. et al. (2011). Colchicine for recurrent pericarditis (CORP): a randomized trial. *Annals of Internal Medicine* 155: 409–414.

## Further Reading

An excellent reference resource for guiding management of all pericardial diseases is: Maisch, B., Seferovic, P.M., Ristic, A.D. et al. (2004). Guidelines on the diagnosis and management of pericardial diseases. Executive summary. The task force on the diagnosis and management of pericardial diseases of the European Society of Cardiology. *European Heart Journal* 25: 587–610.

# Aortic Diseases

**19**

**19.1.** A 50-year-old male with a history of a heart murmur for most of his adult life sees you in the clinic with symptoms of dyspnea on minimal effort and chest pain with minimal effort. Blood pressure (BP) is 130/80 mmHg, heart rate is 72 bpm. Grade III/VI harsh systolic ejection murmur is heard in the right upper sternal border. Echocardiogram showed a bicuspid valve with aortic valve area of 0.6 cm². What is the lifetime risk of aortic dissection in this patient?

A. 2–4%  
B. 4–6%  
C. 6–7%  
D. 10–12%

**19.2.** Aortopathy associated with bicuspid aortic valve is due to which of the following?

A. Abnormal fibrillin  
B. Vascular smooth muscle cell apoptosis  
C. Matrix metallopeptidase 9  
D. All of the above  
E. A and C only

**19.3.** The right/left fusion pathology in a bicuspid valve is seen commonly. What is its incidence?

A. 20%  
B. 40%  
C. 60%  
D. 80%

**19.4.** The sites of aortic dissection may be (a) just past the left subclavian artery, (b) 3 cm distal to the aortic valve, and (c) at the aortic arch. Which of the following options matches the aortic dissection sites in decreasing order?

A. a, b, c  
B. b, c, a  
C. b, a, c  
D. a, c, b

**19.5.** The treatment of choice in a 49-year-old male with acute type III aortic dissection, minimally dilated aorta with no leak, good flow in false lumen, BP of 200/100 mmHg, severe interscapular pain, pallor, and tachycardia is which of the following?

A. Emergency surgery  
B. Endovascular graft implantation with fenestration  
C. Intravenous (IV) nitroprusside  
D. IV esmolol

*Cardiology Board Review*, Second Edition. Ramdas G. Pai and Padmini Varadarajan.
© 2023 John Wiley & Sons Ltd. Published 2023 by John Wiley & Sons Ltd.

19.6. A 70-year-old patient with a history of three-drug hypertension and tobacco use presents to the emergency room with acute onset of substernal chest pain and electrocardiogram showing ST elevation in inferior leads. His BP is 80 mmHg systolic in the left arm and 150 mmHg systolic in right arm. What is your test of choice?

A. Emergency coronary angiography

B. Echocardiography

C. Computed tomography (CT) of the chest without contrast

D. CT of the chest with contrast

19.7. The angiogram in Figure 19.7 is most likely to be associated with which of the following?

A. 70-year-old African American woman

B. 38-year-old Asian Indian woman

C. 35-year-old Polish male

D. 60-year-old Peruvian male

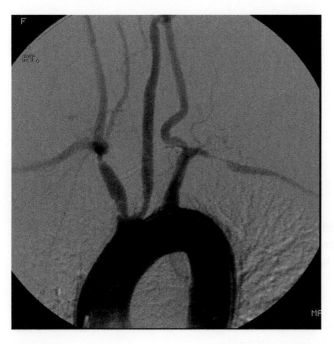

Figure 19.7

19.8. An 80-year-old woman presents with 20 lb. weight loss over the last six months. She also reports nausea and diarrhea and states she has to eat small meals as she has abdominal pain if she eats normal portions. She has a history of coronary artery bypass grafting, done 10 years previously. She had traveled to India six months ago. Which test will have the highest yield?

A. Esophagogastroduodenoscopy

B. Colonoscopy

C. Infectious disease consultation

    **D.** CT with contrast of the chest and abdomen
    **E.** None of the above

**19.9.** The patient in Figure 19.9 has history hypertension and shortness of breath. Which of the following does the patient have?
    **A.** Hyperparathyroidism     **C.** Prostate cancer
    **B.** Lymphoma     **D.** None of the above

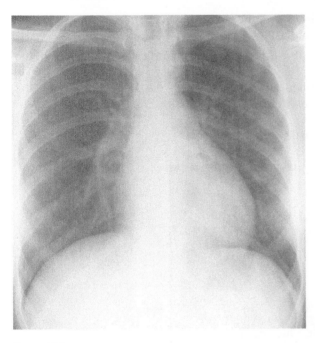

Figure 19.9

**19.10.** A patient presents with "trash foot" after a cardiac catheterization with the TEE image shown in Figure 19.10. There is a palpable pulse and the foot is warm. Which of the following would you order?
    **A.** IV prostaglandin     **D.** IV nitroglycerine
    **B.** IV steroids     **E.** None of the above
    **C.** IV heparin

**19.11.** What is your test of choice to make the diagnosis of the patient in Question 19.10?
    **A.** Arterial duplex of the lower extremities
    **B.** Venous duplex study of the lower extremities
    **C.** CT of the abdomen
    **D.** Abdominal ultrasound

**19.12.** A 53-year-old male presents with symptoms of progressive hoarseness. Figure 19.12 shows the TEE (long-axis view) done. What is the best next step?
    **A.** IV vancomycin and gentamicin
    **B.** Repeat echocardiography in two weeks
    **C.** Esmolol drip
    **D.** CT of the chest with contrast

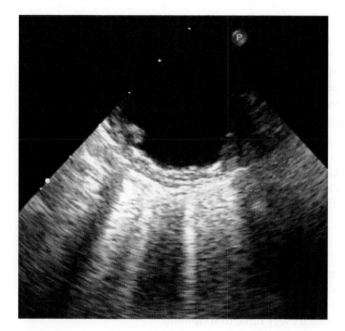

Figure 19.10

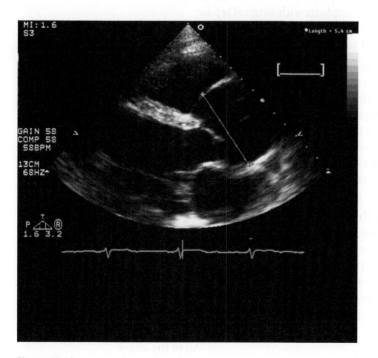

Figure 19.12

**19.13.** A 58-year-old male is known to have Marfan syndrome. His echocardiogram shows an ascending aortic aneurysm 4.1 cm in size. What is the next step?
A. CT every six months
B. Echocardiogram every six months
C. Annual CT or magnetic resonance imaging (MRI)
D. Echocardiogram every three months

**19.14.** A 43-year-old male had recent surgery for a dissecting aortic aneurysm. Which of the following is/are recommended?
A. CT or echocardiogram at 6 and 12 months after surgery
B. Lifelong beta blockade
C. Use of homografts to replace infected prostheses is contraindicated
D. Control BP to less than 135/80 mmHg
E. B and D
F. A and D

**19.15.** A 60-year-old male was diagnosed with infrarenal abdominal aortic aneurysm (AAA) of 5.5 cm. What should this patient have?
A. CT every 6–12 months
B. Should undergo repair
C. Monitored by ultrasound every three to six months
D. Only A and C

**19.16.** Endovascular repair of the aneurysm of the descending thoracic aorta is associated with which of the following complications compared with open surgical repair?
A. Higher risk of paraplegia with endovascular repair
B. Lower risk of paraplegia with surgical repair
C. Higher risk of respiratory failure with open repair
D. Higher risk of respiratory failure with endovascular repair

**19.17.** A 50-year-old woman presents to your office with 6-month history of hypertension that has been difficult to control, headaches, fatigue of the lower extremities on minimal effort, and claudication if she pushes herself. She has had malaise, low-grade fevers, and night sweats. Her BP is 200/105 mmHg in both upper extremities and 100/60 mmHg in both of her ankles. What is the diagnosis?
A. Takatsubo's syndrome
B. Coarctation of the aorta
C. Mid-aortic syndrome
D. Bilateral iliac artery stenosis

**19.18.** With which of the following is 45,X chromosomal anomaly associated?
A. Development of complete heart block
B. Ventricular septal defect
C. Aortic aneurysm and dissections
D. Tall stature and a violent personality

**19.19.** "Bamboo" spine is associated with which of the following?
A. Ascending aortic aneurysm
B. Uveitis
C. Arthritis
D. Ulcerative colitis
E. A, B, and C
F. A, C, and D
G. All of the above

19.20. Leriche syndrome is associated with which of the following?
   A. Impotence
   B. Buttock claudication
   C. Atrophy of the lower extremities
   D. All of the above
   E. A and B only

19.21. Which of the following describes collateral arterial pathways around total occlusions of the infrarenal aorta?
   A. Inferior epigastric artery to the internal mammary artery
   B. Lumbar artery to the hypogastric artery
   C. Inferior mesenteric artery to the hypogastric artery
   D. The sacral artery to the hypogastric artery
   E. A and B only
   F. All of the above
   G. A, B, and C only

19.22. A 68-year-old woman presents with severe anterior unrelenting chest pain that radiates to her back. BP is 200/110 mmHg. She has a CT scan of the chest, shown in Figure 19.22a. Which of the following is the next best step?
   A. Medical therapy
   B. Transthoracic echocardiogram
   C. Cardiothoracic surgery consultation and proceed to the operating room with intra operation TEE
   D. MRI of the chest

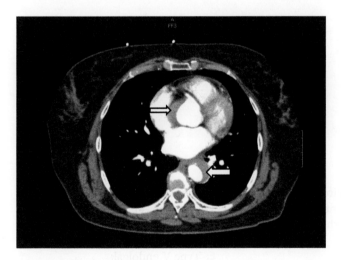

Figure 19.22a

19.23. Which of the following is the treatment of choice in the 80-year-old patient in Figure 19.23a with advanced chronic obstructive pulmonary disease (COPD) and hypertension? She is status post mastectomy three years ago with no residual disease.
   A. Endovascular repair
   B. Open surgical repair
   C. Risk factor modification with conservative therapy

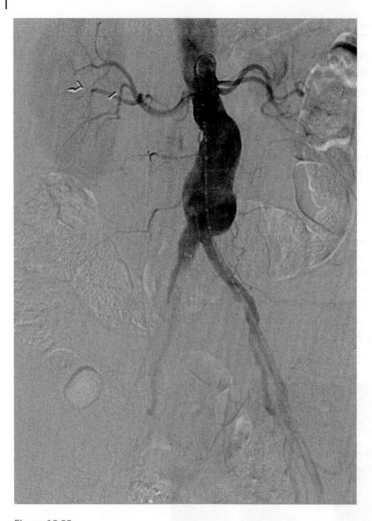

**Figure 19.23a**

19.24. You successfully repaired a 6.5 cm infrarenal aortic aneurysm one year previously. The aneurysm has continued to grow by 1 cm on a follow-up CT scan. There is no contrast seen within the sac of the aneurysm. What is this an example of?
   A. Type I endoleak
   B. Type II endoleak
   C. Type III endoleak
   D. Type IV endoleak
   E. Type V endoleak

19.25. True or false, "sartans" slow the growth of aneurysms in Marfan syndrome?
   A. True
   B. False

19.26. Which of the following might 45,X0 be associated with?
   A. Brachiofemoral delay
   B. Bicuspid aortic valve
   C. Dilatation of the aorta
   D. Impaired glucose tolerance
   E. All of the above

19.27. A bifid uvula is seen in which of the following?
   A. Ehlers-Danlos syndrome (EDS)
   B. Loeys-Dietz syndrome (LDS)
   C. Aneurysms-osteoarthritis syndrome (AOS)
   D. Arterial tortuosity syndrome (ATS)
   E. Marfan syndrome

19.28. The non-syndromic forms of thoracic aortic aneurysm and dissection (nsTAAD) may be associated with bicuspid aortic valve and/or persistent ductus arteriosus and display typical cystic medial necrosis on pathologic examination. Mutations in genes (*FBN1, TGFBR1,* and *TGFBR2*) are frequently seen.
   A. True
   B. False

19.29. The most characteristic and frequently reported clinical presentation of an intimal angiosarcoma of the aorta is the embolic occlusion of the mesenteric or peripheral artery. Leiosarcomas and fibrosarcomas originate from the media or adventitia of the aortic wall. Which rare tumor of the aorta is most common?
   A. Angiosarcoma
   B. Leiosarcoma
   C. Fibrosarcoma

19.30. What structures are the long and short arrows in Figure 19.30 pointing to?
   A. Aorta and lateral epigastric artery
   B. Aorta and the inferior epigastric artery
   C. Aorta and intercostal artery
   D. None of the above

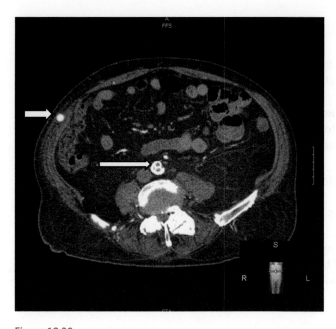

Figure 19.30

19.31. The risk of paraplegia with endovascular thoracic aneurysm repair (Figure 19.31a) is which of the following?

A. 20%

B. 25%

C. 5%

D. 10%

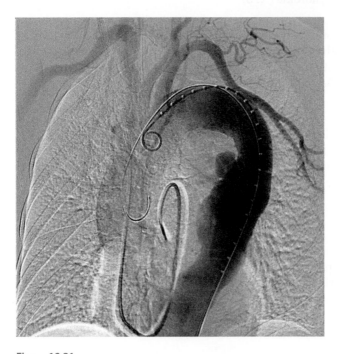

Figure 19.31a

19.32. A 30-year-old Asian female presents with fever, fatigue, and syncopal episode. Examination reveals absent radial pulses. What is the most accurate diagnostic test?

A. Erythrocyte sedimentation rate/C-reactive protein

B. Antineutrophil cytoplasmic antibody (ANCA), antinuclear antibody (ANA)

C. Magnetic resonance angiography (MRA)

D. All of the above

19.33. Takayasu's arteritis affects which of the following?

A. Aorta

B. Pulmonary arteries

C. Renal arteries

D. All of the above

E. A, B, and C

19.34. Treatment of Takayasu's arteritis includes which of the following?

A. Steroid 1 mg/kg of body weight per day

B. Mycophenolate and tocilizumab

C. Bypass grafting

D. Stenting

E. All of the above

19.35. Which of the following is the most accurate to diagnose dissecting ascending aortic aneurysm?
A. TEE
B. CT angiogram
C. MRA
D. All of the above

19.36. Which of the following is/are associated with ascending aortic dissection?
A. Blunt trauma
B. Marfan syndrome
C. Aortic regurgitation
D. Syphilis
E. A, B, and D
F. All of the above

19.37. Severe hypotension at presentation is a grave prognostic indicator in ascending aortic dissection, and is due to which of the following?
A. Pericardial tamponade
B. Severe aortic insufficiency
C. Rupture of the aorta
D. A, B, and C
E. None of the above

19.38. Ascending aortic dissection and aortic regurgitation can be explained by which of the following?
A. The dissection may dilate the annulus of the aortic valve
B. The dissection may extend into the aortic root and detach the aortic valve leaflets
C. Both A and B
D. None of the above

19.39. Which of the following is/are correct regarding myocardial infarction in ascending aortic dissection?
A. Due to involvement of coronary arteries
B. Incidence rate 1–2%
C. Right coronary more commonly involved than left coronary
D. Thrombolytics are indicated
E. A and B
F. A, B, and C

19.40. Pleural effusion in ascending aortic dissection is caused by which of the following?
A. Due to inflammation of the pleura
B. Due to blood from rupture
C. Due to fluid from inflammation around the aorta
D. B and C
E. None of the above

19.41. Aortic dissection is more common in males.
A. True
B. False

19.42. Anatomic reporting of aortic dissection by society of vascular surgeons and thoracic surgeons classify dissection based on which of the following?
A. Location of Entry Tear (A vs B)
B. Proximal Extent (0–12)
C. Distal extent (0–12)
D. A and C
E. A, B, and C

Chapter 19

19.43. Which of the following is true about penetrating aortic ulcer?
  A. Involves presence of a tear in intima and false lumen having blood externally bound only by the outer third of media and adventitia
  B. Lacks an identifiable direct communication between true and false lumen, and is best seen on non-contrast-enhanced computed tomography
  C. Penetrating Aortic Ulcer (PAU) is atherosclerotic penetration of internal elastic lamina of aortic wall and can co-exist with or without IMH.
  D. All of the above

19.44. What segment of ascending aorta is difficult to examine or is invisible on Transesophageal Echocardiogram?
  A. Short segment of the distal ascending aorta, just before the innominate artery
  B. Proximal ascending aorta, near the sino-tubular junction
  C. Proximal descending aorta
  D. Distal descending aorta
  E. A and B

19.45. A 42-year-old male smoker presents to cardiology clinic after incidental diagnoses of aortic dilatation on CT abdomen. Patient is 6 ft 4 in tall and has history of flexible joints. Which of the following, when used prophylactically, reduce the progression of aortic dilatation or occurrence of complications in this patient?
  A. Beta-blockers
  B. Statins
  C. Angiotensin receptor blockers
  D. Diuretics
  E. A, B, and C
  F. All of the above

19.46. Mr. Jones underwent carotid-femoral pulse wave velocity measurement during comprehensive evaluation for hypertension. His results showed carotid-femoral pulse wave velocity of 14 m/s. Aortic stiffness has independent predictive value for all-cause and cardiovascular mortality
  A. True
  B. False

19.47. A 68-year-old male with history of smoking underwent endovascular aortic repair complicated by an Endoleak requiring immediate re-intervention. Which of the following statements is true about endoleaks following EVAR?
  A. Types I and III endoleaks are treatment failures and warrant further treatment
  B. Type II endoleak can be managed conservatively – "wait and watch approach"
  C. Types IV and V endoleaks are indirect and benign except when aneurysm is enlarging
  D. A and B
  E. A, B, and C

19.48. Which of the following statement is a class recommendation about TEVAR?
  A. Proximal and distal landing zones of at-least 2 cm are considered optimal
  B. Stent with a 10–15% larger diameter than aorta is required for aortic aneurysms
  C. Preventive cerebrospinal fluid drainage should be considered for high-risk cases
  D. All of the above

**19.49.** A 55-year-old male with a history of uncontrolled hypertension and smoking presents with precordial chest pain and syncope. BP 90/60 mmHg and HR 130/min. Which of the following is true?
  A. Syncope is associated with an increased risk of in-hospital mortality
  B. Cardiac tamponade and supra-aortic vessel dissection should be ruled out
  C. TTE followed by TOE or ECG gated CT should be performed
  D. B and C
  E. A and C
  F. A, B, and C

**19.50.** An 84-year-old male with a history of hypertension, CKD 4, and stage 4 COPD develops sharp chest pain. Gated CT chest showed 49 mm ascending aorta and type A intramural hematoma (thickness 10 mm) (Kitai et al. 2009). Which of the following is the best management option?
  A. Emergent surgery is indicated for Type A acute aortic syndrome
  B. Optimal medical therapy with "wait and watch strategy"
  C. Send to Hospice
  D. All of the above
  E. Neither of the above

**19.51.** Frozen elephant trunk involves which of the following
  A. Ascending aorta replacement
  B. Aortic arch replacement
  C. Descending aorta replacement
  D. Integrated stent grafting of descending aorta
  E. A, B, C
  F. A, B, D

**19.52.** "Cobweb" sign and "Mercedes-Benz" sign are seen in which of the following conditions
  A. Aortic aneurysm
  B. Aortic dissection
  C. Ruptured aortic aneurysm
  D. Renal artery stenosis
  E. Polyarteritis nodosa

**19.53.** A 64-year-old male presented to emergency room with acute chest pain. CT chest with contrast showed highly mobile linear intraluminal filling defect mimicking an intimal flap. Which of the following are true about "pulsation artifact"?
  A. Pulsation artifact is most common cause of misdiagnosis of aortic dissection
  B. Pulsation artifact is caused by movement of ascending aorta between end-diastole and end-systole
  C. It can be eliminated by ECG gating or 180° linear interpolation reconstruction algorithm
  D. A and B
  E. A, B, and C

**19.54.** A 71-year-old male with history of hypertension presented to the hospital with chest discomfort. He was diagnosed with Type B aortic dissection. His pain resolved and blood pressure came under control with initiation of medical therapy. Which of the following holds true for TEVAR in comparison to medical therapy for uncomplicated aortic dissection?

Chapter 1

A. TEVAR provides no survival benefit over medical therapy
B. TEVAR has lower aorta-related mortality and disease progression at five years
C. TEVAR leads to higher rates of aortic remodeling at two years
D. A, B, and C
E. A and B

19.55. A 55-year-old male with history of hyperlipidemia and hypertension presented to the ED with chest pain radiating to the back. CT scan showed a Type B aortic dissection. He is currently chest-pain free and denies any recurrence. CT did not show early aortic expansion, malperfusion, hemothorax, or hematoma formation. Blood pressure and HR with maximal medication are 136/90 mmHg and 62 per minute, respectively. What would be the treatment of choice?
A. Medical therapy
B. TEVAR
C. Surgery with deep hypothermic circulatory arrest
D. Wait and watch

19.56. Penetrating aortic ulcers most commonly involve mid and lower descending aorta.
A. True
B. False

19.57. A 24-year-old married female with some Marfanoid features was found to have 4.9 cm aortic root aneurysm. What will be the best next course?
A. Medical management with one year follow up of on repeated CT scan
B. TEVAR
C. Surgery
D. A and B

19.58. Which of the following is true about Mycotic aneurysms?
A. Majority of mycotic aneurysms are caused by fungus
B. Majority of mycotic aneurysms are caused by bacteria
C. Mortality related to infected aortic aneurysm is lower when medical and surgical therapies are combined compared with medical treatment alone
D. Following debridement of an infected infrarenal aortic aneurysm, extra-anatomic reconstruction (e.g. axillofemoral bypass) is generally preferred
E. A, C, and D
F. B, C, and D

19.59. Which of the following apply to non-infectious aortitis?
A. 0.5–1 mg/kg prednisone daily is recommended dose
B. One to two years of corticosteroid treatment is required with initiation of dose tapering after two to three months
C. About 50% patients relapse requiring additional immunosuppression
D. Dilations of the aortic root and ascending aorta are common and can lead to dissection or rupture
E. A comprehensive vascular examination and periodic imaging for the development of thoracic or abdominal aortic aneurysm, given the known risk of these complications

19.60. Which of the following statements is true about follow up after EVAR or TEVAR?
  A. Surveillance is recommended after 1 month, 6 months, 12 months, and then yearly
  B. CT is recommended as the first-choice imaging technique for follow-up
  C. If neither endoleak nor AAA sac enlargement is documented during first year, then color DUS, with or without contrast agents, should be considered for annual postoperative surveillance, with non-contrast CT imaging every five years
  D. All of the above

## Answers

19.1. C. 6–7%.
  See Losenno et al. (2012).

19.2. D. All of the above.
  All of the factors are part of the extracellular matrix and are abnormal causing cystic medial necrosis.

19.3. C. 60%.
  Right and left cusp fusion is seen 70% of the time, followed by right and non-coronary cusps 15–25%, and left/noncoronary cusps 5% of the time.

19.4. C. b, a, c.
  The most common site of dissection is the first few centimeters of the ascending aorta, with 90% occurring within 10 cm of the aortic valve. The second most common site is just distal to the left subclavian artery. Between 5% and 10% of dissections do not have an obvious intimal tear. These are often attributed to rupture of the aortic vasa vasorum, as first described by Krukenberg in 1920.

19.5. D. IV esmolol.
  IV beta blockade is to decrease the shear force on the wall of the aorta. If the BP is not controlled on IV beta blockade (first drug of choice per American College of Cardiology guidelines) add other agents to lower BP.

19.6. D. CT of the chest with contrast.
  Or emergency transesophageal echocardiogram (TEE). Acute ascending aortic dissection can cause right coronary artery compromise and pericardial tamponade. Unrecognized, the mortality is 1–2% per hour.

19.7. B. A 38-year-old Asian Indian woman.
  Takayasu's arteritis, or pulseless disease, is most commonly seen in Japan and Asia. Neurologic and ophthalmologic symptoms are common. Fever, malaise, and loss of upper extremity pulse and a low BP in the upper extremity are common. The angiogram in Figure 19.7 shows severe left subclavian artery stenosis and right innominate artery origin stenosis (Rizzi et al. 1999).

19.8. D. CT Chest and abdomen.
  The history is consistent with abdominal angina with weight loss, history of atherosclerosis (see Box 19.1), fear of food, and abdominal pain. Generally, two of the three mesenteric vessels are compromised to manifest these symptoms.

Chapter 19

The vascular supply of the gut is extensive with robust collateral supply (Hovenwalter 2009).

**19.9.** D. None of the above.

There is rib notching due to intercostal artery collateral formation seen with coarctation of the aorta.

**19.10.** E. None of the above.

**19.11.** C. CT of the abdomen.

This is "trash foot" from atheroemboli likely from an abdominal aortic aneurysm, though the image shown is from the thoracic aorta, which shows only moderate aortic atheroma without debris. The triad of pain, livedo reticularis, and intact peripheral pulses is pathognomonic for cholesterol embolization. No single therapy has been shown to be clinically beneficial. CT is the most accurate for diagnosing and sizing the abdominal aortic aneurysm prior to repair.

**19.12.** D. CT of the chest with contrast.

The echocardiogram in Figure 19.12 exhibits a large proximal ascending aortic aneurysm that may require surgery. Stretch of the recurrent laryngeal nerve by the aortic arch causes hoarseness. The CT will exactly size the aneurysm.

**19.13.** C. Annual CT or magnetic resonance imaging (MRI).

See guidelines in Table 19.1.

**19.14.** E. B and D.

See European Society of Cardiology guidelines in Table 19.2.

**19.15.** B. Should undergo repair.

See Table 19.3. The risk of rupture goes up exponentially as the size of the aneurysm increases.

**19.16.** C. Higher risk of respiratory failure with open repair.

As the open repair requires a thoracotomy, there is a higher risk of respiratory failure. Thoracic aneurysms should be repaired when the size is >6 cm. If a thoracic aneurysm is detected, the rest of the aorta should be imaged to rule out other aneurysms; this applies to aneurysms of the aorta in any location.

Table 19.1

| Etiology/location | Size (cm) | Time interval/modality |
|---|---|---|
| Root or ascending aorta | | |
| • Degenerative | 3.5–4.4 | Annual CT or MRI |
| | 4.5–5.4 | Echocardiogram to follow valve disease (if needed) Biannual CT or MRI |
| Root or ascending aorta | 3.5–4.4 | Echocardiogram to follow valve disease (if needed) Annual CT or MRI |
| • Marfan syndrome | | Echocardiogram to follow valve disease |
| • Bicuspid aortic valve | | (if needed) |
| • Other genetically mediated disorder | 4.5–5.0 | Biannual CT or MRI |

Table 19.2

| Intervention | Recommendations | Level of evidence |
|---|---|---|
| Medical therapy | Lifelong beta blockade | Class II |
| | Control of BP to <135/80 mmHg (130/80 mmHg for Marfan syndrome) | Class I |
| Surveillance | Imaging at 1, 3, 6, and 12 months, then yearly thereafter (by MRI, CT, or TEE) | Class I |
| Repeat aortic surgery | Surgery for secondary aneurysm in dissected aorta remote from initial repair | Class I |
| | Surgery for recurrent dissection or aneurysm formation at previous intervention site | Class I |
| | Use of homografts to replace infected prostheses | Class IIa |
| | Endovascular stenting instead of surgery if anatomy is suitable | Class IIa |

Table 19.3

| Intervention | Recommendations | Level of evidence |
|---|---|---|
| Screening | Men >60 years who are either the siblings or offspring of patients with AAA should undergo physical examination and screening abdominal ultrasound | Class I |
| | Men 65–75 years who have ever smoked should undergo physical examination and screening abdominal ultrasound | Class IIa |
| Surveillance | Patients with AAA 4.0–5.4 cm in diameter should be monitored by ultrasound or CT scans every 6–12 months to detect expansion | Class I |
| | Patients with AAA <4.0 cm in diameter should be monitored by ultrasound every 2–3 years | Class IIa |
| Repair | Patients with infrarenal or juxtarenal AAA >5.4 cm in diameter should undergo repair | Class I |
| | Repair can be beneficial in patients with infrarenal or juxtarenal AAA measuring 5.0–5.4 cm in diameter | Class IIa |
| | Repair may be indicated in patients with suprarenal or thoracoabdominal AAA measuring 5.5–6.0 cm | Class IIa |

Chapter 1

The popliteal arteries should be palpated and imaged with ultrasound to rule out aneurysms. Popliteal aneurysms do not rupture but present with acute limb ischemia. Risk of paraplegia is higher with open surgical repair.

**19.17.** C. Mid-aortic syndrome.

In this patient, this is likely a sequel to Takayasu's syndrome with near occlusion of the mid-abdominal aorta. Repair is endovascular if focal, otherwise surgical (Delis and Gloviczki 2005).

19.18. C. Aortic aneurysm and dissections.

Turner syndrome is associated with aortic aneurysm and dissection (Matura et al. 2007).

19.19. E. A, B, and C.

Ankylosing spondylitis is associated with aneurysm of the ascending aorta, uveitis, and arthritis of the spine and the sacroiliac joint. A radiograph shows fusion of the vertebrae and has the appearance of a bamboo tree on X-ray.

19.20. D. All of the above.

Leriche syndrome is due to atherosclerotic total occlusion of the terminal aorta. The triad of symptoms are as noted.

19.21. G. A, B, and C only.

19.22. C. Aortic hematomas are treated like a dissection. Type A aortic dissection carries with it a mortality of 1–2% per hour. This patient had a tear in the lesser curve of the arch of the aorta opposite the takeoff from the right innominate artery (Figure 19.22b). The hematoma then advanced in an antegrade and retrograde fashion. Such patients need to be taken to surgery with intraoperative TEE.

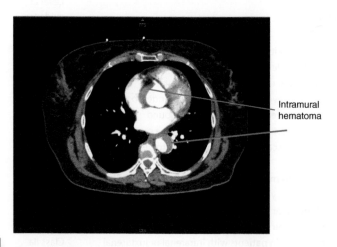

Intramural
hematoma

Figure 19.22b

19.23. A. Endovascular repair.

The patient has a life span of more than one year. There is more than 15 mm of infrarenal aortic neck and she is well suited for endovascular aneurysm repair (Figure 19.23b). Open repair carries with it a 4–5% 30-day mortality as opposed to 3% by endovascular repair. The need for re-intervention is higher in the endovascular group.

19.24. E. Type V endoleak.

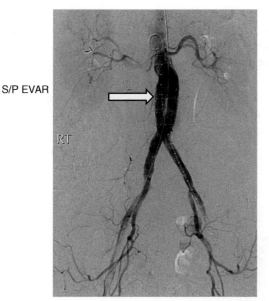

S/P EVAR

RT

Figure 19.23b

Type I is a leak from either end of the graft due to a gap between the graft and the aorta; type II is filling of the sac via collaterals – most commonly lumbar; type III is a break in the components of the graft; type IV is leak from the fabric of the graft material; type V is no cause (White et al. 2000).

**19.25.** A. True.

See Erbel et al. (2014).

**19.26.** E. All of the above.

See Erbel et al. (2014).

**19.27.** B. Loeys-Dietz syndrome (LDS).

These are part of the chromosomal and inherited syndromic thoracic aortic aneurysms and dissection. Type IV EDS has significantly shortened life spans (50% mortality rate by 48 years) due to the spontaneous rupture of visceral organs (colon, uterus) and blood vessels; it affects the entire vascular system and the heart. Fusiform aneurysms are reported. LDS is a triad of arterial tortuosity and aneurysms throughout the arterial tree, hypertelorism, and bifid uvula, as well as features shared with Marfan syndrome. AOS is an autosomal dominant condition combining early-onset joint abnormalities (including osteoarthritis and osteochondritis dissecans) and aortic aneurysms and dissections. ATS is characterized by arterial tortuosity, elongation, stenosis, and aneurysm of the large- and middle-sized arteries; ATS is a very rare autosomal recessive disease.

See Erbel et al. (2014).

**19.28.** A. False.

The first part of the statement is true. The second part is true for the genetic syndrome associated TAAD. Genes for the nsTAAD are not as well defined.

**19.29.** A. Angiosarcoma.

*En bloc* resection of the aorta with clean margins is the therapy of choice. Prognosis is poor.

Chapter 19

**19.30.** D. None of the above.

The long arrow points to the aorta with occluded prosthetic graft in it, and the short arrow points to an extra-anatomic Dacron bypass graft – axillofemoral bypass. This was done in a patient with Leriche syndrome.

**19.31.** C. 5%.

With spinal cord protection, the incidence in contemporary studies shows a risk of cord injury of 5%. As shown in the Figure 19.31b, endovascular repair was performed with a covered stent.

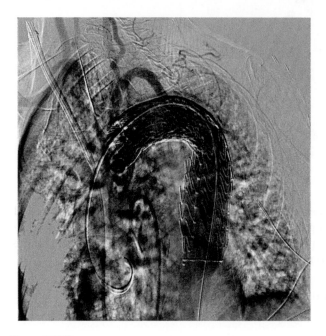

Figure 19.31b

**19.32.** C. Magnetic resonance angiography (MRA).

This patient has Takayasu's arteritis (pulseless disease, aortic arch syndrome, nonspecific aortoarteritis), which affects young Asian females and is characterized by large-vessel granulomatous vasculitis with massive intimal fibrosis and vascular narrowing. Diagnosis can be made by MRA, CT angiogram, and aortography. It is not associated with ANCA, rheumatoid factor, ANA, or anti-cardiolipin antibodies.

**19.33.** E. A, B, and C.

Takayasu's arteritis affects the aorta and its branches, the pulmonary arteries, and the renal arteries that can cause renovascular hypertension. It is characterized by segmental and patchy granulomatous inflammation of the aorta and branches, leading to arterial stenosis, thrombosis, and aneurysms.

**19.34.** E. All of the above.

**19.35.** D. All of the above.

TEE, CT angiogram, and MRA have equal sensitivity and specificity to diagnose dissecting ascending aortic aneurysm.

**19.36.** F. All of the above.

Blunt trauma, Marfan syndrome, EDS, congenital bicuspid aortic valve, history of aortic dissection, Turner syndrome, aortic regurgitation, cardiac catheterization, intra-aortic balloon pump, and tertiary syphilis are associated with ascending aortic dissection.

**19.37.** D. A, B, and C.

Severe hypotension at presentation is a grave prognostic indicator in ascending aortic dissection, and is associated with pericardial tamponade, severe aortic insufficiency, and rupture of the aorta.

**19.38.** C. Both A and B.

Ascending aortic dissection and aortic regurgitation can be due to the following:

- the dissection may dilate the annulus of the aortic valve;
- the dissection may extend into the aortic root and detach the aortic valve leaflets;
- in extensive intimal tear, the intimal flap may prolapse into the left ventricular outflow tract, causing intimal intussusception into the aortic valve, thus preventing proper valve closure.

**19.39.** F. A, B, and C.

Myocardial infarction in ascending aortic dissection is due to involvement of coronary arteries, with the right coronary more commonly involved than the left coronary with incidence rate 1–2%. Thrombolytics are absolutely contraindicated, as mortality increases to over 70%, mostly due to bleeding into the pericardial sac causing pericardial tamponade.

**19.40.** D. B and C.

Pleural effusion in ascending aortic dissection is caused by blood from rupture and fluid from inflammation around the aorta. More commonly in the left hemithorax.

**19.41.** A. Men are more frequently affected by acute aortic dissection (Atkins et al. 2006).

**19.42.** E. A, B, and C (Lombardi et al. 2020)

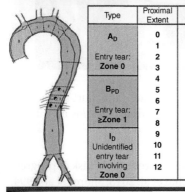

**Society for Vascular Surgery and Society of Thoracic Surgery Reporting Standards for Type B Aortic Dissections**

| Type | Proximal Extent | Distal Extent |
|------|-----------------|---------------|
| $A_D$ | 0 | 0 |
| | 1 | 1 |
| Entry tear: | 2 | 2 |
| Zone 0 | 3 | 3 |
| | 4 | 4 |
| $B_{PD}$ | 5 | 5 |
| | 6 | 6 |
| Entry tear: | 7 | 7 |
| ≥Zone 1 | 8 | 8 |
| $I_D$ | 9 | 9 |
| Unidentified | 10 | 10 |
| entry tear | 11 | 11 |
| involving Zone 0 | 12 | 12 |

**Anatomic Reporting of Aortic Dissections are based on:**

✓ Location of Entry Tear (A vs B)
✓ Proximal & Distal Extent

**EXAMPLES**

Type $A_9$: Entry tear identified in zone 0 (A), Distal extent in zone 9.

Type $B_{4,10}$: Entry tear is identified > zone 0 (B) Proximal extent in zone 4, Distal extent in zone 10.

JVS Journal of Vascular Surgery — Official Publication of the Society for Vascular Surgery

Lombardi et al. *J Vasc Surg, March 2020*

Copyright © 2020 by the Society for Vascular Surgery®

🐦 @JVascSurg
f @TheJVascSurg

Chapter 1

19.43. C. A is aortic dissection, B refers to Intramural hematoma, and C is definition for PAU (Lombardi et al. 2020)

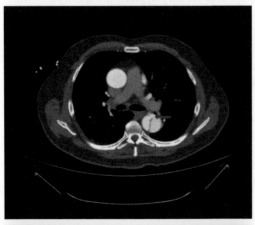

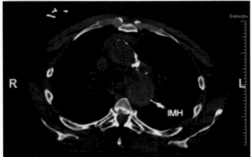

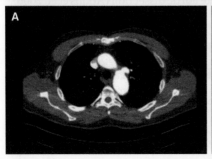
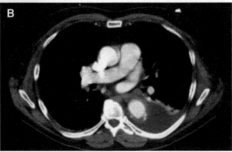

19.44. A. Owing to interposition of the right bronchus and trachea, a short segment of the distal ascending aorta, just before the innominate artery, remains invisible (a "blind spot").

19.45. E. A, B, and C
    Betablockers, ARB's and statins have been shown to reduce the risk of progression of aortic aneurysms (Groenink et al. 2013; Chiu et al. 2013; Shores et al. 1994; Jovin et al. 2012; Stein et al. 2013).

19.46. A. True
    Aortic stiffness measured by aortic pulse wave velocity predicts all cause and cardiovascular mortality, fatal and non-fatal coronary events, and fatal strokes in

patients with various levels of cardiovascular risk, with a higher predictive value in subjects with a higher baseline cardiovascular risk (Ben-Shlomo et al. 2013; Vlachopoulos et al. 2010). According to The Expert Consensus Statement in the 2013 European Society of Hypertension (ESH)/ESC Guidelines, a threshold for the pulse wave velocity of 10 m/s has been suggested. Increased arterial stiffness results an increased speed of the pulse wave in the artery. Carotid-femoral pulse wave velocity is the "gold standard" for measuring aortic stiffness, given its simplicity, accuracy, reproducibility, and strong predictive value for adverse outcomes.

19.47. E. A, B, and C (Grabenwoger et al. 2012)

19.48. D. A and B are class I C recommendations, and C is Class IIa level C- See Erbel et al. (2014)

19.49. F. All of the above. See Erbel et al. (2014)

Unstable patient means very severe pain, tachycardia, tachypnoea, hypotension, cyanosis, and/or shock

19.50. B. In elderly patients or those with significant comorbidities, initial medical treatment with a "wait-and-watch strategy" (optimal medical therapy with blood pressure and pain control and repetitive imaging) may be a reasonable option, particularly in the absence of aortic dilation (<50 mm) and IMH thickness < 11 mm. In medically treated patients, maximum aortic diameter was the only predictor of early and late progression of ascending IMH (hazard ratio, 4.43; 95% CI, 2.04–9.64; P<0.001). Aortic diameter ≥50 mm predicted progression of ascending IMH with the positive and negative value of 83% and 84%, respectively.

19.51. F. **(Sherstha et al. 2015)**

19.52. B. The cobweb sign is seen in cases of arterial dissection (usually aortic dissection) on CT angiogram (CTA) examinations and represents strands or ribbons of media crossing the false lumen, and appearing as thin filiform filling defects.

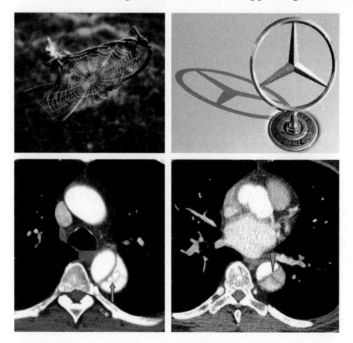

*Source:* Yudin et al. (2014) / with permission of Springer Nature.

Chapter 19

After IV enhancement, intimal flaps in the false channel of the dissected aorta may create a view of a network or a web, the "cobweb" sign (↑), or a symbol of the Mercedes-Benz company, the "Mercedes-Benz" sign (Δ). These signs always coexist with the "beak sign."(Yudin 2014).

**19.53.** E.

It is important to recognize the highly mobile linear intraluminal filling defect, which may mimic an intimal flap on CT. The so-called "pulsation artifact" is the most common cause of misdiagnosis. It is caused by pulsatile movement of the ascending aorta during the cardiac cycle between end-diastole and end-systole. The potential problem of pulsation artifacts can be eliminated with ECG-gating, or else by a 180° linear interpolation reconstruction algorithm. See Erbel et al. (2014).

**19.54.** D. A, B, and C

INSTEAD and INSTEAD-XL trial by Nienaber CA, et al.

The Investigation of Stent Grafts in Patients with Type B AD (INSTEAD) trial randomized a total of 140 patients with sub-acute (0.14 days) uncomplicated Type B AD. Two-year follow-up results indicated that TEVAR is effective (aortic remodeling in 91.3% of TEVAR patients versus 19.4% of patients receiving medical treatment; P, 0.001); however, TEVAR showed no clinical benefit over medical therapy (survival rates: 88.9% + 3.7% with TEVAR versus 95.6%+2.5% with optimal medical therapy; P ¼ 0.15). Extended follow-up of this study (INSTEAD-XL) recently showed that aorta-related mortality (6.9% vs. 19.3%, respectively; P ¼ 0.04) and disease progression (27.0% vs. 46.1%, respectively; P ¼ 0.04) were significantly lower after five years in TEVAR patients compared with those receiving medical therapy only. No difference was found regarding total mortality.

**19.55.** B. Class 1 recommendation in cases of complicated Type B AD

The term "complicated" means persistent or recurrent pain, uncontrolled hypertension despite full medication, early aortic expansion, malperfusion, and signs of rupture (hemothorax, increasing periaortic and mediastinal hematoma). Additional factors, such as the FL diameter, the location of the primary entry site, and a retrograde component of the dissection into the aortic arch, are considered to significantly influence the patient's prognosis.

**19.56.** A.

PAU is often encountered in the setting of extensive atherosclerosis of the thoracic aorta, may be multiple, and may vary greatly in size and depth within the vessel wall. The most common location of PAU is the middle and lower descending thoracic aorta (Type B PAU). Erbel et al. (2014).

**19.57.** C.

Surgery should be performed in patients with Marfan syndrome, who have a maximal aortic diameter ≥50 mm. A lower threshold of 45 mm can be considered in patients with additional risk factors, including family history of dissection, size increase 0.3 mm/year (in repeated examinations using the same technique and confirmed by another technique), severe aortic regurgitation, or desire for pregnancy. Erbel et al. (2014).

**19.58.** F. B, C, and D

**19.59.** ESC guidelines.

**19.60.** ESC guidelines for post intervention follow up.

---

**Box 19.1   Clinical Pearls**

---

**Conditions Affecting the Aorta**

- Hypertension
- Atherosclerosis: atheromatous debris
- Genetic conditions such as Marfan syndrome and bicuspid aortic valve
- Infectious causes such as syphilis, mycotic aneurysm
- Trauma
- Inflammatory: vasculitis or arteritis
- Aneurysm, dissection, aortic ulcer, intramural hematoma, aortic rupture, abscess
- Mural thrombi

**Aneurysms of the Aorta**

- Associated with bicuspid aortic valve and Marfan syndrome due to a defect in fibrillin 1 and other components of the arterial medial wall.
- Operate when ascending and abdominal aorta diameter is >5 cm and thoracic aneurysm diameter is >6 cm. Need close follow-up post repair.
- When one aneurysm is detected, look for others, including berry aneurysm of the cerebral arteries and popliteal artery aneurysms.
- Rupture and dissection are the most dreaded complication.
- Stanford type A dissections (entry point proximal to the left subclavian) carries with it mortality of 1–2% per hour and is a surgical emergency. Type B dissections are managed medically with IV beta blockers being the first line of therapy followed by IV vasodilators. Type B dissections require surgery if complicated by organ malperfusion or rupture. CT and TEE are good initial imaging modalities.
- 15–20% of patients may present with intramural hematoma. Intramural hematoma was found to progress to frank dissection in 45% of patients.

**Aortitis**

- Inflammation of the aorta. Causes are syphilis, mycotic, giant-cell arteritis, Takayasu's, ankylosing spondylitis, rheumatoid arthritis, and relapsing polychondritis.
- Thickness of the wall is increased and may be difficult to differentiate from intramural hematoma.
- Thoracic aortic stenosis is most commonly seen in Takayasu's aortitis; syphilis affects the ascending aorta. Ankylosing spondylitis affects the ascending aorta – thickening of the root and nodularities of the aortic valve.

**Atherosclerosis**

- Associated with stroke and embolic events. >4 mm plaques are prone to emboli. Aortic penetrating ulcers can lead to intramural hematoma. Most are hypertensive and present with chest or back pain.

# References

Atkins, M.D. Jr., Black, J.H. 3rd, and Cambria, R.P. (2006). Aortic dissection: perspectives in the era of stent-graft repair. *Journal of Vascular Surgery* 43 (Suppl A): 30A–43A. https://doi.org/10.1016/j.jvs.2005.10.052. PMID: 16473168.

Ben-Shlomo, Y., Spears, M., Boustred, C. et al. (2013). Aortic pulse wave velocity improves cardiovascular event prediction: an individual participant meta-analysis of prospective observational data from 17635 subjects. *Journal of the American College of Cardiology* 93.

Chiu, H.H., Wu, M.H., Wang, J.K. et al. (2013). Losartan added to beta-blockade therapy for aortic root dilation in Marfan syndrome: a ran-domized, open-label pilot study. *Mayo Clinic Proceedings* 88: 271–276. ESC Guidelines 2923 Downloaded from https://academic.oup.com/eurheartj/article/35/41/2873/407693 by Johns Hopkins University user on 26 September 2021.

Delis, K.T. and Gloviczki, P. (2005). Middle aortic syndrome: from presentation to contemporary open surgical and endovascular treatment. *Perspectives in Vascular Surgery and Endovascular Therapy* 17 (3): 187–203.

Erbel, R., Aboyans, V., and Boileau, C. (2014). 2014 ESC guidelines on the diagnosis and treatment of aortic diseases: document covering acute and chronic aortic diseases of the thoracic and abdominal aorta of the adult. The task force for the diagnosis and treatment of aortic diseases of the European Society of Cardiology (ESC). *European Heart Journal* 35: 2873–2926.

Grabenwoger, M., Alfonso, F., Bachet, J. et al. (2012). Thoracic Endovascular Aortic Repair (TEVAR) for the treatment of aortic diseases: a position statement from the European Association for Cardio-Thoracic Surgery (EACTS) and the European Society of Cardiology (ESC), in collaboration with the European Association of Percutaneous Cardiovascular Interventions (EAPCI). *European Heart Journal* 33: 1558–1563.

Groenink, M., den Hartog, A.W., Franken, R. et al. (2013). Losartan reduces aortic dilatation rate in adults with Marfan syndrome: a randomized controlled trial. *European Heart Journal* 34: 3491–3500.

Hovenwalter, E.J. (2009). Chronic mesenteric ischemia: diagnosis and treatment. *Seminars in Interventional Radiology* 26 (4): 345–351.

Jovin, I.S., Duggal, M., Ebisu, K. et al. (2012). Comparison of the effect on long-term outcomes in patients with thoracic aortic aneurysms of taking versus not taking a statin drug. *The American Journal of Cardiology* 109: 1050–1054.

Kitai, T., Kaji, S., Yamamuro, A. et al. (2009). Clinical outcomes of medical therapy and timely operation in initially diagnosed type A aortic intramural hematoma: a 20-year experience. *Circulation* 120: S292–S298.

Lombardi, J.V., Hughes, G.C., Appoo, J.J. et al. (2020). Society for Vascular Surgery (SVS) and Society of Thoracic Surgeons (STS) reporting standards for type B aortic dissections. *Journal of Vascular Surgery* 71 (3): 723–747. https://doi.org/10.1016/j.jvs.2019.11.013. Epub 2020 Jan 27. PMID: 32001058.

Losenno, K.L., Goodman, R.L., and Chu, M.W.A. (2012). Bicuspid aortic valve disease and ascending aortic aneurysms: gaps in knowledge. *Cardiology Research and Practice* 2012: 145202.

Matura, L.A., Ho, V.B., Rosing, D.R., and Bondy, C.A. (2007). Aortic dilatation and dissection in turner syndrome. *Circulation* 116: 1663–1670.

Rizzi, R., Bruno, S., Stellacci, C., and Dammacco, R. (1999). Takayasu's arteritis: a cell-mediated large-vessel vasculitis. *International Journal of Clinical and Laboratory Research* 29 (1): 8–13.

Shores, J., Berger, K.R., Murphy, E.A., and Pyeritz, R.E. (1994). Progression of aortic dilatation and the benefit of long-term beta-adrenergic blockade in Marfan's syndrome. *The New England Journal of Medicine* 330: 1335–1341.

Shrestha, M., Bachet, J., Bavaria, J. et al. (2015). Current status and recommendations for use of the frozen elephant trunk technique: a position paper by the Vascular Domain of EACTS. *European Journal of Cardiothoracic Surgery* 47 (5): 759–769.

Stein, L.H., Berger, J., Tranquilli, M., and Elefteraides, J.A. (2013). Effect of statin drugs on thoracic aortic aneurysms. *The American Journal of Cardiology* 112: 1240–1245.

Vlachopoulos, C., Aznaouridis, K., O'Rourke, M.F. et al. (2010). Prediction of cardiovascular events all-cause mortality with central haemodynamics: asystematic review, meta-analysis. *European Heart Journal* 31: 1865–1871.

White, G.H., May, J., and Petrasek, P. (2000). Specific complications of endovascular aortic repair. *Seminars in Interventional Cardiology* 5: 35–46.

Yudin, A. (ed.) (2014). Cobweb Sign and Mercedes-Benz Sign. In: *Metaphorical Signs in Computed Tomography of Chest and Abdomen*, 71–72. Cham: Springer International Publishing.

# Carotid and Vertebral Artery Disease

# 20

20.1. The arch angiogram in Figure 20.1a demonstrates which type of aortic arch morphology?
   A. Type I
   B. Type II
   C. Type III
   D. Type IV

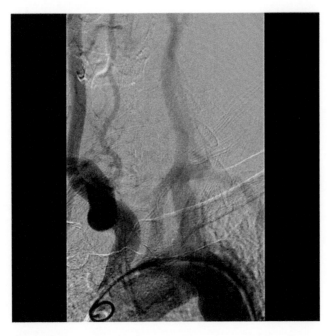

Figure 20.1a

20.2. What does the term "bovine" arch refer to?
   A. The aortic arch morphology in cattle
   B. A shared common origin of the brachiocephalic and left common carotid arteries
   C. A shared common origin of the left subclavian and common carotid arteries
   D. A shared common origin of the left and right common carotid arteries

*Cardiology Board Review*, Second Edition. Ramdas G. Pai and Padmini Varadarajan.
© 2023 John Wiley & Sons Ltd. Published 2023 by John Wiley & Sons Ltd.

20.3. Which of the following is the most frequent cause of extracranial cerebrovascular disease?
   A. Fibromuscular dysplasia
   B. Cystic medial necrosis
   C. Atherosclerosis
   D. Arteritis

20.4. A 74-year-old man presents for a routine clinical follow-up. He has a 20 pack-year smoking history, having quit smoking 10 years previously, hypertension, and diabetes mellitus. He is clinically asymptomatic and functionally independent. Physical examination is normal with the exception of an audible bruit over the right carotid artery. Which of the following is the most appropriate recommendation?
   A. Medication optimization and continued abstinence from cigarette smoking
   B. Medication optimization and continued abstinence from cigarette smoking and a carotid duplex ultrasound
   C. Medication optimization and continued abstinence from cigarette smoking and a magnetic resonance angiography (MRA) of the head and neck
   D. Medication optimization and continued abstinence from cigarette smoking and a computed tomography (CT) of the head and neck

20.5. A 50-year-old woman presents for a routine clinical evaluation. She has a past medical history of gastroesophageal reflux disease and bipolar disorders. She is a nonsmoker. Physical examination is normal with the exception of an audible bruit over the right carotid artery. An electrocardiogram demonstrates sinus rhythm with nonspecific ST-T wave changes. Which of the following is the most appropriate recommendation?
   A. Medication optimization and routine healthcare maintenance
   B. Medication optimization and routine healthcare maintenance and carotid duplex ultrasonography
   C. Medication optimization and routine healthcare maintenance and MRA of the head and neck
   D. Medication optimization and routine healthcare maintenance and CT of the head and neck

20.6. An 80-year-old right-handed woman with a past medical history of coronary artery disease, sinus node dysfunction status post pacemaker implantation, and hypertension presents to the emergency department. Her laboratory assessment and electrocardiogram are essentially normal. Her daughter reports that she noted her mother was having some word-finding difficulty on the telephone. She also appeared to be bumping into objects to her left and appeared as though she had not seen them. Ischemia or infarction in which arterial distribution most likely explains this patient's deficits?
   A. Left vertebral artery
   B. Left internal carotid artery
   C. Right vertebral artery
   D. Right internal carotid artery

20.7. Bilateral carotid duplex ultrasonography is performed in the patient in Question 20.6. Which criteria are most commonly utilized in assessing the severity of internal carotid artery stenosis by ultrasonography?
A. Visual estimation of the degree of internal carotid stenosis and comparison with the normal-caliber vessel distal to the stenotic segment
B. Measurement of the peak systolic velocity in the internal carotid artery and its ratio with the peak systolic velocity in the external carotid artery
C. Measurement of the peak systolic velocity in the internal carotid artery and its ratio with the peak systolic velocity in the common carotid artery
D. Measurement of the end-diastolic velocity in the internal carotid artery

20.8. The carotid duplex ultrasound performed on the patient in Question 20.6 has equivocal results due to conflicting velocity and ratio data. Which of the following would be the most appropriate next step?
A. MRA
B. Repeat carotid duplex ultrasonography with pre-sedation
C. Conventional catheter-based angiography
D. CT

20.9. Which of the following treatment strategies is not effective in stroke prevention given the current evidence-based literature?
A. Intensive glucose control and hemoglobin A1c reduction in a patient with diabetes mellitus type 2
B. Interventions aimed at lowering blood pressure below 140/90 mmHg
C. Initiation of high-dose statin medication in patients with recent stroke or transient ischemic attack (TIA)
D. Smoking cessation

20.10. Which of the following antiplatelet regimens is not indicated in reduction of stroke risk in an asymptomatic patient with carotid or vertebral artery atherosclerosis?
A. Aspirin 75–325 mg daily
B. Clopidogrel 75 mg daily
C. Aspirin 75–325 mg plus clopidogrel 75 mg daily
D. Aspirin plus extended-release dipyridamole twice daily
E. Aspirin plus low-dose (2.5 mg twice daily) rivaroxaban

20.11. Which of the following is the recommended method of assessing stenosis severity on angiography?
A. Minimal residual lumen through the zone of stenosis is compared with the estimated diameter of the carotid bulb
B. Minimal residual lumen through the zone of stenosis is compared with the estimated diameter of the common carotid artery
C. Minimal residual lumen through the zone of stenosis is compared with the French size of the diagnostic catheter used during angiography
D. Minimal residual lumen through the zone of stenosis is compared with the diameter of the distal internal carotid artery

20.12. A 68-year-old patient with a past medical history of hypertension and dyslipidemia presents to the hospital with left motor deficit for seven hours. He has a 20 pack-year smoking history. He was previously active. He does not have any active cardiopulmonary disease. A carotid duplex ultrasound demonstrates >70% right internal carotid artery stenosis. Carotid angiography is shown in Figure 20.12. Which of the following is the most effective treatment?

A. Optimization of medical therapy with a target blood pressure less than 130/80 mmHg and initiation of statin therapy in addition to smoking cessation counseling

B. Optimization of medical therapy with a target blood pressure less than 130/80 mmHg and initiation of statin therapy in addition to smoking cessation counseling plus carotid endarterectomy within two weeks

C. Optimization of medical therapy with a target blood pressure less than 130/80 mmHg and initiation of statin therapy in addition to smoking cessation counseling plus carotid artery stenting within two weeks

D. Optimization of medical therapy with a target blood pressure less than 130/80 mmHg and initiation of statin therapy in addition to smoking cessation counseling and discharge after stabilization; revascularization only if recurrent events

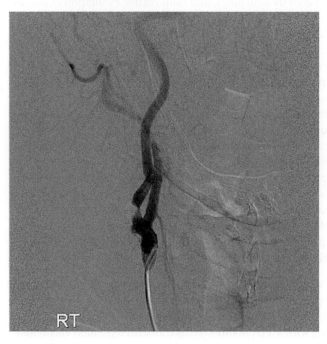

Figure 20.12

20.13. Which of the following patients would not be considered high risk for a carotid endarterectomy?

A. An 84-year-old man with a prior history of stroke. Carotid angiography now demonstrates a complete occlusion of the right internal carotid artery and a high-grade stenosis in the proximal left internal carotid artery

B. A 75-year-old woman with a prior history of head and neck radiation for previous cancer now presents two weeks after an ischemic stroke. Carotid angiography demonstrates a high-grade right internal carotid artery stenosis. The left internal carotid artery is widely patent.

C. A 68-year-old man with a history of inferior wall myocardial infarction one year previously which was treated with implantation of a drug-eluting stent in the right coronary artery. He also has a history of diet-controlled diabetes mellitus type 2. He now presents with a left middle cerebral artery territory ischemic stroke. MRA demonstrates a high-grade left internal carotid artery stenosis. The right internal carotid artery is widely patent.

D. A 76-year-old man with a history of coronary artery disease, hypertension, and chronic left ventricular systolic dysfunction presents with dysarthria and right-sided motor deficit. MRI demonstrates an ischemic stroke. He was discharged from the hospital three weeks previously after undergoing coronary artery bypass graft surgery. His post-surgical course was uncomplicated. His estimated left ventricular ejection fraction prior to discharge was 30%.

20.14. A 72-year-old man with a past medical history of hypertension, dyslipidemia, and diabetes mellitus type 2 presents to the hospital with transient left-sided hemiparesis. He is evaluated by neurology, and noninvasive evaluation confirms a high-grade stenosis of the right internal carotid artery. He undergoes carotid endarterectomy with an uncomplicated post-operative course. He now presents to the outpatient clinical for post-discharge follow-up. Which of the following is correct regarding his ongoing management?

A. He should be on aspirin in addition to his antihypertensive and lipid-lowering medication and should have a follow-up carotid ultrasound in one month.

B. He should be continued on antihypertensive and lipid-lowering medication and have a follow-up carotid duplex ultrasound in one month. Aspirin is not indicated as he does not have a documented history of coronary artery disease and the bleeding risk is too high.

C. He should be on aspirin in addition to antihypertensive medications. A carotid duplex ultrasound should be performed in one month. Lipid-lowering medication is not indicated as he has had a successfully uncomplicated carotid endarterectomy unless he has markedly elevated lipid levels.

D. He should be on aspirin in addition to his antihypertensive and lipid-lowering medications. Carotid duplex ultrasound is not indicated for one year.

20.15. An 81-year-old man with a prior history of coronary artery disease, chronic obstructive pulmonary disease, hypertension and diabetes mellitus presents to the clinical for post-discharge follow-up. He was recently discharged from the hospital after presenting with a TIA manifested as transient left-sided vision loss. He is dependent on 2l of oxygen via nasal cannula but is otherwise functioning independently. He had a coronary artery bypass graft surgery about 10 years previously and has not had recurrent angina. Examination reveals a left carotid bruit and carotid duplex ultrasound demonstrates a greater than 70% left internal carotid artery stenosis confirmed by MRA. What would be the best treatment recommendation?

A. Start aspirin, optimize medical therapy, and follow with serial duplex ultrasound; no carotid intervention is indicated given his age and comorbidities
B. Start aspirin, optimize medical therapy, and refer for carotid endarterectomy
C. Start aspirin, optimize medical therapy, and refer for carotid artery stenting
D. Start aspirin, optimize medical therapy only; order a CT angiogram of the head and neck

20.16. An 85-year old man with a past medical history of hypertension, coronary artery bypass graft surgery, oxygen-dependent chronic obstructive pulmonary disease, and a TIA is referred for carotid angiography. The results are shown in Figure 20.16. He is deemed high risk for carotid endarterectomy and a decision is made to proceed with carotid artery stenting. Which of the following statements is true regarding peri-procedural management?
  A. Hemodynamic instability is rare because you are not working on the coronary circulation; therefore, any issues can be addressed on an *ad hoc* basis as the procedure should be performed quickly
  B. If bradycardia develops, a temporary pacemaker should be immediately inserted, as it is likely to be persistent
  C. If persistent hypotension develops, intravenous phenylephrine should be easily accessible and immediately administered
  D. The patient should be heavily sedated to facilitate rapid completion of the procedure

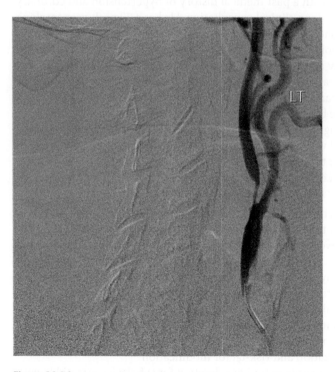

Figure 20.16

20.17. The patient in Question 20.16 has an uncomplicated post-procedure course and is discharged home the following day. He now presents to the clinic for a follow-up visit. Which of the following is the appropriate post-procedural management strategy?

A. Aspirin and clopidogrel for at least 30 days in addition to antihypertensive medication

B. Aspirin alone in addition to antihypertensive medication

C. No antiplatelet therapy is indicated given the large caliber of the stent and the fact that it is not a drug-eluting device; continue antihypertensive medication

D. Aspirin and clopidogrel for at least 30 days; hold antihypertensive medication to allow systolic hypertension given the history of TIA and carotid stenting

20.18. Which of the following has been demonstrated in the literature regarding the comparative efficacy of carotid artery stenting and carotid endarterectomy?

A. Carotid endarterectomy has a lower risk for death and stroke, while carotid artery stenting has a shorter length of stay and myocardial infarction

B. Carotid artery stenting has a lower risk of myocardial infarction and stroke

C. Carotid endarterectomy and carotid artery stenting have been shown to be equivalent across all endpoints as long as patient selection is performed diligently

D. Carotid endarterectomy is associated with a lower rate of peri-procedural stroke, while carotid artery stenting is associated with a lower rate of peri-procedural myocardial infarction or cranial nerve injury

20.19. A 68-year-old patient with a past medical history of hypertension and coronary artery disease presents for a clinical consultation. He has a 20 pack-year smoking history. He reports that he has intermittent episodes of dizziness and sometimes feels that he has double vision. He thinks that his symptoms are from cervical arthritis because they are more noticeable when he turns his head. He has also noted ringing in his years. These symptoms have been present for several months. He has been seen by an ENT specialist and the evaluation was negative. Which of the following is the best diagnostic test?

A. He likely has benign positional vertigo; therefore, empiric medical therapy should be initiated without any further imaging

B. CT angiography of the head and neck

C. Duplex ultrasound of the great vessels

D. Referral to another ENT specialist for a second opinion

20.20. A 75-year-old man with a past medical history of hypertension, dyslipidemia, and diabetes mellitus type 2 presents to establish himself as a new patient. He quit smoking about five years previously but has a 40 pack-year smoking history. He is physically active and has no complaints of chest pain or disproportionate dyspnea. He denies any dizziness or lightheadedness. He is an avid tennis player and denies any limitations during his game. Physical examination demonstrates a loud left infraclavicular bruit. A duplex ultrasound demonstrates a left subclavian artery stenosis with flow reversal in the ipsilateral vertebral artery? What is the most appropriate treatment strategy?

A. Medication optimization and risk-factor modification

B. Referral to a vascular surgeon for consideration for subclavian-carotid bypass

C. Referral to an endovascular specialist for consideration for percutaneous intervention on the subclavian artery

D. Instruct him to limit left-arm utilization to prevent disease progression

20.21. A 35-year-old patient presents with severe right-sided neck discomfort after a bout of coughing. She also thinks that she may have had transient blindness in the right eye. She has no known past medical history. Physical examination reveals that her right eyelid is drooping. Which of the following is the most appropriate next step in her management?

A. Immediate referral to an ophthalmologist as she likely has a detached retina

B. Reassurance, as she likely has whiplash with self-limiting symptoms

C. CT angiography of the head and neck

D. Catheter-based angiography of the great vessels

20.22. The patient in Question 20.21 undergoes a CT angiography which demonstrates a right carotid artery dissection. Which is the most appropriate initial therapeutic modality?

A. Surgical bypass

B. Carotid stenting

C. Anticoagulation with heparin followed by warfarin

D. No specific therapy is indicated as, in an otherwise young healthy individual, the dissection will heal over time

20.23. Which one of the following factors is not known to be associated with increased risk of stroke in asymptomatic patients?

A. Concomitant left main coronary artery disease

B. Contralateral TIA/stroke

C. Intra-plaque hemorrhage noted on MRA

D. Ipsilateral silent infarction on cerebral imaging

E. Large, echolucent plaque noted on arterial duplex imaging

20.24. What is the optimal timing of carotid endarterectomy (CEA) of a significant carotid stenosis (>70%) after an admission for ipsilateral ischemic stroke?

A. Within 24 hours of admission

B. Between 24 and 48 hours of admission

C. Between 48 hours and two weeks after admission for stroke

D. More than six weeks after admission for stroke

20.25. Which of the following antithrombotic regimens are not recommended for secondary prevention of stroke in a patient with ipsilateral severe carotid stenosis and recent TIA/stroke?

A. Aspirin 325 mg daily

B. Warfarin with a target INR of 2–3

C. Combination of aspirin 81 daily and clopidogrel 75 daily for up to 90 days

D. Combination of aspirin 81 daily and ticagrelor 90 twice daily for up to 30 days

20.26. A 52-year-old woman presents to the ER with complaints of left-sided headache with "dizziness" and "floaters" in her left visual field that started about an hour previously. These symptoms were associated with nausea, generalized weakness and a near-syncopal episode. CT/MRI head did not show evidence for an acute stroke. A left carotid bruit is heard on auscultation and a carotid duplex demon-

strated 50–69% stenosis in the left internal carotid artery and <50% stenosis in the right internal carotid artery. What is the next best step?
A. Aggressive cardiovascular risk factor modification alone
B. Refer for carotid angiography to confirm diagnosis
C. Refer for carotid endarterectomy
D. Refer for carotid artery stenting

20.27. A 75-year-old man with a history of hypertension, diabetes, dyslipidemia, and coronary artery disease with stent placement last year presents to the ER with complaints of left-sided weakness and word-finding difficulties that started about eight hours prior to presentation. He is also a chronic smoker with a 45 pack-year smoking history. An urgent non-contrast CT of the brain revealed a large ischemic infarction involving the right middle cerebral artery. CT of the neck showed an occluded right internal carotid artery and a 50–69% stenosis in the left internal carotid artery. What is the next best step?
A. Revascularization of the right internal carotid artery
B. Revascularization of the left internal carotid artery
C. Revascularization of both internal carotid arteries
D. Aggressive cardiovascular risk factor modification alone

20.28. What percentage of ischemic stroke are attributed to cervical carotid disease?
A. <10%
B. 10–30%
C. 50–70%
D. >90%

20.29. Cerebral hyper-perfusion syndrome (CHS) is a clinical syndrome seen after carotid revascularization procedures. The following is true about CHS.
A. It is seen following carotid artery stenting but not after carotid endarterectomy
B. Patients usually present with headache contralateral to the intervention side
C. Cerebral blood flow studies such as transcranial doppler, perfusion CT or quantitative MRI aid in diagnosis of CHS
D. Pacemaker placement is required to treat severe sinus bradycardia

20.30. The following is true about intracranial endovascular therapy (EVT) for acute stroke interventions:
A. It can only be offered to patients presenting within six hours
B. Administration of tPA precludes further EVT
C. EVT usually includes mechanical thrombectomy but intracranial stenting is generally not recommended
D. Patients should be loaded with antiplatelets immediately after the procedure

## Answers

20.1. B. Type II.
   The three types of aortic arch morphologies are determined by the relationship of the brachiocephalic trunk to the aortic arch. In type I morphology, the origin of all three great vessels originates from the same linear plane (defined by

the outer curvature of the arch). In type II, the brachiocephalic trunk originates from a plane between the outer and inner curvatures of the aortic arch as demonstrated in Figure 20.1b. In type III, it originates below the inner curvature of the aortic arch.

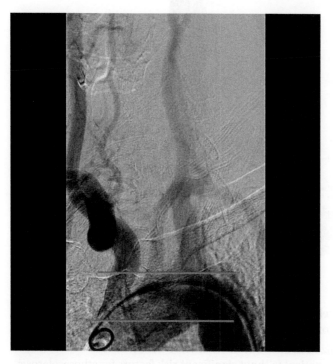

Figure 20.1b

20.2. B. A shared common origin of the brachiocephalic and left common carotid arteries.

The bovine arch is a variant of normal arch anatomy in which the brachiocephalic artery (black arrow in Figure 20.2) and the left common carotid (brown arrow in Figure 20.2) artery share a common origin from the aortic arch. This term is a misnomer as this common anatomic variant noted in humans bears no resemblance to the aortic arch of ruminant animals such as cows and buffalo.

20.3. C. Atherosclerosis.

Systemic atherosclerosis remains the most frequent cause of extracranial cerebrovascular disease. Other causes, such as fibromuscular dysplasia, cystic medial necrosis, arteritis, and dissection, are much less prevalent.

Chapter 2

20.4. B. Medication optimization and continued abstinence from cigarette smoking and a carotid duplex ultrasound.

In a patient with multiple atherosclerotic risk factors and an asymptomatic carotid bruit, a carotid duplex ultrasound should be performed in addition to medication optimization and risk-factor modification. However, it should be

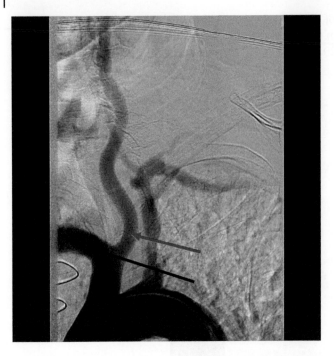

Figure 20.2

noted that a bruit itself is more likely a marker of the systemic atherosclerosis rather than a marker of significant carotid artery stenosis.

20.5. A. Medication optimization and routine healthcare maintenance.

In an asymptomatic patient without significant risk factors for atherosclerosis, there is no indication for further diagnostic evaluation of a carotid bruit. The positive predictive value for a significant carotid stenosis in such a patient is relatively low. Therefore, the best course of action is to continue with medication optimization and routine healthcare maintenance.

20.6. B. Left internal carotid artery.

Ischemia in the left internal carotid artery may lead to right-sided motor and sensory deficit. It may also cause aphasia, often manifested as word-finding difficulty. Left-sided monocular blindness is another manifestation. Vertebrobasilar system insufficiency most often results in ataxia, a lack of coordination, dizziness, and cranial nerve deficits. Right internal carotid artery ischemia may lead to left-sided motor and sensory deficits, monocular blindness affecting the right eye, and left-sided neglect, among other symptoms. Aphasia may be seen in patients with right internal carotid ischemia, and in those who are left-handed or ambidextrous.

20.7. C. Measurement of the peak systolic velocity in the internal carotid artery and its ratio with the peak systolic velocity in the common carotid artery.

The consensus is that peak velocity in the internal carotid artery, the ratio of the systolic velocities in the internal and *common* carotid artery, *as well as* the end-diastolic velocity in the internal carotid artery can be used in estimating the degree of stenosis within the internal carotid artery. Table 20.1 provides a rough guideline.

Table 20.1 Society for Radiologists in Ultrasound (SRU) Consensus Criteria to assess severity of ICA stenosis using duplex ultrasound.

| Degree of stenosis (%) | Peak systolic velocity ICA (cm/s) | ICA: CCA ratio | End-diastolic velocity ICA (cm/s) |
|---|---|---|---|
| Normal | <125 | <2 | <40 |
| <50 | <125 | <2 | <40 |
| 50–69 | 125–230 | 2–4 | 40–100 |
| >70 | >230 | >4 | >100 |

CCA: common carotid artery; ICA: internal carotid artery.

20.8. D. CT.

Though carotid duplex ultrasonography is the most cost-effective first diagnostic test in evaluating carotid stenosis, the possibility of equivocal results often necessitates further testing. Alternatives include conventional catheter-based angiography, MRA, and computed angiography. The choice of testing modality is often dependent on institutional availability and expertise. MRA provides a highly sensitive and specific alternative in assessing the carotid vasculature for stenosis. However, its use is limited in patients with implantable devices such as pacemakers and defibrillators, and those with morbid obesity and claustrophobia. In addition, there is a tendency for overestimation of stenosis severity. CT angiography also provides an excellent alternative and would be the test of choice in this individual given the presence of a pacemaker. Its sensitivity and specificity are comparable to conventional angiography. Heavy calcification leads to a decrease in sensitivity and specificity. In addition, the requirement for use of iodinated contrast material limits its use in those with significant renal dysfunction. Catheter-based conventional angiography remains the gold standard for vascular imaging, but it should be used as the last option given its associated costs and the risks associated with an invasive procedure. It may be used when the aforementioned contraindications preclude the use of noninvasive modalities.

20.9. A. Intensive glucose control and hemoglobin A1c reduction in a patient with diabetes mellitus type 2.

Intensive glucose control and reduction of hemoglobin A1c levels below 7% has not been shown to reduce the risk to stroke in patients with diabetes mellitus type 2 in several contemporary clinical trials. The other modalities stated in this question, including blood pressure reduction, high-dose statin, and smoking cessation, have in fact been associated with significant reductions in strokes. Hyperhomocysteinemia is another biochemical abnormality associated with increased risk of stroke. The administration of vitamins, mainly B vitamins, does lower plasma homocysteine levels, but without an effect of stroke risk.

20.10. C. Aspirin 75–325 mg plus clopidogrel 75 mg daily.

Aspirin plus clopidogrel has not been shown to be more effective than either therapy alone in the reduction of stroke risk in clinical trials. Aspirin alone, clopidogrel alone, and the combination of aspirin plus extended-release dipyridamole or aspirin and low-dose rivaroxaban (COMPASS trial), on the other hand, have demonstrated efficacy in the reduction in stroke risk.

20.11. D. Minimal residual lumen through the zone of stenosis is compared with the diameter of the distal internal carotid artery.

The North American Symptomatic Carotid Endarterectomy Trial (NASCET) criteria, which compare the zone of stenosis with the diameter of the distal normal segment of internal carotid artery, are the most commonly used criteria for estimating the degree of stenosis. These criteria have led to the delineation of cutoffs of degrees of stenosis most likely to benefit from carotid revascularization.

20.12. B. Optimization of medical therapy with a target blood pressure less than 130/80 mmHg and initiation of statin therapy in addition to smoking cessation counseling plus carotid endarterectomy within two weeks.

In patients with symptomatic carotid stenosis of greater than 70% by noninvasive assessment and >50% by invasive assessment, revascularization after 48 hours but within two weeks is indicated in addition to medical optimization if the perioperative morbidity and mortality risk is estimated to be <6%. The rates of death, stroke, or TIA are significantly higher with medical therapy alone in this group of patients.

20.13. C. A 68-year-old man with a history of inferior wall myocardial infarction one year previously which was treated with implantation of a drug-eluting stent in the right coronary artery. He also has a history of diet-controlled diabetes mellitus type 2. He now presents with a left middle cerebral artery territory ischemic stroke. MRA demonstrates a high-grade left internal carotid artery stenosis. The right internal carotid artery is widely patent.

Clinical characteristics considered high risk for a carotid endarterectomy include contralateral carotid occlusion or stenosis greater than 50%, significant cardiopulmonary disease, a history of radical neck surgery or radiation, prior history of coronary artery bypass graft, age greater than 80 years, and New York Heart Association class III/IV heart failure. Previous carotid endarterectomy or carotid stenting is also among high-risk features.

20.14. A. The patient should be on aspirin in addition to his antihypertensive and lipid-lowering medication and should have a follow-up carotid ultrasound in one month.

Aggressive secondary prevention measures are indicated in all patients after successful carotid revascularization. This includes antiplatelet therapy with aspirin and continued medical optimization of cardiovascular risk factors. Carotid duplex ultrasonography is recommended at intervals of one month, six months, and annually thereafter until serial examinations demonstrate stability.

20.15. C. Start aspirin, optimize medical therapy, and refer for carotid artery stenting.

Revascularization is clearly indicated in this symptomatic patient with demonstration of carotid stenosis in the area of cerebral ischemia. Given his multiple risk factors, he would be a candidate for carotid artery stenting.

20.16. C. If persistent hypotension develops, intravenous phenylephrine should be easily accessible and immediately administered.

Transient hemodynamic instability in the form of bradycardia or hypotension is not rare during the carotid stenting procedure. Atropine and phenylephrine should be readily available in the catheterization laboratory and immediately administered in the event of hemodynamic instability. A temporary pacemaker should only be inserted in the event of persistent bradycardia not responsive to intravenous atropine. The patient should be minimally sedated so that neurologic status can be assessed throughout the procedure.

20.17. A. Aspirin and clopidogrel for at least 30 days in addition to antihypertensive medication.

Dual antiplatelet therapy with aspirin and clopidogrel is recommended for at least 30 days, as there is a risk for stent thrombosis while the stent endothelializes. In addition, after the acute hospital course, risk factors should be managed as per national guidelines, and there is no role for permissive hypertension after the acute hospitalization.

20.18. D. Carotid endarterectomy is associated with a lower rate of peri-procedural stoke, while carotid artery stenting is associated with a lower rate of peri-procedural myocardial infarction or cranial nerve injury.

Meta-analysis has demonstrated that carotid endarterectomy and stenting have comparable rates of stroke, death, or myocardial infarction over the 30-day and 1-year periods. However, carotid endarterectomy has been associated with a lower risk of peri-procedural stroke, which has translated to a high risk of peri-procedural mortality. Carotid artery stenting, on the other hand, is associated with a lower risk of peri-procedural myocardial infarction and cranial nerve injury.

20.19. B. CT angiography of the head and neck.

This patient's symptoms may be stemming from vertebrobasilar insufficiency. Symptoms of dizziness, diplopia, and tinnitus, though not specific, can be attributable to the vertebrobasilar system when taken together. Ultrasound has a lower sensitivity and specificity for detecting significant vertebral artery disease. The test of choice should be a CT angiogram or MRA. Catheter-based angiography may be needed prior to consideration for revascularization to reliably identify the origin of the vertebral arteries.

20.20. A. Medication optimization and risk-factor modification.

This patient has asymptomatic subclavian artery stenosis with steal syndrome as demonstrated by flow reversal in the ipsilateral vertebral artery. There is no indication for revascularization in such a patient, whether surgical or endovascular, unless the ipsilateral internal mammary artery is required for surgical myocardial revascularization. Medical optimization and risk-factor modification should continue to prevent acute cardiovascular events.

20.21. C. CT angiography of the head and neck.

Chapter 2

This patient's symptoms are concerning for spontaneous carotid artery dissection and should be further evaluated with a CT angiogram.

20.22. C. Anticoagulation with heparin followed by warfarin.

Initial therapy for a spontaneous carotid dissection is usually anticoagulation with heparin followed by warfarin for three to six months. Revascularization is reserved for patients who continue to exhibit recurrent symptoms despite adequate anticoagulation.

20.23. A. Concomitant left main coronary artery disease.

Concomitant left main coronary artery disease is considered a risk factor for identification of carotid artery disease in asymptomatic patients, however, this does not predict occurrence of a future stroke/TIA. Findings of clinical contralateral stroke/TIA, ipsilateral silent infarction on cerebral imaging, duplex findings of large, echolucent plaques and MRA finding of intraplaque hemorrhage or lipid-rich necrotic core are considered high risk factors for stroke in asymptomatic patients.

20.24. C. Between 48 hours and two weeks after admission for stroke.

Most professional societies recommend CEA of a culprit ipsilateral carotid stenosis (70–99% stenosis) to be performed within the first two weeks after a TIA or non-disabling stroke. However, a large study (Stromberg et al. 2012) reported high perioperative risk when CEA is performed within the first 48 hours after a stroke. So, the ideal time to perform CEA would be between day 3 and 14 after the index event.

20.25. B. Warfarin with a target INR of 2–3.

As per the 2021 AHA/ASA Guidelines for Prevention of Stroke in Patients with stroke and TIA (Kleindorfer et al. 2021), aspirin 325 mg is recommended over warfarin (Class I recommendation) for secondary prevention. A combination of aspirin and clopidogrel for up to 90 days carries a Class IIA recommendation and a combination of low-dose aspirin and ticagrelor for 30 days (based on results of the THALES trial) carries a Class IIB recommendation.

20.26. A. Aggressive cardiovascular risk-factor modification alone.

It is particularly important to differentiate symptomatic from asymptomatic carotid artery stenosis as this will change the management strategy. A patient is considered symptomatic if he/she experiences a transient or permanent loss of vision in the ipsilateral eye with or without focal neurologic symptoms (weakness/numbness) in the contralateral cerebral hemisphere within the previous six months. Based on the dominant hemisphere, patients may also present with aphasia, dysarthria, or visual field defects. Non-specific symptoms such as headache, "dizziness," syncopal episodes, or positive visual phenomena such as floaters in the visual field do not qualify as symptomatic carotid artery stenosis even in the presence of high-grade stenosis (>70%). Initial management of asymptomatic carotid artery stenosis should focus on modifying cardiovascular risk by starting antiplatelet therapy with aspirin, encouraging smoking cessation, regular exercise, weight loss and dietary modification, as well as aggressive control of vascular risk factors (Hassani and Fischer 2022).

20.27. D. Aggressive cardiovascular risk-factor modification alone.

Both the American and European guidelines recommend best medical therapy alone for patients with near-total or total occlusion of an ipsilateral internal carotid artery as a Class I recommendation. The contralateral moderate internal carotid artery stenosis in this patient is an incidental finding that does not require revascularization.

20.28. B. 10–30%.

Approximately 10–30% of ischemic strokes are attributed to cervical carotid disease. Some small observational studies quote ranges somewhat higher or lower than this, but overall the incidence is generally within this range. This concept is important to understand vis-à-vis coronary artery disease whereby nearly 90% of angina or myocardial infarction is caused by epicardial coronary artery disease.

20.29. C. Cerebral blood flow studies such as transcranial Doppler, perfusion CT or quantitative MRI aid in diagnosis of CHS.

Cerebral hyper-perfusion syndrome (CHS) is a rare but potentially lethal complication that could be seen after either carotid endarterectomy or carotid artery stenting. The typical risk profile includes treatment of high-grade stenosis in a patient with history of hypertension and contralateral occlusion. Impaired cerebral vascular autoregulation is believed to be the underlying pathophysiology. Patients usually present with ipsilateral or diffuse headache in the setting of uncontrolled HTN but may also have severe symptoms of focal neurologic deficits or seizures. Imaging modalities listed are typically used for diagnosis. Treatment strategies are directed toward BP control.

20.30. C. EVT usually includes mechanical thrombectomy but intracranial stenting is not generally recommended.

Endovascular therapy for acute ischemic stroke has evolved in recent years and is now considered the gold standard in select patients with large vessel occlusion. It was initially offered to patients presenting within six hours but now can be offered up to 24 hours in patients with mismatch between deficit and infarct as evaluated by perfusion imaging. It can also be offered to patients who have received tPA. This includes mechanical thrombectomy but intracranial stenting is not routinely done. For the same reason (no intracranial stent placement), antiplatelets are not started within the first 24 hours after a stroke.

## References

Hassani, S. and Fisher, M. (2022). Management of atherosclerotic carotid artery disease: a brief overview and update. *American Journal of Medicine* 135 (4): 430–434.

Kleindorfer, D.O., Towfighi, A., Chaturvedi, S. et al. (2021). Guideline for the prevention of stroke in patients with stroke and transient ischemic attack: a guideline from the American Heart Association. *Stroke* 52 (7): e3643–e3467.

Strömberg, S., Gelin, J., Osterberg, T. et al. (2012). Very urgent carotid endarterectomy confers increased procedural risk. *Stroke* 43 (5): 1331–1335.

# Peripheral Vascular Disease

# 21

**21.1.** Cigarette smoking increases the odds ratio of peripheral vascular disease by which of the following?
- A. Sevenfold
- B. Threefold
- C. Ninefold
- D. Twofold
- E. None of the above

**21.2.** The underlying mechanism(s) of peripheral vascular disease is/are which of the following?
- A. Atherosclerosis
- B. Hypoperfusion
- C. Artery spasm
- D. A and C

**21.3.** The highest incidence worldwide of peripheral vascular disease is seen in which of the following populations?
- A. Asian Indians
- B. Native American Indians
- C. Indo-Caribbeans
- D. Eskimo Indians

**21.4.** Which of the following is/are correct about peripheral vascular disease (PVD)?
- A. Framingham risk score >10% has a higher incidence of PVD
- B. Aspirin does not appear to help those with mild disease
- C. Leg pain worsened by standing in one place but better with walking
- D. Age over 70 years is associated with higher prevalence of PVD
- E. All of the above

**21.5.** A 30-year-old male 6 ft. 8 in tall, myopic, presents with left-sided transient ischemic attack. This patient is at high risk for what other conditions or what features?
- A. High incidence of venous thromboembolism in postoperative state
- B. Abnormal lower extremity pulse examination
- C. Bony abnormalities
- D. Shortened life span
- E. Autosomal recessive inheritance
- F. Autosomal dominant inheritance
- G. A, B, C, D, and E
- H. A, B, C, D, and F

**21.6.** Which of the following statements regarding smoking cannabis is/are correct?
- A. Causes arteritis picture similar Burger's disease
- B. 8–8- and £-9-tetrahydrocanabinols cause severe vasospasm
- C. May cause strokes
- D. Venous thrombosis may occur
- E. All of the above

*Cardiology Board Review*, Second Edition. Ramdas G. Pai and Padmini Varadarajan.
© 2023 John Wiley & Sons Ltd. Published 2023 by John Wiley & Sons Ltd.

**21.7.** Which of the following statement(s) is/are true regarding ankle brachial index (ABI)?
A. An ABI of 1.5 is associated with high cardiovascular mortality
B. Is the first-line study upon suspicion peripheral arterial disease (PAD)
C. A decrease in ABI of 15–20% after exercise would be diagnostic of PAD
D. An ABI of 0.4 is associated with high cardiovascular mortality
E. All of the above

**21.8.** A 60-year-old male has a history of smoking and hypertension and complains of intermittent claudication. His ABI is 0.7. What is the best next step?
A. Computed tomography (CT) of lower extremities
B. Magnetic resonance angiography (MRA) of lower extremities
C. Doppler ultrasound of lower extremities
D. Angiography
E. Cardiac risk-factor modification and a supervised exercise regimen

**21.9.** Which of the following is used for PAD classification?
A. Trans-Atlantic Inter-Society Consensus (TASC) II
B. Wound, ischemia, and foot infection (WIfI)
C. Fontaine stages
D. Robert B. Rutherford
E. All of the above

**21.10.** Which of the following is/are correct?
A. Individuals with PAD have an exceptionally elevated risk for cardiovascular events
B. The majority will eventually die of a cardiac or cerebrovascular etiology
C. Prognosis is correlated with the severity of the PAD as measured by the ankle-brachial pressure index (ABPI)
D. Large-vessel PAD increases mortality from cardiovascular disease significantly
E. PAD carries a greater than 20% risk of a coronary event in 10 years
F. All of the above

**21.11.** Which of the following is the commonest clinical presentation of PAD in patients >50 years of age?
A. Asymptomatic          C. Classic claudication
B. Atypical leg pain      D. Threatened limb

**21.12.** A 57-year-old male with a 30-year smoking history and diabetes mellitus presents with buttock pain on walking and erectile dysfunction. He also reports that his legs look thinner than in the past. On examination, there is an extremely weak femoral pulse bilaterally. What is the most likely diagnosis?
A. Coarctation of the aorta          C. Lumbar spinal stenosis
B. Leriche syndrome                   D. All of the above

**21.13.** A 56-year-old male with history of smoking and diabetes mellitus presents with calf pain on walking that resolves with resting. Bedside ABI is 0.91. What is the best next step?
A. Doppler ultrasound          C. MRA
B. CT                          D. Exercise testing

Chapter 2

**21.14.** A 56-year-old male with history of smoking and diabetes presents with a right cold foot. Ultrasound shows a thrombosed popliteal artery aneurysm. What is the treatment of choice?

A. Tissue plasminogen activator infusion followed by stent implantation

B. Direct covered stent implantation

C. Tissue plasminogen activator infusion of the aneurysm followed by surgical bypass

D. None of the above

**21.15.** What is/are the indication for popliteal artery aneurysm repair?

A. All popliteal aneurysms should be repaired

B. All symptomatic aneurysms that present with acute limb ischemia regardless of size

C. Patients with patent popliteal aneurysms >2.0 cm in diameter

D. B and C

**21.16.** A 25-year-old female with no significant medical history presents with calf pain upon competitive bicycling. Bedside ABI is 0.91. The popliteal pulse is diminished upon plantar flexion of the foot against the floor. What is the most likely diagnosis?

A. Popliteal aneurysm

B. Popliteal arteritis

C. Popliteal entrapment syndrome

D. None of the above

**21.17.** A 40-year-old obese male with no medical problem presents complaining of chronic intermittent claudication. ABI is 1.0, and Doppler ultrasound normal. Angiogram shows obstruction of right popliteal artery. What is the most likely diagnosis?

A. Atherosclerosis of the popliteal artery

B. Popliteal artery spasm

C. Adventitial cystic disease

D. Buerger's disease

**21.18.** A 45-year-old male heavy smoker presents with black skin discoloration and pain in both hands and feet. What is the strongest risk factor?

A. Diabetes mellitus

B. Cigarette smoking

C. Hypertension

D. Hyperlipidemia

**21.19.** Which of the following is/are an indication for intervention to the infrageniculate arteries?

A. Rest pain

B. Nonhealing ulcerations

C. Severe pain on walking

D. A and B

**21.20.** Which of the following is/are true about an arterial ulcer?

A. It occurs at tips of toes, heel, and lateral ankle

B. Painful

C. Edema

D. A and B

**21.21.** Which of the following is/are a feature of a venous ulcer?

A. Minimal pain

B. Large punched-out ulcer

C. Capillary refill >3.0 second

D. None of the above

**21.22.** A 69-year-old male with history of smoking, diabetes mellitus, hypertension, and paroxysmal atrial fibrillation on aspirin presents with acute severe right foot pain. Examination reveals delayed capillary refill, weakness, decreased sensation, and inaudible arterial Doppler. What is the best next step?

A. Angiography

B. Thrombolysis

C. Emergency embolectomy

D. Intravenous heparin

**21.23.** A 56-year-old female presents complaining of leg pain and heaviness. Examination shows varicose veins, with pigmentation and edema. No ulcer. What is the clinical, etiologic, anatomic, and pathophysiological (CEAP) class in this patient?

A. C1

B. C2

C. C3

D. C4a

**21.24.** Which of the following is/are a risk factor for chronic venous disease?

A. Increased body mass index

B. Smoking

C. Presence of arteriovenous shunt

D. Flat feet

E. All of the above

**21.25.** A 25-year-old obese female with no significant medical history presents with recurrent left lower extremity deep vein thrombosis. Antithrombin III, protein C, protein S, factor V Leiden, and prothrombin G20210A are all normal. What is the most accurate confirmatory diagnostic test?

A. Intravascular ultrasound

B. Venography

C. Venous/interstitial pressure measurement

D. Plethysmography

**21.26.** Which of the following is/are a contraindication to lower extremity venous ablation?

A. Acute deep vein thrombosis

B. Joint disease that interferes with mobility

C. Klippel-Trenaunay syndrome

D. All of the above

**21.27.** Which of the following is/are a complication of varicose veins?

A. Stasis dermatitis

B. Pulmonary embolism

C. Carcinoma

D. A, B, and C

**21.28.** A 78-year-old diabetic male with history of a quadruple coronary artery bypass graft eight years ago is referred to you by his primary care doctor for difficult-to-control blood pressure (BP). He was admitted to the hospital three months ago with acute pulmonary edema. He is currently on benazepril 40 mg/day, amlodipine 10 mg/day, metoprolol 50 mg BID. His BP is 180/110 mmHg. You add clonidine 0.1 mg TID. The creatinine is 1.9 mg/gl. What is the next most appropriate step?

A. Renal vein renin sampling

B. CT angiography

C. Abdominal angiography using carbon dioxide

D. MRA

**21.29.** What is the gold standard for diagnosing renal artery stenosis (RAS)?
A. CT angiography
B. MRA
C. Renal arteriography
D. Duplex Doppler ultrasonography

**21.30.** Which of the following describes superior mesenteric artery syndrome?
A. A clinical entity characterized by a decreased acuity of the angle between the aorta and superior mesenteric artery due to the loss of mesenteric fat between the superior mesenteric artery and aorta resulting in compression of the third portion of the duodenum.
B. Present with symptoms consistent with a proximal small bowel obstruction.
C. An aortomesenteric artery angle of <40° is the most sensitive measure of diagnosis
D. A and B
E. A, B, and C

**21.31.** An 80-year-old female presents with chronic postprandial abdominal pain and weight loss of 30 lb. over the last six months. She can only eat small portions due to severe abdominal pain. She has prior percutaneous coronary intervention to the left anterior descending and right coronary arteries. She also had a right superficial femoral artery stent eight months previously. There is a history of a transient ischemic attack in the past, and she has a left carotid bruit. Abdominal examination detects an abdominal bruit. Abdominal ultrasound is normal. What is the most likely clinical diagnosis?
A. RAS
B. Chronic pancreatitis
C. Celiac artery compression syndrome
D. None of the above

**21.32.** Which of the following is/are types of varicosities?
A. Reticular veins
B. Telangiectasia
C. Varicose veins
D. Venulectasia
E. All of the above

**21.33.** ACC/AHA guidelines recommend which of the following in critical limb ischemia (CLI)?
A. Patients with CLI in whom open surgical repair is anticipated should undergo assessment of cardiovascular risk
B. Patients with CLI and features to suggest athero-embolization should not be evaluated for aneurysmal disease
C. Systemic antibiotics should be initiated promptly in patients with CLI, skin ulcerations, and evidence of limb infection
D. A and C

**21.34.** In PAD diagnosis, which of the following is/are correct?
A. Exercise treadmill tests are recommended to provide the most objective evidence of the magnitude of the functional limitation of claudication and to measure the response to therapy
B. Duplex ultrasound of the extremities is useful to diagnose anatomic location and degree of stenosis of PAD

C. Duplex ultrasound of the extremities can be useful to select patients as candidates for endovascular intervention

D. Duplex ultrasound can be useful to select patients as candidates for surgical bypass and to select the sites of surgical anastomosis

E. All of the above

**21.35.** In treatment of PAD, which of the following is correct?

A. Beta-adrenergic blocking drugs are effective antihypertensive agents and are not contraindicated in patients with PAD

B. Antiplatelet therapy is indicated to reduce the risk of myocardial infarction (MI), stroke, or vascular death in individuals with atherosclerotic lower extremity PAD

C. A therapeutic trial of cilostazol should be considered in all patients with lifestyle-limiting claudication (in the absence of heart failure)

D. All of the above

**21.36.** Which of the following is/are indications for percutaneous revascularization of RAS?

A. Patients with hemodynamically significant RAS

B. Recurrent, unexplained congestive heart failure

C. Sudden, unexplained pulmonary edema

D. A and B

E. A, B, and C

**21.37.** Which of the following statements regarding chronic intestinal ischemia is/are true?

A. Should be suspected in patients with abdominal pain and weight loss without other explanation, especially those with cardiovascular disease

B. Only duplex ultrasound, but not CT angiography, and gadolinium-enhanced MRA are useful initial tests for supporting the clinical diagnosis of chronic intestinal ischemia

C. Surgical revascularization is indicated for patients with asymptomatic intestinal arterial obstructions

D. Percutaneous endovascular treatment of intestinal arterial stenosis is not indicated in patients with chronic intestinal ischemia

**21.38.** An 80-year-old male undergoes endovascular aneurysm repair uneventfully. The next day he develops severe abdominal pain and a "trash" foot. The next best step is which of the following?

A. Duplex sonography of the abdomen is an appropriate diagnostic tool for suspected acute intestinal ischemia

B. Surgical consultation

C. Angiography

D. CT angiography

**21.39.** A 23-year-old female presents with symptoms of hypertension, intermittent claudication, and renal failure. What is the most likely diagnosis?

A. RAS   C. Midaortic syndrome
B. Pheochromocytoma   D. Renal vein thrombosis

**21.40.** A 70-year-old female presents with several near-syncopal spells and chest pain followed by vigorous mopping. She is status post-coronary artery bypass grafting 10 years previously (Figure 21.40a). The right arm systolic BP is 140 mmHg; the left arm systolic BP is 110 mmHg. She smokes one pack per day. The next best step is which of the following?

   **A.** CT angiography of the chest and neck
   **B.** Ultrasound of the carotid and subclavian arteries
   **C.** MRA of the chest and neck
   **D.** Coronary and subclavian angiography and intervention

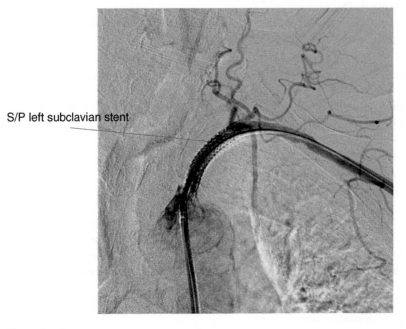

S/P left subclavian stent

**Figure 21.40a**

**21.41.** Which of the following is not part of the "6 P's" of acute limb ischemia?

   **A.** Pain
   **B.** Pallor
   **C.** Pulselessness
   **D.** Petechiae
   **E.** Parasthesias
   **F.** Paralysis
   **G.** Poikilothermia

**21.42.** Which of the following will place a limb in the "threatened" category of acute limb ischemia?

   **A.** No muscle weakness
   **B.** Profound sensory loss
   **C.** Audible arterial and venous Doppler
   **D.** Audible venous Doppler, inaudible arterial Doppler

**21.43.** An inter-arm blood pressure difference of how much is considered abnormal and suggestive of subclavian artery stenosis?

A. 0–5 mmHg

B. 5–10 mmHg

C. 10–15 mmHg

D. >15 mmHg

**21.44.** Given the following measurements, what is the ABI of the right lower extremity?

Left arm = 148/90. Right arm = 155/89. Left dorsalis pedis = 142/75. Left posterior tibial = 149/78. Right dorsalis pedis = 131/69. Right posterior tibial = 134/71.

A. 0.85

B. 0.86

C. 0.89

D. 0.90

E. 0.96

F. 1.01

**21.45.** Screening all patients with PAD for asymptomatic atherosclerosis is indicated for which arterial bed?

A. Renal arteries

B. Carotid arteries

C. Cerebral arteries

D. Coronary arteries

E. None of the above

**21.46.** Which of the following medications has shown proven benefit for the treatment of claudication?

A. Cilostazol

B. Pentoxyfylline

C. Chelation therapy (EDTA acid)

D. B-complex vitamins

**21.47.** What is the goal of revascularization in patients with claudication?

A. Prolong length of life

B. Reduce symptoms

C. Reduce hospitalizations

D. Limb salvage

**21.48.** What factors related to femoropopliteal disease reduce durability of revascularization procedures?

A. Long disease segment

B. Poor quality runoff

C. Diabetes mellitus

D. Renal failure

E. Smoking

F. All of the above

**21.49.** Acute limb ischemia is a condition that requires emergent recognition and intervention. What is the approximate length of time that skeletal muscle can tolerate ischemia?

A. 2–4 hours

B. 4–6 hours

C. 6–8 hours

D. 8–12 hours

**21.50.** The evaluation of an embolic cause for acute limb ischemia includes which of the following tests?

A. EKG

B. Prolonged heart rhythm monitoring

C. Echocardiography

D. All of the above

**21.51.** A 52-year-old woman with a history of diabetes and smoking presents with a painful left leg since last four days. She initially had pain with ambulation but now has rest pain. On examination, her left leg is pale and cool to touch. She has diminished sensation but normal strength. There are no palpable distal pulses on left leg. Right leg examination is normal. What is the next best step in management?

A. Smoking cessation counseling

B. Supervised exercise program

C. Aspirin and statin therapy

D. Lower extremity angiogram

21.52. IVC filter placement is supported by most clinical societal guidelines in which of the following patient/s?

A. A 45-year-old male with submassive pulmonary embolism after a long flight

B. A 78-year female with acute DVT and metastatic colon CA

C. A 22-year-old female with acute DVT and antiphospholipid syndrome

D. A 36-year-old male with acute ilio-femoral DVT and small intracranial hemorrhage

E. All of the above

21.53. You are asked to see a 56-year-old female patient for IVC filter placement. What can you tell the patient about the potential risks and benefits associated with the procedure based on clinical trials?

A. It may reduce her risk of future pulmonary embolism

B. It may reduce her risk of future DVT

C. It will provide her with mortality benefit

D. A and B

E. A and C

F. A, B, and C

21.54. Screening for peripheral arterial disease with Ankle-brachial Index (ABI) is indicated in which of the following situations?

A. Non-healing wounds

B. Exertional leg symptoms

C. Age >65 years

D. Age 50–64 years with risk factors

E. Age <50 years with diabetes and one other risk factor

F. All of the above

21.55. A 69-year-old woman with history of tobacco smoking and diabetes mellitus comes in to your office for vascular evaluation of exertional leg cramps that has been getting worse over last six months. An ankle-brachial index done in the primary care physician's office by a mobile vascular laboratory was reported as normal at 1.3. What would you recommend for her?

A. Tell her she has no peripheral arterial disease based on ABI report

B. Repeat ABI with toe-brachial index

C. Schedule for lower extremity invasive angiogram

D. Schedule for lower extremity CT angiogram

21.56. Which of the following patients should be offered peripheral revascularization?

A. A 45-year woman with leg cramps after walking that subside with rest

B. An 89-year-old man who develops calf pain after climbing three flight of stairs

C. A 57-year-old woman who develops leg pain after standing in the kitchen for long time

D. A 47-year-old man with diabetes who has an ulcer on the base of great toe that has not been healing for three months despite wound care

**21.57.** Cilostazol is effective in the treatment of claudication symptoms and has shown to improve walking distances. It is contraindicated in
A. Heart failure  C. Liver failure
B. Renal failure  D. COPD

**21.58.** Renal artery angiogram should be considered in which of the following situations?
A. Patient who develops hyperkalemia after starting ACE-inhibitors
B. Routinely at the end of the coronary angiogram
C. Patient with hypertension and peripheral arterial disease
D. All of the above
E. None of the above

**21.59.** Which of the following is true about inferior epigastric artery?
A. It is a branch of external iliac artery
B. It marks the upper limit of "safe-zone" for femoral arterial access
C. It can provide important collateral pathway in case of aorto-iliac occlusion
D. It is an important anatomic landmark which outlines the site of the occurrence of direct inguinal hernias
E. All of the above

**21.60.** Which of the following is true about drug-coated balloons (DCB) for percutaneous interventions?
A. DCB are widely used in the United States for coronary interventions
B. DCB have shown decreased amputation rates for infra-popliteal interventions
C. DCB have been shown to decrease clinically driven revascularizations in femoral-proximal popliteal interventions
D. All of the above

## Answers

**21.1.** A. Sevenfold.
Cigarette smoking increases the odds ratio for peripheral vascular disease by 7.3-fold. Other risk factors include diabetes mellitus, hypertension, and hyperlipidemia (Shammas 2007).

**21.2.** D. A and C.
The underlying mechanisms of peripheral vascular disease are atherosclerosis and artery spasm.

**21.3.** A. Asian Indians.
See Fowkes et al. (2013).

**21.4.** E. All of the above.

**21.5.** G. A, B, C, D, and E.
Features are suggestive of hyperhomocysteinemia: autosomal recessive inheritance (most enzymatic defects) with Marfanoid features, premature atherosclerosis, downward lens dislocation, and mental retardation. It is a defect of methionine metabolism. Pyridoxine, at a dose of 100–500 mg/day, is the drug of choice for treatment.

Chapter 2

**21.6.** E. All of the above.

    See Disdier et al. (2001).

**21.7.** D. An ABI of 0.4 is associated with high cardiovascular mortality.

    The first-line study in patient with PAD is the ankle-brachial pressure index (ABPI/ABI). Normal ABI range is 1.00–1.40. The patient is diagnosed with PAD when the ABI is ≤0.90. ABI values of 0.91–0.99 are considered "borderline," and values >1.40 indicate noncompressible arteries. PAD is graded as mild to moderate if the ABI is between 0.41 and 0.90, and an ABI <0.40 is suggestive of severe PAD. See Box 21.1 and Figure 21.7.

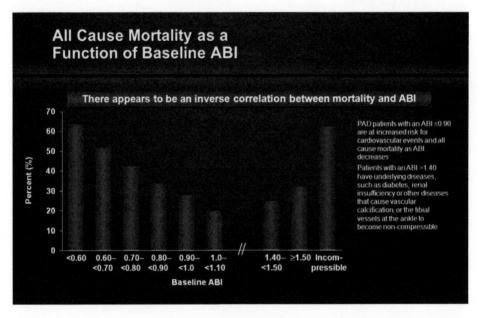

Figure 21.7 All-cause mortality as a function of baseline ABI. *Source:* Adapted from Resnick et al. (2004).

**21.8.** E. Cardiac risk-factor modification and a supervised exercise regimen.

    If ABIs are abnormal, the next best step is cardiovascular risk-factor modification and a supervised walking regimen.

**21.9.** E. All of the above.

    See Tables 21.9a, 21.9b, and 21.9c.

Table 21.9a Fontaine stages.

| Stage | Clinical |
| --- | --- |
| I | Asymptomatic |
| IIa | Mild claudication |
| IIb | Moderate-tosevere claudication |
| III | Ischemic rest pain |
| IV | Ulceration or gangrene |

**Table 21.9b** Rutherford.

| Grade | Category | Clinical |
|-------|----------|----------|
| 0 | 0 | Asymptomatic |
| I | 1 | Mild claudication |
| I | 2 | Moderate claudication |
| I | 3 | Severe claudication |
| II | 4 | Ischemic rest pain |
| III | 5 | Minor tissue loss |
| III | 6 | Major tissue loss |

**Table 21.9c** TASC II classification of superficial femoral artery occlusion.

| Type | Clinical |
|------|----------|
| A | Single occlusion <5 cm in length |
| B | Single occlusion <5 cm but heavily calcified, or multiple occlusions each <5 cm, or single occlusion <15 cm |
| C | Multiple occlusion >15 cm |
| D | Chronic total occlusion >20 cm |

**21.10.** F. All of the above.

**21.11.** A. Asymptomatic.

The 2005 American College of Cardiology (ACC)/American Heart Association (AHA) guidelines on PAD suggested the following distribution of clinical presentation of PAD in patients >50 years of age:
- asymptomatic, 20–50%;
- atypical leg pain, 40–50%;
- classic claudication, 10–35%;
- threatened limb, 1–2%.

**21.12.** B. Leriche syndrome.

Leriche syndrome is the triad of buttock claudication, atrophy of the lower extremities, and erectile dysfunction. Lesion involves truncation of the terminal aorta with collateral formation via the inferior mesenteric artery, the sacral artery, and the iliolumbar arteries (Figure 21.12a). The internal mammary artery can also anastomose with the inferior epigastric artery to supply collaterals. The infrarenal aorta is occluded. Inferior mesenteric artery and lumbar collaterals are seen (arrows in Figure 21.12b).

Chapter 21

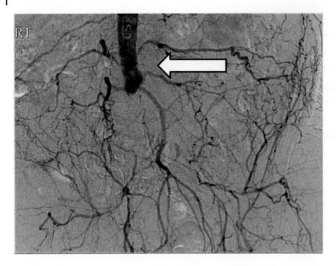

**Figure 21.12a** Total occlusion of the infrarenal aorta.

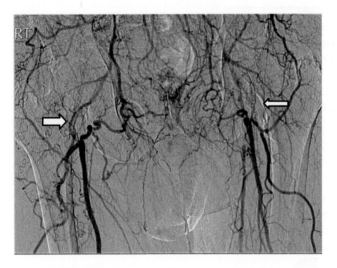

**Figure 21.12b** Bilateral superficial femoral arteries filling via collaterals.

**21.13.** D. Exercise testing.

In people with suspected PAD but normal resting ABIs, exercise testing of ABI can be done. A baseline ABI is obtained prior to exercise. The patient is then asked to exercise (usually patients are made to walk on a treadmill at a constant speed) until claudication pain occurs (or a maximum of five minutes), following which the ankle pressure is again measured. A decrease in ABI of 15–20% would be diagnostic of PAD.

**21.14.** C. Tissue plasminogen activator infusion of the aneurysm followed by surgical bypass.

Graft patency is improved if thrombus burden is reduced prior to bypass. Also, three-vessel runoff improves long-term graft patency. The popliteal artery is the most common site of a peripheral artery aneurysm that causes symptoms of lower extremity ischemia, which is due to aneurysm thrombosis. The presence of a peripheral aneurysm should prompt evaluation for other aneurysms (Carpenter et al. 1994).

**21.15.** D. B and C.

The indications for popliteal artery repair are: all symptomatic aneurysms that present with acute limb ischemia regardless of size, to relieve symptoms and minimize the risk of limb loss, and patients with patent popliteal aneurysms >2.0 cm in diameter, as these patients have a 30–40% risk of developing acute ischemic complications which are associated with a high risk for limb loss.

**21.16.** C. Popliteal entrapment syndrome.

This entity results from a developmental defect in which the popliteal artery passes medial to and beneath the medial head of the gastrocnemius muscle or a slip of that muscle, with consequent compression of the artery. Rarely, an anomalous fibrous band or the popliteus muscle deep to the medial head of the gastrocnemius is the compressing structure. Treatment is surgical release of the artery.

**21.17.** C. Adventitial cystic disease.

Adventitial cystic disease is a rare entity that can lead to arterial obstruction related to mucoid degeneration of the artery due to cyst formation in the adventitia and compression of the popliteal artery. When it occurs in the femoral or popliteal artery, claudication symptoms are indistinguishable from atherosclerotic popliteal disease. Patients tend to be younger, and typical risk factors for cardiovascular disease are often absent. Etiology is unknown.

**21.18.** B. Cigarette smoking.

Thromboangiitis obliterans (Buerger's disease) is a nonatherosclerotic, segmental, inflammatory disease that most commonly affects the small- to medium-sized arteries and veins of the extremities. Patients are younger than the typical patients with atherosclerotic vascular disease, and are heavy smokers. Digit ischemia is the most common presentation; and though larger artery involvement is uncommon, claudication can occur but is nearly always associated with signs of distal ischemia.

**21.19.** D. A and B.

Both rest pain and nonhealing ulcer are indication for intervention. Above the knee, intervention is indicated for claudication.

**21.20.** D. A and B.

Arterial ulcer characterized by
- being painful
- decreased/absent pulses
- pallor on elevation, rubor on dangling
- thin shiny skin with hair loss
- located at tips of toes, heel, lateral ankle, dorsum of the feet
- punched out and well defined
- covered with slough and necrotic tissue

- no edema
- capillary refill >3 seconds
- ABI <0.75

**21.21.** A. Minimal pain.

Features of venous ulcer include:
- painless/minimal pain
- pulses present
- brown varicose vein/pigmentation
- thick, hardened skin
- located at medial gaiter region
- sloping and gradual, covered with slough
- edema present
- capillary refill <3 seconds
- ABI >0.9.

**21.22.** A. Angiography.

This patient needs angiography to define the location and extent of the thrombus, and then procced with emergency surgery. See Table 21.22.

**Table 21.22** Classification of acute limb ischemia.

|  | Viable | Threatened | Nonviable |
|---|---|---|---|
| Pain | Mild | Severe | Variable |
| Capillary refill | Intact | Delayed | Absent |
| Motor deficit | None | Partial | Complete |
| Sensory deficit | None | Partial | Complete |
| Arterial Doppler | Audible | Inaudible | Inaudible |
| Venous Doppler | Audible | Audible | Inaudible |
| Treatment | Urgent work-up | Emergency surgery | Amputation |

**21.23.** D. C4a.

CEAP clinical classification:
C0 – no visible or palpable signs of venous disease
C1 – telangiectasias or reticular veins
C2 – varicose veins
C3 – edema
C4a – pigmentation or eczema
C4b – lipodermatosclerosis or atrophie blanche
C5 – healed venous ulcer
C6 – active venous ulcer

**21.24.** E. All of the above.

The risk factors for chronic venous disease include advanced age, family history of venous disease, smoking, sedentary lifestyle, lower extremity trauma, prior venous thrombosis (superficial or deep), ligamentous laxity (e.g. hernia, flat feet), prolonged standing, increased body mass index, the presence of arteriovenous shunt, high estrogen states, and pregnancy.

**21.25.** A. Intravascular ultrasound.

This is because the flattened vein may not be noticed on conventional venography.

This patient has May-Thurner syndrome (iliac vein compression syndrome) is a rare condition of compression of the left common iliac vein (Figure 21.25) by the overlying right common iliac artery which causes stasis of blood, predisposing the individual to the formation of blood clots. Severe May-Thurner syndrome may require thrombolysis if there is a recent onset of thrombosis, followed by angioplasty and stenting of the iliac vein.

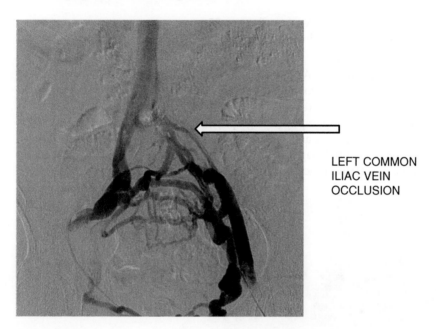

LEFT COMMON
ILIAC VEIN
OCCLUSION

**Figure 21.25**

**21.26.** D. All of the above.

Contraindications to lower extremity venous ablation are pregnancy, acute superficial or deep vein thrombosis, moderate-to-severe peripheral artery disease, joint disease that interferes with mobility, Klippel-Trenaunay syndrome, and advanced generalized systemic disease that limits quality-of-life improvements expected following venous intervention.

**21.27.** D. A, B, and C.

Varicose veins complications are:
- Pain, tenderness, heaviness, stasis dermatitis, venous ulcers. Development of carcinoma or sarcoma in long-standing venous ulcers is about 0.4–1%.
- Severe bleeding from minor trauma; superficial thrombophlebitis, which is frequently isolated to the superficial veins, but can extend into deep veins, becoming a more serious problem.
- Acute fat necrosis can occur, especially at the ankle of overweight patients with varicose veins.

Chapter 21

**21.28.** C. Abdominal angiography using carbon dioxide.

A CO2 angiogram is the safest to define anatomy and intervention in this diabetic patient. The following are suggestive of reno-vascular disease:

- An acute elevation in serum creatinine of at least 30% after administration of angiotensin-converting enzyme inhibitor or angiotensin II receptor blocker.
- Moderate-to-severe hypertension in a patient with diffuse atherosclerosis, a unilateral small kidney, or asymmetry in renal size of more than 1.5 cm that cannot be explained by another reason.
- Moderate-to-severe hypertension in patients with recurrent episodes of flash pulmonary edema.
- Onset of stage II hypertension after age 55 years.
- Systolic or diastolic abdominal bruit.

**21.29.** C. Renal arteriography.

The gold standard for RAS diagnosis is renal arteriography, but duplex Doppler ultrasonography, CT angiography, and MRA are noninvasive tests and reasonable alternatives for initial testing.

Captopril renal scintigraphy (renography), selective renal vein renin measurements, and plasma renin activity (in isolation or after captopril administration) are not useful as initial diagnostic tests for RAS, though renography is useful to determine the relative function of each kidney.

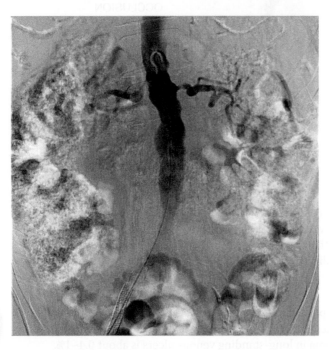

**Figure 21.29** Bilateral RAS.

**21.30.** D. A and B.

Superior mesenteric artery syndrome (Cast syndrome, Wilkie syndrome, arteriomesenteric duodenal obstruction, and chronic duodenal ileus) is an unusual cause of proximal intestinal obstruction, characterized by compression of the third portion of the duodenum due to narrowing of the space between the superior mesenteric artery and aorta and is primarily attributed to loss of the intervening mesenteric fat pad.

The diagnostic imaging criteria for superior mesenteric artery syndrome are:

- Duodenal obstruction with an abrupt cutoff in the third portion and active peristalsis.
- An aortomesenteric artery angle of <25° is the most sensitive measure of diagnosis, particularly if the aortomesenteric distance is <8 mm.
- High fixation of the duodenum by the ligament of Treitz, abnormally low origin of the superior mesenteric artery, or anomalies of the superior mesenteric artery.

**21.31.** D. None of the above.

The patient has mesenteric artery ischemia. Two of the three abdominal branches to the gut are usually compromised to cause these symptoms. CT angiography will usually define these branches and location of stenosis. The treatment is either stent implantation or surgical bypass. Differential includes celiac artery compression syndrome (also known as celiac axis syndrome, median arcuate ligament syndrome, and Dunbar syndrome) which is a chronic, recurrent abdominal pain related to compression of the celiac artery by the median arcuate ligament. It is an uncommon disorder characterized clinically by the triad of postprandial abdominal pain, weight loss, and sometimes an abdominal bruit.

**21.32.** D. All of the above.

**21.33.** D. A and C.

ACC/AHA guidelines recommend the following (see Box 21.2). Patients with CLI in whom open surgical repair is anticipated should undergo assessment of cardiovascular risk. Patients with CLI and features to suggest athero-embolization should be evaluated for aneurysmal disease. Systemic antibiotics should be initiated promptly in patients with CLI, skin ulcerations, and evidence of limb infection.

**21.34.** E. All of the above.

**21.35.** D. All of the above.

See Box 21.1.

**21.36.** E. A, B, and C.

ACC/AHA guidelines recommend percutaneous revascularization of RAS in the following (see Box 21.2):

- Patients with hemodynamically significant RAS
- Recurrent, unexplained congestive heart failure
- Sudden, unexplained pulmonary edema
- Percutaneous revascularization may be considered for patients with RAS and chronic renal insufficiency with unilateral RAS.
- Accelerated hypertension, resistant hypertension, malignant hypertension, hypertension with an unexplained unilateral small kidney, and hypertension with intolerance to medication.

Chapter 2

**21.37.** A. Should be suspected in patients with abdominal pain and weight loss without other explanation, especially those with cardiovascular disease.

ACC/AHA guidelines (see Box 21.2):
- Duplex ultrasound, but not CT angiography, and gadolinium-enhanced MRA are useful initial tests for supporting the clinical diagnosis of chronic intestinal ischemia.
- Surgical revascularization is indicated for patients with asymptomatic intestinal arterial obstructions.
- Percutaneous endovascular treatment of intestinal arterial stenosis is not indicated in patients with chronic intestinal ischemia.

**21.38.** B. Surgical consultation.

Acute intestinal ischemia ACC/AHA guidelines (see Box 21.2):
- In contrast to chronic intestinal ischemia, duplex sonography of the abdomen is not an appropriate diagnostic tool for suspected acute intestinal ischemia.
- Patients who develop acute abdominal pain after arterial interventions in which catheters traverse the visceral aorta or any proximal arteries or who have arrhythmias (such as atrial fibrillation) or recent MI should be suspected of having acute intestinal ischemia.
- Percutaneous interventions (including transcatheter lytic therapy, balloon angioplasty, and stenting) are appropriate in selected patients with acute intestinal ischemia caused by arterial obstructions who are not surgical candidates.

**21.39.** C. Midaortic syndrome.

Midaortic syndrome is a condition characterized by segmental narrowing of the abdominal/distal descending thoracic aorta, and frequently accompanied by ostial stenosis of the aorta's branches. If left untreated, it can result in life-threatening complications secondary to severe hypertension.

It can be congenital, caused by a developmental anomaly in the fusion and maturation of the paired embryonic dorsal aortas, or acquired secondary to neurofibromatosis, fibromuscular dysplasia, retroperitoneal fibrosis, Williams syndrome, mucopolysaccharidosis, and giant-cell arteritis.

**21.40.** D. Coronary and subclavian angiography and intervention.

Subclavian steal occurs when the left upper extremity is exercised and blood flows retrograde in the left vertebral artery to supply the arm (Figure 21.40b). The blood also flows retrograde in the left internal mammary artery to supply the demands of the left arm (Figure 21.40c). These are the classic indications to intervene. A BP difference in the two upper extremities without symptoms of angina, dizziness, or syncope is not an indication to intervene.

**21.41.** D. Petechiae.

Pain, pallor, pulselessness, parasthesias, poikilothermia and paralysis are described as the 6"P" of acute limb ischemia. Petechiae is typically not a feature of acute limb ischemia.

**21.42.** D. Audible venous Doppler, inaudible arterial Doppler.

The "threatened" category of acute limb ischemia includes mild-to-moderate sensory or motor loss, inaudible arterial Doppler and audible venous Doppler. The other categories are "viable" and "irreversible."

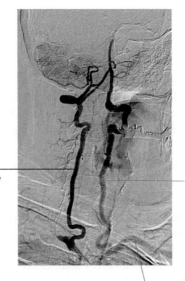

Right vertebral artery injection

Left vertebral artery fills retrograde to supply the left subclavian artery

Left subclavian artery

Figure 21.40b

Left vertebral artery

Occluded left subclavian artery

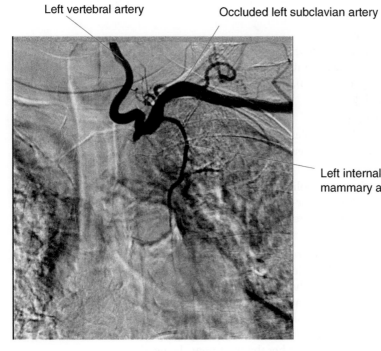

Left internal mammary artery

Figure 21.40c

**Chapter 21**

**21.43.** D. >15 mmHg.

An inter-arm blood pressure difference of >15–20 mmHg is abnormal and suggestive of subclavian artery stenosis.

**21.44.** B. 0.86.

The calculation of ankle-brachial index (ABI) is done by dividing the higher systolic blood pressure of the dorsalis pedis artery or posterior tibial artery in the desired extremity by the higher of the two arm pressures. So to calculate the ABI of the right lower extremity, we would divide 134 by 155 to get 0.86.

**21.45.** E. None of the above.

Currently, there is no evidence that screening all patients with PAD for asymptomatic atherosclerosis in other arterial beds improves clinical outcomes.

**21.46.** A. Cilostazol

Cilastazol is the only medication listed that has been proven as an effective therapy agent to improve symptoms and increase walking distance in patients with claudication symptoms. However, the most effective strategy to improve symptoms and claudication distance is a supervised exercise program (not listed as an option). This should be the initial choice for treatment of claudication before pharmacological options are pursued.

**21.47.** B. Reduce symptoms.

A minority of patient with limb claudication will progress to chronic limb ischemia. Thus, the role of revascularization in claudication is improvement in symptoms, functional status, and quality of life rather than mortality, hospitalization rate, or limb salvage.

**21.48.** F. All of the above.

For femoropopliteal disease, factors that reduce durability include greater lesion length, occlusion rather than stenosis, presence of multiple or diffuse lesions, poor-quality runoff, diabetes mellitus, chronic renal disease, renal failure, and smoking.

**21.49.** B. Four to six hours.

Skeletal muscle will tolerate ischemia for roughly four to six hours. Thus, prompt recognition and treatment of acute limb ischemia is crucial.

**21.50.** D. All of the above.

To evaluate for an embolic etiology of acute limb ischemia, it is important to obtain an EKG to assess for MI, prolonged cardiac rhythm monitoring to assess for AFib, and echocardiogram to assess for valve vegetations, LA/LV thrombus, and intracardiac shunting.

**21.51.** D. Lower extremity angiography.

It is important to be able to identify acute limb ischemia and distinguish it from other forms of peripheral vascular disease presentation due to high morbidity and mortality associated with this condition. This patient has Rutherford Stage 2a acute limb ischemia. While she may eventually benefit from the other therapies listed, an urgent lower extremity angiography is the next best step in management to promptly get her the treatment she needs.

**21.52.** D. A 36-year-old male with acute ileo-femoral DVT and small intracranial hemorrhage.

There are multiple overlapping but somewhat distinctly phrased recommendations and guidelines for IVC filter placement from different clinical societies such as American College of Chest Physicians (ACCP), American Heart Association (AHA), American College of Radiology (ACR) and Society of Interventional Radiology (SIR). Acute Venous thromboembolism (VTE) and inability to anti-coagulate remains the most widely agreed upon indication in societal guidelines.

**21.53.** A. It may reduce her risk for future pulmonary embolism.

Most studies evaluating the clinical efficacy of vena cava filters have been observational. Two important randomized control trials are PREPIC (Prévention du Risque d'Embolie Pulmonaire par Interruption Cave Study Group) and PREPIC 2. The PREPIC study showed that IVC filter placement reduced recurrent PE but increased DVT and had no mortality benefit. PREPIC 2 study confirmed lack of mortality benefit with vena cava filter implantation.

**21.54.** F. All of the above.

AHA/ACC recommends screening for peripheral arterial disease in all of the scenarios described. On the other hand, the United States Preventive Services Task Force (USPSTF) concludes that the current evidence is insufficient to assess the balance of benefits and harms of screening for peripheral artery disease (PAD) and cardiovascular disease (CVD) risk with the ankle-brachial index (ABI) in asymptomatic adults.

**21.55.** B. Repeat ABI with toe-brachial index.

This patient with significant atherosclerotic risk factors presents with classical claudication symptoms. Diabetes vasculopathy can make vessels stiff and non-compressible causing spuriously elevated ABI. Toe vessels are less susceptible to this process making Toe-brachial index (TBI) a useful tool in such cases. Typically toe-brachial index is considered when ABI is >1.4; but it should also be considered in patients with high suspicion of PAD but falsely "normalized" ABI due to non-compressible vessels. A cut-off of 0.7 has been described below which TBI is considered abnormal.

**21.56.** D. A 47-year-old man with diabetes who has an ulcer on the base of the great toe that has not been healing for three months despite wound care.

Revascularization is typically offered to patients with lifestyle limiting claudication or critical limb ischemia (CLI). CLI patients may present with resting claudication or non-healing wounds/ulcers. Though the patient described in options A, B, and C may also have peripheral vascular disease, conservative treatment is recommended for early stages of disease.

**21.57.** A. Heart failure.

Cilostazol is an FDA-approved medication with a class I indication for intermittent claudication. It carries a black box warning due to concerns for increased cardiovascular mortality. It is contraindicated in patients with heart failure of any severity. Phosphodiesterase inhibitors have caused decreased survival compared with placebo in patients with class III or IV heart failure.

Chapter 2

**21.58.** E. None of the above.

Routine "drive-by" renal angiograms were widely reported along with coronary angiograms in the past but have declined now largely due to advent of radial approach and also due to lack of consistent benefit of renal artery interventions in randomized controlled trials.

**21.59.** E. All of the above.

Inferior epigastric artery can collateralize with superior epigastric artery which is a branch of internal thoracic artery and provide an important pathway for blood supply to leg in case of aorto-iliac occlusion. The inferior epigastric artery, together with its accompanying veins, forms the lateral border of the Hesselbach's triangle which is an important anatomic landmark for the occurrence of direct inguinal hernias.

**21.60.** C. DCB have shown to decrease clinically driven revascularization in femoral–proximal popliteal interventions.

Drug-coated coronary balloons are not available in United States. IN.PACT SFA trial showed decrease in clinically driven target lesion revascularizations in superficial femoral artery-proximal popliteal interventions. However, IN.PACT DEEP trial failed to show similar benefit in infra-popliteal interventions. On the contrary, there was statistically non-significant but numerically higher rates of amputation in the cohort treated with DCBs at 12 months. However, many criticisms of the trial design exist.

---

**Box 21.1   Clinical Pearls**

- Any vascular disease that results in arterial stenosis or occlusion can cause symptoms of extremity pain or tissue loss.
- PAD differential diagnosis: arterial aneurysm, arterial dissection, embolism, popliteal entrapment syndrome, adventitial cystic disease, Buerger's disease, limb trauma, radiation arteritis, vasculitis, and ergot use for migraines.
- Risk factors for PAD are similar to those that promote the development of coronary atherosclerosis (i.e. hyperlipidemia, smoking, hypertension, diabetes).
- Classic claudication is characterized by leg pain that is consistently reproduced with exercise and relieved with rest. The degree of symptoms of claudication depends upon the severity of stenosis, the collateral circulation, and the vigor of exercise.
- To confirm the diagnosis of arterial stenosis or occlusion, which is most commonly due to PAD, the resting ABI should be performed in patients with lower extremity exertional symptoms and in those patients with risk factors for PAD.
- An ABI of <0.90 has a high degree of sensitivity and specificity for a diagnosis of PAD.
- Visibly dilated lower extremity veins (i.e. telangiectasias, reticular veins, or varicose veins) may be indicative of underlying venous reflux.
- The goals of treatment are improved symptoms and appearance. Initial treatment for most patients with chronic venous disease is conservative and includes leg elevation, exercise, and compression therapy.
- Laser therapy is the only option for treatment of telangiectasias too small to access.

---

**Box 21.2  ACC/AHA Clinical Guidelines**

- Individuals with asymptomatic lower extremity PAD should be identified by examination and/or measurement of the ABI so that therapeutic interventions known to diminish their increased risk of MI, stroke, and death may be offered.
- Smoking cessation, lipid lowering, and diabetes and hypertension treatment, according to current national treatment guidelines, are recommended for individuals with asymptomatic lower extremity PAD.
- Antiplatelet therapy is indicated for individuals with asymptomatic lower extremity PAD to reduce the risk of adverse cardiovascular ischemic events.
- Angiotensin-converting enzyme inhibition may be considered for individuals with asymptomatic lower extremity PAD for cardiovascular risk reduction.
- Patients with CLI in whom open surgical repair is anticipated should undergo assessment of cardiovascular risk.
- Patients with a prior history of CLI or who have undergone successful treatment for CLI should be evaluated at least twice annually by a vascular specialist owing to the relatively high incidence of recurrence.
- Patients with CLI and features to suggest athero-embolization should be evaluated for aneurysmal disease (e.g. abdominal aortic, popliteal, or common femoral aneurysms).
- Systemic antibiotics should be initiated promptly in patients with CLI, skin ulcerations, and evidence of limb infection.
- Duplex ultrasound of the extremities is useful to diagnose anatomic location and degree of PAD stenosis.
- Duplex ultrasound is recommended for routine surveillance after femoropopliteal or femoral-tibial pedal bypass with a venous conduit. Minimum surveillance intervals are approximately 3, 6, and 12 months, and then yearly after graft placement.

---

## References

Carpenter, J.P., Barker, C.F., Roberts, B. et al. (1994). Popliteal artery aneurysms: current management and outcome. *Journal of Vascular Surgery* 19 (1): 65–72.

Disdier, P., Granel, B., Serratrice, J. et al. (2001). Cannabis arteritis revisited – ten new case reports. *Angiology* 52 (1): 1–5.

Fowkes, F.G.R., Rudan, D., Rudan, I. et al. (2013). Comparison of global estimates of prevalence and risk factors for peripheral artery disease in 2000 and 2010: a systematic review and analysis. *Lancet* 382 (9901): 1329–1340.

Resnick, H.E., Lindsay, R.S., McGrae McDermott, M. et al. (2004). Relationship of high and low ankle brachial index to all-cause and cardiovascular disease mortality. *Circulation* 109 (6): https://doi.org/10.1161/01.CIR.0000112642.63927.54.

Shammas, N.W. (2007). Epidemiology, classification, and modifiable risk factors of peripheral arterial disease. *Vascular Health and Risk Management* 3 (2): 229–234.

**Chapter 21**

## Suggested Reading

Brand, F.N., Dannenberg, A.L., Abbott, R.D., and Kannel, W.B. (1988). The epidemiology of varicose veins: the Framingham study. *American Journal of Preventive Medicine* 4: 96–101.

Callam, M.J. (1994). Epidemiology of varicose veins. *British Journal of Surgery* 81: 167–173.

Cooper, C.J., Murphy, T.P., Cutlip, D.E. et al. (2014). Stenting and medical therapy for atherosclerotic renal-artery stenosis. *The New England Journal of Medicine* 370: 13–22. [947 patients were randomized. Median f/u 43 months. No difference in composite endpoint consisting of death from cardiovascular or renal causes, MI, stroke, hospitalization for congestive heart failure or renal replacement therapy (35% in each group). Systolic BP was lower in stent group by 2.3 mmHg (p = 0.03).].

Gerhar-Herman, M.D., Gornik, H.L., Barrett, C. et al. (2017). 2016 AHA/ACC guideline on the management of patients with lower extremity peripheral artery disease: executive summary: a report of the American College of Cardiology/American Heart Association Task Force on Clinical Practice Guidelines. *Circulation* 135: e686–e725.

Hirsch, A.T., Criqui, M.H., Treat-Jacobson, D. et al. (2001). Peripheral arterial disease detection, awareness, and treatment in primary care. *Journal of the American Medical Association* 286: 1317–1324.

Layden, J., Michaels, J., Bermingham, S. et al. (2012). Diagnosis and management of lower limb peripheral arterial disease: summary of NICE guidance. *British Medical Journal* 345: e4947.

McDermot, M.M., Greenland, P., Liu, K. et al. (2001). Leg symptoms in peripheral arterial disease: associated clinical characteristics and functional impairment. *Journal of the American Medical Association* 286: 1599–1606.

Porter, J.M. and Moneta, G.L. (1995). Reporting standards in venous disease: an update. International Consensus Committee on Chronic Venous Disease. *Journal of Vascular Surgery* 21: 635–645.

Rooke, T.W., Hirsch, A.T., Misra, S. et al. (2013). Management of patients with peripheral artery disease (compilation of 2005 and 2011 ACCF/AHA Guideline Recommendations): a report of the American College of Cardiology Foundation/American Heart Association Task Force on Practice Guidelines. *Journal of the American College of Cardiology* 61: 1555–1570.

# Cardiac Arrhythmias

# 22

**22.1.** A 45-year-old woman is admitted with syncope while standing in the mall. No premonitory symptoms, no other significant past medical history, and is on no medications except the contraceptive pill. Her physical examination, electrocardiogram (ECG), and echocardiogram are normal, as is the tilt table test. What is the most likely cause of her syncope?
   **A.** Neurocardiogenic
   **B.** Pulmonary embolism due to hormone-induced hypercoagulable state
   **C.** Catecholaminergic polymorphic ventricular tachycardia
   **D.** Long QT syndrome

**22.2.** A 55-year-old man with prior myocardial infarction (MI) and coronary stenting three years previously is admitted with sudden loss of consciousness while sitting at a desk. He was on aspirin, statin, angiotensin-converting-enzyme inhibitor, and Coreg. Heart rate was 65 bpm, blood pressure 110/72 mmHg, normal jugular venous pressure, and no murmurs. ECG showed poor R wave progression, echo showed an ejection fraction (EF) of 30% with anterior and apical akinesis and thinning. Left anterior descending artery stent was patent on coronary angiogram. What is the next logical step?
   **A.** Discharge with event monitor
   **B.** Do electrophysiology (EP) testing for inducible arrhythmias
   **C.** Implant an implantable cardioverter-defibrillator (ICD)
   **D.** Perform a stress test for ventricular tachycardia (VT)

**22.3.** Carotid sinus hypersensitivity is more common in which of the following?
   **A.** 20-year-old female
   **B.** 40-year-old male
   **C.** 40-year-old female
   **D.** 75-year-old man

**22.4.** Mortality in long QT syndrome depends upon which of the following?
   **A.** Specific genetic defect
   **B.** QT interval
   **C.** History of syncope
   **D.** All of the above

**22.5.** In a patient with type I Brugada syndrome presenting with syncope, the two-year risk of sudden death is which of the following?
   **A.** 2%            **C.** 30%
   **B.** 10%           **D.** 80%

*Cardiology Board Review*, Second Edition. Ramdas G. Pai and Padmini Varadarajan.
© 2023 John Wiley & Sons Ltd. Published 2023 by John Wiley & Sons Ltd.

**22.6.** Which of the following statements about Brugada syndrome is correct?
  **A.** It is a genetically determined sodium channelopathy
  **B.** Mortality risk is independent of amount of ST elevation
  **C.** The ECG changes are stable and do not change over time
  **D.** They have an underlying left ventricular (LV) dysfunction

**22.7.** A 78-year-old patient with no prior medical history, not on any medications, is noted to be bradycardic at a routine physical examination. ECG shows complete heart block. Upon further questioning, the patient denies complaining of dizziness, near syncope, or syncope. He admits to noticing a gradual decline in exercise capacity over the previous year. What is the next step in the management of this patient?
  **A.** Holter monitor
  **B.** EP test
  **C.** Exercise treadmill test
  **D.** Dual-chamber pacemaker implant

**22.8.** A 37-year-old patient presents with symptoms of palpitations. Holter monitoring revealed episodes of atrial tachycardia and atrial fibrillation. He was prescribed flecainide 100 mg BID and metoprolol succinate 50 mg daily. He noticed an improvement in symptoms of palpitations but complains of fatigue and inability to return to work as a firefighter. What is the best option for this patient?
  **A.** Continue present management
  **B.** Switch to sotalol
  **C.** EP studies and catheter ablation
  **D.** Lower dose of flecainide and metoprolol

**22.9.** A 72-year-old woman with a history of coronary artery disease, ischemic cardiomyopathy, and paroxysmal atrial fibrillation of five years' duration has noticed an increase in frequency and duration of episodes over the previous year. Her medications include Tikosyn® 250 µg BID, Coreg 25 mg BID, enalapril 10 mg daily, aspirin 81 mg daily, and rivoroxaban 20 mg daily. She would like to consider pulmonary vein antrum isolation procedure if she will be taken off rivoroxaban after the procedure. What do you tell her?
  **A.** She can expect to continue taking aspirin and discontinue rivoroxaban
  **B.** She will need to continue taking rivoraxaban and discontinue aspirin
  **C.** Both medications can be stopped
  **D.** Both medications will be continued

**22.10.** An ECG (Figure 22.10) is done on a 35-year-old male who is scheduled to undergo knee surgery. The patient has no symptoms of palpitations. What is the next step in the management?
  **A.** No further work-up is indicated
  **B.** Exercise treadmill test
  **C.** Echocardiogram
  **D.** EP studies and ablation

**22.11.** A 60-year-old patient with history of dilated cardiomyopathy, LVEF 35%, on optimal medical therapy is noted to have frequent premature ventricular complexes (PVCs) on ECG with left bundle branch block (LBBB) morphology and

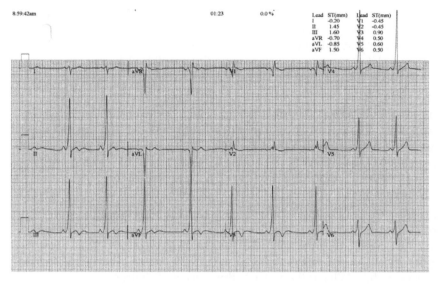

**Figure 22.10**

inferior axis. She denies symptoms of palpitations. On a 24-hour Holter monitor, the PVC burden is 22%. Which of the following options would you offer next?

A. Start amiodarone

B. Repeat echo in six months

C. EP studies and catheter ablation

D. ICD implant

**22.12.** A 40-year-old patient with a history of supraventricular tachycardia (SVT) wishes to undergo EP studies and catheter ablation. What is the expected success rate?

A. 70–75%    C. 90–95%

B. 80–85%    D. 100%

**22.13.** A 65-year-old patient presents with a history of prior MI and a five-year history of recurrent palpitations associated with near syncope. He has been on metoprolol and simvastatin. The 12-lead ECG is suggestive of atrioventricular nodal reentrant tachycardia (AVNRT). Which of the following would you recommend next?

A. Continue metoprolol    C. Amiodarone

B. Flecainide    D. EP study/ablation

**22.14.** A 35-year-old patient presents to the emergency department with a two-hour history of rapid heartbeat associated with dizziness. The blood pressure is 90/60 mmHg; ECG shows atrial fibrillation with ventricular preexcitation. What is the best treatment option?

A. Intravenous (IV) metoprolol

B. IV digoxin

C. Cardioversion

D. IV amiodarone

**22.15.** A 60-year-old patient with chronic kidney disease on dialysis has recurrent episodes of palpitations requiring cardioversion. ECG shows counterclockwise atrial flutter. What is the best treatment option?
A. Metoprolol
B. Sotalol
C. Dofetilide (Tikosyn)
D. EP study/ablation

**22.16.** A 66-year-old female with a history of ischemic cardiomyopathy, status post-ICD implant, hypertension, and diabetes is detected to have three episodes of paroxysmal atrial fibrillation lasting from one to two hours during a routine device check. She denies symptoms of palpitations. What is the next step in the management of this patient?
A. Observation
B. Holter monitor
C. Echocardiogram
D. Anticoagulation

**22.17.** A 70-year-old male with a history of ischemic cardiomyopathy, hypertension, hospitalized for congestive heart failure exacerbation three months previously has four episodes of paroxysmal atrial fibrillation lasting from 8 to 12 hours. He reports symptoms of palpitations and fatigue. He has been taking metoprolol and rivaroxaban. What is the antiarrhythmic agent of choice?
A. Dronaderone
B. Dofetelide
C. Flecainide
D. Propafenone

**22.18.** A 42-year-old patient with no prior medical history presents with palpitations of five days' duration. ECG reveals atrial fibrillation with ventricular rate of 120 bpm. He is placed on IV heparin and undergoes transesophageal echocardiography-guided cardioversion the following day. What does this patient have?
A. Lone atrial fibrillation
B. Paroxysmal atrial fibrillation
C. Persistent atrial fibrillation
D. Long-standing persistent atrial fibrillation

**22.19.** What is the appropriate anticoagulation management for the patient in Question 22.18?
A. Aspirin 75 mg daily for one month
B. Aspirin 325 mg daily for one month
C. Warfarin for one month
D. No aspirin or warfarin are needed

**22.20.** A 55-year-old patient who is status post-coronary artery bypass grafting three days previously is noted to be in atrial flutter. He is placed on metoprolol and warfarin and discharged home. He has been followed by his primary care physician. You see him in the office three months later. He feels well. He is in atrial flutter with ventricular rate 90 bpm. What would be the next step in the management of this patient?
A. Continue rate control
B. Sotalol
C. Cardioversion
D. EP study/ablation

**22.21.** A 68-year-old female patient status post-mechanical valve four years previously on warfarin develops paroxysmal atrial fibrillation. She would like to pursue anticoagulation with a novel oral anticoagulant because of labile international normalized ratio (INR) after she was started on amiodarone. Which of the following do you recommend?

**A.** Pradaxa      **C.** Apixaban
**B.** Rivaroxaban      **D.** None of the above

**22.22.** Which of the following is not a factor Xa inhibitor?

**A.** Apixaban      **C.** Rivaroxaban
**B.** Dabigatran      **D.** Edoxaban

**22.23.** A 70-year-old patient with paroxysmal atrial fibrillation was started on flecainide 100 mg BID. She has been doing well. An ECG done one week later reveals sinus rhythm with LBBB. Which of the following is the appropriate next step?

**A.** No change
**B.** Reduce dose of flecainide to 50 mg BID
**C.** Discontinue flecainide
**D.** Recommend pacer implant

**22.24.** A 72-year-old patient with history of atrial fibrillation is on warfarin and digoxin. He was started on dronedarone. The serum creatinine at baseline was 1.3; one week later it was 1.7. Which of the following statements is false?

**A.** The INR is not affected
**B.** The serum digoxin is unchanged
**C.** Renal tubular secretion of creatinine is inhibited by dronedarone
**D.** Reduction in glomerular filtration rate

**22.25.** When initiating therapy with amiodarone, a reduction in the dose is needed for all of the following agents except which?

**A.** Digoxin
**B.** Warfarin
**C.** Metoprolol
**D.** Apixaban

**22.26.** Which of the following statements regarding Tikosyn is false?

**A.** The dose is determined by creatinine clearance
**B.** It is contraindicated in patients with heart failure
**C.** Inpatient monitoring is mandatory while initiating therapy
**D.** ECG is monitored for QT prolongation

**22.27.** A 57-year-old patient with no prior cardiac history with symptoms of exercise-induced palpitations undergoes an exercise treadmill test. Sustained wide QRS tachycardia at a rate of 170 bpm occurs during recovery. The ECG is shown in Figure 22.27. The patient is hemodynamically stable. She is given 5 mg of IV metoprolol. Sinus rhythm is restored five minutes later. Echocardiogram reveals normal left and right ventricle function. What is the most likely diagnosis?

**A.** Ischemic VT
**B.** Idiopathic RVOT VT
**C.** Catecholaminergic VT
**D.** Idiopathic LVVT

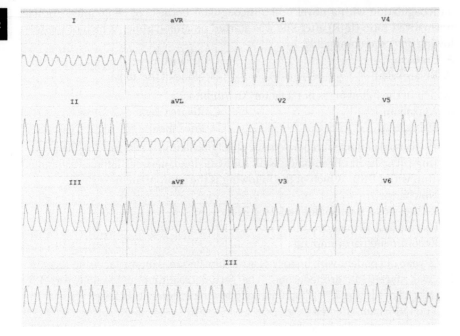

**Figure 22.27**

**22.28.** A 67-year-old female patient with a history of atrial fibrillation, hypertension, and St Jude aortic valve replacement is scheduled to undergo hip replacement. What is the best option for management of anticoagulation?

   **A.** Discontinue warfarin five days prior to procedure, bridge with low molecular weight heparin (LMWH) when INR is 2.0, resume warfarin on day of surgery
   **B.** Discontinue warfarin five days prior to procedure, no bridging with LMWH is needed, resume warfarin on day of surgery
   **C.** Continue warfarin
   **D.** Discontinue warfarin two days prior to procedure, bridge with LMWH after surgery, resume warfarin on day of surgery

**22.29.** A 70-year-old male patient with a history of ischemic cardiomyopathy, status post-ICD implant, atrial fibrillation, hypertension, and diabetes is scheduled for ICD generator replacement. What is the best option for management of anticoagulation?

   **A.** Discontinue warfarin five days prior to procedure, bridge with LMWH when INR is 2.0, resume warfarin on day of surgery
   **B.** Discontinue warfarin five days prior to procedure, no bridging with LMWH is needed, resume warfarin on day of surgery
   **C.** Continue warfarin
   **D.** Discontinue warfarin two days prior to procedure, bridge with LMWH after surgery, resume warfarin on day of surgery

**22.30.** A 55-year-old female patient with history of atrial fibrillation, hypertension, and diabetes is scheduled to undergo biopsy of breast mass. Her renal function is normal. She is on apixaban 5 mg BID. What is the best option for management of anticoagulation?
  **A.** Discontinue apixaban 24 hours prior to procedure
  **B.** Discontinue apixaban 48 hours prior to procedure
  **C.** Continue apixaban
  **D.** Reduce dose of apixaban to 2.5 mg BID

**22.31.** A 22-year-old patient is hospitalized with abdominal pain. She has no cardiac symptoms. Her ECG is shown in Figure 22.31. What does it demonstrate?
  **A.** Intraventricular conduction disturbance
  **B.** Right bundle branch block (RBBB)
  **C.** WPW syndrome
  **D.** Right ventricular hypertrophy

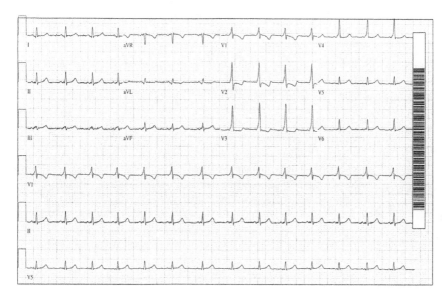

**Figure 22.31**

**22.32.** A 28-year-old female patient has had symptoms of palpitations since the age of 5. They are infrequent, occurring once a year, and are brought on by physical activity. Her ECG, done in the office, is shown in Figure 22.32. What is the most likely explanation for her palpitations?
  **A.** AVNRT
  **B.** Orthodromic atrioventricular reciprocating tachycardia (AVRT)
  **C.** Atrial tachycardia
  **D.** Antidromic AVRT

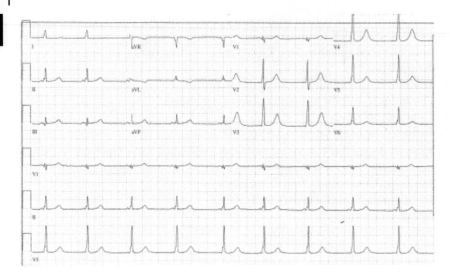

**Figure 22.32**

**22.33.** The ECG in Figure 22.33 demonstrates which of the following?
   **A.** Sinus rhythm with PVC
   **B.** Sinus rhythm with premature atrial complex with aberrant ventricular conduction
   **C.** Sinus rhythm, WPW syndrome with PVC
   **D.** Sinus rhythm, WPW syndrome with two accessory pathways

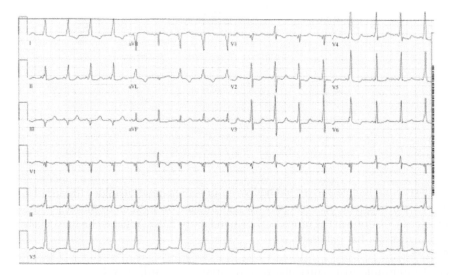

**Figure 22.33**

**22.34.** The intracardiac tracing shown in Figure 22.34a demonstrates which of the following?

    **A.** RBBB

    **B.** Short HV interval

    **C.** Normal HV interval

    **D.** Prolonged HV interval

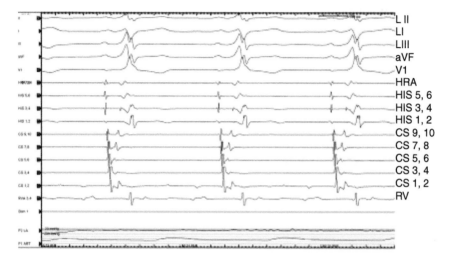

**Figure 22.34a**

**22.35.** The wide QRS beats (beats 1–6) seen in the tracing in Figure 22.35a are due to which of the following?

    **A.** RBBB

    **B.** Aberrant ventricular conduction

    **C.** Preexcitation

    **D.** Idioventricular rhythm

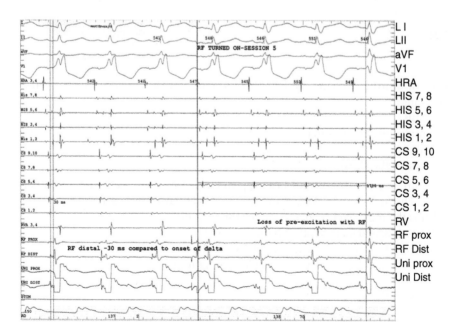

**Figure 22.35a**

**22.36.** The 12-lead ECG shown in Figure 22.36 is consistent with which of the following?

**A.** RBBB

**B.** Antidromic tachycardia

**C.** VT

**D.** None of the above

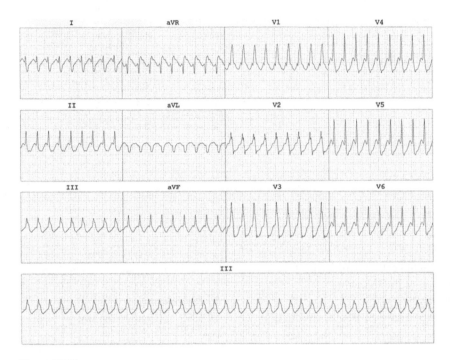

**Figure 22.36**

**22.37.** The intracardiac tracing in Figure 22.37a is consistent with which of the following?

**A.** RBBB

**B.** Antidromic tachycardia

**C.** VT

**D.** None of the above

**22.38.** In Figure 22.38a, the second beat appears different compared with the other beats. The intracardiac electrograms on this beat have a well-defined His spike. What is the most likely explanation for this finding?

**A.** Beats 1, 3, and 4 are ventricular in origin

**B.** There is loss of preexcitation on the second beat

**C.** Beats 1, 3, and 4 are supraventricular in origin with aberrant ventricular conduction

**D.** None of the above

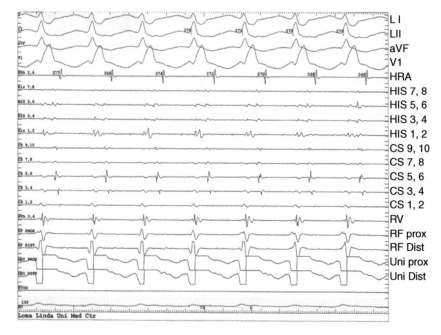

**Figure 22.37a**

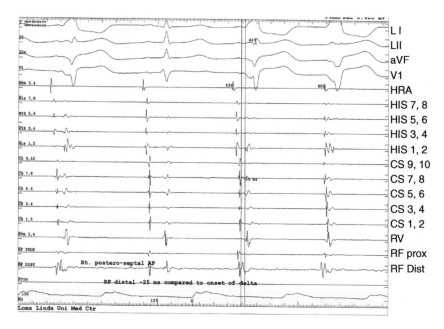

**Figure 22.38a**

**22.39.** The intracardiac signals during ventricular pacing are shown in Figure 22.39a. The mapping catheter (RF 1, 2) is positioned at a right postero-septal location. The retrograde atrial activation is most consistent with which of the following?

**A.** Retrograde VA conduction via AV node
**B.** Retrograde VA conduction via accessory pathway
**C.** Atrial signal is not recorded on RF 1, 2
**D.** None of the above

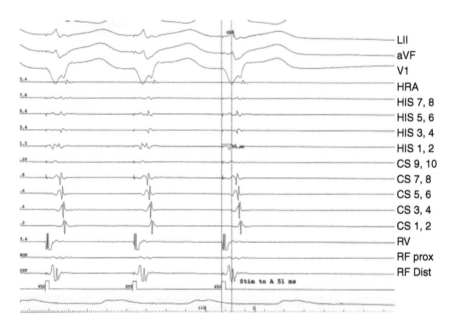

**Figure 22.39a**

**22.40.** Intracardiac signals during sinus rhythm are shown in Figure 22.40. The mapping catheter (RF 1, 2) is positioned in close proximity to poles 3, 4 of the coronary sinus catheter (CS 3, 4). This corresponds to a left lateral position on the mitral annulus. Which of the following statements is correct?

**A.** A left lateral accessory pathway is present.
**B.** There is no evidence of an accessory pathway
**C.** The HV interval is prolonged
**D.** None of the above

**22.41.** In Figure 22.41, the first four beats are ventricular paced beats and the last four beats are SVT beats. The intracardiac signals with ventricular pacing and SVT are identical. What is the most likely mechanism of SVT?

**A.** AVNRT
**B.** AVRT
**C.** Atrial tachycardia
**D.** None of the above

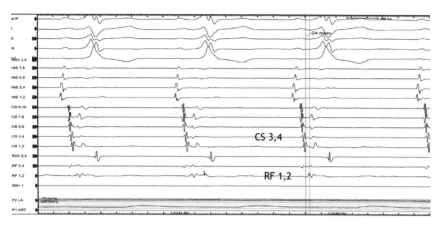

**Figure 22.40**

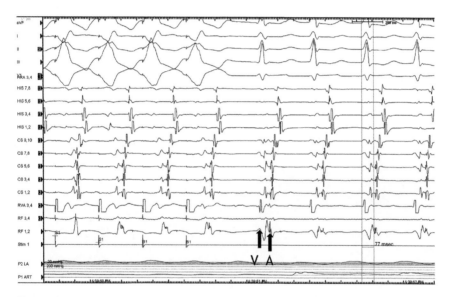

**Figure 22.41**

**22.42.** The 12-lead ECG shown in Figure 22.42 is consistent with which of the following?

A. SVT with aberrant conduction

B. VT

C. Paced rhythm

D. Antidromic tachycardia

**22.43.** What is the most likely underlying cardiac condition in the patient whose 12-lead ECG is shown in Figure 22.43?

A. Prior MI

B. Structurally normal heart

C. WPW syndrome

D. None of the above

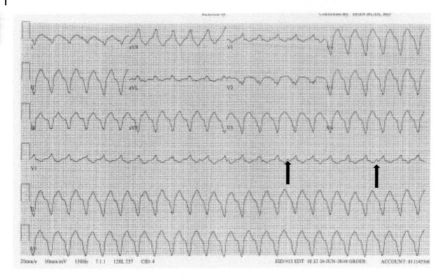

**Figure 22.42**

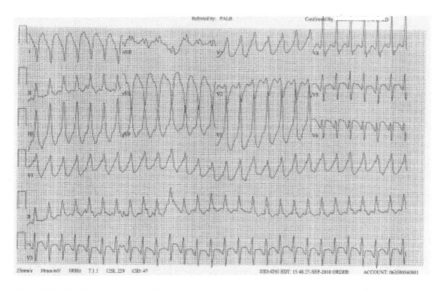

**Figure 22.43**

**22.44.** The rhythm strip in Figure 22.44 was obtained in a 25-year-old female patient with symptoms of palpitations and dizziness. The echocardiogram was normal. During a stress test, the patient developed sustained wide QRS tachycardia at a rate of 170 bpm with an LBBB morphology and inferior axis which terminated spontaneously. What is the likely diagnosis?

**A.** Verapamil-sensitive VT

**B.** Idiopathic RVOT VT

**C.** Catecholaminergic VT

**D.** Long QT syndrome

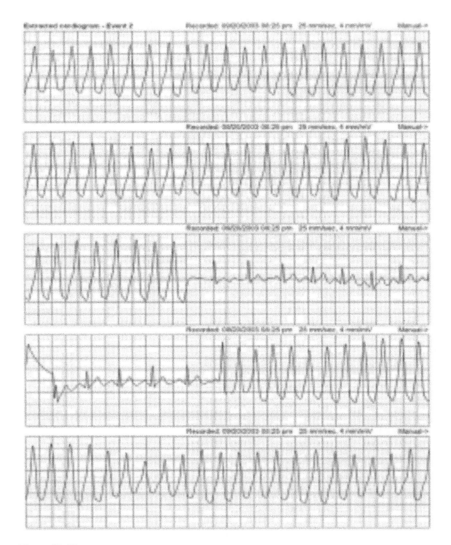

**Figure 22.44**

**22.45.** The intracardiac tracing in Figure 22.45 was obtained during an EP study on a patient with complaints of palpitations and runs of wide QRS tachycardia on an event monitor. What is the likely diagnosis?
  **A.** Idiopathic RVOT
  **B.** Idiopathic LV VT
  **C.** Junctional tachycardia
  **D.** None of the above

**22.46.** The 12-lead ECG in Figure 22.46 demonstrates wide QRS tachycardia. What is the likely diagnosis?
  **A.** SVT with aberrant conduction
  **B.** SVT with underlying bundle branch block
  **C.** VT
  **D.** None of the above

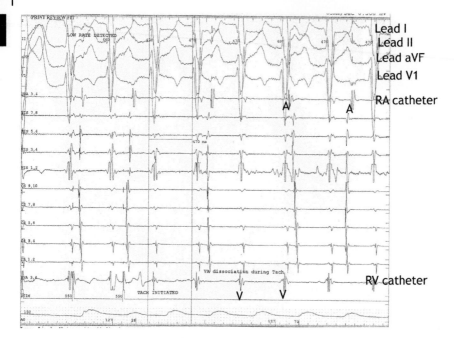

Lead I
Lead II
Lead aVF
Lead V1
RA catheter

RV catheter

**Figure 22.45**

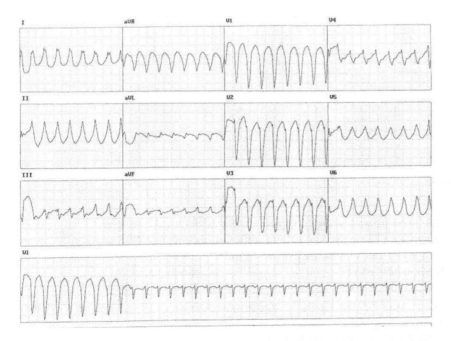

**Figure 22.46**

**22.47.** The intracardiac tracing in Figure 22.47 demonstrates wide QRS tachycardia changing to a narrow QRS tachycardia. The cycle length is longer during wide QRS tachycardia. What is this finding consistent with?
**A.** AVNRT
**B.** AVRT with bundle branch block ipsilateral to accessory pathway
**C.** AVRT with bundle branch block contralateral to accessory pathway
**D.** None of the above

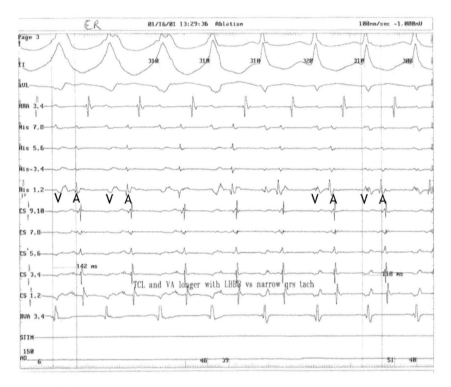

**Figure 22.47**

**22.48.** What is the intracardiac tracing shown in Figure 22.48 consistent with?
**A.** VT
**B.** Bundle branch reentry
**C.** SVT with aberrant conduction
**D.** None of the above

**22.49.** On the intracardiac tracing shown in Figure 22.49, the first four beats are ventricular paced beats followed by SVT. Which of the following statements is false?
**A.** The retrograde atrial activation with ventricular pacing is occurring only via the AV node
**B.** The retrograde atrial activation during SVT is via an accessory pathway
**C.** The retrograde atrial activation with ventricular pacing and during SVT is via an accessory pathway
**D.** A left lateral accessory pathway is present

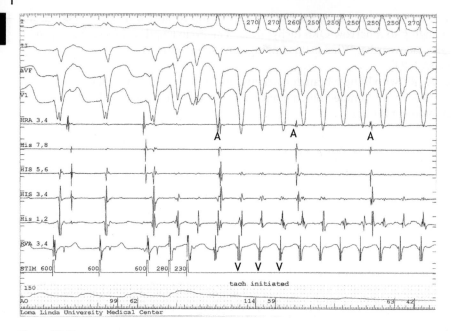

**Figure 22.48**

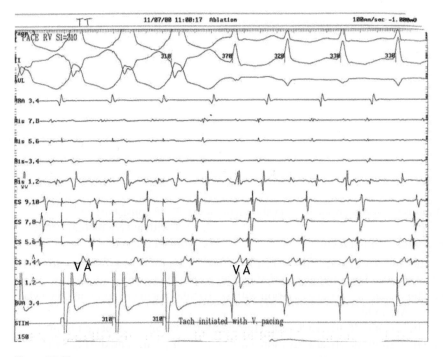

**Figure 22.49**

**22.50.** Following the first three atrial paced beats, an atrial extra-stimulus induces tachycardia. The intracardiac tracing shown in Figure 22.50 demonstrates all of the characteristics *except* which of the following?
  **A.** Long AH interval with the extra-stimulus
  **B.** Short VA interval during tachycardia
  **C.** A His spike preceding the ventricular electrogram
  **D.** Short HV interval on the atrial paced beats

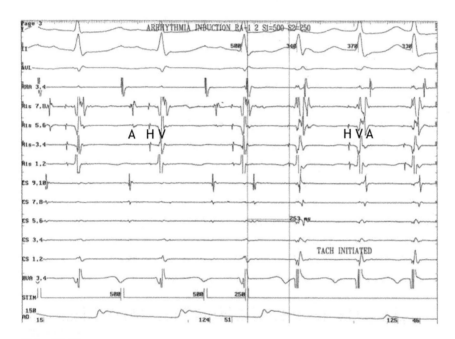

**Figure 22.50**

**22.51.** The ECG shown in Figure 22.51 was obtained during an EP study while positioning a catheter in the His bundle region. Which of the following statements is incorrect?
  **A.** The most likely explanation for this ECG pattern is catheter-induced trauma to the right bundle
  **B.** The conduction through right bundle is likely to recover
  **C.** The conduction system is unlikely to recover and a permanent pacemaker implant is indicated
  **D.** A similar situation can be encountered while placing a right ventricular pacing lead in a patient with a preexisting LBBB

**22.52.** The intracardiac tracing in Figure 22.52 was obtained in a patient with AV block. It demonstrates which of the following?
  **A.** Block at the level of the AV node      **C.** Intra-His block
  **B.** Infra-His block                        **D.** None of the above

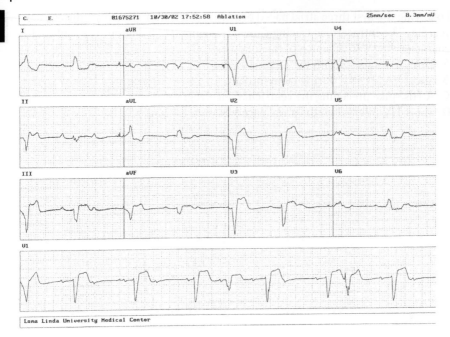

**Figure 22.51**

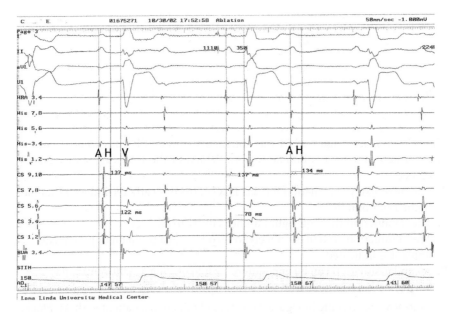

**Figure 22.52**

# Answers

**22.1.** A. Neurocardiogenic.

Statistically, this is the most common cause of syncope in the middle-aged, even if the tilt table test is negative. The tilt table test has a sensitivity of about 60% and specificity of 90% for the diagnosis of neurocardiogenic or vasovagal syncope. In patients with high pretest probability, a negative test is of limited value. The right ventricle was normal, ruling out submassive pulmonary embolism. Cate-cholaminergic arrhythmias occur with physical or emotional stress.

**22.2.** C. Implant an ICD.

A patient with prior MI and extensive scarring with syncope has a high probability of VT as a cause of syncope. Hence, an ICD is indicated and there is no need for arrhythmia monitoring or EP testing to identify the mechanism of syncope. In addition, his EF is <35% on a good medical regimen, and even without syncope would be an indication for ICD for primary prevention.

**22.3.** D. A 75-year-old man.

It occurs in elderly subjects.

**22.4.** D. All of the above.

The longer the QTc, the higher is the arrhythmic mortality, being about 5% in those with QTc of 450 ms, and 50% in those with QTc >500 ms over lifetime. Syncope in these patients is likely due to runs of polymorphic VT.

**22.5.** C. 30%.

An ICD is also indicated.

**22.6.** A. It is a genetically determined sodium channelopathy.

The ECG changes could be dynamic and come and go and can be provoked with procainamide challenge. Type I Brugada with ST elevation of >10 mm has a very high risk of sudden death.

**22.7.** D. Dual-chamber pacemaker implant.

Complete heart block is a class I indication for permanent pacer implant. A dual-chamber device is indicated in the presence of intact sinus mechanism.

**22.8.** C. EP studies and catheter ablation.

The patient has side effects related to his current medication regimen. He is likely to have breakthrough episodes of arrhythmia on a lower dose of flecainide and metoprolol. Trial with a different agent could be tried but is likely to be ineffective. EP studies and ablation is potentially curative.

**22.9.** D. Both medications will be continued.

Her $CHA_2DS_2$–VASc score is 4.

**22.10.** B. Exercise treadmill test.

If there is loss of preexcitation on an exercise treadmill test, accessory pathway conduction is weak and risk of rapid ventricular response if atrial fibrillation occurs is low.

**22.11.** C. EP studies and catheter ablation.

The PVC burden is high. Morphology is suggestive of right ventricular outflow tract (RVOT) origin of PVCs, which is very amenable to catheter ablation. The LVEF is likely to improve after successful ablation.

**22.12.** C. 90–95%.

**22.13.** D. EP study/ablation.

Ablation has a success rate of 90–95%. Patient has history of MI, hence, flecainide is contraindicated. Long-term side effects have to be considered with amiodarone.

**22.14.** C. Cardioversion.

In a patient with Wolff-Parkinson-White (WPW) syndrome and atrial fibrillation, cardioversion is indicated. All other options are contraindicated.

**22.15.** D. EP study/ablation.

In the presence of chronic kidney disease, options B and C are contraindicated. Metoprolol will not prevent recurrence of atrial flutter.

**22.16.** D. Anticoagulation.

Her $CHA_2DS_2$-VASc score is 5; hence, she is a candidate for oral anticoagulation.

**22.17.** B. Dofetilide.

Choices A, C, and D are contraindicated.

**22.18.** B. Paroxysmal atrial fibrillation.

As the duration is less than seven days.

**22.19.** C. Warfarin for one month.

Because atrial mechanical function may take 2–21 days to normalize after cardioversion due to atrial stunning. Stunning also occurs with chemical or spontaneous cardioversions.

**22.20.** C. Cardioversion.

The patient developed postoperative atrial flutter; it is unlikely to recur after successful cardioversion. Therapeutic anticoagulation for three to four weeks is essential before cardioversion.

**22.21.** D. None of the above.

The patient has a mechanical valve, which is a contraindication for novel anticoagulants. She will need to continue taking warfarin.

**22.22.** B. Dabigatran.

This is a direct thrombin inhibitor.

**22.23.** B. Reduce the dose of flecainide to 50 mg BID.

The development of LBBB is due to flecainide. Monitor ECG for prolongation of QRS duration for an increase by >25% over baseline.

**22.24.** D. Reduction in glomerular filtration rate.

The glomerular filtration rate is not affected by dronedarone; it inhibits creatinine secretion, which accounts for the higher serum creatinine.

**22.25.** D. Apixaban.

Dose of apixaban is determined by age, body weight, and serum creatinine.

**22.26.** B. It is contraindicated in patients with heart failure.

Patients with heart failure *are* candidates for Tikosyn.

**22.27.** B. Idiopathic RVOT VT.

ECG of VT of LBBB with inferior axis consistent with RVOT origin.

**22.28.** A. Discontinue warfarin five days prior to procedure, bridge with low molecular weight heparin (LMWH) when INR is 2.0, resume warfarin on day of surgery.

$CHA_2DS_2$-VASc score is 3. Bridging is recommended to reduce risk of thromboembolism.

**22.29.** C. Continue warfarin.

Bridging is associated with increased risk of pocket hematoma. The procedure can be safely performed while patient is still on warfarin (Birnie et al. 2013).

**22.30.** A. Discontinue apixaban 24 hours prior to procedure.

In the presence of normal renal function, hold apixaban for 24 hours.

**22.31.** C. WPW syndrome.

The delta wave is positive in lead V1, suggestive of a left-sided accessory pathway.

**22.32.** B. Orthodromic atrioventricular reciprocating tachycardia (AVRT).

The sinus rhythm ECG shows WPW syndrome. The most likely mechanism of SVT in this patient is orthodromic AVRT utilizing the atrioventricular (AV) node for antegrade conduction and accessory pathway for retrograde conduction.

**22.33.** D. Sinus rhythm, WPW syndrome with two accessory pathways.

The delta wave axis is negative in V1 on the majority of the beats; it is positive on the 6th, 11th, 15th, and 16th beats. The patient had right postero-septal and left lateral accessory pathways.

**22.34.** B. Short HV interval.

This patient has WPW syndrome with antegrade conduction through the AV node as well as accessory pathway. The HV interval is negative due to conduction through the accessory pathway (see Figure 22.34b).

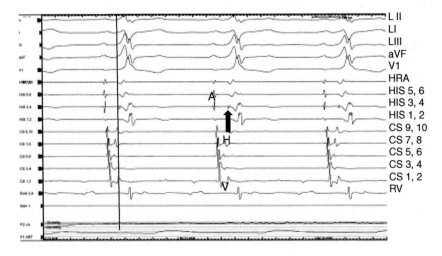

**Figure 22.34b**

**22.35.** C. Preexcitation.

The HV interval on beats 1–6 is short. Following radiofrequency energy application, on beat 7 there is loss of preexcitation (Figure 22.35b). The QRS is narrow and the HV interval is longer. A and V signals are shown on beat 6 (AV 6) and 7 (AV 7) – note that there is greater separation of A and V in beat 7 compared with beat 6.

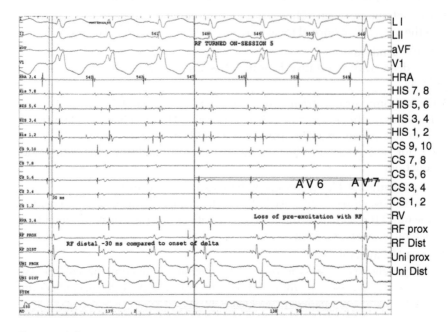

**Figure 22.35b**

**22.36.** A. RBBB.

The wide QRS tachycardia is due to the presence of RBBB, which could be present in the baseline state or may occur as a result of rate-related aberrant ventricular conduction. The morphology criteria – rsR in lead V1 and rs pattern in leads 1 and V6 – favor supraventricular origin. With antidromic tachycardia, antegrade conduction occurs via the accessory pathway which inserts into the ventricular myocardium. Subsequent conduction through the ventricular myocardium would be similar to tachycardia which originates in the ventricular myocardium.

**22.37.** A. RBBB.

A His spike is seen on His 1, 2 (arrow in Figure 22.37b). It precedes the onset of QRS; hence, the rhythm is supraventricular in origin. The retrograde atrial activation is concentric with earliest atrial activation occurring on His leads, likely due to conduction via the AV node.

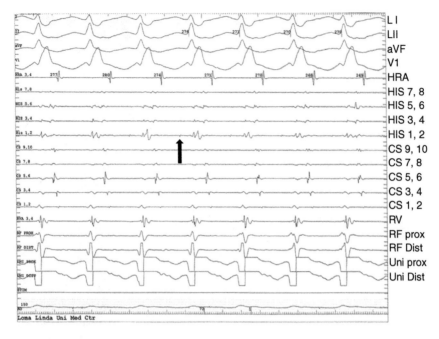

**Figure 22.37b**

**22.38.** B. There is loss of preexcitation on the second beat.

Intermittent preexcitation is present. The QRS is narrow and the HV interval is normal with loss of preexcitation on the second beat (see Figure 22.38b).

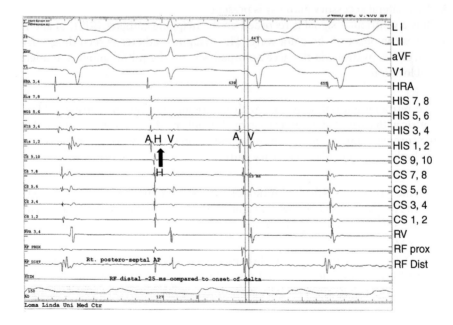

**Figure 22.38b**

**22.39.** B. Retrograde VA conduction via accessory pathway.

The ventricular and atrial signals are fused on RF 1, 2. This is due to retrograde activation via the postero-septal accessory pathway (see Figure 22.39b).

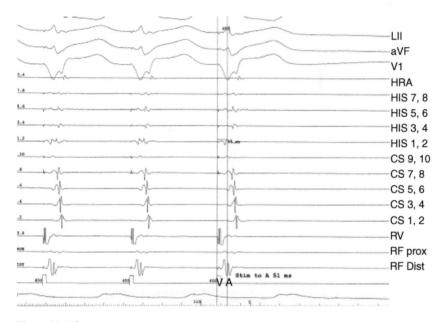

**Figure 22.39b**

**22.40.** A. A left lateral accessory pathway is present.

Only a ventricular signal is recorded on the mapping catheter (RF 1, 2) and it precedes the onset of the delta wave. The mapping catheter is recording early ventricular activation via the accessory pathway on the mitral annulus at a left lateral location.

**22.41.** B. AVRT.

The retrograde atrial activation with ventricular pacing and during SVT is eccentric with earliest atrial activation on the mid and distal coronary sinus poles of the coronary sinus catheter. The antegrade limb is the AV node and the retrograde limb is the left-sided accessory pathway.

**22.42.** B. VT.

The morphology is RBBB with monophasic R wave in lead V1. There is evidence of AV dissociation (arrows in Figure 22.42 point to P waves). The axis is in the northwest (left superior) quadrant.

**22.43.** A. Prior MI.

The ECG is suggestive of VT (wide complex tachycardia with monophasic R in V1 with RBBB morphology, slurred upstroke of QRS). The patient likely had a prior MI.

**22.44.** B. Idiopathic RVOT VT.

Repetitive monomorphic VT in the absence of structural heart disease and LBBB with inferior axis VT morphology is consistent with RVOT origin.

**22.45.** B. Idiopathic LV VT.

The tachycardia has RBBB morphology with left-axis deviation suggestive of origin in the left ventricle in the region of the posterior fascicle.

**22.46.** A. SVT with aberrant conduction.

On the rhythm strip, the tachycardia changes from wide to narrow QRS. Rate-related aberrant conduction during SVT is responsible for wide QRS tachycardia.

**22.47.** B. AVRT with bundle branch block ipsilateral to accessory pathway.

In the presence of bundle branch block ipsilateral to the accessory pathway, the circuit is larger, which increases the cycle length of the tachycardia. For example, in the presence of LBBB with a left-sided accessory pathway, the impulse travels down the AV node, His bundle to right ventricle then left ventricle which then engages the accessory pathway and activates the atrium.

**22.48.** A. VT.

There is VA dissociation during tachycardia and no His spike recorded in front of the V-signal.

**22.49.** A. The retrograde atrial activation with ventricular pacing is occurring only via the AV node.

This statement is not accurate. The retrograde atrial activations with ventricular pacing and during SVT are identical. The earliest atrial activation is in the coronary sinus poles 3, 4 of the coronary sinus catheter, which is located at a left lateral site.

**22.50.** D. Short HV interval on the atrial paced beats.

This is not accurate. All other statements are correct. The HV interval on the first three atrial paced beats is normal. All other findings are present on this tracing obtained from a patient with AVNRT.

**22.51.** C. The conduction system is unlikely to recover and a permanent pacemaker implant is indicated.

This statement is incorrect. This patient has an underlying LBBB. The development of RBBB from catheter-induced trauma results in transient heart block and does not require a permanent pacemaker implant.

**22.52.** B. Infra-His block.

On the P wave following the third ventricular beat, the distal poles of the His bundle catheter (His 1,2) has an atrial electrogram followed by a His spike. There is no ventricular electrogram following the His spike.

## Reference

Birnie, D.H., Healey, J.S., Wells, G.A. et al. (2013). Pacemaker or defibrillator surgery without interruption of anticoagulation. *The New England Journal of Medicine* 368: 2084–2093.

# Pacemakers and Defibrillators

# 23

23.1. A 50-year-old patient gives a history of four dizzy spells in the previous month, occurring once a week. When she is seen in the clinic, she is not on any medications, is asymptomatic, and pulse is 45 bpm. Thyroid function is normal. What is the next step in the management?
A. Observe
B. 48-hours Holter monitor
C. Event monitor
D. Permanent pacer implant

23.2. A 65-year-old obese male patient with history of hypertension was monitored following colonoscopy. He had sinus bradycardia with a heart rate of 45 bpm. A Holter monitor was placed which revealed episodes of second-degree atrioventricular (AV) block with 2 : 1 conduction. The patient did not have any symptoms while he wore the monitor. What is the next step in the management of this patient?
A. Event monitor
B. Sleep studies
C. Electrophysiology (EP) studies
D. Pacer implant

23.3. A 42-year-old patient has noticed fatigue after returning from a trip to the East Coast. He had been hiking in the woods. He denies history of syncope. His ECG shows complete heart block. Which of the following options should be considered next?
A. Observe
B. Lyme serology
C. Temporary pacer
D. Permanent pacer

23.4. A 35-year-old asymptomatic patient with myotonic muscular dystrophy has evidence of first-degree AV block on a routine ECG. Which option should be considered next?
A. Schedule follow up in six months
B. Holter monitor
C. EP studies
D. Permanent pacer implant

*Cardiology Board Review*, Second Edition. Ramdas G. Pai and Padmini Varadarajan.
© 2023 John Wiley & Sons Ltd. Published 2023 by John Wiley & Sons Ltd.

**23.5.** In a patient with history of syncope and evidence of right bundle branch block with left anterior fascicular block on one ECG and a right bundle branch block with left posterior fascicular block on an ECG done the following day, what is the next appropriate step?
A. Event monitor
B. EP studies
C. Loop recorder
D. Permanent pacer implant

**23.6.** A 44-year-old patient is status post-cardiac transplant two days previously. He develops junctional rhythm at 40 bpm. Of the following treatment options, which one is indicated next?
A. Transcutaneous pacing
B. Temporary trans-venous pacing
C. Permanent pacer implant
D. Observe

**23.7.** In patients with cardiac sarcoidosis, which of the following statements is not true?
A. Patients are at risk for developing complete heart block
B. Patients are at risk for developing VT
C. Myocardial involvement occurs in less than 5% of patients
D. Usually affects individuals aged 20–40 years

**23.8.** Which of the following statements regarding carotid sinus hypersensitivity is not true?
A. Elderly patients may present with unexplained falls without loss of consciousness
B. The reflex has a cardio-inhibitory component
C. There is no vasodepressor component
D. Permanent pacing is indicated in patients who develop pause greater than 3.0 s with carotid sinus massage

**23.9.** Which of the following statements regarding the role of pacing in neurocardio-genic syncope is not true?
A. It is not the first-line therapy for most patients.
B. It is indicated if there is no prodrome before syncopal event
C. It is indicated in patients with profound bradycardia or asystole during an episode
D. Those patients in whom other therapies are effective, but patient prefers to undergo pacer implant

**23.10.** In patients with long QT syndrome, which of the following is not an indication for permanent pacer implant?
A. Prevent pause-dependent VT, with or without QT prolongation
B. In high-risk patients with congenital long QT
C. Torsades de pointes VT due to reversible causes
D. Combination of pacing and beta blockade shortens QT interval and reduces risk of sudden cardiac death

**23.11.** In a patient with ischemic cardiomyopathy, ejection fraction (EF) 30%, and New York Heart Association (NYHA) class I, all of the following characteristics are contraindications for cardiac resynchronization therapy (CRT) *except* for which option?
A. Left bundle branch block (LBBB) with QRS duration 120–149 ms
B. Non-LBBB with QRS duration 120–149 ms
C. LBBB with QRS duration >150 ms
D. Non-LBBB with QRS duration >150 ms

**23.12.** A 75-year-old patient with history of sick sinus syndrome, status post-pacer implant is scheduled to undergo generator replacement. Pacer diagnostics revealed that the patient was V-paced 50% of the time. ECG done with pacer inhibited revealed sinus bradycardia with PR interval of 320 ms, QRS duration 110 ms, and QT interval 420 ms. The left ventricular (LV) EF is 35%. What is the next step in the management of this patient?
A. Replace pacer generator
B. Upgrade to CRT pacer
C. Upgrade to dual-chamber implantable cardioverter-defibrillator (ICD)
D. Upgrade to CRT defibrillator

**23.13.** A 78-year-old patient with history of nonischemic cardiomyopathy, EF 20%, and permanent atrial fibrillation was recently hospitalized with congestive heart failure exacerbation. In the office, she is noted to be in atrial fibrillation with ventricular rate 130 bpm at rest. The patient has been on carvedilol 50 mg BID and digoxin 0.125 mg daily. What is the best treatment option?
A. Single-chamber ICD
B. Dual-chamber ICD
C. Biventricular pacer/ICD and AV node ablation
D. Subcutaneous ICD

**23.14.** A 55-year-old patient presents with symptoms of epigastric discomfort of one hour's duration. An ECG revealed acute inferior myocardial infarction with complete AV block. The ventricular rate is 50 bpm, and blood pressure is 80/50 mmHg. He undergoes stent to proximal right coronary artery with resolution of symptoms. The rhythm is unchanged. What is the next step in the management?
A. Observe
B. Transcutaneous pacer
C. Temporary transvenous pacer
D. Permanent pacer implant

**23.15.** A 48-year-old female patient with no prior cardiac history has an out-of-hospital cardiac arrest. After undergoing prolonged resuscitation measures, including four external shocks, she makes a full recovery. The LVEF is 50%. The cardiac enzymes are mildly elevated, and the coronary anatomy is normal. The cardiac magnetic resonance image is normal. Of the following options, which would you recommend?
A. Beta blockers
B. Life vest
C. Amiodarone
D. ICD implant

**23.16.** A 64-year-old patient with history of remote myocardial infarction 10 years previously, LVEF 50%, and with inferior wall infarct on echocardiogram gives history of episodes of palpitations associated with dizziness for the previous month. He presents to the emergency room following an episode of palpitation of a half-hour's duration. ECG reveals wide QRS tachycardia consistent with VT. What is the most appropriate treatment choice for this patient?

    A. Metoprolol

    B. Sotalol

    C. Amiodarone

    D. ICD implant

**23.17.** A 72-year-old patient with history of myocardial infarction 15 years previously is brought to the emergency room following a syncopal spell. He had no warning symptoms. Echocardiogram revealed LVEF 45%, antero-apical infarct. Occluded mid-left anterior descending artery is seen on coronary angiogram. EP studies are performed. Sustained monomorphic VT is induced with programmed ventricular stimulation with the introduction of two extra stimuli. What is the next step in the management of this patient?

    A. Metoprolol

    B. Amiodarone

    C. Life vest

    D. ICD implant

**23.18.** A 47-year-old patient is seen by his cardiologist for follow-up. He had an anterior myocardial infarction six weeks previously and received thrombolytics. He has been doing well. An echocardiogram is done. The LVEF is 35%, and anterior wall is akinetic. The patient is on aspirin, atorvastatin, metoprolol, and enalapril. Which of the following is recommended for this patient?

    A. Spironolactone

    B. Amiodarone

    C. EP studies

    D. ICD implant

**23.19.** A 65-year-old patient with history of nonischemic cardiomyopathy, diagnosed one year previously, and LVEF 30% on recent echo is seen in the office for a routine visit. He has shortness of breath when he walks up an incline. On physical examination, he is euvolemic. Current medications include carvedilol and benazepril. Which of the following therapies would you recommend next?

    A. Lasix

    B. Digoxin

    C. Spironolactone

    D. ICD implant

**23.20.** An ICD implant for primary prevention is indicated in which of the following patients?

    A. A 50-year-old patient with history of myocardial infarction six weeks previously, NYHA class I symptoms, and LVEF 30%

    B. A 40-year-old asymptomatic male with ECG suggestive of Brugada syndrome, whose brother died suddenly

    C. A 45-year-old asymptomatic patient with history of hypertrophic cardiomyopathy, LV thickness 2.0 cm

    D. An 18-year-old female with lightheaded spells and QT prolongation on ECG

**23.21.** A 64-year-old patient with history of myocardial infarction 12 years previously is hospitalized following elective hip surgery. He has an eight-beat run of nonsustained VT at a rate of 130 bpm. He denies symptoms of palpitations or dizziness. An echocardiogram was done; the LVEF was 40%. He is on metoprolol and enalapril. What is the next step in the management of this patient?

A. Mexilitene

B. Sotalol

C. Amiodarone

D. EP studies

## Answers

**23.1.** C. Event monitor.

It is important to determine that dizzy spells are brought on by bradycardia. As the episodes are not every day, Holter recording may not be fruitful.

**23.2.** B. Sleep studies.

The patient most likely has obstructive sleep apnea, which is known to be associated with AV block.

**23.3.** B. Lyme serology.

Lyme disease is a reversible cause of heart block.

**23.4.** D. Permanent pacer implant.

As the risk of progression of AV block is known to be high.

**23.5.** B. EP studies.

These are indicated to determine if the patient has inducible ventricular tachycardia (VT), which could account for syncope. Trifascicular disease is indicative of possible diffuse myocardial disease which provides a substrate for VT. If an EP study is negative, trifascular block is the likely cause of syncope and pacer would be appropriate.

**23.6.** B. Temporary trans-venous pacing.

There is a good chance AV conduction will recover.

**23.7.** C. Myocardial involvement occurs in less than 5% of patients.

About 25% of patients with sarcoid have myocardial involvement, of which 30% develop complete heart block.

**23.8.** C. There is no vasodepressor component.

In 10–20% of patients, a vasodepressor component is present.

**23.9.** D. Those patients in whom other therapies are effective, but patient prefers to undergo pacer implant.

Pacer implant is contraindicated (class III) in patients who respond to other therapies.

**23.10.** C. Torsades de pointes VT due to reversible causes.

Pacing is contraindicated (class III) in patients with torsades de pointes VT due to reversible causes.

**23.11.** C. LBBB with QRS duration >150 ms.

In other situations, patients have to be more symptomatic. The greatest benefit is in those with LBBB with QRSd >150 ms.

**23.12.** D. Upgrade to CRT defibrillator.

As EF is 35% and percentage ventricular pacing is >40%.

**23.13.** C. Biventricular pacer/ICD and AV node ablation.

This is a class IIA indication with near 100% biventricular pacing likely following AV node ablation.

**23.14.** C. Temporary transvenous pacer.

The AV block is likely to resolve in the setting of inferior myocardial infarction.

**23.15.** D. ICD implant.

For secondary prevention of sudden cardiac death. The patient was defibrillated several times, which explains mild elevation of cardiac enzymes.

**23.16.** D. ICD implant.

Sustained VT is a class I indication for ICD implant.

**23.17.** D. ICD implant.

Inducible VT in this patient is a class I indication for ICD implant.

**23.18.** D. ICD implant.

Class I indication for ICD implant for primary prevention as patient is 40 days post-myocardial infarction with LVEF 35%.

**23.19.** D. ICD implant.

Class I indication.

**23.20.** A. A 50-year-old patient with history of myocardial infarction six weeks previously, NYHA class I symptoms, LVEF 30%.

Class I indication for ICD implant.

**23.21.** D. EP studies.

If VT is induced, it is a class I indication for ICD implant.

# Cardiac Masses

# 24

**24.1.** An 85-year-old female came in with complaints of chest pain. Her past history is significant for coronary artery disease, diabetes mellitus, and partial left mastectomy for a stage 2 breast cancer six years previously. Her lab work was negative for any acute process. She has a history of drug-eluting stent placement to her left circumflex artery six months prior to this admission. She has a nuclear stress test which was negative for ischemia. She also underwent an echocardiogram as part of her workup. What does the image in Figure 24.1 show?

A. Normal

B. Enlarged liver

C. Cysts in the kidneye

D. Mass in the liver

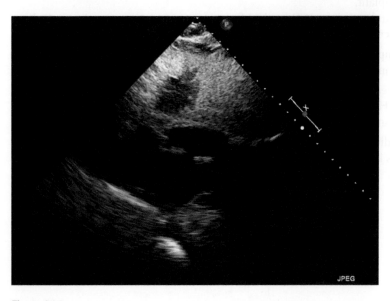

**Figure 24.1**

**24.2.** What is the next best step for the patient in Question 24.1?

A. Nothing at this time, as she has no abdominal complaints

B. Aspiration biopsy of the liver mass

C. Ultrasound of the liver

D. CT scan of the liver

*Cardiology Board Review*, Second Edition. Ramdas G. Pai and Padmini Varadarajan.
© 2023 John Wiley & Sons Ltd. Published 2023 by John Wiley & Sons Ltd.

24.3. A 33-year-old female presented with complaints of shortness of breath, choking sensation, and facial swelling. She has a history of a vaginal delivery four weeks prior to this presentation. She denies any other previous medical problems. An echocardiogram was performed. What does the image in Figure 24.3 show?
A. Normal echocardiogram from the suprasternal window
B. An artifact
C. Large mass in the superior mediastinum
D. Cannot tell

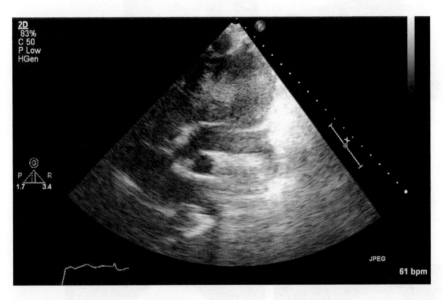

Figure 24.3

24.4. What is the next step for the patient in Question 24.3?
A. Diagnostic imaging with computed tomography (CT) scan
B. Ultrasound of the neck
C. No need for additional imaging
D. PET scan

24.5. A CT scan, shown in Figure 24.5, was ordered for the patient in Question 24.3. What does the image show?
A. Mass in the anterior mediastinum
B. Mass in the posterior mediastinum
C. Mass in the lung
D. Nothing abnormal is seen

24.6. What is the next best step for the patient in Question 24.3?
A. Biopsy of the mass
B. Ultrasound of the mass
C. Consultation with a surgeon
D. Nothing at this time

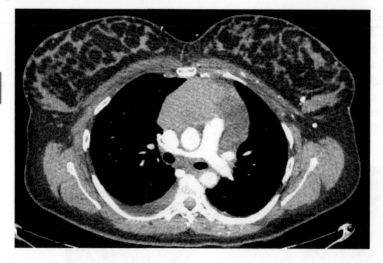

Figure 24.5

24.7. A 31-year-old male is admitted to the hospital for complaints of hemoptysis. He is a prisoner and has a remote history of tuberculosis that was treated. An echocardiogram was performed. What does the still frame obtained from parasternal long axis view and subcostal view in Figure 24.7a show?

A. Mass in the left atrium
B. Mass in the right atrium
C. Large artifact
D. No abnormality is noted

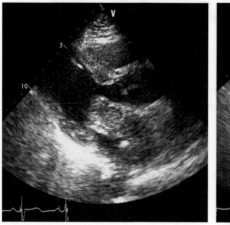
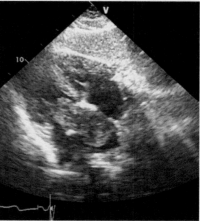

Figure 24.7a

24.8. The patient in Question 24.7 then underwent cardiac magnetic resonance imaging. The SSFP image is shown in Figure 24.8a. What does this image show?

A. Mass in the left atrium
B. Mass in the left atrium with filling defect in the right lower pulmonary vein and bilateral pleural effusions

C. No cardiac abnormality is noted

D. Mass in the right atrium

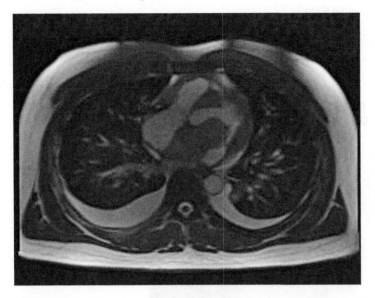

Figure 24.8a

24.9. The patient in Question 24.7 also then started having hemoptysis, for which a CT scan was done. What does the image in Figure 24.9a show?

A. Normal CT scan of the chest

B. A mass encircling the right bronchus

C. Mass in the pulmonary artery

D. Mass in the liver

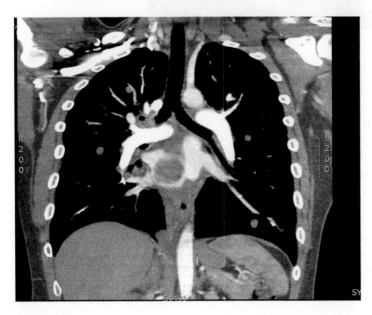

Figure 24.9a

**24.10.** The patient in Question 24.7 then started complaining of left thigh pain and swelling. A CT scan of the lower extremities was completed; see Figure 24.10a. What does the image show?

A. A normal CT scan

B. Normal right thigh and a large mass in the left thigh

C. A large mass in the lower abdomen

D. Mass in the right thigh

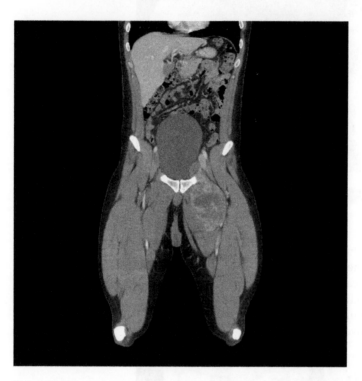

Figure 24.10a

**24.11.** What is the next best step for the patient in Question 24.7?

A. Consultation with the surgeons to remove the left atrial tumor

B. Biopsy of the left thigh mass

C. Biopsy of the left atrial mass

D. Surgical consultation to remove the left thigh mass

**24.12.** A 72-year-old male presented with a history of mechanical mitral valve replacement for rheumatic heart disease. He was on a therapeutic dose of warfarin and had subdural hemorrhage. Warfarin was discontinued by his treating physicians. The cardiologist paged late Friday evening for assistance as the patient went into flash pulmonary edema, atrial fibrillation with rapid ventricular response, was intubated emergently and imaging was performed; see Figure 24.12a. What does the image show?

A. Vegetations

B. Pannus

C. Tumor masses

D. Thrombus

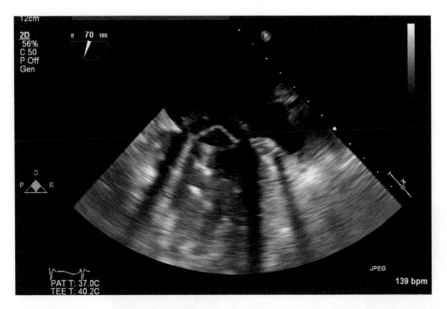

Figure 24.12a

24.13. A 74-year-old male was being evaluated for complaints of shortness of breath. His echo was unremarkable except for the image shown in Figure 24.13a. What does the image show?
A. Normal subcostal view
B. Artifact in the inferior vena cava (IVC)
C. Discrete masses in the IVC
D. Discrete masses in the aorta

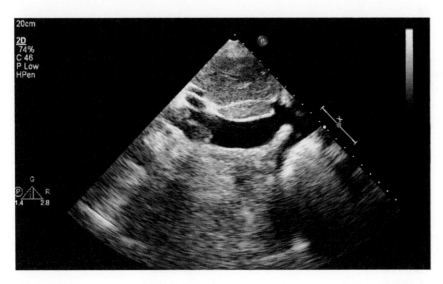

Figure 24.13a

24.14. What is the next best step for the patient in Question 24.12?
   A. Do nothing
   B. Ultrasound of the abdomen
   C. Magnetic resonance imaging of the abdomen
   D. Initiate anticoagulation

24.15. A 64-year-old male was admitted to hospital with complaints of fever, fatigue, and night sweats. He had a transthoracic echocardiogram; see Figure 24.15a. What does this left-sided subcostal image show?
   A. Normal structures                  C. Hepatomegaly
   B. Nephromegaly                       D. Splenomegaly

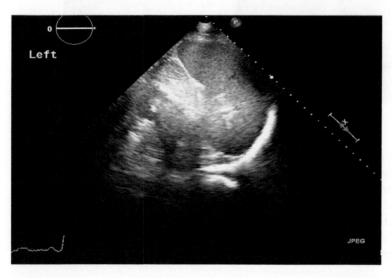

Figure 24.15a

24.16. A 20-year-old male presents to the hospital with complaints of fever, chills, and loss of appetite. He has a history of endocarditis and had a history of tricuspid valve replacement about two years prior to this admission. On examination, he was febrile and tachycardiac. He had an echocardiogram; see Figure 24.16a. What does the image show?
   A. Normal native tricuspid valve
   B. Vegetations on the bioprosthetic valve
   C. Tumor masses
   D. Thrombus on the valve

24.17. A 34-year-old male presents with complaints of malaise and shortness of breath on exertion. Physical examination is otherwise unremarkable. He had an echocardiogram; see Figure 24.17a (LA: left atrium; LV: left ventricle; RA: right atrium; RV: right ventricle). What does the image show?
   A. Thrombus                           C. Sarcoma
   B. Myxoma                             D. Vegetation

Chapter 2

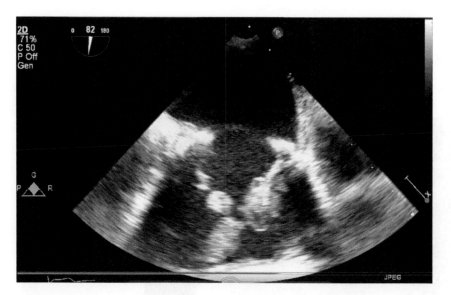

Figure 24.16a

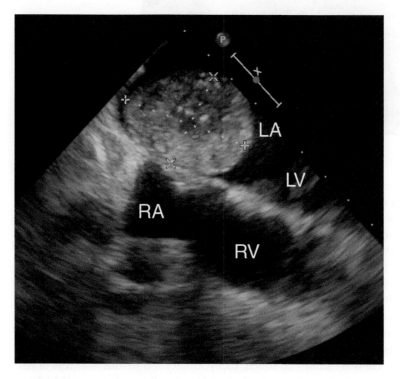

Figure 24.17a

24.18. A 45-year-old female had sudden onset of palpitations and had near syncope. She had no significant past medical history. She had an echocardiogram; see Figure 24.18a (LV: left ventricle; RV: right ventricle). What does the image show?

A. Myxoma                    C. Fibroma

B. Rhabdomyoma         D. Lymphoma

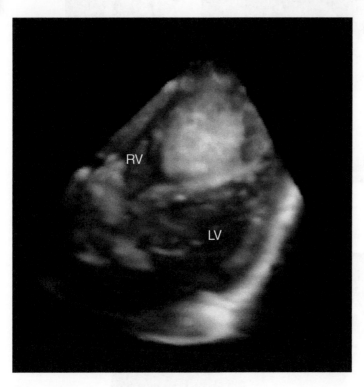

Figure 24.18a

24.19. A 56-year-old male presents to the hospital with a history of transient ischemic attack. On examination, he has no motor or sensory deficits. His cardiac examination is normal. He had an echocardiogram; see Figure 24.19a. What does the image show?

A. Vegetation on the mitral valve

B. Papillary fibroelastoma of the aortic valve

C. Papillary fibroelastoma of the mitral valve

D. Thrombus on the aortic valve

24.20. A 35-year-old male with a history of long-standing type 2 diabetes mellitus, hypertension, and end-stage renal disease started dialysis two months previously. He presents to the hospital complaining of fever, chills, malaise, nausea, and loss of appetite. He was clammy to touch, tachycardiac, and febrile. The rest of his physical examination was normal. He had blood cultures drawn and had an echocardiogram; see Figure 24.20a. What does the image show?

A. Vegetation on the catheter       C. Tumor mass

B. Thrombus                       D. Nothing abnormal is detected

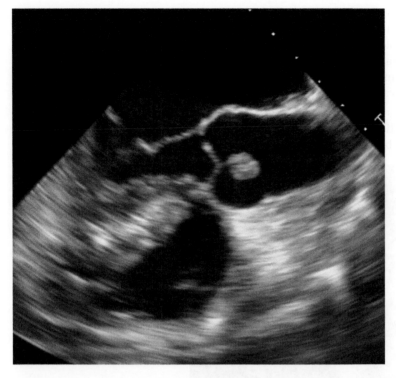

Figure 24.19a  *Source:* Reproduced with permission of Dr. Natesa G. Pandian.

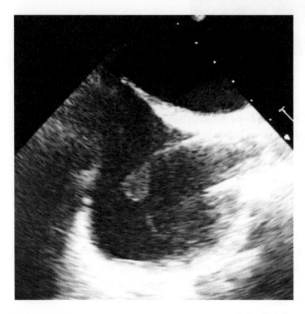

Figure 24.20a

24.21. What is the initial management strategy for the patient in Question 24.20?
   A. Start antibiotics
   B. Draw blood cultures, one from the periphery and one from the line, and then start antibiotics
   C. CT scan of the chest
   D. Observation

24.22. What does the image in Figure 24.22a show?
   A. Vegetation          C. Blood cyst
   B. Thrombus            D. Tumor

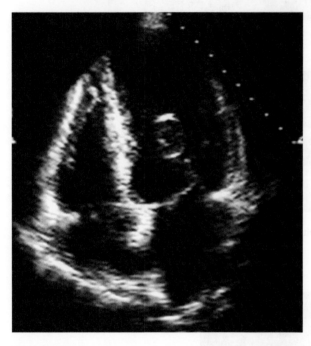

Figure 24.22a

24.23. A 75-year-old patient with a history of hypertension had an echocardiogram at an outside hospital. The patient was referred to this hospital for evaluation of a right atrial mass. What does the image in Figure 24.23a (LA: left atrium; RA: right atrium) show?
   A. Lymphoma
   B. Sarcoma
   C. Thrombus
   D. Lipomatous hypertrophy of the interatrial septum

24.24. A 65-year-old female with a history of hypertension came to the hospital with complaints of right-sided weakness. Her cardiac examination was remarkable for an irregularly irregular pulse. She had an echocardiogram; see Figure 24.24a (LA: left atrium; LV: left ventricle). What does the image show?
   A. Normal left atrial appendage
   B. Mass in the left atrial appendage which is likely to be a thrombus
   C. Coumadin ridge
   D. No abnormality is seen

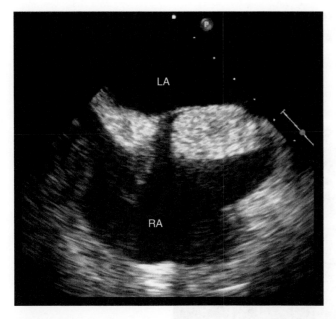

Figure 24.23a

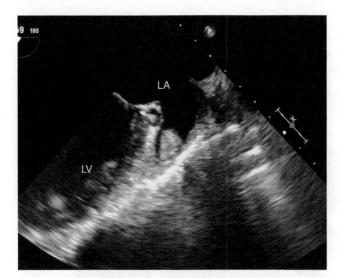

Figure 24.24a

24.25. A 37-year-old male patient had an echocardiogram. What does the subcostal image in Figure 24.25a show?
  A. Sarcoma
  B. Rhabdoma
  C. Pericardial cyst
  D. Lymphoma

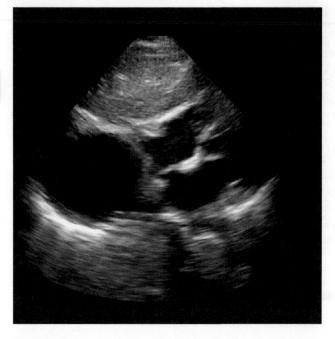

Figure 24.25a

24.26. A newborn baby was diagnosed with tuberous sclerosis. She has seizures. She had an echocardiogram; see Figure 24.26a. What does the image show?
   A. Multiple small tumors, likely rhabdomyoma
   B. Lipomas
   C. Sarcoma
   D. Fibroma

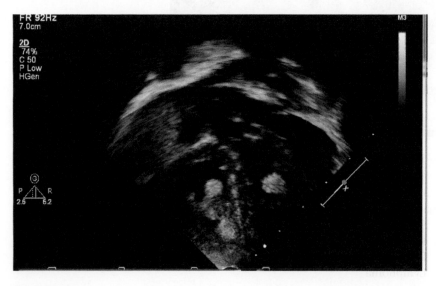

Figure 24.26a

24.27. What is the recommended management strategy for the patient in Question 24.26?
   A. Refer for surgery
   B. Chemotherapy
   C. Do nothing, manage seizures
   D. Radiation

24.28. A 59-year-old male presents to the hospital with complaints of acute onset of 9/10 central chest pressure. A 12-lead electrocardiogram showed anterior ST elevation and he was rushed to the cardiac catheterization laboratory. He was found to have a 100% mid-left anterior descending artery stenosis for which he had successful coronary intervention and placement of a drug-eluting stent. He then had an echocardiogram the next day, which showed akinesis of the left anterior descending artery territory. What does the apical four chamber image in Figure 24.28a (LA: left atrium; LV: left ventricle; RA: right atrium; RV: right ventricle) show?
   A. Tumor in the left ventricular apex
   B. A thrombus in the left ventricular apex
   C. Artifact from overlying ribs
   D. Obliterative myocarditis

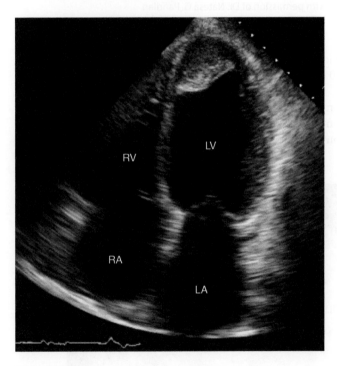

Figure 24.28a

24.29. A 32-year-old male with a previous history of HIV infection is on antiretroviral therapy. He presents to the hospital with complaints of fever, night sweats, loss of appetite, and unintentional weight loss of 12 lb. in two months. He had an echocardiogram; see Figure 24.29. What is the most likely explanation?
   A. Thrombus in the right atrium
   B. Renal cell carcinoma
   C. Sarcoma
   D. Lymphoma

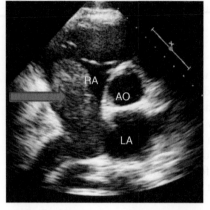
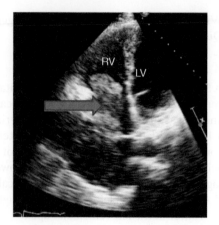

RA-right atrium     RV-right ventricle
LA-left atrium      LV-left ventricle
AO-aorta

Figure 24.29 *Source:* Reproduced with permission of Dr. Natesa G. Pandian.

24.30. A 67-year-old male had a routine echocardiogram. What does the subcostal view shown in Figure 24.30 demonstrate?
A. Normal findings
B. A mass arising from the superior pole of the right kidney
C. A mass arising from the liver
D. A mass arising from the spleen

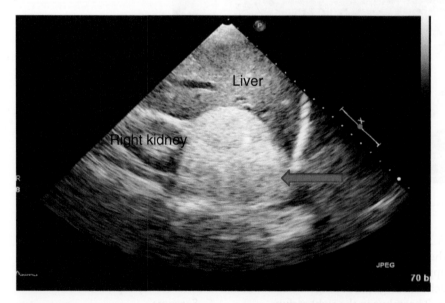

Figure 24.30

24.31. A 28-year-old male has a history of systemic lupus erythematosus and chronic kidney disease stage 2. He had a routine echocardiogram. What does the parasternal long axis view in Figure 24.31a demonstrate?
A. Normal looking mitral valve
B. Inflammatory changes of the mitral valve suggestive of Libman-Sacks endocarditis
C. Papillary fibroelastoma
D. Rheumatic changes of the mitral valve

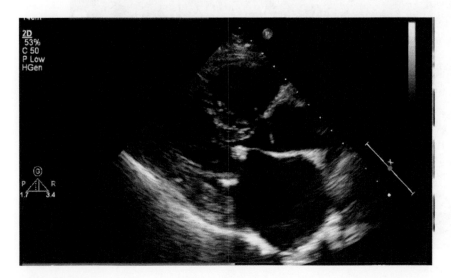

Figure 24.31a

24.32. What does the subcostal view in Figure 24.32a demonstrate?
A. Renal stones　　　　　　　　　　C. Hepatic stones
B. Gall stones　　　　　　　　　　　D. None of the above

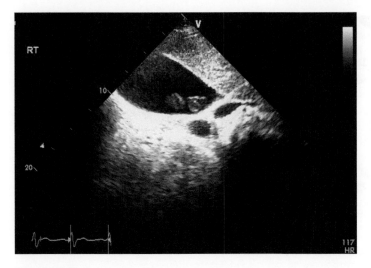

Figure 24.32a

24.33. A 72-year-old male was admitted to the hospital with complaints of fever, chills, night sweats, weight loss of 10 lb. in one month. He had a routine echocardiogram. What does the subcostal view in Figure 24.33a show?

A. Normal appearance of the liver      C. Right renal mass

B. Cystic lesions in the liver      D. None of the above

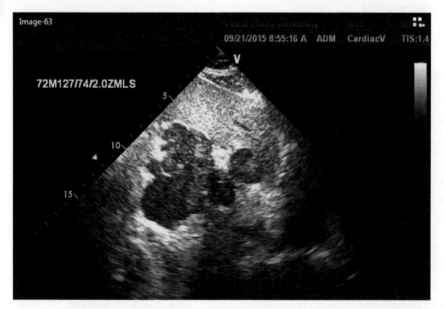

Figure 24.33a

24.34. A 63-year-old male with a history of end-stage renal disease and type 2 diabetes mellitus was admitted to the hospital to manage his dialysis catheter. He underwent a routine echocardiogram. What do the images in Figure 24.34a (LA: left atrium; LV: left ventricle; RV: right ventricle) and Figure 24.34b show?

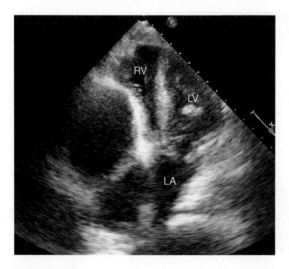

Figure 24.34a

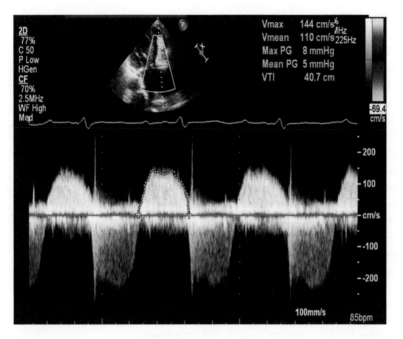

Chapter 24

**Figure 24.34b**

A. Normal apical four-chamber view
B. Apical four-chamber view showing extrinsic compression of the tricuspid valve
C. Apical four-chamber view showing intrinsic compression of the tricuspid valve
D. Apical four-chamber showing compression of the mitral valve

## Answers

24.1. D. Mass in the liver.
There is a hypoechoic mass seen in the liver on this subcostal view. The mass measures 45 mm × 34 mm.

24.2. B. Aspiration biopsy of the liver mass.
The liver mass is hypoechoic and is not cystic. She has a previous history of breast carcinoma, which heightens the suspicion for a metastatic mass. She underwent a biopsy of the liver mass which showed metastasis from breast origin. It was positive for both estrogen and progesterone receptors but was negative for HER2 protein.

24.3. C. Large mass in the superior mediastinum.
The image in Figure 24.3 is from the suprasternal window and it shows a large mass in the superior mediastinum. The mass is probably compressing the superior vena cava (SVC), causing SVC syndrome. The mass may also be compressing

her airways, which is probably contributing to her sensation of choking. The mass is seen above the arch of the aorta. Differential diagnosis includes goiter, thymoma, lymphoma, and germ cell tumors. The echocardiogram also showed a medium-sized pericardial effusion with no tamponade, raising the suspicion for malignancy.

**24.4.** A. Diagnostic imaging with computed tomography (CT) scan.

This patient needs additional diagnostic imaging to ascertain the location and extent of the mass. A CT scan is very appropriate and will help in assessing the size and location of the mass.

**24.5.** A. Mass in the anterior mediastinum.

There is a large mass in the anterior mediastinum. This mass measured 9.3 mm × 6.4 cm. The mass is seen surrounding the SVC and the airways. This probably represents a large tumor.

**24.6.** A. Biopsy of the mass.

The patient has a large anterior mediastinal mass, with SVC syndrome. She is symptomatic from this mass. The next best step is to biopsy the mass to characterize it further. The patient underwent a needle biopsy of the mass. The biopsy (Figure 24.6) showed sparse lymphocytic population with features suspicious for mediastinal large B-cell lymphoma. She had further cytologic studies and the mass was deemed to be a primary large B-cell lymphoma.

She had other work-up and was negative for metastasis. She was started on R-EPOCH chemotherapy and responded well. Her symptoms of facial swelling and choking sensation had resolved at the time of discharge from the hospital.

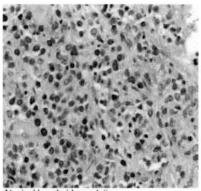
Atypical lymphoid population
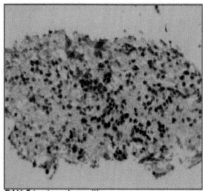
PAX-5 is strongly positive

Figure 24.6

**24.7.** A. Mass in the left atrium.

The parasternal long-axis image and the subcostal four-chamber image show a large mass that is probably attached to the interatrial septum and is prolapsing through the mitral valve (Figure 24.7b). Differential diagnosis includes a myxoma.

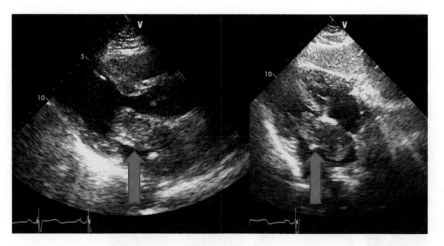

Figure 24.7b

**24.8.** B. Mass in the left atrium with filling defect in the right lower pulmonary vein and bilateral pleural effusions.

There is a large mass in the left atrium with filling defects in the right lower pulmonary vein (Figure 24.8b). Though the mass appears to be attached to the interatrial septum, this could be a distant metastasis through the pulmonary vein.

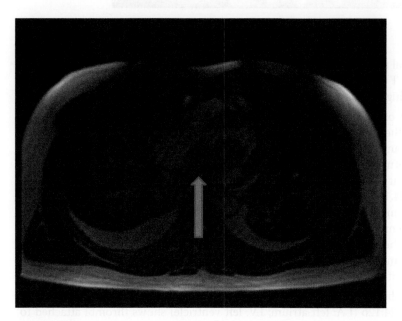

Figure 24.8b

24.9. B. A mass encircling the right bronchus.

There is an abnormal mass seen encircling the right main bronchus (Figure 24.9b). The mass (arrowed) is also seen at the carina infiltrating the airways. This probably is giving rise to hemoptysis.

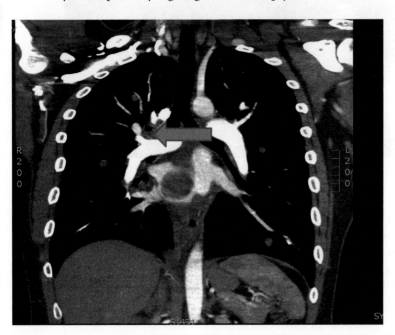

Figure 24.9b

24.10. B. Normal right thigh and a large mass in the left thigh.

This CT scan shows no abnormality in the right thigh. A large mass is seen in the left thigh in the adductor group (arrowed in Figure 24.10b).

24.11. B. Biopsy of the left thigh mass.

Since the patient has a mass in the left atrium, in the chest surrounding the airways, and in the left thigh, a biopsy of the thigh mass should be undertaken first. This mass is more easily accessible and would provide a tissue diagnosis. He underwent a biopsy of the thigh mass which showed a high-grade sarcoma (Figure 24.11).

His primary tumor was the high-grade sarcoma in his left thigh, which probably then metastasized to the heart though the pulmonary veins and to the chest through the blood. The mass in the chest was also biopsied, which showed evidence of metastasis from his sarcoma. Though the left atrial mass mimicked a myxoma, it was essentially a metastasis from the thigh.

24.12. D. Thrombus.

Figure 24.12b (LA: left atrium; LV: left ventricle) shows thrombi attached to the mitral valve sewing ring (blue arrows). The thrombi are preventing the prosthetic valve from opening. The red arrows are pointing to prosthetic valve leaflets.

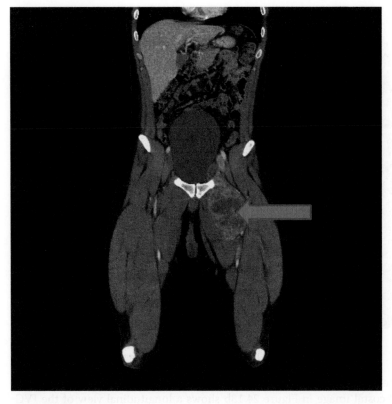

Figure 24.10b

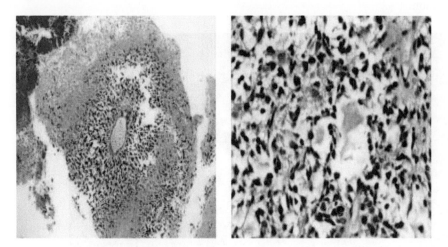

Figure 24.11  Left: Spindled tumor cells surrounding vessel. Right: Spindled and round cells with occasional mitosis.

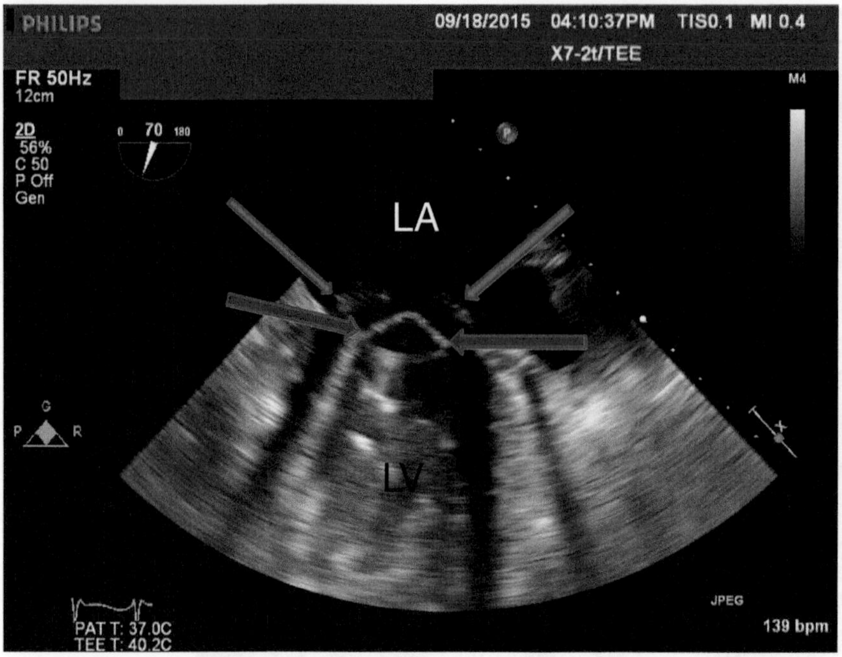

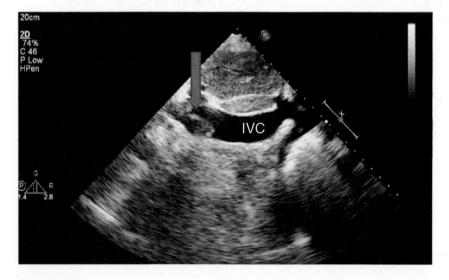

Figure 24.12b

24.13. C. Discrete masses in the IVC.

  The subcostal image in Figure 24.13b shows a longitudinal view of the IVC with at least two masses (blue arrow). Differential includes thrombus and tumor masses. The masses are more rounded and discrete and favor thrombi more than tumor.

Figure 24.13b

**24.14.** B. Ultrasound of the abdomen.

The patient underwent an ultrasound of the abdomen, which demonstrated the masses in the IVC. The masses were suggestive of thrombi. The patient then had ultrasound of his lower extremities and was positive for a thrombus in the right popliteal vein. The patient was then initiated on anticoagulants. Though he complained of shortness of breath, he had a negative CT of the pulmonary arteries.

## Chapter 2

**24.15.** D. Splenomegaly.

The subcostal image is obtained from the left side. Usual structures seen are the left kidney and spleen when it is enlarged. Figure 24.15b shows an enlarged spleen (blue arrow) and a normal-sized kidney (red arrow). This patient was subsequently diagnosed with acute myeloid leukemia.

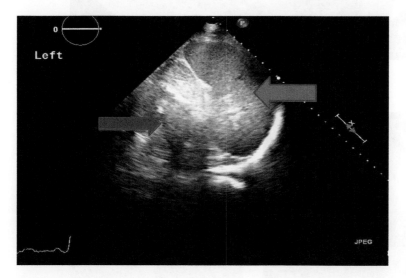

Figure 24.15b

**24.16.** B. Vegetations on the bioprosthetic.

There is a bioprosthetic tricuspid valve. There are numerous masses on the valve leaflets. Given his clinical picture, he probably has recurrent endocarditis. The blue arrow in Figure 24.16b (RA: right atrium; RV: right ventricle) shows the sewing ring of the prosthetic valve. The red arrow points to the masses seen on the valve leaflets.

**24.17.** B. Myxoma.

Figure 24.17b (RA: right atrium; RV: right ventricle) shows a large mass in the left atrium (blue arrow), probably attached to the interatrial septum. This is the most common location for a myxoma. The patient had surgery and the mass was removed. On histology, it was proven to be a myxoma.

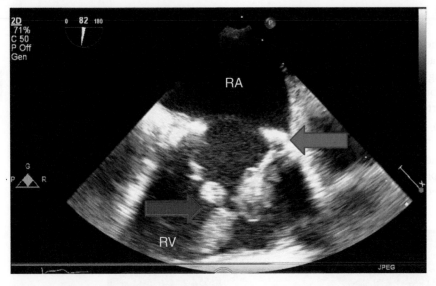

Figure 24.16b

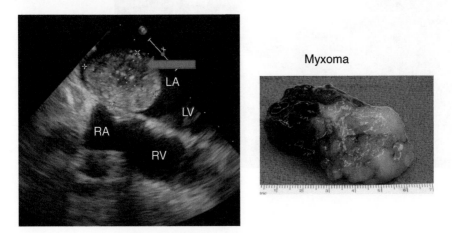

Figure 24.17b *Source:* Reproduced with permission of Dr. Natesa G. Pandian.

24.18. C. Fibroma.

There is a large mass seen in the right ventricle (arrowed in Figure 24.18b). The mass is occupying most of the right ventricle, is discreet and single. It is seen to be extending from the right ventricular wall. Fibromas are known to cause arrhythmias especially ventricular arrhythmias. The arrow points to the fibroma.

24.19. B. Papillary fibroelastoma of the aortic valve.

Figure 24.19 (LA: left atrium; LV: left ventricle) shows a small mass that appears like a frond arising from a thin stalk from the aortic valve (arrow). This is a characteristic appearance of a papillary fibroelastoma and has been shown to cause a stroke.

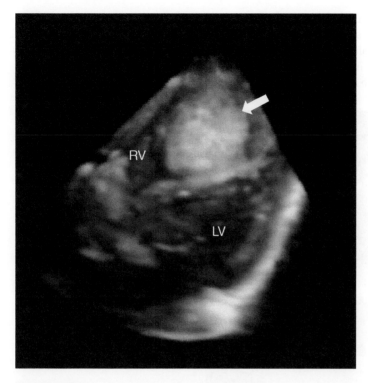

Figure 24.18b

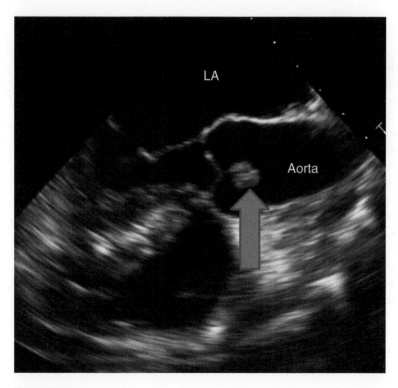

Figure 24.19

**24.20.** A. Vegetation on the catheter.

There is a mass attached to the end of the catheter in the SVC. The patient's presentation points to endocarditis. This mass is most probably a vegetation. The blue arrow in Figure 24.20b (LA: left atrium; RA: right atrium) points to the catheter and the red arrow shows the mass.

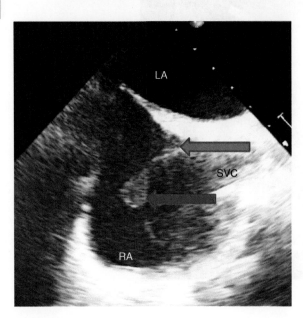

Figure 24.20b

**24.21.** B. Draw blood cultures, one from the periphery and one from the line, and then start antibiotics.

Since the mass is suspicious for a vegetation, blood cultures should be the initial step. It is recommended that peripheral cultures also be sent along with blood from the suspicious line. Antibiotics can then be initiated and narrowed depending on the organism. This patient probably has endocarditis due to gram-positive bacteria. The line should then be removed and a new dialysis catheter should be inserted.

**24.22.** C. Blood cyst.

This small cystic appearing mass (arrow in Figure 24.22b – LA: left atrium; LV: left ventricle; RA: right atrium; RV: right ventricle) is a blood cyst attached to the mitral valve.

**24.23.** D. Lipomatous hypertrophy of the interatrial septum.

Figure 24.23b (LA: left atrium; RA: right atrium) shows the interatrial septum, which is like a dumbbell. There is a thin fossa ovalis with lipomatous hypertrophy of the interatrial septum on either side. This is a normal finding. When there is extreme lipomatous hypertrophy, it can be mistaken for a tumor mass. The red arrow points to the thin fossa and the blue arrow shows the lipomatous hypertrophy of the septum.

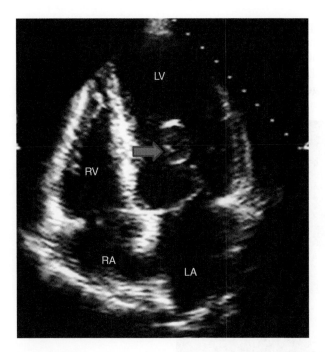

Figure 24.22b

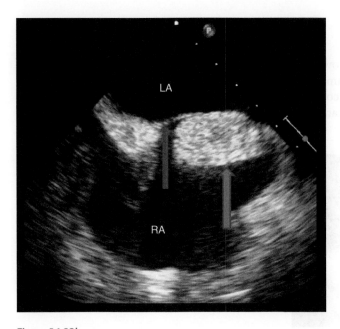

Figure 24.23b

24.24. B. Mass in the left atrial appendage which is likely a thrombus.

The patient probably has underlying atrial fibrillation which predisposed her to form a clot in the left atrial appendage. This potentially was the cause for her stroke. In Figure 24.24b (LA: left atrium; LV: left ventricle), the red arrow points to the left atrial appendage and the blue arrow shows the left atrial thrombus.

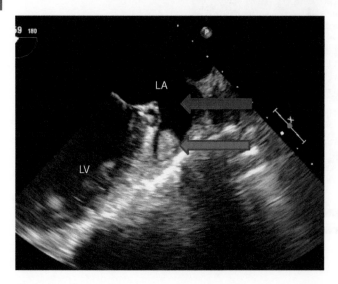

Figure 24.24b

24.25. C. Pericardial cyst.

Figure 24.25b (arrow, left image) shows a large cystic mass outside the right atrium (LA: left atrium; RA: right atrium). This probably represents a large pericardial cyst. The accompanying CT scan (Figure 24.25b, right) confirms the presence of the pericardial cyst.

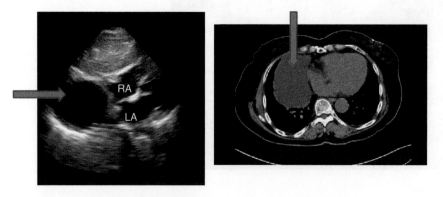

Figure 24.25b *Source:* Reproduced with permission of Dr. Natesa G. Pandian.

24.26. A. Multiple small tumors, likely rhabdomyoma.

    Figure 24.26b is a representative four-chamber view (apex down) showing multiple masses (arrows) in the right ventricle, left ventricle, and right atrium. The patient carries a diagnosis of tuberous sclerosis. Rhabdomyoma, which occurs as multiple small tumors in the heart, is a common association with tuberous sclerosis and most of them are diagnosed at an early age as they present with seizures.

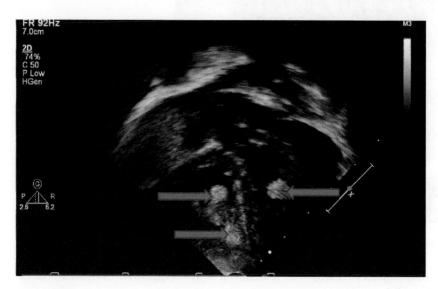

Figure 24.26b

24.27. C. Do nothing, manage seizures.

    Rhabdomyomas present as multiple tumors in the heart. They are benign tumors and usually regress as the child grows. The most common strategy is to do nothing for the tumors. When contrast-enabled studies are undertaken, the tumors will not take up the contrast, suggestive of a lesser amount of vascularity, unlike malignant tumors.

24.28. B. A thrombus in the left ventricular apex.

    This patient has presented with an acute ST elevation myocardial infarction involving the left anterior descending artery. The echocardiogram (Figure 24.28b) (LA: left atrium; LV: left ventricle; RA: right atrium; RV: right ventricle) showed akinesis of the LV segments subtended by the left anterior descending artery, which then is a good set up for formation of a thrombus (arrow).

24.29. D. Lymphoma.

    The echocardiogram shows masses in the right atrium (Figure 24.29, arrow). This patient has HIV infection. These patients are at risk of developing lymphoma. Biopsy from the tumor mass proved to be lymphoma of B cell origin.

24.30. B. A mass arising from the superior pole of the right kidney.

    The subcostal view (Figure 24.30) was obtained from the right side of the abdomen. The liver appears to be normal. The kidney on the right is well visualized. There is a homogeneous mass (arrow) arising from the superior pole of the right kidney, probably from the adrenal gland.

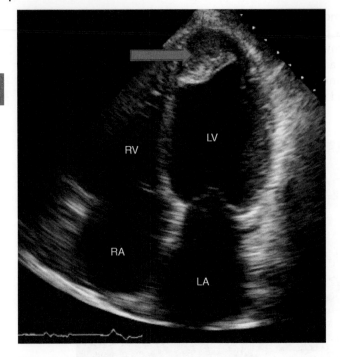

Figure 24.28b

24.31. B. Inflammatory changes of the mitral valve suggestive of Libman-Sacks endocarditis.

This patient with systemic lupus erythematosus is at risk for developing inflammation and development of nonbacterial endocarditis. The mitral leaflet tips are abnormal, probably a result of post-inflammatory changes. Figure 24.31b shows significant mitral regurgitation and a moderate amount of mitral stenosis.

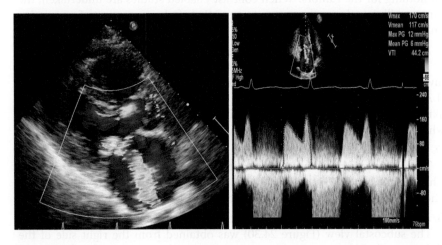

Figure 24.31b

**24.32. B. Gall stones.**

The subcostal view demonstrates a gall bladder with some gall stones (arrow in Figure 24.32b).

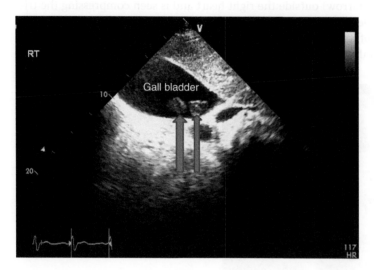

Figure 24.32b

**24.33. B. Cystic lesions in the liver.**

The cystic lesions in the liver are indicated by the arrow in Figure 24.33b. This patient has a presentation which is suggestive of lymphoma. The subcostal view shows the liver, most of which is replaced by numerous cystic lesions. The patient had a biopsy which proved to be B cell lymphoma.

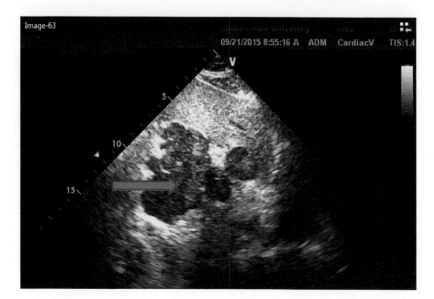

Figure 24.33b

24.34. **B.** Apical four-chamber view showing compression of the tricuspid valve.

The right side is seen to be compressed. The arrow in Figure 24.34c (LA: left atrium; LV: left ventricle; RV: right ventricle; TV: tricuspid valve) points to a large cystic structure (arrow) outside the right heart and is seen compressing the tricuspid valve. The mean gradient across the tricuspid valve is noted to be 5 mmHg at a heart rate of 85 bpm. This patient has polycystic kidney disease. The cyst is probably a manifestation of his polycystic kidney disease.

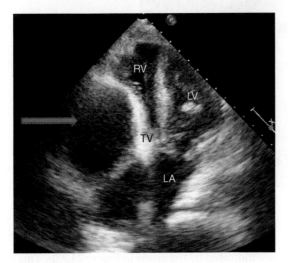

**Figure 24.34c**

25.1. Cardiovascular effects of acromegaly include which of the following?
  A. Left ventricular hypertrophy
  B. Hypertension
  C. Insulin resistance and diabetes mellitus
  D. All of the above

25.2. With which of the following is Cushing's syndrome not associated with?
  A. Hypertension
  B. Diabetes mellitus
  C. Atrial myxomas
  D. Mitral regurgitation

25.3. What is the triad of hyperpigmentation, low blood pressure, and hyperkalemia suggestive of?
  A. Addison's disease
  B. Conn's disease
  C. Hypopituitarism
  D. Cushing's syndrome

25.4. Cardiac effects of hyperthyroidism include which of the following?
  A. Atrial fibrillation
  B. High-output heart failure
  C. Higher blood volume
  D. All of the above

25.5. Which of the following could be cardiac effects of hypothyroidism?
  A. Pericardial effusion
  B. Cardiomyopathy
  C. Elevated serum cholesterol level
  D. Low cardiac output and elevated peripheral vascular resistance
  E. All of the above

25.6. Which of the following endocrine disorders may be associated with cardiomyopathy?
  A. Hyperthyroidism
  B. Hypothyroidism
  C. Pheochromocytoma
  D. All of the above

25.7. Which of the following statements about pheochromocytoma are accurate?
  A. About 75% are discovered at autopsy and are commonly missed antemortem
  B. Most are >1 cm in size and unilateral
  C. 10% could be familial and in such cases may be multicentric and extra-adrenal
  D. There is an association with neurofibromatosis
  E. All of the above

25.8. Which of the following statements is not true regarding diagnosis of pheochromocytoma?
- A. Plasma catecholamines or 24-hours urine metanephrines are good screening tests
- B. Clonidine suppression test is positive with pheochromocytoma with >50% suppression of serum norepinephrine
- C. Magnetic resonance imaging (MRI) is the more specific imaging modality compared with computed tomography (CT) scan
- D. Metaiodobenzylguanidine (MIBG) scan is helpful to show that the discovered mass is indeed producing hormones

25.9. Deficiency in the enzyme methionine synthase may result in severe hyperhomo-cysteinemia manifested by which of the following?
- A. Premature atherosclerosis
- B. Venous thrombosis
- C. Both A and B
- D. Neither A nor B

25.10. Which of the following is not a major Jones criterion for the diagnosis of rheumatic fever?
- A. Carditis
- B. Chorea
- C. Erythema nodosum
- D. Subcutaneous nodules

25.11. Which of the following is not an acceptable prophylactic antibiotic regimen for rheumatic fever?
- A. Benazathine penicillin 1.2 million units once a month
- B. Penicillin V 250 mg BID
- C. Sulfadiazine 1 g once a week
- D. Erythromycin 250 mg BID

25.12. Which of the following statements regarding duration of secondary prevention of rheumatic fever is true?
- A. For carditis with residual valvular disease, at least 10 years from last episode and till the age of 40 years
- B. For carditis with no residual valvular disease, at least 10 years from last episode and till the age of about 21 years
- C. For those with no carditis, at least 10 years from last episode and till the age of about 21 years
- D. All of the above

25.13. Patients with giant-cell arteritis are more likely to have which of the following?
- A. Thoracic aortic aneurysm
- B. Abdominal aortic aneurysm
- C. Subclavian artery stenosis
- D. All of the above
- E. None of the above

25.14. Cardiac involvement in ankylosing spondylitis may include which of the following?
- A. Atrioventricular conduction blocks
- B. Aortitis and aortic root dilation
- C. Aortic leaflet nodules and aortic regurgitation
- D. All of the above

25.15. Which of the following options is not a cardiac manifestation of scleroderma?
A. Pericarditis and effusion
B. Pulmonary hypertension
C. Patchy myocardial fibrosis and increased risk of sudden death
D. Aortic valve fibrosis resulting in stenosis

25.16. Cardiovascular manifestations of sarcoid do not include which of the following?
A. Complete heart block
B. Myocardial scarring with increased risk of sudden death
C. Cardiomyopathy
D. Pulmonary hypertension
E. Aortic regurgitation

25.17. Which of the following is not a cardiac manifestation of myotonia dystrophica?
A. Conduction blocks such as atrioventricular block and right bundle branch block
B. Myocardial fibrosis and fatty metaplasia
C. Cardiomyopathy
D. Mitral valve prolapse

25.18. Which of the following can occur with acute subarachnoid hemorrhage?
A. Giant T-wave inversion
B. Takatsubo-like syndrome with cardiac dysfunction and troponin release
C. Neurogenic pulmonary edema due to capillary leak syndrome
D. QT prolongation and torsades
E. All of the above

## Answers

25.1. D. All of the above.

25.2. D. Mitral regurgitation.
This is not an association; the others are. Association with myxoma is called Carney complex. The myxoma generally occurs in the left atrium but may be multicentric.

25.3. A. Addison's disease.
Hyperpigmentation is due to elevated adrenocorticotropic hormone level. Conn's disease is primary hyperaldosteronism and results in hypertension and hypokalemic alkalosis. Addison's syndrome can occur because of autoimmune disorder, tuberculosis, adrenal bleeding in sepsis, chronic suppressive doses of corticosteroids (prednisone >10 mg/day for >1 month), and so on. Diagnosis is made with the adrenocorticotropic hormone stimulation test.

25.4. D. All of the above.
They also have low peripheral vascular resistance. Increased cardiac output may also precipitate angina. Chronic elevation of heart rate can also result in a myopathic process leading to left ventricular systolic dysfunction.

25.5. E. All of the above.

25.6. D. All of the above.

25.7. E. All of the above.

In addition, they could be part of multiple endocrine neoplasia type 2 (with hyperparathyroidism and medullary carcinoma of thyroid) or multiple endocrine neoplasia type 2B (medullary thyroid cancer and mucosal neurofibromatosis of lips and tongue).

25.8. B. Clonidine suppression test is positive with pheochromocytoma with >50% suppression of serum norepinephrine.

This is not accurate. Norepinephrine suppression occurs in essential hypertension and not in pheochromocytoma. A computed tomography scan is more sensitive than MRI.

25.9. C. Both A and B.

25.10. C. Erythema nodosum.

This is not a major criterion, but erythema marginatum is. Polyarthritis is the other major criterion. Minor criteria include arthralgia, fever, elevated erythrocyte sedimentation rate or C-reactive protein. Two major or one major and two minor criteria make the diagnosis of rheumatic fever very likely.

25.11. C. Sulfadiazine 1 g once a week.

This- is not accurate. It must be once a day.

25.12. D. All of the above.

25.13. D. All of the above.

25.14. D. All of the above.

25.15. D. Aortic valve fibrosis resulting in stenosis.

This is not accurate. There is no significantly increased risk of valvular abnormalities. Treatment of pericarditis with corticosteroids may increase the risk of scleroderma renal crisis.

25.16. E. Aortic regurgitation.

This is not accurate. All other statements are correct. It can also result in aortitis and systemic vasculitis with aneurysm formation. Cardiac involvement may occur in 30% of patients and is grossly underdiagnosed. Sudden death may be the first cardiac manifestation and cardiac MRI with delayed enhancement may help in screening for scar burden and assess the risk of sudden death.

25.17. D. Mitral valve prolapse.

This is not accurate. The other options are accurate.

25.18. E. All of the above.

# Interdisciplinary Consultative Cardiology

# 26

**26.1.** Which is the most common cause of sudden death among young athletes?
   A. Hypertrophic cardiomyopathy
   B. Anomalous origin or coronary arteries
   C. Myocarditis
   D. Commotio cordis

**26.2.** A college basketball athlete is found to have anomalous origin of left coronary artery from right sinus of Valsalva with interarterial course on a computed tomography (CT) of the chest performed for an unrelated reason. He has no cardiac symptoms. What will you recommend?
   A. Continue with competitive sport as he has no symptoms
   B. Perform a stress test and if it is normal allow competitive athletic activity
   C. Advise against further competitive activity and refer for further evaluation and possible surgical reimplantation of left coronary artery
   D. None of the above

**26.3.** For a 72-year-old asymptomatic diabetic man scheduled for cataract surgery, which of the following preoperative tests are indicated?
   A. Resting electrocardiogram (ECG)
   B. Echocardiogram
   C. Stress ECG
   D. None of the above
   E. All of the above

**26.4.** For a patient with moderate asymptomatic aortic stenosis undergoing an elective high-risk surgery, which of the following statements are accurate?
   A. There is a higher risk of perioperative myocardial infarction
   B. There is a higher risk of 30-day cardiac event rate
   C. There is a higher 30-day mortality
   D. All of the above
   E. None of the above

**26.5.** An asymptomatic patient with severe aortic stenosis with normal left ventricular (LV) function and pulmonary artery (PA) pressure is scheduled for knee replacement. What would you recommend?
   A. Aortic balloon valvuloplasty before surgery
   B. Transcatheter aortic valve replacement before surgery
   C. Proceed with surgery with close hemodynamic monitoring
   D. Proceed with surgery with beta blockade

**26.6.** A 76-year-old man with severe symptomatic aortic stenosis is admitted with abdominal pain and diagnosed to have rupture of abdominal aortic aneurysm

*Cardiology Board Review*, Second Edition. Ramdas G. Pai and Padmini Varadarajan.
© 2023 John Wiley & Sons Ltd. Published 2023 by John Wiley & Sons Ltd.

(AAA) deemed to be unsuitable for endovascular aneurysm repair. What is the right course of action?

A. Proceed with AAA repair surgery

B. Perform aortic balloon valvotomy before surgery

C. Treat medically

D. None of the above

26.7. Routine use of beta blockers before surgery may result in higher risk of which of the following?

A. Hypotension

B. Stroke

C. Bradycardia

D. None of the above

E. All of the above

26.8. Which of the following statements are accurate regarding elective surgery after percutaneous coronary intervention?

A. Should be postponed >14 days if aspirin (ASA) needs to be stopped and balloon angioplasty was performed

B. Should be postponed >30 days if dual antiplatelet therapy needs to be stopped and bare-metal stent was implanted

C. Should be postponed >1 year if dual antiplatelet therapy needs to be stopped and drug-coated stent was implanted

D. None of the above

E. A, B, and C

26.9. Based on the 2014 American College of Cardiology/American Heart Association guidelines (Box 26.1), which of the following are class I indications for beta blockade perioperatively?

A. Those on chronic beta blockade

B. Those with moderate or high-risk myocardial ischemia on preoperative stress testing

C. Those with three or more revised clinical risk index (RCRI) risk factors; for example, diabetes mellitus, heart failure, coronary artery disease (CAD), renal insufficiency, cerebrovascular accident

D. All of the above

26.10. Results of the POISE trial addressing perioperative beta blockade yielded which of the following results?

A. Use of beta blocker reduced risk of atrial fibrillation

B. Use of beta blocker reduced risk of myocardial ischemia

C. Beta blocker use resulted in higher risk of stroke and noncardiac death

D. All of the above

26.11. In a patient with stable CAD on ASA, beta blocker, and statin undergoing AAA surgery, which of the following would you recommend to reduce the risk of perioperative myocardial ischemia?

A. Continue beta blocker

B. Continue statin

C. Continue ASA if possible

D. Administer perioperative prophylactic intravenous nitroglycerine

E. All of the above

F. A, B, and C

**26.12.** Which of the following is the predominant cause of mortality in patients with end-stage renal disease (ESRD) on dialysis?
A. Cardiac
B. Hyperkalemia
C. Stroke related to hypertension
D. Progressive renal failure

**26.13.** How does CAD in ESRD differ from patients without ESRD?
A. ESRD patients have more extensive CAD
B. ESRD patients have medial calcification more than intimal calcification
C. ESRD patients have more extensive coronary calcification
D. All of the above
E. None of the above

**26.14.** A 62-year-old ESRD patient with diabetes and hypertension is being evaluated for renal transplant. The resting ECG and LV wall motion on echo are normal. EF is 65%. He had a stress echocardiogram which was negative for ischemia at a heart rate of 136 bpm and 8.7 METs. On the insistence of the renal transplant committee, he had a coronary angiogram which showed a 70% mid left anterior descending (LAD) artery lesion. What has been shown to reduce the risk of peri-operative cardiac events?
A. LAD artery stent drug-eluting stent
B. Left internal mammary artery to LAD artery
C. Perioperative beta blockade
D. None of the above

**26.15.** A 48-year-old patient with ESRD on hemodialysis is seen because of dyspnea. His heart rate is 75 bpm, and blood pressure is 134/80 mmHg. He has no edema, has positive abdominojugular reflux, and no murmurs. Hemoglobin (Hb) is 12.2 g/dl. An echocardiogram shows mild LV hypertrophy, moderate left atrial enlargement, EF of 60% with normal wall motion and normal valves. The calculated PA systolic pressure is 50 mmHg, inferior vena cava is flat, mitral E/A velocity ratio is 1.5, and E/medial Em ratio is 22. Isovolumic relaxation time is 70 ms. What would you recommend?
A. Reduce the dry weight by 4–5 lbs. (1.8–2.3 kg) by dialysis
B. Prescribe Coreg
C. Recommend pulmonary vasodilator
D. Prescribe oral frusemide

**26.16.** Which medications are recommended for a 63-year-old nondiabetic patient with ESRD and normal blood pressure on hemodialysis?
A. ASA
B. Statin
C. Beta blocker
D. Angiotensin-converting-enzyme inhibitor

**26.17.** What echocardiographic findings may you encounter in a patient with end-stage liver disease?
A. LA enlargement
B. Hyperdynamic left ventricle with high cardiac output

C. Elevated pulmonary pressure

D. All of the above

**26.18.** A 46-year-old patient with hepatitis C cirrhosis is short of breath at rest and has an oxygen saturation of 85%. He has normal LV and valvular function and normal PA pressure. What is the most likely cause of dyspnea?

A. Emphysema due to α-1-antitrypsin deficiency

B. Pulmonary arteriovenous fistulae

C. Patient foramen ovale

D. Diastolic heart failure

**26.19.** What is the best way to diagnose hepatopulmonary syndrome?

A. Saline contrast echocardiography

B. Pulmonary CT angiography

C. Contrast pulmonary angiography (invasive)

D. Magnetic resonance angiography

**26.20.** Which cardiac testing has been shown to improve liver transplant outcomes in end-stage liver disease patients?

A. Dobutamine echo

B. Nuclear stress test

C. Routine coronary angiography

D. None of the above

**26.21.** Which is not included in the risk calculation using RCRI?

A. Age

B. Creatinine >2 mg/dl

C. CAD

D. Type of surgery

**26.22.** What is an elevated risk according to RCRI?

A. RCRI ≥2

B. RCRI ≥3

C. RCRI ≥4

D. RCRI ≥5

**26.23.** A 43-year-old man with mechanical mitral valve on warfarin is admitted with melena and Hb of 10 g/dl. What will predict higher risk of rebleed on emergency upper gastrointestinal (GI) endoscopy?

A. Active bleeding

B. Large ulcer with visible vessel at the ulcer base

C. Adherent clot to ulcer base

D. All of the above

E. None of the above

**26.24.** What are the high-risk markers in upper GI bleed?

A. Heart rate >110 bpm

B. Systolic blood pressure <90 mmHg

C. Hb <10g/dl

D. Active bleeding at upper GI endoscopy or rebleed

E. Comorbidities such as CAD and old age

F. All of the above

**26.25.** In the patient in Question 26.23, with a duodenal-ulcer-related GI bleed, what intervention is likely to shorten anticoagulant-free period?

A. Sclerosant injection to ulcer base

B. Stapling the bleeding site

C. Proton pump inhibitor

D. All of the above

**26.26.** What is the prevalence with regard to atrial fibrillation after cardiac surgery?
A. 10%
B. 20%
C. 30–50%
D. 80%

**26.27.** With regard to atrial fibrillation after cardiac surgery, which of the following drugs may not reduce its risk?
A. Beta blocker
B. Sotalol
C. Amiodarone
D. Digoxin

**26.28.** A 72-year-old man is admitted with a TIA and no signs of infarct in head CT. He is in atrial fibrillation and has normal LV function and no visible thrombi. What is a reasonable timing for starting anticoagulation?
A. 0–2 days
B. One week
C. Two weeks
D. There is no need for anticoagulation

**26.29.** A 66-year-old woman is admitted with dense right hemiplegia and a large non-hemorrhagic infarct in the left hemisphere occupying 40% of middle cerebral artery area. The patient is in atrial fibrillation and a gated CT of the chest did not show any left atrial thrombus. When would you start therapeutic anticoagulation?
A. Immediately
B. After one week
C. After two weeks
D. Will not anticoagulate as there is no thrombus

**26.30.** At what level of doxorubicin therapy do cardiotoxic effects increase exponentially?
A. $300\,mg/m^2$
B. $450\,mg/m^2$
C. $600\,mg/m^2$
D. No threshold

**26.31.** What factors compound the toxic effects of doxorubicin on the heart?
A. Radiation to chest
B. CAD
C. Age >65 years
D. All of the above

**26.32.** In addition to Adriamycin®, which other cancer chemotherapeutic agents are potentially cardiotoxic?
A. Herceptin
B. Cyclophosphamide
C. Mitoxantrone
D. All of the above

**26.33.** Which of the following can 5-fluorouracil potentially cause?
A. Coronary vasospasm, especially in those with CAD
B. Myocarditis
C. Pericarditis
D. None of the above

**26.34.** Which anticancer drug is associated with arterial or venous thromboembolism?
A. Cisplatin
B. Cyclophosphamide
C. Adriamycin
D. None of the above

**26.35.** Angiogenesis inhibitors (anti-vascular endothelial growth factor), cancer drugs angiogenesis inhibitors that target vascular endothelial growth factor with either antibodies against vascular endothelial growth factor (bevacizumab) or small molecule tyrosine kinase inhibitors (sunitinib, sorafenib), can produce which of the following side effects?

A. Cardiac dysfunction
B. Heart failure
C. Hypertension
D. All of the above

26.36. Following a hip fracture in the elderly, what is the general consensus regarding recommendation for timing of surgery?

A. Within 48 hours
B. Within four days
C. Within one week
D. Within one month

## Answers

26.1. A. Hypertrophic cardiomyopathy.

This accounts for about 26%. Commotio cordis (ventricular fibrillation with blunt trauma to chest) accounts for about 20%, coronary anomalies about 14%, and myocarditis about 5%. These are the leading causes.

26.2. C. Advise against further competitive activity and refer for further evaluation and possible surgical reimplantation of the left coronary artery.

The risk of sudden death is substantial, accounting for 1/7–1/10 deaths in competitive athletes. However, it is not known what percentage of patients with this coronary anomaly will have sudden death as such data are not available. Lots of patients may be asymptomatic and detected incidentally; hence, the denominator is not known.

26.3. D. None of the above.

No further testing is indicated before a low-risk surgery in an asymptomatic patient.

26.4. D. All of the above.

Though the risk has diminished substantially in recent years with better anesthetic techniques and monitoring, the risk is still about twice as high as those without aortic stenosis.

26.5. C. Proceed with surgery with close hemodynamic monitoring.

This is a class IIa indication in those with severe asymptomatic valve lesions. Options A and B are inappropriate in asymptomatic patients.

26.6. A. Proceed with AAA repair surgery.

Proceed with AAA repair surgery with close hemodynamic monitoring in view of the need for emergency surgery. Balloon valvotomy would have been appropriate in less urgent situations.

26.7. E. All of the above.

26.8. E. A, B, and C.

See Box 26.2.

26.9. A. Those on chronic beta blockade.

See Fleischer et al. (2014). Options B and C are class IIb indications.

**26.10.** D. All of the above.

**26.11.** F. A, B, and C.

Option D is a class III indication in a stable patient. It does not reduce the risk of perioperative ischemia.

**26.12.** A. Cardiac.

Cardiovascular disease is the leading cause of mortality in patients with ESRD. These patients have aggressive forms of CAD, hypertensive heart disease, and heart failure (mostly with preserved ejection fraction [EF]).

**26.13.** D. All of the above.

**26.14.** D. None of the above.

This patient has no inducible ischemia at good workload and hence there is no data that any of the options listed would improve the outcome. ASA, statin, and angiotensin-converting-enzyme inhibitor are likely to be beneficial in view of CAD and diabetes.

**26.15.** A. Reduce the dry weight by 4–5 lbs. (1.8–2.3 kg) by dialysis.

The elevated E/Em ratio indicates elevated left atrial (LA) pressure and this is likely responsible for his pulmonary hypertension. It is not uncommon to have normal right atrial pressure despite high LA pressure in these patients. Pulmonary vasodilator is inappropriate for this patient.

**26.16.** A. ASA.

According to guidelines. Statins have not been shown to improve outcomes in the absence of diabetes or CAD and are not recommended unless low-density lipoprotein >190 mg/dl.

**26.17.** D. All of the above.

Elevated pulmonary pressure is called portopulmonary syndrome and it is theorized that it may be due to some factors reaching the lungs from the gut bypassing the liver. This is due to increased pulmonary vascular resistance, and treatment with pulmonary vasodilators is indicated. This corrects after liver transplant.

**26.18.** B. Pulmonary arteriovenous fistulae.

This is called hepatopulmonary syndrome and can result in profound hypoxemia depending upon the degree of transpulmonary, right-to-left, shunting. Diastolic heart failure is ruled out by normal PA pressure.

**26.19.** A. Saline contrast echocardiography.

Saline contrast echocardiography by late appearance of bubbles on the left side (after four beats) and without Valsalva maneuver. The shunt can be qualitatively graded depending upon the degree of left-sided opacification. This gets better after liver transplant.

**26.20.** D. None of the above.

Despite lack of data, it has been practice to aggressively screen for CAD in these patients in most transplant centers, perhaps because of two reasons: high-risk surgery and the fact that a precious donor organ is used.

**26.21.** A. Age.

Options B, C, and D (if surgery is intra-abdominal, or intrathoracic, or suprainguinal vascular) earn one point each. Other three predictors are heart failure, cerebral vascular accident or transient ischemic attack (TIA), and diabetes mellitus. There are six possible points. These are validated for prediction of peri-operative major cardiac adverse events.

**26.22.** A. RCRI ≥2.

RCRI of 0 or 1 is considered low risk.

**26.23.** D. All of the above.

Upper GI endoscopy is very helpful to address risk of rebleed, for definitive therapy of bleeding source, and deciding on timing of continuation of anticoagulant therapy.

**26.24.** F. All of the above.

**26.25.** D. All of the above.

**26.26.** C. 30–50%.

**26.27.** D. Digoxin.

**26.28.** A. 0–2 days.

As there is no sign of cerebral infarct, it is safe to start anticoagulation right away because of low risk of hemorrhagic transformation. TIA is a risk factor for recurrent stroke in a patient with atrial fibrillation and the patient should be anticoagulated as soon as possible if there is no risk.

**26.29.** C. After two weeks.

The unwritten rule is to anticoagulate in 0–3 days if there is small infarct, in one week if medium-sized infarct, and in two weeks if large infarct unless need for anticoagulation is urgent. CT is good at excluding LA thrombus, similar to transesophageal echocardiography, and there is no urgency to anticoagulate. If the infarct is >1/3 of middle cerebral artery area, the risk of hemorrhagic transformation with anticoagulation is high. However, if a thrombus is present with embolic potential, earlier anticoagulation would be indicated. Immediate anticoagulation may also be indicated in mechanical valves irrespective of cerebral infarct size for fear of valve thrombosis as recurrent embolization despite the risk of hemorrhagic transformation of the infarct. This is a judgment call and there are no guidelines.

**26.30.** A. 300 mg/m².

**26.31.** D. All of the above.

In addition, very young age and administration of other cardiotoxic agents are also risk factors.

**26.32.** D. All of the above.

Cyclophosphamide in large intravenous doses can cause myocardial hemorrhage. Mitoxantrone is an anthracycline.

**26.33.** A. Coronary vasospasm, especially in those with CAD.

**26.34.** A. Cisplatin.

**26.35.** D. All of the above.

**26.36.** A. Within 48 hours.

This is important in terms of presurgical cardiac optimization. The data are only observations supporting this; there are no randomized trials. The stated benefits of early surgery include reduced length of stay and cost, reduction of pressure sores, reduction in morbidity (venous thromboembolism, urinary tract infection, atelectasis) and mortality, and improved functional status. But the observation studies are also conflicting.

**Box 26.1    Management of Coronary Stents as per 2014 ACC/AHA Guidelines**

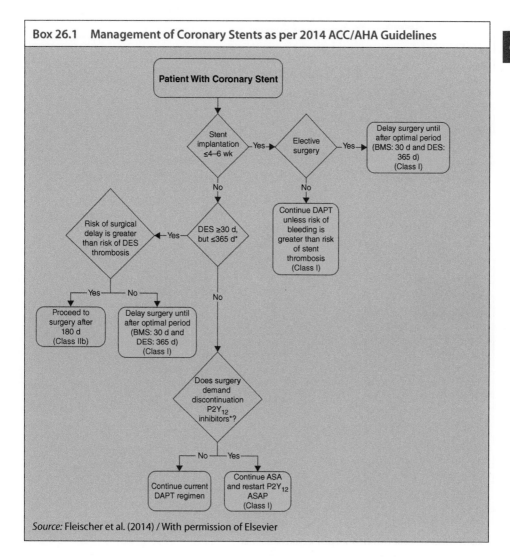

*Source:* Fleischer et al. (2014) / With permission of Elsevier

## Box 26.2  Preoperative Testing Guidelines from 2014 ACC/AHA Guidelines

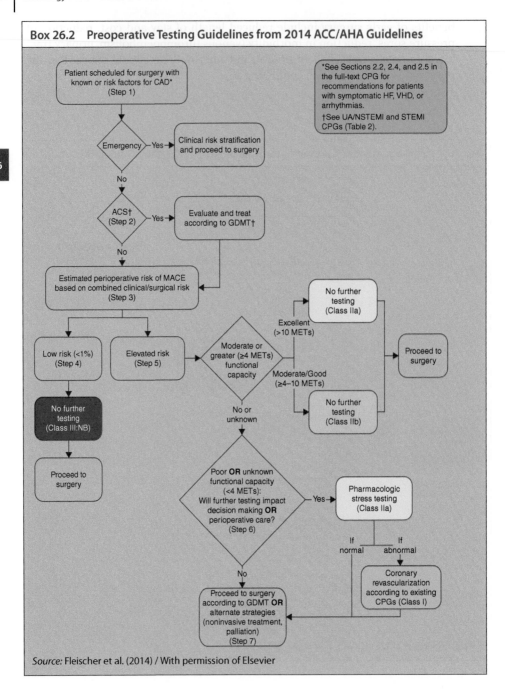

*Source:* Fleischer et al. (2014) / With permission of Elsevier

## Reference

Fleischer, L.A., Fleischmann, K.E., Auerbach, A.D. et al. (2014). 2014 ACC/AHA guideline on perioperative cardiovascular evaluation and management of patients undergoing noncardiac surgery. *Journal of the American College Cardiology* 64 (22): e77–e137. https://doi.org/10.1016/j.jacc.2014.07.944.

# Heart Disease and Pregnancy

27

**27.1.** A 25-year-old female is being seen for genetic counseling. She has a significant family history of Marfan syndrome, with her mother and sister having lens dislocation and aortic aneurysm with dissection. She is asymptomatic, and her aortic root measures 45 mm. She wants to go ahead with pregnancy. What do you recommend?

    **A.** Start a beta blocker before pregnancy
    **B.** Start angiotensin-converting-enzyme inhibitor before pregnancy
    **C.** Avoid pregnancy
    **D.** Start angiotensin-receptor blocker before pregnancy

**27.2.** A 36-year-old African-American female is referred to you. She complains of progressive dyspnea. She denies any prior cardiovascular history. She is 38 weeks pregnant and this is her first pregnancy. On examination, she is tachycardiac, blood pressure (BP) is 110/70 mmHg, jugular venous pressure (JVP) is elevated up to her angle of the mandible, apical impulse is diffuse, she has S3 and S4 gallops, 2/6 apical systolic murmur, and crackles up to middle of the back. Electrocardiogram (ECG) confirms sinus tachycardia. Echocardiogram reveals global left ventricular (LV) hypokinesis and an ejection fraction (EF) of 20%. What is the most likely diagnosis?

    **A.** Viral myocarditis
    **B.** Coronary artery disease
    **C.** Peripartum cardiomyopathy
    **D.** Dissection of the coronary artery

**27.3.** You start the patient in Question 27.2 on diuretics and beta blockers. She complains of persistent shortness of breath. What is your next recommendation?

    **A.** Intra-aortic balloon pump
    **B.** Lisinopril
    **C.** Bromocriptine
    **D.** Ventricular assist device

**27.4.** The patient in Question 27.2 has a successful vaginal delivery. She is now maintained on anti-failure therapy, which includes a diuretic and beta blocker. Her LV function by echocardiogram is now 40%, which has improved from 20%. She evinces interest in a second pregnancy. What do you recommend?

    **A.** To go ahead with pregnancy
    **B.** Recommend reassessing LV function in six months and if normal, then proceed

*Cardiology Board Review*, Second Edition. Ramdas G. Pai and Padmini Varadarajan.
© 2023 John Wiley & Sons Ltd. Published 2023 by John Wiley & Sons Ltd.

**C.** Counsel against pregnancy

**D.** Recommend addition of angiotensin-receptor blocker and then proceed with pregnancy

**27.5.** A 30-year-old female, now 34 weeks pregnant, presents to the hospital with acute onset of severe squeezing chest pressure associated with nausea and diaphoresis. She has a prior history of hypertension and is on medications. She used to smoke up until her pregnancy. In the emergency room, her heart rate is 76 bpm, BP is 160/80 mmHg, and examination is otherwise unremarkable. Her ECG reveals anterior ST elevation. What do you recommend?

**A.** Medical management with heparin, aspirin, nitrates, and beta blocker

**B.** Immediate coronary angiogram with possible intervention

**C.** Thrombolytic therapy

**D.** Colchicine and indomethacin

**27.6.** A 29-year-old Hispanic female is referred to you for complaints of dyspnea. She is 33 weeks pregnant and has recently moved from India. She reports a history of murmur from her childhood. On examination, her heart rate is 110 bpm, BP is 120/80 mmHg, JVP is 14 cmH$_2$O, S1 is increased, S2 is normal with an opening snap, 2/6 diastolic murmur heard along with a holosystolic murmur at the apex. You initiate diuretic therapy. Echocardiogram reveals mitral stenosis with a mean gradient of 17 mmHg. What would your next step would?

**A.** Beta blocker therapy

**B.** Amiodarone

**C.** Synchronized cardioversion

**D.** Percutaneous mitral balloon valvotomy

**27.7.** A 26-year-old G2P2 presents to the hospital with complaints of severe substernal chest pressure. She had a normal vaginal delivery 15 days previously. She describes her chest pressure as severe pressure-like, in the central chest, radiating to her jaw, starting when she was vacuuming her house. She denies any prior medical history. An ECG performed in the emergency room shows 3 mm ST elevations in V1–V6 with ST depression in leads II, III, and aVF. Chest X-ray is unremarkable. What is the most likely diagnosis?

**A.** Acute pulmonary embolus

**B.** Coronary artery disease with plaque rupture

**C.** Spontaneous coronary dissection

**D.** Acute pericarditis

**E.** Aortic dissection

**27.8.** A 27-year-old female is referred to you. She gives a history of murmur from her childhood and is diagnosed with severe aortic stenosis due to a bicuspid aortic valve. She is recommended to undergo aortic valve replacement. She is nulliparous and is planning to have children in the next one to two years. What is the best option for her regarding her aortic valve replacement?

**A.** If she chooses a mechanical valve and is established on daily warfarin of 2.5 mg and achieves a target international normalized ratio (INR) of 2–3, then continuation of warfarin until the 36th week of pregnancy would be an acceptable option

**B.** If she gets a bioprosthetic valve, there is about a 50% chance of valve degeneration at 10 years

    C. The Ross procedure could be an option

    D. If she proceeds with mechanical prosthesis and chooses to go on low molecular weight heparin during pregnancy, then the low molecular weight doses should be adjusted based on anti-Xa levels

    E. All are true

**27.9.** What is the condition associated with the highest maternal mortality with pregnancy?

    A. Marfan syndrome with aortic root measurement of 4.5 cm

    B. Family history of cardiomyopathy

    C. Severe mitral regurgitation

    D. Ventricular septal defect (VSD) with a right-to-left shunt

**Chapter 27**

**27.10.** A 24-year-old female is referred to you for a murmur. She is pregnant, 10 weeks, and asymptomatic at present. She has no prior cardiac events. She has no cardiac risk factors. On examination, heart rate is 76 bpm, BP 110/70 mmHg, and JVP is normal. Apical impulse is undisplaced, normal S1 and S2, and apical S3 present. There is a 3/6 mid peaking ejection systolic murmur with a click and a grade 1 diastolic murmur at the left sternal border. What is the likely cause of her murmur?

    A. Mitral stenosis and mitral regurgitation

    B. Pulmonic stenosis

    C. Bicuspid aortic valve stenosis and regurgitation

    D. Patent ductus arteriosus

**27.11.** A 32-year-old woman, 10 weeks pregnant, was referred for evaluation of murmur. On examination, she had a 5/6 holosystolic murmur at the third left intercostal space with normal S2. No HF. An echocardiogram showed a 4 mm sized perimembranous VSD with normal LV size and PA pressure. What would you recommend?

    A. Termination of pregnancy

    B. Reassure and follow up

    C. Perform cardiac work up during second trimester for shunt ratio

    D. Refer for percutaneous closure

**27.12.** A 24-year-old primigravida is 14 weeks pregnant and has been having repeated episodes of syncope on minimal exertion. An echocardiogram confirms valvular pulmonary stenosis with a peak gradient of 90 mmHg and a mean gradient of 60 mmHg with moderately hypokinetic right ventricle. What will you do?

    A. Recommend termination of pregnancy

    B. Recommend balloon valvotomy of the pulmonary valve

    C. Surgical replacement of pulmonary valve

    D. Treat with pulmonary vasodilators

**27.13.** A 24-year-old woman who had a heart transplant five years earlier is pregnant. What facts would you convey her?

    A. Probability of live birth is about 70%

    B. There is a higher risk of hypertension, eclampsia, and premature birth

    C. Cardiac rejection is rare

    D. All of the above

**27.14.** Cardiac surgery during pregnancy is associated with approximately what percentage fetal loss?

**A.** 5%

**B.** 30%

**C.** 70%

**D.** 100%

**27.15.** Which of the following disorders are associated with the highest risk with pregnancy?

**A.** Primary pulmonary hypertension with a PA systolic pressure of 110 mmHg

**B.** Surgically corrected tetralogy of Fallot

**C.** Severe pulmonary stenosis

**D.** Large atrial septal defect with a shunt ratio of 3:1 and PA systolic pressure of 50 mmHg

## Answers

**27.1.** C. Avoid pregnancy.

She has a significant family history of Marfan syndrome with dissection. She also has significant aortic root dilatation, which puts her at increased risk for rupture. During preconceptual counseling, if aorta is >45 mm then pregnancy should be discouraged. If aorta is <40 mm, pregnancy might be reasonable if low risk. For aortic sizes between 40 and 45 mm, individualized recommendation should be given.

**27.2.** C. Peripartum cardiomyopathy.

Diagnosis of heart failure due to LV systolic dysfunction that occurs in the last trimester to six months postpartum. It is usually a diagnosis of exclusion. The incidence varies. In the USA, the incidence is 1 in 3200 deliveries, in South Africa it is 1 in 1000, and in Haiti occurrence is 1 in 300. Frequency is increased with advanced maternal age, multiparity, multifetal pregnancy, African-American women, and risk factors such as diabetes mellitus, smoking, and hypertension (Elkayam 2011).

**27.3.** C. Bromocriptine.

One of the pathophysiologies of peripartum cardiomyopathy includes defective antioxidant defense mechanism, wherein levels of cathepsin D and prolactin and angiostatic 16 kDa prolactin levels are increased with increasing oxidative stress. This leads to inhibition of endothelial cell proliferation, migration, increases apoptosis, disrupts capillaries, and causes cardiomyocyte dysfunction. In studies on mice, bromocriptine prevented the onset of peripartum cardiomyopathy (Sliwa et al. 2010a,b).

**27.4.** C. Counsel against pregnancy.

Pregnancy is not recommended when LVEF is <25% at initial presentation or there is persistent decrease in LVEF (Elkayam et al. 2001).

**27.5.** B. Immediate coronary angiogram and intervention.

Incidence of myocardial infarction is about 1 in 35 700 deliveries. Usually occurs in older females (>35 years), multiparous females, white or African-American women, with associated risk factors of hypertension, diabetes mellitus, and smoking (Ladner et al. 2005).

**27.6.** A. Beta blocker therapy.

The best recommendation is initiation of beta blocker therapy as she is tachycardic and mitral mean gradient is dependent on the heart rate. Controlling heart rate will reduce the mitral diastolic gradient.

**27.7.** C. Spontaneous coronary dissection.

Presentation with chest pressure and ST elevations in the anterior leads points to pathology in the left anterior descending artery. Acute aortic dissection usually results in the dissection flap extending into the right coronary artery. This patient has spontaneous dissection of her left anterior descending artery.

**27.8.** E. All are true.

A young woman needing valve surgery such as this patient is usually recommended a bioprosthetic valve, but with the understanding that valve degeneration can occur rapidly and the bioprosthesis may need replacement in 10 years. In the case of a mechanical valve, continuing warfarin is the best strategy to prevent valve thrombosis, which is preferred by the European Society of Cardiology guidelines. Warfarin can cause embryopathy in the first trimester, but that risk is minimized if the daily dose of warfarin is <5 mg. Alternatively, if low molecular weight heparin is chosen, it should be adjusted to achieve an anti-Xa level of 1–1.2 U/ml. This is the option chosen by the American College of Chest Physicians. It has been noted that a small minority of patients with mechanical prosthesis on low molecular weight heparin have suffered valve thrombosis despite therapeutic anti-Xa levels. The Ross procedure can also be an option in this patient.

**27.9.** D. Ventricular septal defect (VSD) with a right-to-left shunt.

In this situation, there is evidence of Eisenmenger syndrome with a right-to-left shunt. This portends a 30–50% maternal mortality rate and pregnancy is absolutely contraindicated. Uncorrected regurgitant valve lesions are usually well tolerated during pregnancy. Family history of cardiomyopathy is not a contraindication for pregnancy. In Marfan syndrome, an aortic root that exceeds 4.5 cm is associated with a maternal mortality rate of 10%. If diagnosed during pregnancy, therapy with beta blocker should be initiated, serial echocardiograms should be performed, and cesarean section should be performed.

**27.10.** C. Bicuspid aortic valve stenosis and regurgitation.

**27.11.** B. Reassure and follow up.

This is a small defect and there is neither significant volume overload (normal LV size) nor pulmonary hypertension. This would be well tolerated during pregnancy. There is no indication for VSD closure, and also perimembranous VSDs are not suitable for percutaneous closure (only muscular VSDs).

**27.12.** B. Recommend balloon valvotomy of the pulmonary valve.

This lesion is very amenable to balloon valvotomy and this should result in good pregnancy outcome.

**27.13.** D. All of the above.

**27.14.** B. 30%.

**27.15.** A. Primary pulmonary hypertension with a PA systolic pressure of 110 mmHg. Eisenmenger's complex is also associated with one of the highest risks.

## References

Elkayam, U. (2011). Clinical characteristics of peripartum cardiomyopathy in the United States: diagnosis, prognosis, and management. *Journal of the American College of Cardiology* 58 (7): 659–670.

Elkayam, U., Tummala, P.P., Rao, K. et al. (2001). Maternal and fetal outcomes of subsequent pregnancies in women with peripartum cardiomyopathy. *The New England Journal of Medicine* 344 (21): 1567–1571. [Erratum: *The New England Journal of Medicine* (2001) 345(7): 552.].

Ladner, H.E., Danielsen, B., and Gilbert, W.M. (2005). Acute myocardial infarction in pregnancy and the puerperium: a population-based study. *Obstetrics and Gynecology* 105 (3): 480–484.

Sliwa, K., Blauwet, L., Tibazarwa, K. et al. (2010a). Evaluation of bromocriptine in the treatment of acute severe peripartum cardiomyopathy: a proof-of-concept pilot study. *Circulation* 121 (13): 1465–1473. https://doi.org/10.1161/CIRCULATIONAHA.109.901496 [Erratum: Circulation (2010) 121(21): e425. Struhman, Ingrid - corrected to Struman, Ingrid].

Sliwa, K., Hilfiker-Kleiner, D., Petrie, M.C. et al. (2010b). Current state of knowledge on aetiology, diagnosis, management, and therapy of peripartum cardiomyopathy: a position statement from the Heart Failure Association of the European Society of Cardiology Working Group on peripartum cardiomyopathy. *European Journal of Heart Failure* 12 (8): 767–778. https://doi.org/10.1093/eurjhf/hfq120.

# Racial and Gender Disparities

# 28

**28.1.** Which of the following statements regarding blacks is not true compared with whites?
A. Age-adjusted cardiovascular death rate is higher in blacks
B. Risk of stroke in blacks is twice as high
C. Blacks are less likely to receive guideline-recommended therapies in heart failure
D. Blacks have a lower risk of left ventricular (LV) hypertrophy

**28.2.** Which of the following statements are accurate?
A. Black adults are far more likely than white adults to be admitted to the hospital for angina and congestive heart failure
B. Blacks are more likely to be admitted to emergency rooms
C. Blacks are less likely to be insured and get regular medical care
D. All of the above

**28.3.** Which of the following statements are correct?
A. American Indians die from heart disease much earlier than expected
B. Alaska Natives die from heart disease much later than expected
C. American Indians / Alaska Natives die from heart disease much earlier than expected
D. None of the above

**28.4.** Which is the leading cause of death in US women?
A. Cancer
B. Heart disease
C. Accidents
D. Alzheimer's disease

**28.5.** Which of the following statements are correct?
A. Among Hispanic women, heart disease and cancer cause roughly the same number of deaths each year
B. For American-Indian or Alaska-Native and Asian- or Pacific-Islander women, heart disease is second only to cancer
C. Two-thirds of women who die suddenly of coronary heart disease have no previous symptoms
D. All of the above

**28.6.** Which ethnic groups have the highest risk of coronary artery disease (CAD)?
A. White Americans
B. Black Americans
C. Japanese Americans
D. People from South Asian origin

**28.7.** Among the Japanese, the risk of CAD has been the highest in which of the following groups?

*Cardiology Board Review*, Second Edition. Ramdas G. Pai and Padmini Varadarajan.
© 2023 John Wiley & Sons Ltd. Published 2023 by John Wiley & Sons Ltd.

A. Japanese in Japan

B. Japanese settled in Hawaii

C. Japanese settled in continental USA

D. Risk is similar

28.8. Compared with men, what are women more likely to describe the ischemic chest pain as?

A. Sharp or burning

B. In neck or jaw

C. In abdomen or back

D. All of the above

28.9. Who have the highest prevalence of diabetes mellitus?

A. Native Americans

B. White Americans

C. Black Americans

D. Hispanics

28.10. Regarding patients undergoing cardiac surgery in the USA (STS database), which of the following statements is not accurate regarding blacks compared with whites?

A. Have higher prevalence of hypertension and diabetes

B. Have higher prevalence of preoperative dialysis

C. Have lower preoperative adverse features, such as LV dysfunction, recent myocardial infarction, and 3 or >4 mitral regurgitations

D. Have higher adjusted operative mortality and morbidity

28.11. Spontaneous coronary artery dissection (SCAD) is most commonly seen in which of the following groups?

A. Young women

B. Young men

C. Elderly women

D. Elderly men

28.12. In a woman with SCAD, all of the following are recommended except which option?

A. Screen other vascular beds, such as femoral, radial, carotid, and intracranial arteries

B. Avoid pregnancy, as it may precipitate recurrent SCAD; avoid oral contraceptives

C. May use aspirin

D. Use high-dose statin

28.13. A 43-year-old overweight woman is being evaluated for exertional central chest pain. She has no other cardiac risk factors. Her echocardiogram was normal. She walked 7 METs during a stress test, experienced the same chest pain associated with 1.5 mm flat ST segment depression in V3 to V6 lasting three minutes into recovery. What would you recommend?

A. Exercise stress nuclear test

B. Coronary angiogram and, if normal, ergonovine challenge

C. Coronary angiography and, if normal, test for coronary flow reserve

D. Stress cardiac magnetic resonance imaging with rest and stress first-pass perfusion

28.14. Microvascular angina in women may be associated with which of the following?

A. Abnormal stress myocardial perfusion

B. Abnormal stress myocardial energy production demonstrated by $^{31}P$ myocardial spectroscopy

C. Higher risk of cardiac events and emergency room admission

D. All of the above

## Answers

28.1. D. Blacks have a lower risk of (LV) hypertrophy.

This statement is wrong; all others are accurate as per American Heart Association statistics.

28.2. D. All of the above.

According to American Heart Association data.

28.3. C. American Indians / Alaska Natives die from heart disease much earlier than expected.

Some 36% of both these populations are under 65 compared with only 17% for the US population overall.

28.4. B. Heart disease.

In both black and white women.

28.5. D. All of the above.

28.6. D. People from South Asian origin.

That is, people from the Indian subcontinent. The risk is about four times white Americans. They also tend to have premature CAD, diffuse disease, central obesity despite lower body mass index, metabolic syndrome, and diabetes mellitus.

28.7. C. Japanese settled in continental USA.

28.8. D. All of the above.

28.9. A. Native Americans.

28.10. C. Have lower preoperative adverse features, such as LV dysfunction, recent myocardial infarction, and 3 or $\geq 4$ mitral regurgitations.

This is wrong. The preoperative adverse features are higher among blacks. The other statements are correct.

28.11. A. Young women.

Mean age is 42 years. This is not atherosclerotic but may be associated with fibromuscular dysplasia. There could be genetic and hormonal factors; may occur during pregnancy.

28.12. D. Use high-dose statin.

This is not accurate as the lesions are not atherosclerotic and are due to fibromuscular dysplasia. Also avoid heavy exertion. The artery may remodel, and about 80% of the lesions disappear. Intravascular ultrasound and CT are very useful in making a diagnosis.

28.13. C. Coronary angiography and, if normal, test for coronary flow reserve.

If epicardial coronary arteries are normal, it is likely to be microvascular angina. The microvasculature is best evaluated with coronary flow reserve. The ergonovine challenge is rarely used, and it is a test for coronary spasm which would be nonexertional and is associated with ST elevation rather than depression. Angina in women is microvascular in about 30%.

28.14. D. All of the above.

# Pharmacologic Principles of Cardiac Drugs

# 29

29.1. JT is a 45-year-old male who presents to your outpatient clinic for a routine follow-up. His medical history is significant for atrial fibrillation. Upon examination, you learn that JT has been skipping dinner for the previous several weeks due to work-related time restraints. The efficacy of which of the following on JT's current medication list will be *least* affected if administered on an empty stomach?
   A. Rivaroxaban 20 mg once daily at 1900
   B. Carvedilol CR 20 mg once daily at 1900
   C. Dronedarone 400 mg twice daily at 0700 and 1900
   D. Diltiazem 24H ER 120 mg once daily at 1900

29.2. PJ is a 56-year-old male who is admitted to a percutaneous coronary intervention (PCI)-capable hospital for an ST elevation myocardial infarction (STEMI). Intravenous (IV) cangrelor is bolused prior to PCI, followed immediately by a cangrelor infusion throughout the duration of PCI. An oral $P2Y_{12}$ platelet inhibitor is administered during the cangrelor infusion. Which of the following $P2Y_{12}$ platelet inhibitors would be best to use concurrently with the cangrelor infusion to prevent stent thrombosis?
   A. Clopidogrel 300 mg
   B. Clopidogrel 600 mg
   C. Prasugrel 60 mg
   D. Ticagrelor 180 mg

29.3. TW is a 77-year-old female with a history of atrial fibrillation, hypertension (HTN), and heart failure with reduced ejection fraction (HFrEF) who is admitted to the hospital for a total prosthetic-hip-associated infection. Vancomycin and rifampin are initiated for empiric antimicrobial therapy. The team would also like to start oral anticoagulation for stroke prevention. Which of the following oral anticoagulants may be recommended in this patient?
   A. Warfarin plus therapeutic enoxaparin
   B. Dabigatran
   C. Rivaroxaban
   D. Edoxaban

29.4. PY is a 42-year-old female admitted to the hospital for worsening dysuria, urinary frequency, flank pain, and intermittent fevers for the past two days. PMH includes paroxysmal atrial fibrillation, HTN, and dyslipidemia. Home medications include simvastatin 40 mg oral (PO) QHS, lisinopril 40 mg PO daily, carvedilol

*Cardiology Board Review*, Second Edition. Ramdas G. Pai and Padmini Varadarajan.
© 2023 John Wiley & Sons Ltd. Published 2023 by John Wiley & Sons Ltd.

12.5 mg PO BID, and dofetilide 500 µg PO BID. Urinalysis reveals cloudy appearance, large leukocytes, ≥100 white blood cells (WBC), plus nitrites, a 3+ leukocyte esterase, and many bacteria. Which of the following antimicrobials is best recommended for this patient?

A. Ceftriaxone
B. Ciprofloxacin
C. Levofloxacin
D. Trimethoprim-sulfamethoxazole

29.5. PT is a 72-year-old male who is admitted for new-onset atrial fibrillation, refractory to diltiazem. The team initiates an amiodarone drip for pharmacologic cardioversion. After four days on the amiodarone drip, the patient has become stable enough to transition to oral therapy. Which of the following is a reasonable strategy for conversion of IV to PO amiodarone?

A. Stop drip. Initiate 200 mg PO daily immediately after
B. May overlap by one day. Initiate 200 mg PO daily
C. May overlap by one day. Initiate 400 mg PO TID
D. Stop drip. Initiate 800 mg PO TID 48 hours after discontinuation of the infusion

Chapter 29

29.6. NM is an 81-year-old female who was started on amiodarone 200 mg PO once daily for maintenance of sinus rhythm approximately nine months ago. She presents to your cardiology clinic for a routine follow-up. Labs are drawn. Which of the following abnormal labs is *least likely* to be caused from her amiodarone?

A. WBC $28 \times 10^9$ cells/l
B. Aspartate aminotransferase 860 U/l
C. Thyroid stimulating hormone 46 mU/l
D. Thyroid stimulating hormone 0.004 mU/l

29.7. A 45-year-old male presents with confusion and visual disturbances. The electrocardiogram (ECG) reveals third-degree heart block. His wife claims that the patient just picked up a 30-day supply of digoxin 250 µg PO daily this morning. Upon review of the medication vial, you note that there are only 24 tablets remaining. How many vials of digoxin immune Fab may be recommended for this patient in the setting of acute digoxin toxicity?

A. 3 vials                          C. 10 vials
B. 6 vials                          D. 20 vials

29.8. Rivaroxaban is started inpatient in a 67-year-old female for stroke prevention in the setting of atrial fibrillation. The patient's creatinine clearance is calculated at 62 ml/min. Which of the following is the appropriate dose of rivaroxaban for this patient?

A. Rivaroxaban 20 mg PO daily         C. Rivaroxaban 10 mg PO daily
B. Rivaroxaban 15 mg PO BID           D. Rivaroxaban 15 mg PO daily

29.9. Which of the following genetic tests could you order as a send-out before initiating warfarin in a patient?

A. *VKORC1* genotype                  C. HLA-B* 1502 allele
B. HLA-B* 5701 allele                 D. *CYP2C19* genotype

29.10. FL is a 77-year-old male who presents to the emergency department with complaints of fatigue, dizziness, and shortness of breath. Upon further examination, the patient admits to melena for the past several days. A computed tomography (CT) scan is concerning for a gastrointestinal (GI) hemorrhage. Of note, the patient has been on chronic anticoagulation therapy with warfarin; INR on admission was found to be 11.2. The team would like to use Kcentra for urgent reversal. Which of the following is the best recommended dose for this patient?
A. 50 units/kg of the factor II component (maximum dose 5000 units)
B. 50 units/kg of the factor VII component (maximum dose 5000 units)
C. 50 units/kg of the factor IX component (maximum dose 5000 units)
D. 50 units/kg of the factor X component (maximum dose 5000 units)

29.11. Which of the following statements is correct?
A. Beta-blockers may cause peripheral vasoconstriction through their beta-1 receptor antagonism effects
B. Beta-blockers may cause peripheral vasoconstriction through their beta-2 receptor antagonism effects
C. Beta-blockers may cause peripheral vasodilation through their beta-1 receptor antagonism effects
D. Beta-blockers may cause peripheral vasodilation through their beta-2 receptor antagonism effects

29.12. LG is a 36-year-old female with HFrEF (left ventricular ejection fraction 30%), HTN, diabetes mellitus, and chronic kidney disease stage III. The patient has a reported allergy to valsartan with a reaction of angioedema. Current medications include carvedilol, insulin glargine, insulin lispro, and amlodipine. The team would like to start a medication to optimize the patient's heart failure therapy. Which of the following medications may be started in this patient?
A. Lisinopril                          C. BiDil®
B. Losartan                           D. Entresto®

29.13. TN is a 40-year-old male with a past medical history that includes asthma and heart failure with preserved ejection fraction (EF). In addition to a rescue inhaler, the patient is currently using fluticasone/salmeterol for maintenance of his asthma. The team would like to start a beta-blocker for this patient but has concerns about concomitant use of a beta-blocker and a beta-agonist. Which of the following beta-blockers would be best to use in this patient?
A. Metoprolol succinate 25 mg PO daily
B. Propranolol 40 mg PO BID
C. Labetalol 100 mg PO BID
D. Carvedilol 6.25 mg PO BID

29.14. Which of the following medications has an active metabolite with the longest half-life?
A. Aspirin                            C. Prasugrel
B. Clopidogrel                        D. Ticagrelor

29.15. A 36-year-old male presents with chest pain, associated with bilateral nipple tenderness and sensitivity. Cardiac enzymes are negative. Which of the following medications in this patient's profile can mostly likely cause these symptoms?

A. Triamterene/hydrochlorothiazide
B. Spironolactone
C. Labetalol
D. Ranolazine

29.16. Which of the following diuretics may be used in a patient with a confirmed Stevens-Johnson reaction to trimethoprim-sulfamethoxazole?
A. Furosemide
B. Hydrochlorothiazide
C. Metolazone
D. Ethacrynic acid

29.17. TJ is a 54-year-old male who is started on immediate-release isosorbide mononitrate for chronic stable angina, refractory to beta-blocker monotherapy. Which of the following regimens is best to start in this patient?
A. 10 mg PO at 0700 and 1400
B. 10 mg PO at 0700 and 1900
C. 10 mg PO at 0700 and 1900 for three days, then 20 mg PO at 0700 and 1900
D. 10 mg PO at 0700 and 1500 and 2300

Chapter 2

29.18. WL is a 68-year-old female who is placed in observation awaiting an adenosine stress test. Which of the following statements is false?
A. Chocolate milk, coffee, tea, brownies, and energy bars should be avoided prior to test
B. Patient must remain NPO four to six hours prior to test
C. The patient is not to take Aggrenox˚ for at least 24 hours prior to test
D. The patient is not to take theophylline-containing medications for at least 12 hours prior to test

29.19. A 65-year-old female presents to the emergency department with severe, sharp, chest pain, weak pulses, altered level of consciousness, and weakness. BP upon admission was 212/126 mmHg. Upon further examination, the team diagnosed the patient with aortic dissection in the setting of hypertensive emergency. Which agent is best to initiate in this patient to lower blood pressure?
A. IV labetalol
B. IV metoprolol
C. IV nicardipine
D. IV diltiazem

29.20. Which of the following has been proven to be most beneficial for initial treatment in pulmonary arterial HTN (World Health Organization functional class II) to reduce clinical failures, such as death, hospitalization, or worsening pulmonary arterial HTN?
A. Epoprostenol IV 5 µg/(kg min)
B. Ambrisentan 10 mg daily
C. Tadalafil 40 mg daily
D. Ambrisentan 10 mg daily and tadalafil 40 mg daily

29.21. EM is a 60-year-old female diagnosed one year previously with HFrEF. Around that time, she began taking enalapril 10 mg PO BID, carvedilol 25 mg PO BID, and furosemide 20 mg PO BID. Upon further discussion with the patient, it is decided to transition the enalapril to Entresto. Which is the best method in transitioning enalapril to Entresto?
A. Stop enalapril and begin Entresto 49/51 mg PO BID at the time the next dose of enalapril was scheduled

B. Overlap enalapril and Entresto 24/26 mg PO BID by 24 hours

C. Overlap enalapril and Entresto 49/51 mg PO BID by 24 hours

D. Stop enalapril 36 hours before starting Entresto 49/51 mg PO BID

29.22. The team wants to start a moderate-intensity HMG-CoA reductase inhibitor for atherosclerotic cardiovascular disease primary prevention in a patient taking the following current medications: lisinopril 20 mg PO daily, verapamil 120 mg PO QID, metformin 1000 mg PO BID, and glipizide 5 mg PO BID. Which of the following is the best HMG-CoA reductase inhibitor to start in this patient?

A. Simvastatin 40 mg PO QHS

B. Rosuvastatin 10 mg PO QHS

C. Atorvastatin 10 mg PO QHS

D. Lovastatin 40 mg PO QHS

29.23. PT is a 58-year-old male who presents with chest pain for the past four months that worsens upon exertion. Vitals include BP of 87/60 mmHg and heart rate of 57 bpm. The team would like to start a medication for chronic stable angina. Which is the best agent to initiate in this patient?

A. Ranolazine

B. Amlodipine

C. Isosorbide mononitrate

D. Nifedipine

29.24. LT is a 24-year-old pregnant female. During her second trimester, she presents complaining of excessive fatigue, shortness of breath, palpitations, and swelling in her ankles. She is found to have developed atrial fibrillation on her ECG and, on echo, her ejection fraction is found to be 25%. Which of the following medications would be deemed safe for the fetus?

A. Enalapril

B. Atorvastatin

C. Digoxin

D. Warfarin

29.25. Which of the following anticoagulants does not require antithrombin III for its anticoagulant effect to work?

A. Heparin

B. Enoxaparin

C. Rivaroxaban

D. Fondaparinux

29.26. XR is an 88-year-old male being treated for a non-STEMI. He is given a 4000-unit bolus of heparin and started at 500 units/h due to his low weight. Six hours after initiating heparin, he develops epistaxis and oozing around the IV site. Upon further investigation, it is found that his heparin drip rate was running at 1000 units/h by accident rather than 500 units/h for the previous six hours since heparin initiation. What dose of protamine is best to reverse the effect of the heparin?

A. 42.5 mg

B. 30 mg

C. 17.5 mg

D. 5 mg

29.27. JG is a 23-year-old patient presenting to the emergency room with palpitations and shortness of breath. An ECG reveals the patient is in atrial fibrillation and delta waves are present. Which of the following agents would be the best choice to help control this patient's atrial fibrillation?

A. Ibutilide

B. Diltiazem

C. Metoprolol

D. Amiodarone

29.28. Which of the following medications would not require monitoring potassium levels in patients?

A. Eplerenone      C. Furosemide

B. Enalapril      D. Amlodipine

29.29. MJ is a 63-year-old patient presenting with acute decompensated heart failure (New York Heart Association [NYHA] class IV), a systolic BP of 84/46 mmHg, and a heart rate of 110 bpm. Which of the following medications would be reasonable to initiate at this time?

A. Dobutamine 2 μg/(kg min)

B. Milrinone 50 μg/kg bolus then 0.75 μg/(kg min)

C. Nesiritide 2 μg/kg bolus, then 0.01 μg/(kg min)

D. Ivabradine 5 mg PO BID

29.30. YT is a 67-year-old female with a past medical history of HFrEF, HTN, diabetes mellitus type 2, atrial fibrillation, and myocardial infarction four years previously. She presents today in atrial fibrillation with rapid ventricular response and acute decompensated heart failure with symptoms at rest. Her home medications are lisinopril 40 mg PO daily, carvedilol 25 mg PO BID, pravastatin 40 mg PO daily, digoxin 0.125 mg PO daily, aspirin 81 mg PO daily, warfarin 5 mg PO daily, pioglitazone 30 mg PO daily, and empagliflozin 10 mg PO daily. An amiodarone drip is started to help control the atrial fibrillation. Which of the following statements are false?

A. Empaglifozin has been found to reduce cardiovascular mortality

B. Pioglitazone should be stopped in patients with NYHA class IV heart failure

C. The patient's INR will likely come back with a marked increase on tomorrow morning's lab draw due to the amiodarone inhibiting warfarin hepatic metabolism

D. The patient's digoxin level will likely come back with a marked increase on tomorrow morning's lab draw due the amiodarone drip's effect on the patient's hepatic metabolism

29.31. ML is a 66-year-old female presenting to the catheterization laboratory with a non-STEMI. During the history and physical examination, the patient mentions that previous genetic testing revealed that she is deficient in the CYP 2C19 enzyme. Which of the following options for antiplatelet therapy during PCI would be best to avoid based upon her genetic profile?

A. Prasugrel 60 mg PO × 1

B. Ticagrelor 180 mg PO × 1

C. Cangrelor 30 μg/kg IV bolus, followed by 4 μg/(kg min) IV continuous infusion

D. Clopidogrel 600 mg PO × 1

29.32. Which of the following antiarrhythmics would require the most dose adjustment when added to a patient already taking a high dose of metoprolol?

A. Propafenone      C. Flecainide

B. Dofetilide      D. Disopyramide

Chapter 29

## Answers

29.1. D. Diltiazem 24H ER 120 mg once daily.

Coadministration of rivaroxaban with food increases the bioavailability of the 15 mg and 20 mg dose. Administration of carvedilol CR with a high-fat meal results in increases (~20%) in area under the curve (AUC) and $C_{max}$. The absolute bioavailability of dronedarone increases from 4% without food to 15% when administered with a high-fat meal. Rivaroxaban 15 mg and 20 mg, carvedilol CR, and dronedarone should all be taken with food.

29.2. D. Ticagrelor 180 mg.

Loading doses of thienopyridines, such as clopidogrel and prasugrel, should not be given until discontinuation of the cangrelor infusion due to a drug interaction related to competitive binding to the $P2Y_{12}$ receptor. However, a loading dose of ticagrelor may be given at any time during or immediately after discontinuation of the cangrelor infusion.

29.3. A. Warfarin plus therapeutic enoxaparin.

Concomitant use of dabigatran, rivaroxaban, or edoxaban with strong dual P-glycoprotein and cytochrome P450 3A4 (CYP3A4) inducers, such as rifampin, should be avoided due to decreased levels of the anticoagulant; it is also unfeasible to determine the extent of reduction of the anticoagulant due to a lack of monitoring assays to test for efficacy. Rifampin may also decrease the effect of warfarin; however, this may be monitored closely through international normalized ratio (INR) readings, and doses may be adjusted accordingly.

29.4. A. Ceftriaxone.

Concomitant use of QT-prolonging agents (i.e. fluoroquinolones) should be avoided with dofetilide. Trimethoprim-sulfamethoxazole has been shown to cause a substantial increase in dofetilide plasma concentrations which, in turn, may cause a dose-dependent QT interval prolongation.

29.5. C. May overlap by one day, initiate 400 mg PO TID.

The optimal dose for changing from IV to PO amiodarone depends on the dose of the IV amiodarone already administered. In patients who have been on an amiodarone drip for less than one week, an initial daily dose of 800–1600 mg of PO amiodarone may be recommended. Amiodarone can cause stomach upset and nausea, which is minimized by giving no more than 400 mg at one time. PO therapy may overlap with IV therapy; however, this is not required. Of note, there are no official recommendations on transitioning from IV to PO amiodarone. Clinical monitoring is recommended.

29.6. A. WBC $28 \times 10^9$ cells/l.

Because amiodarone is a potential source of large amounts of inorganic iodine, it can cause hypothyroidism or hyperthyroidism. Liver enzyme elevations and/or hepatotoxicity are also associated with amiodarone use and should be monitored closely. The incidence of leukocytosis due to amiodarone is unlikely.

29.7. A. Three vials.

Each vial of digoxin immune Fab 40 mg will bind to approximately 0.5 mg of digoxin. The total number of vials required can be calculated by dividing the total body load of digoxin (in milligrams) by 0.5 mg per vial. Total body load is approximately equal to the amount ingested (in milligrams) multiplied by the bioavailability of the tablet preparation, which is 0.8. This patient ingested a total of 1.5 mg of digoxin (0.25 mg × 6 tablets). 1.5 mg × 0.8 = 1.2 mg total digitalis body load 1.2 mg/0.5 = 2.4 vials. Thus, three vials of digoxin immune Fab may be administered. Alternatively, in the setting of acute ingestion of unknown amounts of digoxin and absence of a serum digitalis concentration level, administer 20 vials of digoxin immune Fab; this may be administered as 10 vials initially, followed by another 10 vials, if needed, to avoid a febrile reaction.

29.8. A. Rivaroxaban 20 mg PO daily.

This is the recommended dose for stroke prevention in non-valvular atrial fibrillation in patients with creatinine clearance >50 ml/min.

29.9. A. *VKORC1* genotype.

Warfarin reduces the regeneration of vitamin K epoxide in the vitamin K cycle through inhibition of VKOR, a multiprotein enzyme complex. Certain single nucleotide polymorphisms in the *VKORC1* gene have been associated with variable warfarin dose requirements.

Chapter 2

29.10. C. 50 units/kg of the factor IX component (maximum dose 5000 units).

Kcentra is composed of factors II, VII, IX, and X, as well as proteins C and S. 50 units/kg of the factor IX component is recommended in pretreatment INRs greater than 6. It should be noted that the dose of Kcentra is based on the actual potency as stated on the carton, which will vary from 20 to 31 factor IX units per milliliter. For patients weighing more than 100 kg, the maximum dose should not be exceeded.

29.11. B. Beta-blockers may cause peripheral vasoconstriction through their beta-2 receptor antagonism effects.

29.12. C. BiDil.

BiDil (hydralazine/isosorbide dinitrate). Angiotensin-converting enzyme (ACE) inhibitors and angiotensin receptor blockers (ARBs) can both cause angioedema. In patients with a documented reaction of angioedema to an ARB, it is recommended to avoid ACE inhibitors and other ARBs. Entresto is a newly approved heart failure medication that contains a combination of valsartan and sacubitril.

29.13. A. Metoprolol succinate 25 mg PO daily.

It was once recommended to avoid beta-blockers in patients with asthma. However, it has been shown that cardioselective beta-blockers are unlikely to produce unfavorable respiratory symptoms in patients with asthma. Metoprolol succinate is the only cardioselective beta-blocker listed and is likely to target mainly beta-1 receptors when given at a low daily dose of 25 mg.

29.14. D. Ticagrelor.

Ticagrelor has an active metabolite with the longest half-life of approximately nine hours. See Box 29.1.

29.15. B. Spironolactone.

These symptoms are consistent with gynecomastia, which is a dose- and duration-dependent adverse effect of spironolactone. Gynecomastia may be reversible following discontinuation of therapy, but on rare occasions may persist.

**29.16.** D. Ethacrynic acid.

Ethacrynic acid is the only diuretic listed that does not have a sulfonamide chemical group and may be used in patients with a confirmed sulfonamide allergy.

**29.17.** A. 10 mg PO at 0700 and 1400.

Immediate-release isosorbide mononitrate is dosed twice daily. Tolerance to nitrate effects develops with chronic exposure. Dose escalation does not overcome this effect. Tolerance can only be overcome by short periods of nitrate absence from the body. Two doses given seven hours apart are recommended to decrease tolerance development. Of note, hydralazine has been shown to inhibit the development of tolerance to nitrates, which may explain why the combination of hydralazine and isosorbide dinitrate can be dosed TID and is beneficial in heart failure patients.

**29.18.** C. The patient is not to take Aggrenox for at least 24 hours prior to test.

The patient is not to take the medicine Aggrenox (aspirin/extended-release dipyridamole) for at least 48 hours prior to the test. Aspirin alone is not a problem and should be considered if Aggrenox is held.

**29.19.** A. IV labetalol.

In the setting of acute aortic dissection, BP should be reduced rapidly (generally to a goal systolic BP less than 120 mmHg) with a beta-adrenergic antagonist and a vasodilator within the first 10 minutes of treatment. As a selective alpha-1 adrenergic, and a nonselective beta-adrenergic antagonist, labetalol maintains coronary blood flow, minimizes aortic wall stress, and reduces systemic vascular resistance without reducing total peripheral blood flow.

**29.20.** D. Ambrisentan 10 mg and tadalafil 40 mg daily.

The AMBITION trial was a randomized double-blind, multicenter study that showed the combination of ambrisentan and tadalafil reduced the risk of clinical failure by 50% compared with ambrisentan or tadalafil monotherapy. IV epoprostenol may be considered as first-line therapy in patients with pulmonary HTN and World Health Organization functional class IV.

**29.21.** D. Stop enalapril 36 hours before starting Entresto 49/51 mg PO BID.

Allow a wash-out period of 36 hours if switching from or to an ACE inhibitor. For patients receiving a total daily dose of >10 mg of enalapril (or therapeutically equivalent doses), start Entresto 49/51 mg PO BID. For patients receiving a total daily dose of ≤10 mg of enalapril (or therapeutically equivalent doses), start Entresto 24/26 mg PO BID.

**29.22.** B. Rosuvastatin 10 mg PO QHS.

As a CYP3A4 inhibitor, verapamil may increase the serum concentration of simvastatin, atorvastatin, and lovastatin. Rosuvastatin, on the other hand, is less dependent on CYP3A4-mediated metabolism.

**29.23.** A. Ranolazine.

Ranolazine exerts antianginal and anti-ischemic effects with minimal change in hemodynamic parameters (heart rate, BP). The other antianginal agents may lower BP in this patient, who is already hypotensive.

**29.24.** C. Digoxin.

Digoxin is pregnancy category C but is often used in pregnant women with peripartum cardiomyopathy. Warfarin and atorvastatin are pregnancy category X and would not be recommended in this case. ACE inhibitors, such as enalapril, have been shown to be detrimental to the fetus in all three trimesters.

29.25. C. Rivaroxaban.

Rivaroxaban does not require antithrombin III for its anticoagulation effect. Heparin, enoxaparin, and fondaparinux all require antithrombin III for their anticoagulation effect and the effectiveness is greatly diminished in patients with low antithrombin III levels.

29.26. C. 17.5 mg.

Since heparin has a half-life of around 60–90 minutes, after four hours, the preceding amount of heparin has been eliminated. The calculation is 1 mg of protamine for every 100 units of heparin in the first 30 minutes, 0.5 mg of protamine for every 100 units of heparin given between 30 and 120 minutes, and 0.25 mg of protamine for every 100 units of heparin given between two and four hours.

Ticagrelor has an active metabolite with the longest half-life of approximately nine hours. See Box 29.1.

29.27. A. Ibutilide.

Ibutilide is a IV class III antiarrhythmic which will convert a patient to sinus rhythm without blocking the AV node. Amiodarone, metoprolol, and diltiazem all block the AV node and could worsen symptoms by allowing increased conduction down the accessory pathway.

29.28. D. Amlodipine.

Amlodipine does not affect potassium levels in patients. Furosemide will lower potassium due to blocking of the $Na^+/K^+$ channels in the kidney. Eplerenone and enalapril both increase potassium levels in patients.

29.29. A. Dobutamine 2 pg/(kg min).

Dobutamine, starting at a low dose, should not adversely affect the BP. In fact, it would not be unexpected if the BP were to rise due to the increased cardiac output. Milrinone should not be bolused in patients with a systolic BP less than 90 mmHg due to its vasodilatory effects. Both nesiritide and ivabradine are contraindicated in systolic BP less than 90 mmHg. Ivabradine is also not recommended during an acute heart failure exacerbation.

29.30. D. The patient's digoxin level will likely come back with a marked increase on tomorrow morning's lab draw due the amiodarone drip's effect on the patient's hepatic metabolism.

This is false. Digoxin levels will increase on an amiodarone drip due to the P-glycoprotein pump inhibition, not a reduction in hepatic metabolism. An amiodarone drip will often increase INR levels drastically for patients on a stable dose of warfarin; often, even if warfarin is stopped, the INR can trend up for a few days before it starts to normalize. The Empagliflozin Cardiovascular Outcomes and Mortality in Type 2 Diabetes Mellitus (EMPA-REG) trial demonstrated a reduction in all-cause and cardiovascular mortality in patients using empagliflozin in comparison with placebo. Pioglitazone has a black box warning contraindicating its initiation in patients in NYHA class III or IV heart failure.

**29.31.** D. Clopidogrel 600 mg PO × 1.

Clopidogrel requires a two-step metabolism to be converted into its active metabolite, and CYP 2C19 is one of the main enzymes required for this conversion. Prasugrel, on the other hand, is converted into its active metabolite primarily by the CYP 3A4 and CYP 2B6 enzymes. Ticagrelor is active in its parent form and is metabolized primarily by the CYP 3A4 enzyme. Cangrelor is active in its parent form and is not dependent on either renal or hepatic enzymes for its metabolism.

**29.32.** A. Propafenone.

Propafenone possesses independent beta-blocking activity and can also increase metoprolol serum blood levels up to five times that of normal, increasing the risk of severe hypotension and heart block. If a beta-blocker is needed, one should keep the metoprolol dose low or alternatively use atenolol, since 50% of atenolol is renally cleared.

---

**Box 29.1   Clinical Pearls**

---

Remember that a drug's half-life does not always correlate to how long its effects last in the body. Aspirin has a short half-life, but due to it irreversibly inhibiting platelets, its effect lasts until the body can make new platelets rather that how long the drug remains in the body.

Drugs with a large volume of distribution will have a much shorter effective half-life when they are first initiated due to rapid declines in the blood levels. For example, an IV bolus of amiodarone will have a 90% drop in the blood level 45 minutes afterward due to the drug distributing to the tissues and out of the bloodstream. This is why a drip should be initiated after a bolus dose even though the half-life of the drug is over one month long.

There are many ways drugs can interact: they can have synergistic effects, such as clopidogrel and warfarin; they can affect each other's metabolism, such as metoprolol and propafenone; they can inhibit their excretion through P-glycoprotein pumps, such as with digoxin and amiodarone; and they can both affect similar electrical channels for synergistic QT prolongation, such as methadone and erythromycin.

Drugs can have multiple effects on the body, and it is important to determine which effect will win out. One example are beta-blockers, which cause direct vasoconstriction though blocking beta-2 receptors in blood vessels, reduction of cardiac output through decreases in heart rate, and inhibition of the release of renin from the kidneys, leading to a net effect of lowered BP in patients.

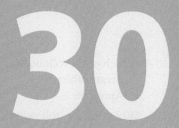
30.1. A 55-year-old male presents with acute onset of shortness of breath. He has a computed tomography angiogram in the emergency room and is noted to have bilateral segmental and subsegmental pulmonary emboli (PEs). His past medical history is significant for non-small cell carcinoma of the lung, for which he is undergoing treatment. He reports nausea and vomiting. Which of the following would be the choice of anticoagulation?
   A. Warfarin
   B. Low molecular weight heparin (LMWH)
   C. Dabigatran
   D. Edoxaban

30.2. In a patient with deep venous thrombosis (DVT) of the leg, not cancer associated, what would not be the choice of anticoagulation for the first three months?
   A. Dabigatran
   B. Rivaroxaban
   C. Apixaban
   D. Edoxaban
   E. Warfarin

30.3. Initial parenteral anticoagulation is a must with what agents, when used to treat non-cancer-associated DVT or PEs?
   A. Rivaroxaban and apixaban
   B. Dabigatran and edoxaban
   C. Rivaroxaban and edoxaban
   D. Dabigatran and apixaban

30.4. A patient is on dabigatran 150 mg BID for paroxysmal atrial fibrillation. He is then prescribed dronedarone for rhythm control. What is the recommendation for dabigatran dosing?
   A. Continue at 150 mg BID
   B. Reduce dosage to 75 mg BID
   C. Stop using dabigatran
   D. Reduce dosage to 75 mg once daily

30.5. A 65-year-old male is on ketoconazole therapy. He has paroxysmal atrial fibrillation and his $CHA_2DS_2$-VASc score is 4. His physician decides on starting a novel anticoagulant, dabigatran. What is the recommendation regarding dabigatran dosing in this patient?
   A. Start on 150 mg BID
   B. Do not use dabigatran
   C. Start on 75 mg BID
   D. Start on 75 mg once daily

30.6. Which of the novel anticoagulants is mostly excreted through the kidneys?
   A. Dabigatran
   B. Rivaroxaban
   C. Apixaban
   D. Edoxaban

*Cardiology Board Review*, Second Edition. Ramdas G. Pai and Padmini Varadarajan.
© 2023 John Wiley & Sons Ltd. Published 2023 by John Wiley & Sons Ltd.

30.7. Which of the following novel anticoagulants is a direct thrombin inhibitor?
A. Rivaroxaban
B. Apixaban
C. Dabigatran
D. Edoxaban

30.8. Which of the following drugs has been approved by the US Food and Drug Administration for use to reverse the effect of dabigatran?
A. Idarucizumab
B. Andexanet alfa
C. Aripazine
D. Protamine

30.9. Which of the following drugs is being studied to reverse the effect of apixaban and rivaroxaban?
A. Idarucizumab
B. Andexanet alfa
C. Aripazine
D. Protamine

30.10. Which of the following drugs is being evaluated as a universal anticoagulant reversal agent (anti-direct thrombin inhibitors, anti-Xa inhibitors, unfractionated heparin, LMWH, and fondaparinux)?
A. Idarucizumab
B. Andexanet alfa
C. Aripazine
D. Protamine

30.11. For patients undergoing major orthopedic surgery, including total hip arthroplasty, total knee arthroplasty, and hip fracture surgery, what is the current recommendation for thromboprophylaxis from the day of surgery?
A. Thromboprophylaxis in the outpatient period for up to 35 days
B. Thromboprophylaxis for 10 days
C. No need for thromboprophylaxis
D. Thromboprophylaxis for 14 days

30.12. In patients undergoing total hip arthroplasty or total knee arthroplasty, irrespective of the concomitant use of an intermittent pneumatic compression device or length of treatment, what is the recommended choice for thromboprophylaxis?
A. Aspirin alone
B. Unfractionated heparin
C. LMWH
D. Vitamin K antagonist

30.13. For patients undergoing total hip arthroplasty, total knee arthroplasty, and hip fracture surgery, what is the recommended time period to start thromboprophylaxis with LMWH?
A. 4 hours preoperatively
B. 4 hours postoperatively
C. 12 hours or more preoperatively or postoperatively
D. 24 hours postoperatively

30.14. For acutely sick hospitalized medical patients who are at increased risk for thrombosis, what is the current recommendation for thromboprophylaxis?
A. LMWH
B. Low-dose unfractionated heparin (LDUH) BID
C. LDUH TID
D. Fondaparinux
E. All of the above
F. None of the above

30.15. Based on the RE-LY trial, which of the following statements is false?
A. Dabigatran 110 mg was noninferior to warfarin in preventing stroke or embolism
B. Dabigatran 150 mg was superior to warfarin in preventing stroke/embolism
C. Dabigatran was associated with more gastrointestinal bleeds
D. Dabigatran was associated with more intracranial bleeds

30.16. Which of the following is not true regarding novel anticoagulants in nonvalvular atrial fibrillation?
   A. Rivaroxaban was noninferior to warfarin in preventing stroke
   B. Edoxaban was noninferior to warfarin in preventing stroke
   C. Apixaban was superior to warfarin in preventing stroke
   D. Apixaban was noninferior to warfarin in preventing stroke

30.17. In a patient with acute isolated distal DVT, what is the current recommendation regarding management?
   A. Serial imaging of the deep veins in two weeks when there are no severe symptoms or risk for extension
   B. Serial imaging in four weeks
   C. No need to image further
   D. Start anticoagulation

30.18. In a patient diagnosed with a distal DVT managed with serial imaging, which of the following statements is not true?
   A. Anticoagulation if the thrombus has not extended
   B. Anticoagulation is recommended if the thrombus has extended but remains confined to distal veins
   C. Anticoagulation is recommended if the thrombus extends into the proximal veins

30.19. Which of the following is not true?
   A. In patients with acute DVT of the leg, use of compression stockings is not recommended
   B. In patients with subsegmental PE (not involving proximal pulmonary arteries) without proximal DVT of legs and a low risk for venous thromboembolism (VTE), clinical surveillance is recommended
   C. In patients with subsegmental PE (not involving proximal pulmonary arteries) without proximal DVT of legs and a high risk for VTE, clinical surveillance is recommended
   D. In patients with low-risk pulmonary embolism, treatment at home or early discharge is recommended (before five days of treatment)

30.20. Which of the following statements are true?
   A. In patients with acute PE being managed by thrombolysis, systemic thrombolytic therapy is recommended over catheter-delivered thrombolysis
   B. In patients with acute PE associated with hypotension, catheter-assisted thrombus removal is recommended when they are at high risk for bleeding, failed systemic thrombolysis, or in shock
   C. In patients with upper extremity DVT involving axillary or more proximal veins, anticoagulation therapy is recommended over thrombolysis
   D. In patients with recurrent DVT on therapeutic doses of warfarin or other NOACS, switching to LMWH for at least one month is recommended
   E. Increasing the dose of LMWH by one-quarter to one-third is recommended if recurrent DVT occurs while on therapeutic dose of long-term LMWH therapy
   F. All of the above
   G. None of the above

## Answers

30.1. B. Low molecular weight heparin (LMWH).

This patient has just been diagnosed with PEs and is related to his underlying cancer. He also reports vomiting. This patient should be treated with LMWH initially (Kearon et al. 2016).

30.2. E. Warfarin.

According to the recent CHEST guidelines (Kearon et al. 2016), in patients with DVT of the leg or PEs, warfarin is not the choice of therapy (for first three months) (evidence grade 2B). See Box 30.1.

30.3. B. Dabigatran and edoxaban.

If novel anticoagulants are chosen to treat a DVT or a PE when not associated with cancer, initial parenteral anticoagulation is recommended with dabigatran and edoxaban and is not needed with rivaroxaban and apixaban and is overlapped with warfarin.

30.4. B. Reduce dosage to 75 mg BID.

Dronedarone inhibits P-glycoprotein and cytochrome P450 3A4 and hence increases the plasma concentration of dabigatran, which may lead to increased bleeding. Hence, the current recommendation is to reduce the dose of dabigatran to 75 mg BID in the USA. See Box 30.2.

30.5. C. Start on 75 mg BID.

Ketoconazole, itraconazole, voriconazole, and posaconazole will increase the serum concentration of dabigatran through P-glycoprotein and breast cancer resistance protein competition and cytochrome P450 3A4 inhibition. Hence, it is recommended to start dabigatran dose at 75 mg BID while on any of the aforementioned antifungals in the USA.

30.6. A. Dabigatran.

Among the drugs listed in the question, dabigatran is cleared through the kidneys (80%), while rivaroxaban (66%), apixaban (25%) and edoxaban (50%) have lower rates of renal clearance.

30.7. C. Dabigatran.

Dabigatran is a direct thrombin inhibitor, while all the other agents are factor Xa (FXa) inhibitors.

30.8. A. Idarucizumab.

Idarucizumab is a humanized, monoclonal, antibody fragment that specifically binds with high affinity to dabigatran, an oral direct thrombin inhibitor. It acts by competitively displacing dabigatran from thrombin to reverse anticoagulation and restore fibrin formation. Dabigatran has an affinity for idarucizumab that is 350 times greater than its affinity for thrombin. The dose currently studied in the phase 3 trial is 5 g. A global phase 3 case series study known as RE-VERSE AD is currently enrolling patients treated with dabigatran who have uncontrolled bleeding or require emergency surgery or procedures. A dose of 5 g idarucizumab will be administered intravenously to reverse the effect of dabigatran. The trial will measure plasma-diluted thrombin time and ecarin clotting time as primary outcome measures. Time to cessation of bleeding will be a secondary outcome. Results from the trial are expected in 2017.

30.9. B. Andexanet alfa.

It is a modified recombinant FXa molecule intended for intravenous (IV) administration. It has been developed as an antidote to reverse anticoagulant activity of oral direct (e.g. apixaban, edoxaban, and rivaroxaban) and injectable indirect (e.g. enoxaparin and fondaparinux) FXa inhibitors. Andexanet alfa acts to target and sequester with high specificity both oral and injectable FXa inhibitors in the blood. Part 1 of the phase 3 ANNEXA-R trial – which was designed to compare the administration of an 800 mg IV bolus of andexanet alfa with placebo in 39 patients pretreated with rivaroxaban 20 mg for four days – were presented at the 2015 American College of Cardiology Scientific Sessions on March 16, 2015. Andexanet alfa produced a statistically significant and rapid reduction in anti-FXa activity from baseline (primary outcome); mean percentage change anti-FXa from baseline to nadir was 92% ($P <$ 0.0001 versus placebo). Normalization of coagulation parameters was achieved within two minutes of completing the IV bolus infusion; the effect lasted one to two hours with the IV bolus dose. Part 2 is ongoing and will investigate IV bolus followed by a two-hours continuous infusion to demonstrate sustained reversal.

30.10. C. Aripazine.

It is a small, synthetic molecule designed with broad reversal activity and administered as a single IV bolus dose. It binds to oral FXa inhibitors and direct thrombin inhibitors, as well as to injectable unfractionated heparin and LMWH via noncovalent bonding and charge–charge interactions to neutralize anticoagulation and bleeding. Currently in phase 2 trials.

30.11. A. Thromboprophylaxis in the outpatient period for up to 35 days.

The current guideline recommendation is to extend thromboprophylaxis to 35 days from the day of surgery.

30.12. C. LMWH.

The guidelines recommend the use of LMWH in preference to the other agents recommended as alternatives: fondaparinux, apixaban, dabigatran, rivaroxaban, low-dose unfractionated heparin (LDUH) (all grade 2B), adjusted-dose vitamin K antagonist (VKA), or aspirin (all grade 2C).

30.13. C. 12 hours or more preoperatively or postoperatively.

For patients undergoing major orthopedic surgery (total hip arthroplasty, total knee arthroplasty, and hip fracture surgery) and receiving LMWH as thromboprophylaxis, the guidelines recommend starting either 12 hours or more preoperatively or postoperatively rather than within four hours or less preoperatively or postoperatively (grade 1B).

30.14. E. All of the above.

Current recommendations are to use any of the following anticoagulants for thromboprophylaxis: LMWH, LDUH BID, LDUH TID, or fondaparinux (grade 1B).

30.15. D. Dabigatran was associated with more intracranial bleeds.

This is false. In the RE-LY trial, dabigatran was associated with 2.71% (110 mg) and 3.11% (150 mg) major bleeding rates compared with warfarin (3.36%) but was associated with lower rates of intracranial bleeding. See Box 30.3.

30.16. D. Apixaban was noninferior to warfarin in preventing stroke.

This is false. Apixaban was superior to warfarin in preventing stroke (ARISTOTLE trial), while ROCKET AF and ENGAGE AF showed rivaroxaban and edoxaban respectively to be noninferior to warfarin in preventing stroke or embolism. See Box 30.3.

30.17. A. Serial imaging of the deep veins in two weeks when there are no severe symptoms or risk for extension.

In a patient with isolated distal DVT without severe symptoms or risk for extension, serial imaging of the deep veins over two weeks is recommended.

30.18. A. Anticoagulation if the thrombus has not extended.

The current recommendation for patients with isolated distal DVT managed by serial imaging is to start anticoagulation if the thrombus has extended into the distal veins or into proximal veins.

30.19. C. In patients with subsegmental PE (not involving proximal pulmonary arteries) without proximal DVT of legs and a high risk for VTE, clinical surveillance is recommended.

This is not true. In patients with subsegmental PE (not involving proximal pulmonary arteries) without proximal DVT of legs and a high risk for venous thromboembolism (VTE), anticoagulation over clinical surveillance is recommended.

30.20. F. All of the above.

See CHEST guidelines (Kearon et al. 2016); Box 30.1.

---

**Box 30.1    CHEST Guideline and Expert Panel Report**

Kearon et al. (2016) updated recommendations on 12 topics that were in the ninth edition of the guidelines and addressed three new topics. The main points taken from Kearon et al. (2016), without altering the original language, are as follows (where the asterisks indicate the newly added or changed recommendations since publication of the 9th edition):

*1. In patients with proximal DVT or pulmonary embolism (PE), we recommend long term (three months) anticoagulant therapy over no such therapy (Grade 1B). For patients with DVT of the leg or PE and no cancer who are not treated with dabigatran, rivaroxaban, apixaban, or edoxaban, we suggest VKA therapy over low-molecular weight heparin (LMWH) (Grade 2C).

*2. In patients with DVT of the leg or PE and no cancer, as long-term (first three months) anticoagulant therapy, we suggest dabigatran, rivaroxaban, apixaban, or edoxaban over vitamin K antagonist (VKA) therapy (all Grade 2B).

Remarks: Initial parenteral anticoagulation is given before dabigatran and edoxaban, is not given before rivaroxaban and apixaban, and is overlapped with VKA therapy. See text for factors that influence choice of therapy.

*3. In patients with DVT of the leg or PE and cancer ("cancer-associated thrombosis"), as long-term (first three months) anticoagulant therapy, we suggest LMWH over VKA therapy (Grade 2C), dabigatran (Grade 2C), rivaroxaban (Grade 2C), apixaban (Grade 2C), or edoxaban (Grade 2C).

*4. In patients with DVT of the leg or PE who receive extended therapy, we suggest that there is no need to change the choice of anticoagulant after the first three months (Grade 2C).

*Remarks:* It may be appropriate for the choice of anticoagulant to change in response to changes in the patient's circumstances or preferences during long-term or extended phases of treatment.

5. In patients with a proximal DVT of the leg or PE provoked by surgery, we recommend treatment with anticoagulation for three months over (i) treatment of a shorter period (Grade 1B), (ii) treatment of a longer time-limited period (e.g. 6, 12, or 24 months) (Grade 1B), or (iii) extended therapy (no scheduled stop date) (Grade 1B).

6. In patients with a proximal DVT of the leg or PE provoked by a nonsurgical transient risk factor, we recommend treatment with anticoagulation for three months over (i) treatment of a shorter period (Grade 1B) and (ii) treatment of a longer time-limited period (e.g. 6, 12, or 24 months) (Grade 1B). We suggest treatment with anticoagulation for three months over extended therapy if there is a low or moderate bleeding risk (Grade 2B), and recommend treatment for three months over extended therapy if there is a high risk of bleeding (Grade 1B).

*Remarks:* In all patients who receive extended anticoagulant therapy, the continuing use of treatment should be reassessed at periodic intervals (e.g. annually).

7. In patients with an isolated distal DVT of the leg provoked by surgery or by a nonsurgical transient risk factor, we suggest treatment with anticoagulation for three months over treatment of a shorter period (Grade 2C), we recommend treatment with anticoagulation for three months over treatment of a longer time-limited period (e.g. 6, 12, or 24 months) (Grade 1B), and we recommend treatment with anticoagulation for three months over extended therapy (no scheduled stop date) (Grade 1B).

*Remarks:* Duration of treatment of patients with isolated distal DVT refers to patients in whom a decision has been made to treat with anticoagulant therapy; however, it is anticipated that not all patients who are diagnosed with isolated distal DVT will be prescribed anticoagulants.

8. In patients with an unprovoked DVT of the leg (isolated distal or proximal) or PE, we recommend treatment with anticoagulation for at least three months over treatment of a shorter duration (Grade 1B), and we recommend treatment with anticoagulation for three months over treatment of a longer time-limited period (e.g. 6, 12, or 24 months) (Grade 1B).

*Remarks:* After three months of treatment, patients with unprovoked DVT of the leg or PE should be evaluated for the risk–benefit ratio of extended therapy. Duration of treatment of patients with isolated distal DVT refers to patients in whom a decision has been made to treat with anticoagulant therapy; however, it is anticipated that not all patients who are diagnosed with isolated distal DVT will be prescribed anticoagulants.

9. In patients with a first VTE that is an unprovoked proximal DVT of the leg or PE and who have a (i) low or moderate bleeding risk (see text), we suggest extended anticoagulant therapy (no scheduled stop date) over three months of therapy (Grade 2B), and (ii) high bleeding risk (see text), we recommend three months of anticoagulant therapy over extended therapy (no scheduled stop date) (Grade 1B).

Chapter 30

*Remarks:* Patient sex and D-dimer level measured one month after stopping anticoagulant therapy may influence the decision to stop or extend anticoagulant therapy (see text). In all patients who receive extended anticoagulant therapy, the continuing use of treatment should be reassessed at periodic intervals (e.g. annually).

10. In patients with a second unprovoked VTE and who have a (i) low bleeding risk (see text), we recommend extended anticoagulant therapy (no scheduled stop date) over three months (Grade 1B); (ii) moderate bleeding risk (see text), we suggest extended anticoagulant therapy over three months of therapy (Grade 2B); or (iii) high bleeding risk (see text), we suggest three months of anticoagulant therapy over extended therapy (no scheduled stop date) (Grade 2B).

    *Remarks:* In all patients who receive extended anticoagulant therapy, the continuing use of treatment should be reassessed at periodic intervals (e.g. annually).

11. In patients with DVT of the leg or PE and active cancer ("cancer-associated thrombosis") and who (i) do not have a high bleeding risk, we recommend extended anticoagulant therapy (no scheduled stop date) over three months of therapy (Grade 1B), or (ii) have a high bleeding risk, we suggest extended anticoagulant therapy (no scheduled stop date) over three months of therapy (Grade 2B).

*12. In patients with an unprovoked proximal DVT or PE who are stopping anticoagulant therapy and do not have a contraindication to aspirin, we suggest aspirin over no aspirin to prevent recurrent VTE (Grade 2B).

    *Remarks:* Because aspirin is expected to be much less effective at preventing recurrent VTE than anticoagulants, we do not consider aspirin a reasonable alternative to anticoagulant therapy in patients who want extended therapy. However, if a patient has decided to stop anticoagulants, prevention of recurrent VTE is one of the benefits of aspirin that needs to be balanced against aspirin's risk of bleeding and inconvenience. Use of aspirin should also be reevaluated when patients stop anticoagulant therapy because aspirin may have been stopped when anticoagulants were started.

13. In patients with acute isolated distal DVT of the leg and (i) without severe symptoms or risk factors for extension (see text), we suggest serial imaging of the deep veins for two weeks over anticoagulation (Grade 2C) or (ii) with severe symptoms or risk factors for extension (see text), we suggest anticoagulation over serial imaging of the deep veins (Grade 2C).

    *Remarks:* Patients at high risk for bleeding are more likely to benefit from serial imaging. Patients who place a high value on avoiding the inconvenience of repeat imaging and a low value on the inconvenience of treatment and on the potential for bleeding are likely to choose initial anticoagulation over serial imaging.

14. In patients with acute isolated distal DVT of the leg who are managed with anticoagulation, we recommend using the same anticoagulation as that for patients with acute proximal DVT (Grade 1B).

15. In patients with acute isolated distal DVT of the leg who are managed with serial imaging, we (i) recommend no anticoagulation if the thrombus does not extend (Grade 1B), (ii) suggest anticoagulation if the thrombus extends but remains

confined to the distal veins (Grade 2C), and (iii) recommend anticoagulation if the thrombus extends into the proximal veins (Grade 1B).

16. In patients with acute proximal DVT of the leg, we suggest anticoagulant therapy alone over CDT (catheter-directed thrombolysis) (Grade 2C).

    *Remarks:* Patients who are most likely to benefit from CDT (see text), who attach a high value to prevention of postthrombotic syndrome (PTS), and a lower value to the initial complexity, cost, and risk of bleeding with CDT, are likely to choose CDT over anticoagulation alone.

17. In patients with acute DVT or PE who are treated with anticoagulants, we recommend against the use of an inferior vena cava (IVC) filter (Grade 1B).

*18. In patients with acute DVT of the leg, we suggest not using compression stockings routinely to prevent PTS (Grade 2B).

*19. In patients with subsegmental PE (no involvement of more proximal pulmonary arteries) and no proximal DVT in the legs who have a (i) low risk for recurrent VTE (see text), we suggest clinical surveillance over anticoagulation (Grade 2C) or (ii) high risk for recurrent VTE (see text), we suggest anticoagulation over clinical surveillance (Grade 2C).

    *Remarks:* Ultrasound (US) imaging of the deep veins of both legs should be done to exclude proximal DVT. Clinical surveillance can be supplemented by serial US imaging of the proximal deep veins of both legs to detect evolving DVT (see text). Patients and physicians are more likely to opt for clinical surveillance over anticoagulation if there is good cardiopulmonary reserve or a high risk of bleeding.

*20. In patients with low-risk PE and whose home circumstances are adequate, we suggest treatment at home or early discharge over standard discharge (e.g. after the first five days of treatment) (Grade 2B).

21. In patients with acute PE associated with hypotension (e.g. systolic BP <90 mmHg) who do not have a high bleeding risk, we suggest systemically administered thrombolytic therapy over no such therapy (Grade 2B).

*22. In most patients with acute PE not associated with hypotension, we recommend against systemically administered thrombolytic therapy (Grade 1B).

*23. In selected patients with acute PE who deteriorate after starting anticoagulant therapy but have yet to develop hypotension and who have a low bleeding risk, we suggest systemically administered thrombolytic therapy over no such therapy (Grade 2C).

    *Remarks:* Patients with PE and without hypotension who have severe symptoms or marked cardiopulmonary impairment should be monitored closely for deterioration. Development of hypotension suggests that thrombolytic therapy has become indicated. Cardiopulmonary deterioration (e.g. symptoms, vital signs, tissue perfusion, gas exchange, cardiac biomarkers) that has not progressed to hypotension may also alter the risk–benefit assessment in favor of thrombolytic therapy in patients initially treated with anticoagulation alone.

*24. In patients with acute PE who are treated with a thrombolytic agent, we suggest systemic thrombolytic therapy using a peripheral vein over CDT (Grade 2C).

    *Remarks:* Patients who have a higher risk of bleeding with systemic thrombolytic therapy and who have access to the expertise and resources required to do CDT are likely to choose CDT over systemic thrombolytic therapy.

*25. In patients with acute PE associated with hypotension and who have (i) a high bleeding risk, (ii) failed systemic thrombolysis, or (iii) shock that is likely to cause death before systemic thrombolysis can take effect (e.g. within hours), if appropriate expertise and resources are available, we suggest catheter-assisted thrombus removal over no such intervention (Grade 2C).

   *Remarks:* Catheter-assisted thrombus removal refers to mechanical interventions, with or without catheter directed thrombolysis.

*26. In selected patients with chronic thromboembolic pulmonary hypertension (CTEPH) who are identified by an experienced thromboendarterectomy team, we suggest pulmonary thromboendarterectomy over no pulmonary thromboendarterectomy (Grade 2C).

   *Remarks:* Patients with CTEPH should be evaluated by a team with expertise in treatment of pulmonary hypertension. Pulmonary thromboendarterectomy is often lifesaving and life-transforming. Patients with CTEPH who are not candidates for pulmonary thromboendarterectomy may benefit from other mechanical and pharmacologic interventions designed to lower pulmonary arterial pressure.

27. In patients with acute upper extremity DVT (UEDVT) that involves the axillary or more proximal veins, we suggest anticoagulant therapy alone over thrombolysis (Grade 2C).

   *Remarks:* Patients who (i) are most likely to benefit from thrombolysis (see text); (ii) have access to CDT; (iii) attach a high value to prevention of PTS; and (iv) attach a lower value to the initial complexity, cost, and risk of bleeding with thrombolytic therapy are likely to choose thrombolytic therapy over anticoagulation alone.

28. In patients with UEDVT who undergo thrombolysis, we recommend the same intensity and duration of anticoagulant therapy as in patients with UEDVT who do not undergo thrombolysis (Grade 1B).

*29. In patients who have recurrent VTE on VKA therapy (in the therapeutic range) or on dabigatran, rivaroxaban, apixaban, or edoxaban (and are believed to be compliant), we suggest switching to treatment with LMWH at least temporarily (Grade 2C).

   *Remarks:* Recurrent VTE while on therapeutic-dose anticoagulant therapy is unusual and should prompt the following assessments: (i) reevaluation of whether there truly was a recurrent VTE; (ii) evaluation of compliance with anticoagulant therapy; and (iii) consideration of an underlying malignancy. A temporary switch to LMWH will usually be for at least one month.

*30. In patients who have recurrent VTE on long-term LMWH (and are believed to be compliant), we suggest increasing the dose of LMWH by about one-quarter to one-third (Grade 2C).

---

| Box 30.2   Clinical Trials |
| --- |

- **RE-LY trial** (Connolly et al. 2009): a noninferiority study randomizing 18 000 patients with nonvalvular atrial fibrillation with moderate or high risk of stroke to either high dose dabigatran, low-dose dabigatran, or warfarin. High-dose dabigatran was associated with reduced incidence of stroke 1.11% versus 1.69% (relative risk [RR] 0.66, 95% confidence interval [CI] 0.53–0.82, $P < 0.001$ for superiority) without any major bleeding increase 3.11% versus 3.36% (P = 0.31) when compared with warfarin. Even though it was a non-inferiority study, the final analysis showed dabigatran to be superior to warfarin. The US Food and Drug Administration approved the high-dose 150 mg BID for stroke prevention in nonvalvular atrial fibrillation. Subsequently, the lower dose of 75 mg BID was approved for use in patients with renal impairment, though not studied in trials. Both low-dose and high-dose dabigatran were associated with a statistically significant increase in rate of myocardial infarction (0.74% versus 0.72% versus 0.53%).

- **ROCKET AF trial** (Patel et al. 2011): randomized 14264 patients with nonvalvular atrial fibrillation to rivaroxaban or warfarin. *Results.* Stroke or embolism: intention-to-treat, 2.1 versus 2.4 events per 100 patient-years (hazard ratio [HR] 0.88, 95% CI 0.75–1.03; $P < 0.001$ for noninferiority, $P = 0.12$ for superiority); per protocol, 1.7 versus 2.2 events per 100 patient-years (HR 0.79, 95% CI 0.66–0.96, $P < 0.001$ for noninferiority). Major bleeding 5.6% versus 5.4% (nonsignificant).
- **ARISTOTLE trial** (Granger et al. 2011): randomized 18201 patients with nonvalvular atrial fibrillation and >1 risk factor for stroke to apixaban or warfarin. Median follow-up 1.8 years, apixaban was superior to warfarin for stroke or systemic embolism reduction (1.27% versus 1.60%, HR 0.79, 95% CI 0.66–0.95; $P = 0.01$ for superiority and $P < 0.001$ for noninferiority). It was also associated with less major bleeding (2.13% versus 3.09%).
- **ENGAGE AF trial** (Giugliano et al. 2013): randomized 21105 patients to either low-dose or high-dose edoxaban or warfarin in patients with nonvalvular atrial fibrillation. Primary outcome of stroke or embolism: 1.50% with warfarin versus 1.18% with high-dose edoxaban (HR 0.79, 97.5% CI 0.63–0.99; $P < 0.001$ for noninferiority) and 1.61% with low-dose edoxaban (HR 1.07, 97.5% CI 0.87–1.31; $P = 0.005$ for noninferiority). The annualized rate of major bleeding was 3.43% with warfarin versus 2.75% with high-dose edoxaban (HR 0.80, 95% CI 0.71–0.91; $P < 0.001$) and 1.61% with low-dose edoxaban (HR 0.47, 95% CI 0.41–0.55; $P < 0.001$).

---

**Box 30.3   April 2014 AHA/ACC/HRS Atrial Fibrillation Guidelines**

Adapted from January et al. (2014).
- In patients with nonvalvular atrial fibrillation with prior stroke, transient ischemic attack, $CHA_2DS_2$-VASc score $\geq 2$, recommend oral anticoagulation with:
  d) warfarin, goal INR 2–3 (class 1, level A)
  e) dabigatran (class 1, level B)
  f) rivaroxaban (class 1, level B)
  g) apixaban (class 1, level B).
- In patients with nonvalvular AF unable to maintain INR 2–3 with warfarin, recommend dabigatran, rivaroxaban, or apixaban (class 1, level C).
- In patients with nonvalvular AF with moderate or severe chronic kidney disease with CHA2DS2-VASc score >2, consider treatment with reduced doses of dabigatran, rivaroxaban, or apixaban, though safety has not been clearly demonstrated (class IIb, level C).
- In patients with ESRD, dabigatran and rivaroxaban are untested and not recommended (class III, level C).
- In patients with mechanical valve, do not use dabigatran (class III, level B).

## References

Connolly, S.J., Ezekowitz, M.D., Yusuf, S. et al. (2009). Dabigatran versus warfarin in patients with atrial fibrillation. *The New England Journal of Medicine* 361: 1139–1151.

Giugliano, R.P., Ruff, C.T., Braunwald, E. et al. (2013). Edoxaban versus warfarin in patients with atrial fibrillation. *The New England Journal of Medicine* 369: 2093–2104.

Granger, C.B., Alexander, J.H., McMurray, J.J.V. et al. (2011). Apixaban versus warfarin in patients with atrial fibrillation. *The New England Journal of Medicine* 365: 981–992.

January, C.T., Wann, L.S., Alpert, J.S. et al. (2014). 2014 AHA/ACC/HRS guideline for the management of patients with atrial fibrillation: executive summary: a report of the American College of Cardiology/American Heart Association task force on practice guidelines and the Heart Rhythm Society. *Circulation* 130 (23): 2071–2104. [Erratum: *Circulation* (2014) 130(23): e270–e271.].

Kearon, C., Akl, E.A., Ornelas, J. et al. (2016). Antithrombotic therapy for VTE disease: CHEST guideline and expert panel report. *Chest* 149 (2): 315–352.

Patel, M.R., Mahaffey, K.W., Garg, J. et al. (2011). Rivaroxaban versus warfarin in nonvalvular atrial fibrillation. *The New England Journal of Medicine* 365 (10): 883–891.

# Aspirin and Antiplatelet Therapy

# 31

**31.1.** CJ is a 64-year-old female who is transferred to the catheterization laboratory for an emergent PCI following an ST elevation myocardial infarction (STEMI). Two drug-eluting stents are placed. Past medical history includes hypertension (HTN), hyperlipidemia, diabetes mellitus type 2, and gastroesophageal reflux disease. The patient's current medications include lisinopril, simvastatin, metformin, glipizide, and pantoprazole. Which of the following antiplatelets would be best to start in combination with aspirin 324 mg in this patient for prevention of stent thrombosis?

A. Clopidogrel 300 mg loading dose, then 75 mg PO daily
B. Clopidogrel 600 mg loading dose, then 75 mg PO daily
C. Prasugrel 60 mg loading dose, then 10 mg PO daily
D. Ticagrelor 180 mg loading dose, then 90 mg PO twice daily

**31.2.** What is the proposed rationale behind avoiding concomitant use of ticagrelor with aspirin doses above 100 mg per day?

A. Concomitant use of ticagrelor and aspirin >100 mg daily may result in decreased efficacy of aspirin
B. Concomitant use of ticagrelor and aspirin >100 mg daily may result in decreased efficacy of ticagrelor
C. Concomitant use of ticagrelor and aspirin >100 mg daily may result in intolerable gastrointestinal adverse events that may lead to drug discontinuation
D. Concomitant use of ticagrelor and aspirin >100 mg daily may result in increased hypersensitivity to aspirin

**31.3.** JP is a 60-year-old female who presents to your outpatient clinic for a check-up. She has been on long-term warfarin therapy for secondary stroke prevention with a history significant for atrial fibrillation and ischemic stroke (2011). From reviewing her electronic profile, it is apparent that JP's warfarin therapy has been difficult to maintain within therapeutic range. You would like to consider transitioning her to rivaroxaban as this is what her insurance company will cover. What is an appropriate method of transitioning JP from warfarin to rivaroxaban?

A. Discontinue warfarin; start rivaroxaban when international normalized ratio (INR) <2
B. Discontinue warfarin; start rivaroxaban when INR <3
C. Discontinue warfarin; start rivaroxaban after three to five days of discontinuation of warfarin
D. Start rivaroxaban three to five days before discontinuing warfarin

*Cardiology Board Review*, Second Edition. Ramdas G. Pai and Padmini Varadarajan.
© 2023 John Wiley & Sons Ltd. Published 2023 by John Wiley & Sons Ltd.

**31.4.** LT is a 48-year-old male presenting with a new STEMI who is transported from the medical intensive care unit to the catheterizatin laboratory for an emergent percutaneous coronary intervention (PCI). Labs from his current admission observe notable increases in blood urea nitrogen/serum creatinine and decreased urine output, suggesting signs of acute kidney injury. Which of the following intravenous antiplatelet inhibitors would be best to use if the patient is found to require emergency coronary artery bypass grafting surgery?

**A.** Abciximab
**B.** Eptifibatide
**C.** Tirofiban
**D.** Cangrelor

**31.5.** RG is a 46-year-old male who presents with swelling, erythema, and pain in his right lower extremity. Past medical history includes HTN, diabetes, and recent hospitalization for a total knee arthroplasty. The patient further admits to a 10-year smoking history. Ultrasound and D-dimer tests suggest that a deep venous thrombosis (DVT) is highly likely. For convenience, the patient indicates that he refuses parenteral agents and wishes to be started on solely an oral anticoagulant for DVT treatment. Which of the following is the best oral anticoagulant for RG?

**A.** Warfarin
**B.** Dabigatran
**C.** Rivaroxaban
**D.** Edoxaban

**31.6.** GT is a 66-year-old male on long-term warfarin therapy with a past medical history of atrial fibrillation, HTN, diabetes mellitus type 2, gastroesophageal reflux disease, ischemic stroke, and cirrhosis. He presented to the hospital with sharp, crushing chest pain, shortness of breath, and fatigue. Cardiac enzymes are positive, and she is later diagnosed with non-STEMI and one drug-eluting stent is placed in the right coronary artery. What is the best antithrombotic therapy for GT post-PCI?

**A.** Stop warfarin. Start aspirin 81 mg daily and clopidogrel 75 mg daily for at least 12 months. Restart warfarin after 12 months
**B.** Continue warfarin (goal INR 2.0–2.5) lifelong. Start aspirin 81 mg daily and clopidogrel 75 mg daily for at least 12 months
**C.** Continue warfarin (goal INR 2.0–2.5) lifelong. Start aspirin 81 mg daily and clopidogrel 75 mg daily for four weeks. After four weeks, stop aspirin and continue clopidogrel 75 mg daily for at least 12 months
**D.** Continue warfarin (goal INR 2.0–3.0) lifelong. Start aspirin 81 mg daily for at least 12 months.

**31.7.** What is the rationale behind overlapping warfarin with a parenteral agent for at least five days when initiating antithrombotic therapy for venous thromboembolism treatment?

**A.** Warfarin's effects are dependent on the half-lives of the clotting factors it inhibits the production of
**B.** It takes approximately 5–10 days for warfarin to inhibit more clotting factors than are being produced

    C. Double therapy with warfarin and a parental agent is necessary because it requires two antithrombotic agents to overcome the clot burden

    D. A parenteral agent must be used to prevent formation of "white clots," whereas warfarin is used to prevent formation of "red clots"

**31.8.** MN is a 45-year-old male who is transferred to the coronary care unit postPCI for a STEMI. Chart review indicates that appropriate doses of heparin, abciximab, and clopidogrel were used in the catheterization laboratory. Hours later, the patient begins to complain of rectal bleeding. Labs are drawn showing hemoglobin/hematocrit 6.2/26.5, platelets $22000/mm^3$, and INR 2.1. The complete blood count prior to PCI the day before was normal. Which of the following statements is true?

    A. Pseudothrombocytopenia is a common occurrence of STEMI patients, and thus these labs are of little concern

    B. Transient thrombocytopenia is a common adverse event associated with dosing doses of clopidogrel

    C. Heparin-induced thrombocytopenia is likely since platelets have dropped suddenly and the patient is exhibiting signs of bleeding

    D. Abciximab is associated with sudden profound thrombocytopenia

**31.9.** TJ is a 59-year-old male who presents with a new STEMI and is transferred to the catheterization laboratory where three drug-eluting stents are placed. Past medical history includes HTN, diabetes mellitus type 2, hyperlipidemia, and transient ischemic attack. Which of the following $P2Y_{12}$ receptor antagonists may not be used with aspirin 81 mg for dual antiplatelet therapy to prevent stent thrombosis?

    A. Clopidogrel

    B. Prasugrel

    C. Ticagrelor

    D. Cangrelor

**Chapter 31**

**31.10.** Which of the following is a common adverse drug reaction to ticagrelor?

    A. Leukocytosis

    B. Hyperkalemia

    C. Weight loss

    D. Dyspnea

**31.11.** Which of the following antiplatelets would be most affected by initiation of phenytoin in a patient with seizures?

    A. Aspirin                        C. Prasugrel

    B. Clopidogrel                D. Ticagrelor

**31.12.** Which of the following glycoprotein IIb/IIIa inhibitors is associated with the longest observed platelet antagonism effects?

    A. Abciximab                  C. Tirofiban

    B. Eptifibatide               D. Orbofiban

**31.13.** Which of the following antiplatelets requires a two-step CYP enzyme = dependent metabolism to become an active drug?

    A. Aspirin                        C. Prasugrel

    B. Clopidogrel                D. Ticagrelor

**31.14.** Which of the following antiplatelets reversibly binds to platelet receptors on the platelet surface?

**A.** Aspirin                      **C.** Prasugrel

**B.** Clopidogrel                **D.** Ticagrelor

**31.15.** WM is a 36-year-old male with a past medical history of uncontrolled HTN, diabetes mellitus type 2, and non-STEMI (2014, 2015). He presents to the emergency department with atrial fibrillation with rapid ventricular response, in which intravenous diltiazem is ordered for rate control. Recent labs show Na 135 mEq/l, K 4.1 mEq/l, Cl 100 mmol/l, $CO_2$ 22 mmol/l, blood urea nitrogen 16 mg/dl, and serum creatinine 0.8 mg/dl. Most recent weight is 90 kg and height is 6 ft. The team is considering novel oral anticoagulants that may be started for primary stroke prevention. Which agents may not be used in this patient?

**A.** Dabigatran

**B.** Rivaroxaban

**C.** Apixaban

**D.** Edoxaban

## Answers

**31.1.** C. Prasugrel 60 mg loading dose, then 10 mg PO daily.

Clopidogrel, prasugrel, and ticagrelor may all be used in this patient for dual antiplatelet therapy; however, significant benefit was seen with prasugrel, particularly in patients with STEMI and diabetes mellitus.

**31.2.** B. Concomitant use of ticagrelor and aspirin >100 mg daily may result in decreased efficacy of ticagrelor.

Currently, there is a US black box warning to avoid use of aspirin >100 mg with ticagrelor.

**31.3.** B. Discontinue warfarin; start rivaroxaban when INR <3.

It should be noted that this specific recommendation is provided in Xarelto's package insert. To date, there is little evidence to show better efficacy and safety outcomes with one method of transition over another method. In contrast, when transitioning from warfarin to either apixaban or dabigatran, the novel oral anticoagulant may be started when INR <2.

**31.4.** D. Cangrelor.

Eptifibatide and tirofiban are renally cleared and require dose adjustment in renal impairment. Abciximab is metabolized via proteolytic cleavage and its clearance is not dependent on renal function, but its antiplatelet effects can last up to 7–14 days. Cangrelor is not dependent on renal or hepatic function and its antiplatelet effect wears off after one hour.

**31.5.** C. Rivaroxaban.

Rivaroxaban is the only agent listed that may be started for DVT treatment and does not require overlap therapy with a parenteral agent. Warfarin, dabigatran, and edoxaban must be started concomitantly with at least five days of a parenteral agent, such as enoxaparin or heparin.

**31.6.** C. Continue warfarin (goal INR 2.0–2.5) lifelong. Start aspirin 81 mg daily and clopidogrel 75 mg daily for four weeks. After four weeks, stop aspirin and continue clopidogrel 75 mg daily for at least 12 months.

Triple versus dual antithrombotic therapy in patients with atrial fibrillation undergoing PCI remains a controversial topic. There are several different recommendations regarding optimal antithrombotic therapy after stent placement. However, answer "A" is incorrect because warfarin has been shown to be superior over aspirin plus clopidogrel to prevent thromboembolism. Answer "B" is not ideal because triple antithrombotic for over a year puts this patient at increased risk for bleeding. From the information provided in the question, this patient's HASBLED score is at least 3, indicating a high bleed risk. Answer "D" is incorrect because it has been shown that the combination of warfarin plus aspirin after PCI puts patients at increased risk for stent thrombosis.

**31.7.** A. Warfarin's anticoagulant effects are dependent on the half-lives of the clotting factors it inhibits the production of.

Warfarin inhibits the vitamin K-dependent synthesis of factors II, VII, IX, X and proteins C and S. Because the half-life of factor II may be as long as 48–72 hours, it is recommended to overlap initial warfarin therapy with a faster-acting parenteral agent.

**31.8.** D. Abciximab is associated with sudden profound thrombocytopenia.

This is typically seen within minutes to hours of abciximab administration and is generally associated with bleeding.

**31.9.** B. Prasugrel.

Of the listed $P2Y_{12}$ receptor antagonists, prasugrel is contraindicated in patients with a history of transient ischemic attack or stroke due to increased risk of significant or fatal bleeding.

**31.10.** D. Dyspnea.

The incidence of dyspnea associated with the use of ticagrelor has been reported to be as high as 14%. This must be taken into consideration as it may result in noncompliance of the medication and has been found to contribute to hospital readmissions.

**31.11.** D. Ticagrelor.

Concomitant use of ticagrelor and strong cytochrome P450 (CYP)3A4 inducers, such as phenytoin, must be avoided as it may lead to decreased serum concentrations of ticagrelor.

**31.12.** A. Abciximab.

Dissociation of abciximab from the glycoprotein IIb/IIIa receptor occurs through proteolytic cleavage, resulting in slow elimination and consequently profound platelet antagonism that can last up to 12 hours post-infusion. Platelet function may remain abnormal up to 7–14 weeks after infusion.

**31.13.** B. Clopidogrel.

Clopidogrel is metabolized extensively via two oxidative steps that are dependent predominantly on CYP2C19 to an active drug. CYP2C19 inhibitors, such as proton pump inhibitors, may lead to reduced serum concentrations of clopidogrel's active metabolite.

Chapter 3

**31.14.** D. Ticagrelor.

Ticagrelor reversibly binds to the $P2Y_{12}$ receptors on the platelet surface, and thus recovery of platelet function is likely dependent on serum concentrations of ticagrelor. Aspirin irreversibly inhibits the cyclooxygenase- (COX)-1 and COX-2 enzymes, and clopidogrel and prasugrel irreversibly bind to the $P2Y_{12}$ receptors. Thus, aspirin, clopidogrel, and prasugrel inhibit coagulation for the lifespan of the platelet.

**31.15.** D. Edoxaban.

Edoxaban should not be used in patients with a creatinine clearance (calculated using the Cockcroft-Gault equation) greater than 95 ml/min. In the ENGAGE AF-TIMI 48 trial, patients with creatinine clearance >95 ml/min observed increased rates of ischemic stroke with edoxaban 60 mg daily in comparison with warfarin.

**32.1.** What is the arithmetic average of observations belonging to a continuous variable?

    **A.** Mean            **C.** Mode

    **B.** Median          **D.** None of the above

**32.2.** Which of the following are measures of dispersion around the mean?

    **A.** Standard deviation (SD)     **D.** Interquartile range (IQR)

    **B.** Variance              **E.** All of the above

    **C.** Range

**32.3.** What proportion of values lie between 1SD around the mean in normal distribution?

    **A.** 34%            **C.** 95%

    **B.** 68%            **D.** 99%

**32.4.** Which of the options in Figure 32.4 is likely to have the smallest SD?

    **A.** P              **C.** R

    **B.** Q              **D.** All have same SD

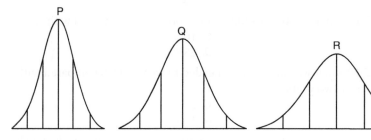

**Figure 32.4**

**32.5.** What would be the best test to decide if the mean age of two groups is different?

    **A.** Unpaired i-test        **C.** Chi squared test

    **B.** Paired i-test          **D.** Linear regression

**32.6.** A group of 40 patients is given a treatment. Measurements of heart rate are taken before and after. What would be the appropriate test to determine if the treatment was effective?

A. Unpaired i-test
B. Paired i-test
C. Chi squared test
D. Linear regression

**32.7.** Treatment "A" cured 40% of the patients and treatment "B" cured 70% of the patients. What would be the appropriate test to determine if the two treatments are different?

A. Unpaired i-test
B. Paired i-test
C. Chi squared test
D. Linear regression

**32.8.** The relationship between age and E/A velocity ratio can be studied best with which test?

A. Unpaired i-test
B. Paired i-test
C. Chi squared test
D. Linear regression

**32.9.** Measures of population description include which of the following?

A. Measures of central tendency and dispersion
B. Mean and median
C. IQR and range
D. Median and SD

**32.10.** The effects of treatments A and B are compared on mortality in a randomized trial. At the end of two years the mortality with treatment A was 15% and treatment B was 12%. What was the relative risk reduction with treatment B?

A. 3%
B. 20%
C. 10%
D. 25%

**32.11.** In Question 32.10, what was the absolute reduction with B compared with A?

A. 3%
B. 20%
C. 10%
D. 25%

**32.12.** In Question 32.10, what was the number needed to treat with B compared with A to save a life over two years?

A. 33
B. 7
C. 8
D. 100

**32.13.** A noninvasive diagnostic test to sort out a symptom is most productive in which patient groups?

A. Low probability of disease
B. Intermediate probability of disease
C. High probability of disease
D. All of these groups

**32.14.** A group of 100 patients with documented disease and 100 without disease received a diagnostic test to detect that disease. Among those with disease 80 had a positive test, and among those without disease 20 had a positive test. What is the sensitivity of the test?

A. 80%
B. 20%
C. 40%
D. 50%

**32.15.** In the example in Question 32.14, what is the specificity of the test?

A. 80%
B. 20%
C. 40%
D. 50%

**32.16.** In the example in Questions 32.14 and 32.15, what is the positive predictive value?

A. 80%  C. 40%

B. 20%  D. 50%

**32.17.** In the example in Questions 32.14 and 32.15, what is the negative predictive value?

A. 80%  C. 40%

B. 20%  D. 50%

**32.18.** Which of the following measures are affected by pretest probability of disease prevalence in which the test is performed? More than one choice may be correct.

A. Sensitivity  D. Negative predictive value

B. Specificity  E. All of the above

C. Positive predictive value  F. None of the above

**32.19.** Which of the following test characteristics are ideal for screening of disease?

A. High sensitivity, low cost, minimal risk

B. High specificity, low cost, minimal risk

C. Either A or B

D. Neither A nor B

**32.20.** Which test characteristics are ideal for confirming the presence of a disease?

A. High sensitivity, low cost, minimal risk

B. High specificity, low cost, minimal risk

C. Either A or B

D. Neither A nor B

**32.21.** Which of the following will false positives increase with?

A. Higher pretest probability  C. Intermediate pretest probability

B. Lower pretest probability  D. None of the above

**32.22.** As the test positivity criterion gets more stringent (e.g. increasing ST depression requirement to 2 mm instead of 1 mm), which of the following will happen to the test?

A. Increase in sensitivity and specificity

B. Decrease in sensitivity and specificity

C. Decrease in sensitivity and increase in specificity

D. Increase in sensitivity and decrease in specificity

**32.23.** What is the positive likelihood ratio (LR+) of a test with 90% sensitivity and 90% specificity?

A. 1  C. 9

B. 5  D. 90

**32.24.** The pretest probability of disease based on risk factors and presentation in an individual is 10%. If the test described in Question 32.23 is positive, what would be the probability of disease?

A. 30%  C. 90%

B. 50%  D. 99%

**32.25.** You want to test if treatment "X" prolongs survival in a disease under study. What would be the best study design?

**A.** A double-blind randomized controlled clinical trial with power > 0.8, an outcome adjudication committee, and safety monitoring committee

**B.** Single blind trial so that you can monitor to make sure that the patient is not harmed

**C.** A smaller trial with outcome surrogates

**D.** A nonrandomized trial with propensity score matching

**32.26.** In the trial in Question 32.25 1800 patients were enrolled, 900 in the active treatment arm and 900 in the placebo arm. At two years there were 200 deaths in the treatment arm and 250 in the placebo arm. The groups are well balanced in terms of baseline characteristics. What is the best approach for outcome analysis?

**A.** Kaplan–Meier analysis
**B.** Student's i-test
**C.** Chi squared test
**D.** None of the above

**32.27.** A large registry of patients with aortic stenosis was analyzed to see if aortic valve replacement (AVR) would prolong survival in patients with severe aortic stenosis with low gradient and normal ejection fraction. What would be the best statistical approach?

**A.** Kaplan–Meier analysis
**B.** Cox regression analysis
**C.** Propensity score analysis
**D.** None of the above

**32.28.** Some of the measures of imprecision or uncertainty around point estimates include which of the following?

**A.** The 95% confidence interval
**B.** The SD
**C.** The standard error of the mean (SEM)
**D.** All of the above

**32.29.** Two treatments for BP reduction are tested. The range of systolic BPs qualifying for trial entry is 160–220 mmHg. What will be the best way to analyze the results?

**A.** Analysis of covariance (ANCOVA)
**B.** Paired i-test
**C.** Unpaired i-test
**D.** Kaplan-Meir analysis

**32.30.** Which of the following statements regarding subset analysis of trial results is not true?

**A.** All subgroup analysis should be prespecified in a statistical analysis plan
**B.** It is used to look at trends in prespecified subsets and interactions
**C.** Any deviation from expected trend is hypothesis generating rather than conclusive
**D.** When the trial is negative and one of the subsets shows a positive result, it confirms benefits in that subset because it is a randomized trial

## Answers

**32.1. A.** Mean.

Median is the middle value, and mode is the most frequent value. All are measures of central tendency. In a normal distribution with number of observations >30, mean, median, and mode are expected to be the same. When the distribution is not normal, the mean, median, and mode are different, as shown in Figure 32.1.

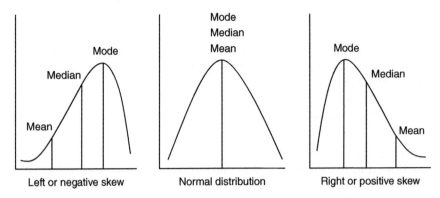

Mode
Median

Mode
Median
Mean

Mode

Mean

Median

Median

Mean

Mean

Left or negative skew          Normal distribution          Right or positive skew

**Figure 32.1**

**32.2.** E. All of the above.

The SD is the root-mean-square deviation; that is, the deviation from the mean of each observation that is squared, summed, averaged, and square rooted. Variance is the square of the SD. Range is the difference between maximum and minimum observation. IQR is the difference between observations at the 75th percentile and 25th percentile. All are measures of spread of the observations.

Chapter 32

**32.3.** B. 68%.

See Figure 32.3.

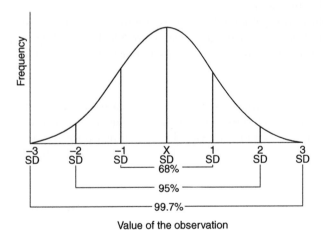

Frequency

$-3$ SD    $-2$ SD    $-1$ SD    X SD    1 SD    2 SD    3 SD
68%
95%
99.7%

Value of the observation

**Figure 32.3**

**32.4.** A. P.

A has the smallest SD. C has greater SD and dispersion.

**32.5.** A. Unpaired i-test.

This is the test to compare two group means. Total number and SD are needed for this calculation. Examples: comparisons of age of two groups or ejection fraction of two groups.

**32.6.** B. Paired t-test.

This is because the same group is compared and a change in the same group is analyzed; that is, delta heart rate. Example: heart rate at baseline and after exercise in a group of people.

**32.7.** C. *Chi* squared test.

This is used to compare proportions (and not means). Means are compared using a t-test.

**32.8.** D. Linear regression.

This is used to test the relationship between two continuous variables. For example, height and weight, age and blood pressure (BP), age and low-density lipoprotein cholesterol.

**32.9.** A. Measures of central tendency and dispersion.

A description of any population should include two measures: central tendency (mean, median, or mode) and dispersion (SD, variance, range, or IQR).

**32.10.** B. 20%.

Relative risk reduction is 3/15 or 20%.

**32.11.** A. 3%.

This is absolute and relative, over the period of study.

**32.12.** A. 33.

Treating 100 patients over two years saves three lives; hence, to save one life, you have to treat 33 patients.

**32.13.** B. Intermediate probability of disease.

A positive versus negative test gives the best separation in terms of post-test probability. Example: chest pain and stress test. See Figure 32.13. According to threshold theory of decision making, you test this population (Pauker and Kassirer 1980).

**32.14.** A. 80%.

Sensitivity is the percentage of patients with disease who have a positive test. That is, true positives divided by all those with disease. The denominator is all those with disease. Among the 100 people with disease, 80 had positive tests (true positive, TP); 20 had negative tests despite the presence of disease (false negative, FN). Hence:

$$\text{Sensitivity} = \frac{\text{TP}}{\text{TP}+\text{FN}} = \frac{80}{100} = 80\%$$

Sensitivity is how well a positive test can detect disease.

**32.15.** A. 80%.

Specificity is the percentage of subjects without disease who have a negative test. That is, true negatives divided by all those without disease. The denominator is those *without* disease. Among the 100 people without disease, 80 had negative tests (true negative, TN); 20 had positive tests despite no disease (false positive, FP). Hence:

$$\text{Specificity} = \frac{\text{TN}}{\text{TN} + \text{FP}} = \frac{80}{100} = 80\%$$

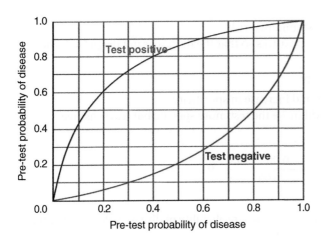

Figure 32.13

Specificity is how well a negative test can detect the absence of disease. To recap: TP is a positive test in those *with* disease ($n = 80$); FP is a positive test in those *without* disease ($n = 20$); TN is a negative test in those *without* disease ($n = 20$); FN is a negative test in those *with* disease ($n = 80$).

**32.16.** A. 80%.

Positive predictive value (PPV) is the true positives divided by all the positives:

$$\text{PPV} = \frac{\text{TP}}{\text{TP} + \text{FP}} = \frac{80}{80 + 20} = 80\%$$

in this example and population, which is 50% *with* disease (100 out of 200).

**32.17.** A. 80%.

Negative predictive value (NPV) is the true negatives divided by all the negatives:

$$\text{NPV} = \frac{\text{TN}}{\text{TN} + \text{FN}} = \frac{80}{80 + 20} = 80\%$$

in this example and population, which is 50% *without* disease (100 out of 200).

**32.18.** C. and D. Positive predictive value and negative predictive value.

Sensitivity and specificity are unique test characteristics and are not affected by the population on which they are tested.

**32.19.** A. High sensitivity, low cost, minimal risk.

The goal is to avoid false negatives so that disease is not missed when it is present.

**32.20.** B. High specificity, low cost, minimal risk.

The goal is to avoid false positives so that the disease is not diagnosed when it is not present.

**32.21.** B. Lower pretest probability.

**32.22.** C. Decrease in sensitivity and increase in specificity.

A stringent criterion will make the test more specific but less sensitive.

**32.23.** C. 9.

$$LR+ = \frac{\text{Sensitivity}}{1-\text{Specificity}} = \frac{0.90}{1-0.90} = \frac{0.9}{0.1} = 9$$

An LR+ of 1 indicates that the post-test probability of disease will be higher than the pretest probability of disease.

**32.24.** C. 90%.

Post-test probability = Pre-test probability $\times$ LR+ $= 10\% \times 9 = 90\%$

**32.25.** A. A double blind randomized controlled clinical trial with power >0.8, an outcome adjudication committee, and safety monitoring committee.

This is the best design. With a single blind trial, bias could be introduced.

**32.26.** A. Kaplan–Meier analysis.

This takes into consideration not only number of deaths, but time to those events, unlike the chi squared test. As the groups are well balanced, adjustment for baseline characteristics using a Cox regression model is not needed.

**32.27.** C. Propensity score analysis.

Propensity score is a score developed through logistical regression analysis to estimate the probability of performing AVR even in those without AVR by using data from patients with AVR. Then, one can match the AVR population with those without AVR based on the propensity score to make sure that similar populations with and without AVR are compared. This type of analysis can remove about 80% of the bias that might have gone into treatment selection. Hence, it cannot replace a randomized trial, which evens out baseline characteristics of patients with and without AVR.

**32.28.** D. All of the above.

The 95% confidence interval encompasses the limit inside which the point estimates is likely to lie 95% of the time; this could be for the mean or single estimate. The mean plus/minus 2SD encompasses the 95% confidence interval for all observations in the sample, and the mean plus/minus 2SEM encompasses the 95% confidence interval for the mean of the sample. The SEM is smaller than the SD, and SEM $= SD/n^{1/2}$, where $n$ is the number of observations.

**32.29.** A. Analysis of covariance (ANCOVA).

As the BP drop also depends upon initial BP, this also has to be considered. Generally, the BP reduction is greater in those with higher baseline BPs than those with lower BP (regression to the mean). Treatment comparison as a function of baseline BP is analyzed by ANCOVA. The *t*-tests do not take baseline BP into analysis. Kaplan-Meir analysis is for time to events.

**32.30.** D. When the trial is negative and one of the subsets shows a positive result, it confirms benefits in that subset because it is a randomized trial.

This statement is wrong. By doing multiple subset analysis, one can find a result just by chance. If you do 20 subset analyses, one should be positive with a *p* value of 0.05 by chance alone. The other three statements are correct.

## Reference

Pauker, S.G. and Kassirer, J.P. (1980). The threshold approach to clinical decision making. *The New England Journal of Medicine* 302 (20): 1109–1117.

# Genetics

33.1. Long QT3 is characterized by a defect in which of the following?
A. *KCNQ1*-encoded slow component of the delayed rectifier potassium current (IKs)
B. KCNH2-encoded rapid component of the delayed rectifier potassium current (IKr)
C. *SCN5A*-encoded sodium channel
D. None of the above

33.2. Brugada syndrome is associated with a mutation in which of the following?
A. Voltage-gated sodium channel
B. L-type calcium channel
C. *SCN5A*-encoded sodium channel
D. Potassium channel

33.3. Which of the following is not an indication for an implantable cardioverter-defibrillator (ICD) in a patient with long QT syndrome?
A. Aborted cardiac arrest (regardless of genotype)
B. Episode of ventricular tachycardia (VT) despite being on optimal medical therapy
C. Symptomatic with a QTc of greater than 550 ms
D. Symptomatic long QT2, diagnosed with cancer with a life expectancy of six months

33.4. A 40-year-old male is being evaluated for symptoms of syncope. He has had three episodes of witnessed syncope. His electrocardiogram (ECG) shows normal sinus rhythm with an incomplete right bundle branch pattern and coved ST segment elevation in the right precordial leads. His father was diagnosed with Brugada syndrome at age 30. His father's ECG was also characteristic for right bundle branch block pattern with coved ST elevation in the right precordial leads. What should his management at this time be?
A. Reassurance and ask to come back for a follow-up in one year
B. Beta-blocker therapy
C. Implantable-defibrillator therapy
D. Genetic testing

33.5. A 20-year-old female is being evaluated for syncope. She gives a history of passing out with exercise. Her maternal aunt, who is aged 35 years, also has a history of syncope. Her aunt's symptoms started soon after she delivered her first baby. She also had an aborted cardiac arrest and had an ICD placed. Her cousin, who

*Cardiology Board Review*, Second Edition. Ramdas G. Pai and Padmini Varadarajan.
© 2023 John Wiley & Sons Ltd. Published 2023 by John Wiley & Sons Ltd.

is aged 25 years, also has a history of syncope. She passes out whenever she hears the doorbell or telephone ring. Her history and physical examination are otherwise unremarkable. What is the best therapy at this time?

A. Implantable defibrillator
B. Beta-blocker therapy
C. Mexiletine
D. Reassurance and follow-up in one year

33.6. Which of the following regarding symptomatic catecholamine-induced polymorphic VT (CPVT) is not true?

A. Type 1 CPVT results from mutations in *RYR2-encoded* cardiac ryanodine receptor
B. Type 2 CPVT results from mutations in CASQ2-encoded calsequestrin
C. Characterized by stress-induced syncope with structurally normal heart and normal QT interval
D. First line of therapy is beta blocker or calcium channel blockers

33.7. The mechanism of medications that prolong QT as a cause for acquired long QT syndrome is which of the following?

A. *SCN5A*-encoded sodium channel
B. Voltage-gated sodium channel
C. Inhibition of *KCNH2-encoded* HERG potassium channel
D. Inhibition of calcium channel

33.8. What is the channel most commonly affected in long QT syndrome?

A. Potassium channel
B. Sodium channel
C. Calcium channel
D. Transient outward potassium channel

**Chapter 3**

33.9. A 14-year-old male patient gives a history of near drowning. His ECG shows a QTc of 600 ms. What is the most likely cause?

A. Gain of function mutation in the *SCN5A*-encoded sodium channel
B. Loss of function mutation in the *SCN5A*-encoded sodium channel
C. Loss of function mutation in the *KCNQ1*-encoded IKs potassium channel
D. Gain of function mutation in the *KCNQ1*-encoded IKr potassium channel

33.10. A 20-year-old female has symptoms of syncope. Her 12-lead ECG shows notching of the T wave, with a corrected QT of 580 ms. What is the most common genotype associated with this?

A. LQT1
B. LQT2

C. LQT3
D. LQT5

33.11. An 18-year-old male is seen at your clinic for a routine evaluation. He has a history of recurrent viral and bacterial infections. Examination shows an underdeveloped chin and low set ears. He attests to having a learning disorder. His chem panel shows evidence of hypocalcemia. You suspect a genetic disorder in which of the following genes?

A. 22q11.2 deletion
B. Trisomy 21

C. 7q11.23 deletion
D. 47 XXY

**33.12.** A 20-year-old male patient is seen in the clinic for a routine examination. He has a history of atrial septal defect. His X-ray of the forearm is significant for absent radial bone. You suspect mutation in which of the following?

A. 45 X

B. TBX5

C. Trisomy 18

D. Trisomy 15

E. None of the above

**33.13.** A 25-year-old male is seen for a routine evaluation. He has evidence of slanted eyes, large tongue, flattened nose, a short neck, low muscle tone, and presence of a single palmar crease. His echocardiogram showed a perimembranous ventricular septal defect (VSD). Which of the following genetic mutations is seen in this patient?

A. 47 XXY

B. 45 XO

C. Trisomy 21

D. PTPN11

**33.14.** Klinefelter syndrome is associated with what genetic abnormality?

A. 45X

B. 47 XXY

C. 47 XXXY

D. 45 XX

**33.15.** A 30-year-old female comes in for a routine follow up. Her physical examination is striking for an unusually short stature and a webbed neck. Her history is also significant for primary amenorrhea. You suspect a genetic mutation in:

A. 45 XX

B. 45 XO

C. 47 XXX

D. 45 XXX

**33.16.** A 21-year-old male is seen in the clinic. He has a characteristic elfin face, and hearing loss. He has a history of hypercalcemia from his infancy. He also has a history of murmur from his childhood. You expect a mutation in:

A. 22 q deletion

B. 7q11.23 deletion

C. KRAS

D. MAP2K1

E. PTPN11

**33.17.** You routinely follow up a patient with known Noonan syndrome in your clinic. Which of the following genetic abnormalities is seen in Noonan syndrome?

A. NOTCH1

B. PTPN11

C. 45XO

D. Fibrillin gene

**33.18.** A 21-year-old male patient comes in your clinic for an initial screening evaluation. He is of very tall and thin stature with long arms and legs, has pectus excavatum, scoliosis, striae on the abdomen, and flexible joints. His father was also diagnosed with a similar disorder and had aortic dissection and died suddenly. You suspect a genetic mutation in:

A. Fibrillin 1 gene

B. NOTCH 1

C. ACTA

D. TGF-B

E. SCAD

**33.19.** You see a 19-year-old male in your aortopathy clinic. Some of the important features on physical examination include widely spaced eyes, cleft palate, spit uvula. He also bruises very easily. He also complains of frequent chronic abdominal pain, diarrhea, allergies to food. His echocardiogram is significant for dilatation of aortic sinuses measuring at 5 cm. You suspect a genetic mutation in:

A. TGFBR1

B. PTPN11

C. ACTA gene

D. COL 3

**33.20.** A 40-year-old male is seen in your clinic for an evaluation. His family history is significant for thoracic aortic aneurysm. His father underwent thoracis aortic aneurysm repair at age 41. He denies any other past history. Examination is unremarkable, BP is normal. A 2D echocardiogram reveals ascending aortic aneurysm measuring 6 cm. Which of the following genetic abnormalities is associated with this condition?

A. SMAD 3  
B. Fibrillin 1  
C. ACTA 2  
D. NOTCH 1

**33.21.** A 70-year-old African-American male is being evaluated for dyspnea on exertion. His ECG in the clinic reveals sinus rhythm with low voltage. His echocardiogram reveals severe biatrial enlargement, concentric left ventricular hypertrophy, thickened atrial septum and valves. Left ventricular ejection fraction is 50%. Filling pressures are elevated with evidence of bilateral pleural effusions. Current guidelines recommend genetic screening for which mutation in this condition?

A. KCNQ1  
B. KCNH2  
C. LDLR  
D. TTR p.Val142lle

**33.22.** A 22-year-old male is seen in the clinic. He has thin translucent skin, with thin lips, small chin, thin nose and large eyes. His history includes surgery for intestinal perforation. He also has increased propensity for bleeding. His family history includes his father and grandfather dying suddenly at age 39. You suspect a heritable syndrome and order an echocardiogram which revealed dilated aortic root. In addition, a genetic panel is sent out. The most common genetic mutation seen in this condition is:

A. ACTA 2  
B. MYH 7  
C. SCN5A  
D. Col3A1

**33.23.** Catecholaminergic polymorphic ventricular tachycardia is associated with:

A. RYR2 mutation  
B. MYL3 mutation  
C. SCN5A mutation  
D. KNCH2 mutation

**33.24.** A 20-year-old female is being evaluated in your clinic for complaints of syncope. ECG shows normal sinus rhythm with Epsilon waves. A 14-day monitor shows evidence of non-sustained ventricular tachycardia. Echocardiogram was performed which showed a normally functioning left ventricle. Right ventricle was not well visualized. Cardiac MRI was then performed which showed a dilated, thin right ventricle. The lateral free wall of the right ventricle was scarred on delayed enhancement imaging. You order a genetic test to evaluate this patient and help in screening other family members (Musunuru et al. 2020). Which of the following gene mutation is most common in this condition:

A. PKP2  
B. MYH7  
C. TPM1  
D. ACTC1

**33.25.** A 25-year-old male is evaluated in the clinic for complaints of dyspnea on exertion. He has a family history of several family members with congestive heart failure and sudden death at a young age. ECG was unremarkable. HR 75 beats/minute, blood pressure 100/65 mmHg, oxygen saturation was 97% room air. An echocardiogram performed in the clinic shows severe dilatation of the left ventricle measured at 6.8 cm, with a reduced ejection fraction of 20%. The right ventricle is also dilated with reduced function. Both atria are moderately dilated with moderate-to-severe mitral regurgitation and moderate tricuspid regurgitation. You suspect a genetic variant of dilated cardiomyopathy and get a genetic panel. Which of the genes is most commonly implicated in dilated cardiomyopathy?

A. RYR2
B. TTN
C. KCNH2
D. LDLR

## Answers

33.1. C. SCN5A-encoded sodium channel.

Long QT3 channelopathy occurs due to a mutation in the *SCN5A*-encoded sodium channel (gain of function). Mutation in the *KCNQ1* (IKs) channel is associated with long QT1, and mutation in the *KCNH2* (IKr) channel is associated with long QT2 syndrome.

33.2. C. SCN5A-encoded sodium channel.

Brugada syndrome occurs due to a mutation in the *SCN5A*-encoded sodium channel, and is a loss of function mutation. It should be noted that a gain of function in the same *SCN5A*-encoded sodium channel results in LQT3 syndrome.

33.3. D. Symptomatic long QT2, diagnosed with cancer with a life expectancy of six months.

ICD therapy is not indicated for patients who do not have a reasonable expectation of survival with an acceptable functional status for at least one year. ICD therapy is otherwise indicated in patients with long QT syndrome in the following situations: (i) In aborted sudden death, regardless of the genotype; and as a secondary prevention measure in (ii) breakthrough cardiac events such as VT/ventricular fibrillation, despite being on optimal medical therapy, and (iii) intolerance to primary medical therapy (Epstein et al. 2008).

33.4. C. Implantable-defibrillator therapy.

The patient in question probably has Brugada syndrome. His father was diagnosed with Brugada syndrome at a young age. The patient has an ECG showing a type I pattern (coved ST elevation), has multiple episodes of syncope, and has a first-degree relative with Brugada syndrome. It is reasonable to give the patient an ICD (class IIa, level of evidence C) (Epstein et al. 2008).

33.5. B. Beta-blocker therapy.

The patient in question probably has long QT1 syndrome. Given her symptoms of syncope she should be started on beta blockers. It is reasonable to consider an ICD if she continues to have symptoms or breakthrough cardiac events on betablocker therapy. Mexiletine is a drug of choice in treating long QT3 patients.

**33.6.** D. First line of therapy is beta blocker or calcium channel blockers.

This is not true. Pharmacotherapy with either beta blockers or calcium channel blockers is not protective and all symptomatic CPVT patients should receive an ICD.

**33.7.** C. Inhibition of *KCNH2-encoded* HERG potassium channel.

Most of the medications that prolong QT act by inhibiting the *KCNH2*-encoded HERG potassium channel.

**33.8.** A. Potassium channel.

**33.9.** C. Loss of function mutation in the *KCNQ1*-encoded IKs potassium channel.

This patient probably has congenital long QT1 syndrome. His symptoms occurred while exercising and his ECG shows an abnormal prolongation of QT interval. Long QT1 is associated with a loss of function mutation in the *KCNQ1*-encoded IKs potassium channel.

**33.10.** B. LQT2.

This patient probably has congenital long QT2 syndrome. She has prolongation of her QTc and has notching of her T waves, which is usually seen in LQT2. LQT1 is usually associated with broad-based T waves, and LQT3 is associated with a long isoelectric ST segment with a normal T wave morphology.

**33.11.** A. The patients' features along with a history of recurrent infections and hypocalcemia point toward a diagnosis of DiGeorge syndrome. This syndrome is associated with a small deletion in chromosome 22 at this particular location 22q11.2. These patients have abnormalities in the thymus gland which is often hypoplastic leading to a deficiency in T-cell especially T lymphocytes

Chapter 3

**33.12.** B. This patient has Holt-Oram syndrome which is associated with mutations in the *TBX5* gene. The *TBX5* gene is known to produce a protein that has been shown to be critical for the proper development of heart and upper limbs *in utero*. This syndrome is autosomal dominant.

**33.13.** C. This patient shows features suggestive of Down Syndrome. They are associated with Trisomy 21. These patients typically have the characteristic facial features, intellectual disability and congenital heart defects such as atrial septal defect (ASD), ventricular septal defect (VSD), atrio-ventricular septal defect (AVSD) and Tetralogy of Fallot (TOF).

**33.14.** C. Klinefelter syndrome is associated with 47 XXY(additional copy of X chromosome). These patients have a tall stature, delayed puberty, hypoplastic testes and developmental disability.

**33.15.** B. This patient has Turner's syndrome, where a female is born with only one X chromosome. Up to 30% have congenital heart disease.

**33.16.** B. This patient has features suggestive of Williams syndrome which is associated with an abnormality of chromosome 7, deletion in the particular location 7q11.23

**33.17.** B. Patients with Noonan syndrome have some features similar to Turner syndrome such as short stature and webbed neck. In addition, they also have chest deformities, abnormal lymphatics, bleeding abnormalities. They can have genetic abnormalities in *PTPN11, KRAS, SOS1, RAF1, NRAS, BRAF,* and *MAP2K1*.

**33.18.** A. This patient has the physical features suggestive of Marfan syndrome, which are associated with a mutation in *Fibrillin 1* gene. This genetic mutation results in excess in transforming growth factor B, which leads to connective tissue problems including the heart. This is an autosomal dominant condition.

**33.19.** A. This patient has characteristic features for Loeys-Dietz syndrome. There are five types of Loeys-Dietz syndrome (1–5). LDS 1-is associated with mutation in transforming growth factor receptor 1 (TGFBR) 1, LDS 2-TGFBR2, LDS-3 SMAD-3, LDS-4-TGFB2, and LDS-5-TGFBR3.

**33.20.** C. This patient has features suggestive of familial thoracic aortic aneurysm. About 20% of the patients with this disorder have a mutation in *ACTA 2* gene. About 2.5% are known to have mutations in *TGFBR2*. The *ACTA 2* gene provides instructions for production of smooth muscle alpha-2 actin which is found in the smooth muscle of vessels. This protein is known to form the core of the sarcomere helping to maintain the shape of the arteries and prevents stretching. Due to the mutation is *ACTA 2*, there is development of aneurysms of the aorta in this syndrome, which is autosomal dominant.

**33.21.** D. Patients with evidence for restrictive cardiomyopathy should be evaluated for transthyretin amyloidosis especially in African Americans with congestive heart failure. Genetic testing to evaluate for TTR p.Val142Ile allele should be undertaken along with hypertrophic cardiomyopathy and dilated cardiomyopathy panels.

**33.22.** D. This patient has an inheritable condition and is suggestive of Vascular Ehler Danlos syndrome. This condition is associated with COL3A mutation. These patients are at risk for organ rupture.

**33.23.** A. Catecholaminergic polymorphic ventricular tachycardia is associated with mutation in *RYR2*.

**33.24.** A. *PKP2*. This patient probably has arrhythmogenic right ventricular dysplasia (ARVD). This condition is caused by mutations in the desmosomal proteins. Some of the desmosomal components are: Plakophilin-2 (PKP2), Desmoglein-2 (DSG-2), Desmocollin-2 (DSC-2), Desmoplakin (DSP) and Plakoglobin (JUP). Among these, the most common genetic mutation occurs in Plakophilin-2 (PKP-2). About 30–50% of the patients may have a family history. ARVD can be passed on in autosomal dominant pattern, autosomal recessive pattern or with compound heterozygosity (two different gene changes in the same gene), digenic mutations (mutations can occur in more than one gene i.e. *PKP2* and *DSG2*). It is recommended that to get a full dilated cardiomyopathy (DCM) panel along with the ARVD panel.

**33.25.** B. About half of the cases of DCM have a genetic basis. Mutations in sarcomeric genes are also seen in DCM and in hypertrophic cardiomyopathy (HCM), where the prevalence is close to 60%. It has been shown that the sarcomeric gene *TTN* is most commonly seen in DCM. These are noted as protein truncating mutations in about 25% of familial and 18% of idiopathic DCM. Other genetic mutations seen include *LMNA, MYH7, TNNT2, BAG3, RBM20, TNCC1, TNNI3, TPM1, SCN5A*, and *PLN*. In addition to ordering a DCM panel, testing for HCM and arrhythmogenic right ventricular dysplasia (ARVD) genes are also recommended.

# References

Epstein, A.E., DiMarco, J.P., Ellenbogen, K.A. et al. (2008). ACC/AHA/HRS 2008 guidelines for device-based therapy of cardiac rhythm abnormalities: executive summary. *Circulation* 117: 2820–2840.

Musunuru, K., Hershberger, R.E., Day, S.M. et al. (2020). Genetic testing for inherited cardiovascular diseases. *Circulation: Genomic and Precision Medicine* 13: 373–385.

Chapter 33

# Cardiac Emergencies and Resuscitation

# 34

34.1. After endotracheal (ET) intubation during a witnessed cardiac arrest, which of the following are useful to confirm correct placement of ET tube.
  A. Chest rise with breathing
  B. Auscultation of abdomen and both lung fields
  C. Chest X-ray
  D. Waveform capnography
  E. All of the above

34.2. What does five-point auscultation after ET intubation consist of?
  A. Auscultation of epigastrium, both lung apices, and both axillary areas
  B. Auscultation of mitral, tricuspid, pulmonary, aortic, and Erb's areas
  C. Epigastric area, front of both chests, backs of both chests
  D. None of the above

34.3. In Question 34.1, which is most reliable?
  A. Chest rise with breathing
  B. Auscultation of abdomen and both lung fields
  C. Chest X-ray
  D. Waveform capnography
  E. All of the above

34.4. With waveform capnography, what is the normal expected $p_{CO2}$?
  A. 35–45 mmHg
  B. 20 mmHg
  C. <10 mmHg
  D. 0 mmHg

34.5. With waveform capnography, what is the expected $p_{CO2}$ during adequate cardiopulmonary resuscitation (CPR) in a code setting?
  A. 35–45 mmHg
  B. 20 mmHg
  C. <10 mmHg
  D. 0 mmHg

34.6. With waveform capnography, what is the expected $p_{CO2}$ during CPR in a code setting with a dislodged ET tube?
  A. 35–45 mmHg
  B. 20 mmHg
  C. <10 mmHg
  D. 0 mmHg

34.7. Which of the following statements are correct for a colorimetric exhaled $CO_2$ detector?
  A. It is not as accurate as capnography
  B. Purple means there is $CO_2$
  C. Yellow means no oxygen
  D. All are correct

*Cardiology Board Review*, Second Edition. Ramdas G. Pai and Padmini Varadarajan.
© 2023 John Wiley & Sons Ltd. Published 2023 by John Wiley & Sons Ltd.

34.8. Which of the following are contraindications for an esophageal-tracheal tube?
   A. Height <4 ft
   B. Age <16 years
   C. Intact gag reflex
   D. Ingestion of caustic
   E. All of the above
   F. None of the above

34.9. Which of the following statements regarding ventilation during cardiac arrest are correct?
   A. 30:2 ratio with bag-mask device
   B. 8–10 breaths per minute with advanced airway for a patient with cardiac arrest
   C. 10–12 breaths per minute with advanced airway for a patient with pure respiratory arrest
   D. None of the above
   E. All of the above

34.10. For witnessed out-of-hospital cardiac arrest due to ventricular fibrillation, what is the appropriate energy level for defibrillation?
   A. 120–200 J with a biphasic shock device
   B. 360 J with a monophasic shock device
   C. 2–4 J/kg body weight for a child
   D. All of the above
   E. None of the above

34.11. In a cardiac arrest situation with no access for drug delivery, what is the preferred access?
   A. Peripheral intravenous (IV) device
   B. Central line
   C. ET tube insertion
   D. Intraosseous (IO) access

34.12. For ET drug delivery, which of the following statements are accurate?
   A. Amount of drug should be about twice as much as IV
   B. Dilute in 5–10 cm³ of fluid
   C. Epinephrine, vasopressin, and lidocaine can be given via an ET route during cardiac arrest situation
   D. All are correct
   E. None are correct

34.13. Which of the following can IO access be obtained from?
   A. Medial malleolus
   B. Upper tibia
   C. Iliac crest
   D. Sternum
   E. All of the above
   F. None of the above

34.14. Which of the following are contraindications for basic life support and advanced cardiopulmonary life support?
   A. Rigor mortis
   B. Advance directives not to resuscitate
   C. Clinical futility due to end-stage disease processes
   D. Attempt to resuscitate puts practitioner at risk
   E. All of the above

Chapter 3

**34.15.** What is the desired depth of chest compression in adult CPR?

A. $\geq 2$ in.

B. 1.5–2 in.

C. Enough to produce a pulse

D. Any of the above

E. None of the above

**34.16.** What is the location for chest compression in CPR?

A. Mid sternum

B. Upper sternum

C. Lower sternum

D. Xiphoid process

**34.17.** What is the desired rate of chest compression in adult CPR?

A. At least 100/min

B. 80–100/min

C. 60/min in adult, 100/min in a child, 120/min in an infant

D. All of the above

**34.18.** How often should you rotate the compressors during CPR?

A. two minutes

B. two to five minutes

C. When tired

D. As needed

**34.19.** What is the desired rate of chest compression in a child?

A. At least 100/min

B. At least 120/min

C. At least 140/min

D. None of the above

**34.20.** What is the first thing to do when an unresponsive, nonbreathing person is found?

A. Activate emergency response

B. Start CPR

C. Feel the pulse

D. Defibrillate the patient

**34.21.** In two-rescuer CPR, what is the optimal compression-to-ventilation ratio?

A. 15:2

B. 30:2

C. 5:1

D. 10:2

**34.22.** What do signs of adequate CPR include?

A. End-tidal $CO_2$ >10 mmHg

B. Diastolic blood pressure (BP) >20 mmHg

C. Both A and B

D. Neither A nor B

**34.23.** What is the dose of epinephrine in cardiac arrest?

A. 1 mg every three to five minutes rapid push

B. 0.5 mg every three to five minutes rapid push

C. 1 mg every three to five minutes over two minutes

D. 0.5 mg every three to five minutes over two minutes

**34.24.** What dose of amiodarone can be used in fibrillatory arrest after the first dose of epinephrine?

A. 300 mg IV push

B. 150 mg IV push

C. 300 mg IV slow push over 10 minutes

D. 150 mg IV slow push over 10 minutes

**34.25.** What does a partial pressure of end-tidal $CO_2$ of >40 mmHg during CPR indicate?

A. Adequate chest compression

B. Adequate ventilation

C. Return of spontaneous circulation

D. All of the above

34.26. What is the dose of IV/IO vasopressin during cardiac arrest?
    A. 40 units
    B. 80 units
    C. 1 unit per kilogram body weight
    D. All are correct

34.27. IV/IO vasopressin during cardiac arrest can be substituted for which of the following?
    A. First dose of epinephrine
    B. Second dose of epinephrine
    C. First or second dose of epinephrine
    D. After the second dose of epinephrine

34.28. What is the $O_2$ saturation goal after return of spontaneous circulation?
    A. >90%
    B. ≥94%
    C. 100%
    D. None of the above

34.29. Hypotension post arrest is defined as:
    A. Systolic BP <90 mmHg or mean arterial pressure <65 mmHg
    B. Systolic BP <90 mmHg
    C. Systolic BP <90 mmHg and mean arterial pressure <65 mmHg
    D. Diastolic BP <40 mmHg

34.30. What is the appropriate volume of IV saline or Ringer's lactate bolus in a hypotensive patient?
    A. 250 cm³
    B. 500 cm³
    C. 1–2 l
    D. None of the above

34.31. What is the appropriate dose of dopamine infusion in a hypotensive patient?
    A. 2–10 µg/(kg min)
    B. 7–35 µg/(kg min)
    C. 0.1–0.5 µg/(kg min)
    D. None of the above

34.32. What is the appropriate dose of epinephrine infusion in a hypotensive patient?
    A. 2–10 µg/(kg min)
    B. 7–35 µg/(kg min)
    C. 0.1–0.5 µg/(kg min)
    D. B and C

34.33. What is the appropriate dose of norepinephrine infusion in a hypotensive patient?
    A. 2–10 µg/(kg min)
    B. 7–35 µg/(kg min)
    C. 0.1–0.5 µg/(kg min)
    D. B and C

34.34. The initial drug therapy for a hypotensive, bradycardic patient includes which of the following?
    A. Atropine
    B. Dopamine infusion
    C. Epinephrine infusion
    D. Any of the above

34.35. What is the therapy for VT with no pulse?
    A. Synchronized cardioversion
    B. Defibrillation (nonsynchronized)
    C. Lidocaine bolus IV
    D. Any of the above

34.36. The Cincinnati prehospital stroke scale components include which of the following?
    A. Facial droop
    B. Arm drift
    C. Abnormal, slurred speech
    D. All of the above

Chapter 34

34.37. Which of the following are components of the Glasgow coma scale?
   A. Eye opening
   B. Best verbal response
   C. Best motor response
   D. All of the above

34.38. For ischemic stroke with no contraindications, IV recombinant tissue plasminogen activator can be given in which of the following cases?
   A. Onset of symptoms <3 hours
   B. Onset of symptoms <6 hours
   C. Onset of symptoms <12 hours
   D. Woke up with stroke symptoms after eight hours of sleep

34.39. Recombinant tissue plasminogen activator in acute stroke is contraindicated in which of the following situations?
   A. Head trauma or stroke in the last three months
   B. Systolic BP >185 mmHg or diastolic BP >110 mmHg
   C. International normalized ratio >1.7
   D. Platelet count <100 000/mm³
   E. Any of the above

34.40. Contraindications for nitroglycerin in acute coronary syndrome include which of the following?
   A. Inferior MI with Kussmaul sign
   B. Systolic BP <90 mmHg
   C. Use of Viagra® (sildenafil) in the last 24 hours
   D. Use of Cialis® (tadalafil) in the last 48 hours
   E. All of the above
   F. None of the above

## Answers

34.1. E. All of the above.

34.2. A. Auscultation of epigastrium, both lung apices, and both axillary areas.
   This is to confirm correct ET tube placement.

34.3. D. Waveform capnography.
   It has a sensitivity and specificity of 100%.

34.4. A. 35–45 mmHg.

34.5. B. 20 mmHg.

34.6. D. 0 mmHg.

34.7. D. All are correct.

34.8. E. All of the above.

34.9. E. All of the above.

34.10. D. All of the above.

34.11. A. Peripheral intravenous (IV) device.
   With central cannulation, CPR may have to be halted temporarily and there is risk of pneumothorax – hence not desirable.

34.12. D. All are correct.

34.13. E. All of the above.

34.14. E. All of the above.

34.15. A. ≥2 in.

34.16. C. Lower sternum.

34.17. A. At least 100/min.

34.18. A. Two minutes.

34.19. A. At least 100/min.

34.20. A. Activate emergency response.

34.21. A. 15:2.

34.22. C. Both A and B.

34.23. A. 1 mg every three to five minutes rapid push.

34.24. A. 300 mg IV push.

34.25. C. Return of spontaneous circulation.

34.26. A. 40 units.

34.27. C. First or second dose of epinephrine.

34.28. B. ≥94%.

34.29. A. Systolic BP <90 mmHg or mean arterial pressure <65 mmHg.

34.30. C. 1–2 l.

34.31. A. 2–10 mmHg/(kg min).

34.32. D. B and C.

34.33. D. B and C.

34.34. D. Any of the above.

34.35. B. Defibrillation (nonsynchronized).

34.36. D. All of the above.

    If any of three are present, the probability of a stroke is 72%.

34.37. D. All of the above.

    Total possible is 15. For eye opening: spontaneous 4, in response to speech 3, in response to pain 2, none 1. For best verbal response: oriented conversation 5, confused conversation 4, inappropriate words 3, incomprehensible sounds 2, none 1. For best motor response: obeys 6, localizes 5, withdraws 4, abnormal flexion 3, abnormal extension 2, none 1. Score 14–15 is mild dysfunction; ≤10 is severe dysfunction.

34.38. A. Onset of symptoms <3 hours.

34.39. E. Any of the above.

34.40. E. All of the above

# Index

Note: The numbers in square brackets indicate the questions or answers where the term appears.

*Cardiology Board Review*, Second Edition. Ramdas G. Pai and Padmini Varadarajan.
© 2023 John Wiley & Sons Ltd. Published 2023 by John Wiley & Sons Ltd.

Printed and bound by CPI Group (UK) Ltd, Croydon, CR0 4YY

16/04/2025

14658834-0002